AROMATHERAPY

Basic Mechanisms and
Evidence-Based Clinical Use

Clinical Pharmacognosy Series

Series Editors
Navindra P. Seeram
Luigi Antonio Morrone

Aromatherapy: Basic Mechanisms and Evidence-Based Clinical Use
Giacinto Bagetta, Marco Cosentino,
and Tsukasa Sakurada

Herbal Medicines: Development and Validation of Plant-Derived Medicines for Human Health
Giacinto Bagetta, Marco Cosentino, Marie Tiziana Corasaniti,
and Shinobu Sakurada

Natural Products Interactions on Genomes
Siva G. Somasundaram

Clinical Pharmacognosy Series

AROMATHERAPY
Basic Mechanisms and Evidence-Based Clinical Use

Edited by

Giacinto Bagetta
University of Calabria
Italy

Marco Cosentino
University of Insubria
Varese, Italy

Tsukasa Sakurada
Daiichi University of Pharmacy
Fukuoka, Japan

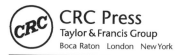

CRC Press
Taylor & Francis Group
Boca Raton   London   New York

CRC Press is an imprint of the
Taylor & Francis Group, an **informa** business

First published in paperback 2024

CRC Press
2385 NW Executive Center Drive, Suite 320, Boca Raton FL 33431

and by CRC Press
4 Park Square, Milton Park, Abingdon, Oxon, OX14 4RN

CRC Press is an imprint of Taylor & Francis Group, LLC

ISBN: 978-1-4822-4663-6 (hbk)
ISBN: 978-1-03-283681-2 (pbk)
ISBN: 978-0-429-17189-5 (ebk)

DOI: 10.1201/b19651

**Visit the Taylor & Francis Web site at
http://www.taylorandfrancis.com**

**and the CRC Press Web site at
http://www.crcpress.com**

Contents

SECTION I   Botanical, Phytochemical, Analytical, and Technological Issues

SECTION II Cell Biological Effects
and Underlying Mechanisms

SECTION III Rational Basis for Aromatherapy

SECTION IV Evidence-Based Clinical Use of Aromatherapy

SECTION V Regulatory Issues

Preface

Aromatherapy is a specialized form of phytotherapy that uses essential oils extracted from diverse parts of aromatic plants more often delivered via inhalation or massage for several minor clinical uses. Essential oils are phytocomplexes made up of several components endowed with a broad spectrum of biological activities, some of which have been deciphered only recently.

A PubMed search on April 13, 2015, using "essential oils" as the keyword phrase resulted in 13,844 articles dating back to 1880, the year of the first article published by H.C. Wood and E.T. Reichut in the prestigious *Journal of Physiology*: "Note on the Action upon the Circulation of Certain Volatile Oils." The reading of this article has an obvious historical meaning, though it anticipates the experimental complexity in studying such phytocomplexes, starting from the important, and not so obvious, qualitative differences in their biological effects in living animals, emerging by changing their route of administration.

In the industrialized countries, the interest in aromatherapy increased a great deal during the second half of the last century for treating stress-induced symptoms of anxiety, mood, and sleep disorders and certain forms of pain, among other disorders. During the last couple of decades, basic research yielded a large body of information in experimental models of diseases, probably not considered enough to provide the rational basis for further research and development of discrete essential oils to be assessed for their efficacy and safety in clinical trials. Instead, controlled clinical trials have been completed in some age-related neurodegenerative diseases where no preclinical data have been generated. Among the most distressing features of dementia are the behavioral and psychological symptoms. Addressing this facet has received particular interest in aromatherapy trials, with a shift in focus from reducing cognitive dysfunction to the reduction of behavioral symptoms in dementia. In fact, some behavioral disorders occurring in demented patients appear to be sensitive to the beneficial action of aromatherapy in a way similar, if not superior, to atypical antipsychotics, at least in some of these trials. Obviously, this is of great importance in view of the lack of major side effects compared to antipsychotics. The notion that olfaction is often dysfunctional in demented people, as well as in other neurodegenerative diseases, is per se a demonstration of the importance of the systemic absorption and distribution of the pharmacologically active components of the phytocomplex for aromatherapy to control disordered behavior, thus minimizing the power of the reported psychological action. For a correct understanding of the latter, however, an entire chapter is dedicated to the transduction mechanisms of odorant signals, immediately after the fascinating historical notes on essential oils and aromatherapy. Along the lines of the previous book in the series, *Herbal Medicines: Development and Validation of Plant-Derived Medicines for Human Health*, (Giacinto Bagetta, Marco Cosentino, Maria Tiziana Corasaniti, Shinobu Sakurada, eds., CRC Press, 2011) in Section I, several chapters are dedicated to botanical, biotechnological, phytochemical, technological, and quality issues concerned with standardization of the natural resource to limit variability of the phytocomplex. Section II reviews the recent growing literature around the cytotoxic and cytoprotective effects of essential oils, together with the underlying mechanisms dissected *in vitro* using mostly tumor cell lines. The rational basis for further research and development of aromatherapy in therapeutic areas in great demand of innovation, such as infectious and inflammatory diseases and control of diverse forms of pain, is reported in Section III. At variance with the latter, research and development of aromatherapy are far from being granted in the cancer area, where more controlled preclinical studies *in vitro* and *in vivo* are needed. As anticipated above, evidence-based information is scarce and available for controlling symptoms associated with neurodegenerative diseases and some pediatric conditions. The use of aromatherapy in dementia care settings is due to increase a great deal because it is one of the few options attractive to practitioners and families, as patients often have reduced insight and ability to verbally communicate adverse reactions. The book ends with important notes on the epidemiology of essential oil utilization in conjunction with the need for pharmacovigilance and phytovigilance for safer use of aromatherapy. Despite limited regulatory issues, together with fundamental aspects of clinical trial planning, performing and reporting are key aspects for the scientifically correct development of this growing area of phytotherapy.

This book should therefore be available to undergraduate and PhD students of pharmacy and health courses and professionals involved in aromatherapy in the clinic for research, regulatory, or therapeutic purposes. The wealth of references collected in the book make it a good venue from which to search for valuable information by scientists dealing with essential oils. Finally, the complete set of knowledge on essential oils and aromatherapy reported herein should be made available to any individual for rationale counseling and competent marketing and to policy makers in health systems worldwide.

The editors are indebted to Hilary LaFoe, whose professional skill made it possible for our venture to come true. Also, we would like to sincerely thank all the people from Taylor & Francis for their highly qualified technical contributions, and all our collaborators. A special thanks goes to Dr. Damiana Scuteri for valuable collaboration during the whole editorial process of the book.

Giacinto Bagetta
Marco Cosentino
Tsukasa Sakurada

Editors

Giacinto Bagetta, MD, (1983), (consultant in pharmacology since 1987) has been a full professor of pharmacology since 1994 in the Department of Pharmacy, Health Science and Nutrition, University of Calabria, Rende, Italy. He is the author of approximately 160 papers (see PubMed) in internationally indexed journals (H-index 40, Citations > 5000, ISI Web of Knowledge; Top Italian Scientist and Top Ten Scientist of the University of Calabria established by Via-Academy), and an editor of eight books produced by Pergamon Press, Elsevier plc, and CRC Press. He has been an invited speaker at prestigious international research institutions such as Imperial College London (UK), the University of Tokyo School of Dentistry, the University of Sendai School of Medicine and Tohoku Pharmaceutical University, Sendai, Department of Pharmacology, University School of Medicine of Wakayama (Japan), Burnham Research Institute, La Jolla (USA), the MRC Toxicology Unit, Leicester (UK), and others. He was awarded the International Galien Prize for Young Investigator. He is a member of the Italian Societies of Pharmacology, Neuroscience and of the International Society for Neurochemistry; a member of the editorial board of high-impact-factor journals such as *Current Opinion in Pharmacology* and a past member of the editorial board of the *Journal of Neurochemistry, Journal of Neuroscience Methods*, and *Journal of Chemotherapy*; a referee for prestigious, internationally recognized scientific journals and research-funding agencies such as The Wellcome Trust (UK), the National Council for Research (CNR, Italy), the Italian Space Agency (ASI), and the Ministry of Scientific Research of the Austrian Government; and a member of the National Health Research Committee at the Ministry of Health from 1996 to December 2010. He was a member of the ethical committees at the Regional General Hospital of Cosenza and IRCCS Mondino Foundation (PV) from 1996 to 2013.

Marco Cosentino, MD, PhD, a professor of medical pharmacology at the University of Insubria (Varese, Italy), earned his MD degree (cum laude) from the University of Pavia and his PhD in pharmacology and toxicology from the University of Turin. He is the director of the Center for Research in Medical Pharmacology and of the School of Specialization in Medical Pharmacology. He is also a coordinator of the PhD program in experimental and clinical medicine and medical humanities. His main research interests include neuro- and immunopharmacology, clinical pharmacology and pharmacogenetics, pharmacoepidemiology and pharmacovigilance, and pharmacology of herbal medicines. He has published more than 100 full-length papers in international scientific journals indexed by ISI-WoS and Scopus, and has served as a referee for more than 50 indexed journals. He is also a reviewer for several public and private funding agencies and academic institutions, including the National Multiple Sclerosis Society (New York, USA), the Slovak Research and Development Agency, the Research Foundation–Flanders (FWO), The Ohio State University (USA), and the University of Southern California (USA). He has served on the editorial board of *Acta Phytotherapeutica* and *Neuroendocrinology Letters*, and is presently on the editorial board of the *Journal of Neuroimmune Pharmacology*, where he has also served as a special issue guest editor. He is on the advisory board of the website Brainimmune. Dr. Cosentino has been invited to give lectures in several academic institutions, including the University of Porto (PT), the University of Regensburg (D), the Instituto de Investigaciones Biológicas Clemente Estable in Montevideo (UY), and the Karolinska Institut in Stockholm (SW). His research activity has been supported by grants from Ministero dell'Istruzione, dell'Università e della Ricerca (PRIN, programmi di internazionalizzazione), Regione Lombardia (UE PIC Interreg IIIA), Fondazione CARIPLO, Fondazione Italiana per la Sclerosi Multipla (FISM; http://www.aism.it), Genova, Italia, Associazione Italiana per la Ricerca sul Cancro (AIRC; http://www.airc.it), and the National Multiple Sclerosis Society (http://www.nmss.org). Together with Giacinto Bagetta, Shinobu Sakurada, and Maria Tiziana Corasaniti, he previously edited for CRC Press, Taylor & Francis Group, the volume *Herbal Medicines: Development and Validation of Plant-Derived Medicines for Human Health* (2012, ISBN 9781439837689).

Tsukasa Sakurada, PhD, is the vice president of Daiichi University of Pharmacy (Fukuoka, Japan), where he is also a professor of pharmacology. He earned his PhD in pharmacology from Tohoku Pharmaceutical University (Sendai, Japan). His main research interests include neuropharmacology in the mechanism of pain and analgesics including herbal medicine. He has published more than 200 research papers in international scientific journals. He has served on the editorial board of the *European Journal of Pharmaceutical Sciences, International Scholarly Research Network* (ISRN), *Pain*, and the *World Journal of Anesthesiology*. Dr. Sakurada has been a member of the council of the Japanese Pharmacological Society and of the Japanese Society for Pharmaceutical Palliative Care and Sciences. He has been invited to give lectures at the University of Uppsala (Uppsala, Sweden) and the University of Calabria (Cosenza, Italy). His research has been supported by a Grant-in-Aid for Scientific Research from the Japanese Ministry of Education, Culture, Sports, Science and Technology. Together with Giacinto Bagetta, Maria Tiziana Corasaniti, and Shinobu Sakurada, he previously edited for the *International Review of Neurobiology—Advances in Neuropharmacology*, vol. 85 (Academic Press, 2009, ISBN-13: 978-0-12-374893-5).

Contributors

Diana Amantea
Department of Pharmacy, Health and
Nutritional Sciences
Section of Preclinical and Translational
Pharmacology
University of Calabria
Rende, Cosenza, Italy

Samaneh Khanpour Ardestani
CARE Program
Department of Pediatrics
Faculty of Medicine and Dentistry
University of Alberta
Edmonton, Alberta, Canada

Giacinto Bagetta
Department of Pharmacy, Health and
Nutritional Sciences
Section of Preclinical and Translational
Pharmacology
and
University Consortium for Adaptive
Disorders and Head Pain (UCADH)
University of Calabria
Rende, Cosenza, Italy

Ivana Beara
Department of Chemistry, Biochemistry
and Environmental Protection
Faculty of Sciences
University of Novi Sad
Novi Sad, Serbia

Laura Berliocchi
Department of Health Sciences
University "Magna Graecia" of
Catanzaro
University Campus "S. Venuta"
Germaneto, Catanzaro, Italy

Raffaella Bombelli
Center for Research in Medical
Pharmacology
University of Insubria
Varese, Italy

Marcella Bracale
Department of Biotechnology and
Life Sciences
University of Insubria
Varese, Italy

Cecilia Bukutu
CARE Program
Department of Pediatrics
Faculty of Medicine and Dentistry
University of Alberta
Edmonton, Alberta, Canada

Gioacchino Calapai
Department of Clinical and
Experimental Medicine
University of Messina
Messina, Italy

Carlo Caltagirone
Department of System Medicine
University of Rome "Tor Vergata"
and
Department of Clinical and
Behavioral Neurology
IRCCS Fondazione Santa Lucia
Rome, Italy

Maria Tiziana Corasaniti
Department of Health Sciences
University "Magna Graecia" of
Catanzaro
University Campus "S. Venuta"
Germaneto, Catanzaro, Italy

Francesco Corica
Department of Experimental and
    Clinical Medicine
University of Messina
Messina, Italy

Andrea Corsonello
Unit of Geriatric
    Pharmacoepidemiology
IRCCS-INRCA
Cosenza, Italy

Donato Cosco
Department of Health Sciences
University "Magna Graecia" of
    Catanzaro
University Campus "S. Venuta"
Germaneto, Catanzaro, Italy

Marco Cosentino
Center for Research in Medical
    Pharmacology
University of Insubria
Varese, Italy

Luca Cravello
Department of Clinical and
    Behavioral Neurology
IRCCS Fondazione Santa Lucia
Rome, Italy

Maria Chiara Cristiano
Department of Health Sciences
University "Magna Graecia" of
    Catanzaro
University Campus "S. Venuta"
Germaneto, Catanzaro, Italy

Rosalia Crupi
Department of Biological and
    Environmental Sciences
University of Messina
Messina, Italy

Salvatore Cuzzocrea
Department of Biological and
    Environmental Sciences
University of Messina
Messina, Italy

and

Manchester Biomedical Research
    Centre
Manchester Royal Infirmary
University of Manchester
Manchester, United Kingdom

Fabio Firenzuoli
University of Florence
Department of Neurosciences,
    Psychology, Drug Research and
    Child Health
Section of Pharmacology and
    Toxicology
Center for Integrative Medicine
Firenze, Italy

Alfredo Focà
Department of Health Sciences
School of Medicine
University "Magna Graecia" of
    Catanzaro
Catanzaro, Italy

Marina Francišković
Department of Chemistry, Biochemistry
    and Environmental Protection
Faculty of Sciences
University of Novi Sad
Novi Sad, Serbia

Sergio Fusco
Unit of Geriatric
    Pharmacoepidemiology
IRCCS-INRCA
Cosenza, Italy

Eugenia Gallo
Department of Neurosciences,
    Psychology, Drug Research and
    Child Health
Section of Pharmacology and
    Toxicology
Center for Integrative Medicine
University of Florence
Firenze, Italy

Soh Katsuyama
Center for Experiential Pharmacy
    Practice
Tokyo University of Pharmacy and Life
    Science
Tokyo, Japan

Takaaki Komatsu
First Department of Pharmacology
Daiichi College of Pharmaceutical
    Sciences
Fukuoka, Japan

Marija Lesjak
Department of Chemistry, Biochemistry
    and Environmental Protection
Faculty of Sciences
University of Novi Sad
Novi Sad, Serbia

Maria Carla Liberto
Department of Health Sciences
School of Medicine
University "Magna Graecia" of
    Catanzaro
Catanzaro, Italy

Anna Loraschi
Center for Research in Medical
    Pharmacology
University of Insubria
Varese, Italy

Franca Marino
Center for Research in Medical
    Pharmacology
University of Insubria
Varese, Italy

Milena Masullo
Dipartimento di Farmacia
Università degli Studi di Salerno
Fisciano, Salerno, Italy

Anna Menini
Neurobiology Group
International School for Advanced
    Studies (SISSA)
Trieste, Italy

Neda Mimica-Dukić
Department of Chemistry, Biochemistry
    and Environmental Protection
Faculty of Sciences
University of Novi Sad
Novi Sad, Serbia

Marco Miroddi
Department of Clinical and
    Experimental Medicine
University of Messina
Messina, Italy

Hirokazu Mizoguchi
Department of Physiology and Anatomy
Tohoku Pharmaceutical University
Sendai, Japan

Paola Montoro
Dipartimento di Farmacia
Università degli Studi di Salerno
Fisciano, Salerno, Italy

Luigi Antonio Morrone
Department of Pharmacy, Health and
    Nutritional Sciences
Section of Preclinical and Translational
    Pharmacology
and
University Consortium for Adaptive
    Disorders and Head Pain (UCADH)
University of Calabria
Rende, Cosenza, Italy

Alessandro Mugelli
Department of Neurosciences,
    Psychology, Drug Research and
    Child Health
Section of Pharmacology and
    Toxicology
Center for Integrative Medicine
University of Florence
Firenze, Italy

Michele Navarra
Department of Drug Sciences and
    Products for Health
University of Messina
Messina, Italy

Dejan Orčić
Department of Chemistry, Biochemistry
    and Environmental Protection
Faculty of Sciences
University of Novi Sad
Novi Sad, Serbia

Donatella Paolino
Department of Health Sciences
University "Magna Graecia" of
    Catanzaro
University Campus "S. Venuta"
Germaneto, Catanzaro, Italy

Sonia Piacente
Dipartimento di Farmacia
Università degli Studi di Salerno
Fisciano, Salerno, Italy

Simone Pifferi
Neurobiology Group
International School for Advanced
    Studies (SISSA)
Trieste, Italy

Cosimo Pizza
Dipartimento di Farmacia
Università degli Studi di Salerno
Fisciano, Salerno, Italy

Alessandra Pugi
Department of Neurosciences,
    Psychology, Drug Research and
    Child Health
Section of Pharmacology and
    Toxicology
Center for Integrative Medicine
University of Florence
Firenze, Italy

Salvatore Ragusa
Department of Health Sciences
University "Magna Graecia" of
    Catanzaro
University Campus "S. Venuta"
Catanzaro, Italy

Laura Rombolà
Department of Pharmacy, Health and
    Nutritional Sciences
Section of Preclinical and Translational
    Pharmacology
University of Calabria
Rende, Cosenza, Italy

Rossella Russo
Department of Pharmacy, Health
    Science and Nutrition
University of Calabria
Rende, Cosenza, Italy

Shinobu Sakurada
Department of Physiology and Anatomy
Tohoku Pharmaceutical University
Sendai, Japan

Tsukasa Sakurada
Drug Innovation Center
Daiichi University of Pharmacy
Fukuoka, Japan

Natasa Simin
Department of Chemistry, Biochemistry
and Environmental Protection
Faculty of Sciences
University of Novi Sad
Novi Sad, Serbia

Giancarlo Statti
Department of Pharmacy, Health
Science and Nutrition
University of Calabria
Rende, Cosenza, Italy

Emilija Svirčev
Department of Chemistry, Biochemistry
and Environmental Protection
Faculty of Sciences
University of Novi Sad
Novi Sad, Serbia

Alfredo Vannacci
Department of Neurosciences,
Psychology, Drug Research and
Child Health
Section of Pharmacology and
Toxicology
Center for Integrative Medicine
University of Florence
Firenze, Italy

Candida Vannini
Department of Biotechnology and
Life Sciences
University of Insubria
Varese, Italy

Sunita Vohra
Integrative Health Institute
CARE Program
Department of Pediatrics
Faculty of Medicine and Dentistry
University of Alberta
Edmonton, Alberta, Canada

Chizuko Watanabe
Department of Physiology and Anatomy
Tohoku Pharmaceutical University
Sendai, Japan

1 Historical Notes on Essential Oils and Aromatherapy with Special Reference to Bergamot Essential Oil

Alfredo Focà and Maria Carla Liberto

CONTENTS

1.1 HISTORICAL NOTES

Before the advent of medical textbooks, and even the written word, we used plants, roots, leaves, and flowers, not only for nutrition, but also as a protection against disease—particularly infection arising as a result of wounds, traumas, and accidents. This instinctive, or folk, medicine has been around as long as we have walked the earth, and officinal plants are still widely used as natural remedies today, the practice evolving alongside progress in scientific understanding. Indeed, primitive preparations of plant matter for medicinal use involving simple processes such as crushing, mastication, and maceration were largely superseded by more complex methods of preparation, such as infusion, digestion, decoction, percolation, distillation, and enfleurage (enfleurage—both hot and cold—is the most ancient "technical" method of obtaining plant-based remedies), made possible by the discovery of fire.

These more advanced methods, many of which are still in use today, furnished more accurate and effective preparations—essential oils, for example, which were prized not only for their medicinal properties, but also as perfumes, and their scope of application continued to evolve alongside further advances in technology. Distillation in particular represented an early but important technological leap, and we know that the Chinese practiced a rudimentary form of distillation 6000 years BCE; they also made use of techniques such as filtration and sublimation. Similar techniques are also thought to have been used by the ancient Sumerians, and fragments of what appears to be primitive distillation equipment have been found at archaeological sites in Mesopotamia—the so-called cradle of civilization—dating back to 5000 years BCE. Evidence of the ancient Egyptians' familiarity with home-made remedies comes in the form of inscriptions on the perimeter wall of the Temple of Horus at Edfu (Behedet). Dating back 2000 years, these inscriptions comprise a kind of medical handbook, a phytopharmaceutical recipe book displayed for all the populace to see and make use of. We also know that the ancient Egyptians were using purpose-designed apparatus for distilling wine and cider even earlier than that, 4000 years BCE.

The oldest literature source we have illustrating the use of distillation apparatus is conserved in the Biblioteca Marciana in Venice (Ms. of St. Mark, gr. 299, fol. 88v) and dates back to around the second century BCE. Attributed to the alchemist (the doctors of the age) known to posterity as Cleopatra, the ancient Greek papyrus document *Chrysopoeia* clearly shows a workable distillation setup of the same name comprising a wide-necked double alembic heated over a water bath and featuring two inclined lateral tubes through which the distilled liquid could be collected (Figure 1.1).

Similar, but less detailed, illustrations can be seen in the alchemical text Ms. 2327 of the Bibliothèque Nationale in Paris, and in the Leyden papyrus, purportedly written at the end of the third century CE. Zosimos of Panopolis, another prominent alchemist, who practiced his art around the turn of the fourth century CE and wrote the oldest known books on the subject, also left us with an illustration of distillation apparatus observed in an ancient temple at Memphis, alongside instructions for preparing the so-called divine waters, that is, distilled liquids of various types, including plant-based essential oils (Figure 1.2). As a condensation system was still lacking at this time, the heated vapors produced during the distillation process were

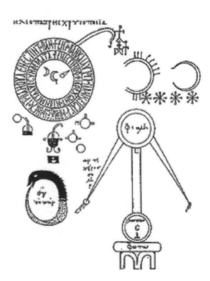

FIGURE 1.1   Cleopatra's *Chrysopoeia*. (From Ms. of St. Mark, gr. 299, fol. 88v.)

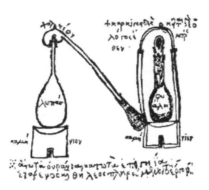

FIGURE 1.2 Distillation apparatus of Zosimos. (From Marcelin Berthelot, *Collection des anciens alchimistes grecs*, 3 vol., Paris, 1887–1888.)

dripped onto fabric pads, which were later squeezed to obtain the few drops of precious liquid produced.

The Arabs, who learned the technique from the ancient Egyptians, became masters of distillation techniques—indeed, the terms *alembic* and *alcohol* are clearly of Arabic origin—and made great strides in the process of extracting essential oils. Khālid al-Qasrī, (?–743 CE), alchemist and governor of Iraq under the Umayyad Caliphate, perfected the distillation technique to produce essential oils from flowers, particularly the rose. Jabir al-Sufi (Geber) (c. 721–c. 815), another Arabic alchemist, classified two extraction techniques, one making use of fire (distillation) and the other without (filtration), which he used to separate two clear liquids by means of a filter. Muhammad ibn Zakariyā Rāzī (854–c. 925), a Persian alchemist, philosopher, and physician, known simply as Razi or Rhazes in the West, and the most eminent chemist of his time, described several methods of distillation: *per ascensum*, *per descensum*, and *per latus*. In his copious works he described the preparation of *aqua vitae*, a concentrated solution of ethanol, and how to concentrate alcohol through distillation, passing alcohol vapors over hot coals or ash, a method he also used to extract perfume from flowers.

The various techniques for obtaining aqua vitae and perfumes developed over the centuries helped scholars to isolate and understand the natural essences derived from plants, and to describe the protective properties of such aromatic substances against infection. The Greek physician, pharmacist, and botanist Dioscorides (Anazarbe, c. 40–c. 90), for example, wrote one of the first written records of the scientific use of therapeutic preparations obtained from plant matter. For distillation, Dioscorides used a piece of equipment that he called the ambic (helmet), from which the Arabic term *alembic* later arose, and his comprehensive encyclopedia of herbal medicine, *De Materia Medica*, was widely circulated throughout the civilized world for centuries after his demise.

Dioscorides himself, not to mention Galen and Hippocrates, is likely to have drawn on the work of Theophrastus (c. 371–c. 287 BCE), a Greek scholar and successor to Aristotle who is today considered the father of botany. Indeed, his *Historia Plantarum*, an encyclopedic work of 10 volumes, classified more than 500 types of plants, focusing on the anatomy and propagation of trees, shrubs, "undershrubs," cereals, legumes, and herbs. The ninth volume of the series described the therapeutic uses of plants and is one of the earliest medicinal herbals to be written. He later expanded upon this theme in his *On the Causes of Plants*, another weighty series of eight volumes.

These texts continued to be relevant in the tenth century (and beyond), when another Persian polymath and father of early modern medicine, Ibn-Sīnā, more widely known in the West as Avicenna (930–1037), introduced a convoluted cooling tube into the distillation apparatus. He described the use of a heating and cooling system for extracting volatile essential oils, which comprised aromatic liquids and what was considered to be their active, antibacterial principle. The conviction that essential oils, and therefore the plants they were obtained from, had antibacterial properties persisted until the Middle Ages (alongside Dioscorides's "pharmacopoeia") and explains why plague doctors wore the distinctive beak-like masks described by Thomas Bartholin in 1661 (Figure 1.3); these masks contained cotton pads soaked in aromatic liquids to filter, and therefore protect them from, the miasma (putrid air), thought to be the means by which the disease was spread.

Avicenna extracted essence of rose by boiling petals of *Rosa centifolia* in a curved alembic and collecting the resulting vapor. The extraction of rose essential oil evidently became fairly commonplace in the Arab world of the early Middle Ages, being described in a number of Byzantine texts. Considered a valuable commodity and exported as far as India and China, Persian rosewater was recommended as a medicament by Theophanes Nonnus, physician to Emperor Michael VIII. It was also immortalized as a toilet water in Constantine Porphyrogenitus's (emperor of the eastern Roman empire) codex of ceremonies, published in 946 CE. Giovanni Plateario, in his *Circa Instans*, tells us that the technique was adopted by the School of Salerno, one of the most influential schools of medicine in eleventh-century Europe and precursor to the universities of today.

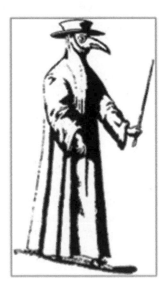

FIGURE 1.3   Thomas Bartholin's plague doctor wearing a "beak" mask filled with aromatic herbs.

Although the use of plant extracts for phytotherapeutic purposes was initially linked to empirical observation, popular customs more likely to be prescribed by shamans and charlatans than by physicians, as the technology evolved, scientific testing has borne out their validity in many cases, granting phytotherapy and aromatherapy a return to respectability, even in the medicine of today. In fact, essential oils from a considerable number of plant species have important applications alongside or as alternatives to better-known natural or synthetic remedies for treating diseases of microbial origin. Although nowadays we can point to the active ingredients and their specific mechanisms of action, the officinal plants from which these essential oils derive are the same used in ancient times, however crude their preparation might first have been.

Modern-day scientific literature contains numerous examples of natural substances with antimicrobial properties (antibacterial, antiviral, antifungal, and antiprotozoal) [1–5], and phytopharmaceuticals also possess certain other advantages, including low toxicity, ease of handling, pleasant smell, and collateral properties, that enhance their effectiveness [6,7] and make them much sought-after remedies even in these enlightened times. Among the substances derived from nature, essential oils are particularly useful for healing purposes, as they possess marked antiseptic and antimicrobial properties, among others. They also possess great evocative power in being able to stimulate the olfactory system (volatile fraction) via a complex synaesthesic process that, although largely unconscious, is exquisitely perceptive and closely linked to memory. Our sense of smell is regulated by a specific area of the brain that has close anatomical ties to the limbic system, specifically the hippocampus, and the olfactory cortex.

Odorant molecules, for example the volatile products of essential oils, are detected by receptors on the olfactory sensory neurons in the mucous lining of the nasal cavity. These sensory neurons project axons to the brain through the olfactory nerve, a cranial nerve that carries electrical signals through the cribiform plate of the ethmoid bone and toward the olfactory bulb, which in turn projects to the olfactory cortex. The olfactory bulb is the site of the so-called olfactive memory, the ability to decipher and discriminate the various aromatic compounds present in the volatile fraction of essential oils. Olfaction develops and is modulated differently in different individuals, but in all cases it enables us to form immediate connections between a particular smell and our own specific memories and emotions. Through its connections to the hypothalamus, the olfactory bulb can stimulate the release of powerful psychoactive mediators and hormones, such as serotonin and noradrenaline, thereby explaining the various sedative, relaxant, euphoric, and stimulant properties of essential oils.

Essential oils are complex substances secreted by plants for various purposes: to attract pollinators, for cell-to-cell communication, and to protect against pests and predators, to name but a few. They are stored in secretory structures located either inside (secretory cavities, ducts, or cells) or on the surface (glandular trichomes) of the plant. Their organoleptic, phytotherapeutic, and psychoactive properties are conferred not only by each of the various chemical constituents, but also by the strong synergistic action they exert. Hence, their characteristics will vary in function depending on the plant species they are extracted from (there is considerable variation between species of the same genus), the part of the plant they are extracted from (fruit, leaf, flower, etc.), the microclimate of the region their parent plants inhabit, the changing of the seasons, and the technique by which they are extracted. There is a wide variety of chemical constituents in the different essential oils [8], and even those from related plant species will exhibit markedly different characteristics. Taking sage, for example, *Salvia sclarea* produces an essential oil of low toxicity and excellent therapeutic properties, while *Salvia officinalis*, common sage, is far more toxic, due to the presence of thujone—a ketone and monoterpene with a menthol odor, also found in wormwood—among its constituents.

At room temperature, essential oils generally form liquids of various densities, although some have a resinous consistency. They are generally pale orange to yellow in color, although those that contain azulene may be green or blue (*Matricaria chamomilla, Helichrysum italicum*). Essential oils tend to darken with age via a process of oxidation, and as the name suggests, they are insoluble in water but soluble in alcohol, organic solvents, and vegetable oils.

Until very recently, the branch of medicine that studies the properties of essential oils, aromatherapy, has been considered a niche speciality, and very few articles on such substances have found their way into the mainstream scientific publications. Gattefossé [9] was the first (1926) to introduce the concept of aromatherapy and indicate some specific healthcare applications for essential oils [10,11]. Since then, however, the majority of studies into the phytotherapeutic benefits of officinal plant extracts, including the essential oils, have been regarded as something of a curiosity and relegated to the status of empirical or alternative medicine. Nevertheless, as laboratory methods advance, more and more repeatable, recognized, and above all, scientific research has been carried out and is beginning to find a wider audience among the readership of accredited journals. Initially such research was focused on globally known (and highly fashionable) plants such as the tea tree (*Melaleuca alternifolia*), but nowadays the scope of aromatherapy has broadened considerably to include a wide variety of plant sources (Table 1.1).

As mentioned, the specific properties of an essential oil will depend on its chemical composition, and therefore the part of the plant it is obtained from and the variety of plant itself. The activity of citrus oils from the leaves of *Citrus aurantium*—the Seville orange—for instance, are high in esters (linalyl acetate), whereas their flowers have a greater preponderance of alcohols (linalool). To give another example, the bark of the cinnamon tree yields an oil rich in cinnaminic aldehyde, while oil from the leaves of the same plant has a high phenol content.

The antiseptic properties of many plants have been recognized empirically for millennia, but the effects of essential oils from common plants used for such purposes are now being confirmed by science. Chamomile (*Chamaemelum nobile*), for example, has long been used to cleanse wounds, burns, and boils, and many other common European plants, including the red fir, silver fir, birch, angelica seeds, basil, and sweet flag (*Acorus calamus*), are also used to produce oils of antiseptic action (Table 1.1). Other, rarer and more exotic, sources of antiseptic oils include sandalwood, myrrh, and the round leaf buchu (*Agathosma betulina*). Cardamom, cinnamon, and caraway oils are antiparasitic as well as antiseptic, and oil of cloves has long been used in dentistry as an analgesic and antiseptic. Rockrose (*Cistus*) yields another powerful antiseptic oil and is one of the first aromatic herbs to be mentioned

TABLE 1.1
Antimicrobial Activities of Essential Oils

Binomial Name	Common Name	AB	AM	AV
Abelmoschus moschatus	Ambrette (seeds)			
Abies alba	White spruce			
Abies balsamea	Balsam fir (needles)	+		
Abies sibirica	Siberian fir			
Achillea millefolium	Yarrow			
Acorus calamus	Sweet flag			
Allium sativum	Garlic			
Amyris balsamifera	Sandalwood			
Anethum gravolens	Dill			
Angelica archangelica	Angelica (seeds)			
Aniba rosaeodora	Brazilian rosewood			+−
Anthemis nobilis	Roman chamomile	+−		
Apium graveolens	Celery			
Aquilaria malaccensis	Agarwood			
Artemisia dracunculus	Tarragon	++	+	
Artemisia pallens	Dhavanam			
Artemisia vulgare	Wormwood			
Barosma betulina	Buchu			
Betula alba	Birch			
Boswellia carterii	Frankincense	++		
Boswellia rivae	Frankincense			
Brassica nigra	Black mustard			
Cananga odorata	Ylang-ylang			
Canarium luzonicum	Elemi			
Carum carvi	Caraway			
Chamaemelum nobile	Roman chamomile	+−		
Cinnamomum canphora	Camphor			
Cinnamomum cassia	Chinese cinnamon			
Cinnamomum verum	Ceylon cinnamon (bark)	+++^	++	+−
Cinnamomun zeylanicum	Ceylon cinnamon (bark)			
Cistus ladaniferus	Brown-eyed rockrose	+	+−	+
Citrus aurantifolia	Lime		+−	+
Citrus aurantium am. (flos)	Neroli	++	+−	
Citrus aurantium am. (fol)	Seville orange	+	+++*	
Citrus aurantium am. (per)	Bitter orange		+−	
Citrus aurantium am. (sinensis)	Sweet orange		+−	
Citrus aurantium dulcis	Citrus dulcis			

(*Continued*)

TABLE 1.1 (CONTINUED)
Antimicrobial Activities of Essential Oils

Binomial Name	Common Name	AB	AM	AV
Citrus bergamia	Bergamot	+++		++
Citrus cedra	Citron			
Citrus grandis	Shaddock/Pomelo			
Citrus limon	Lemon			+
Citrus paradisi	Grapefruit	++		
Citrus reticulata	Mandarin			
Commiphora erythraea	African myrrh			
Commiphora myrrha	Myrrh			+
Copaifera officinalis	Copaiba			
Coriandrum sativum	Coriander	++	+--	
Corymbia citriodora	Spotted gum			
Cuminum cyminum	Cumin		+-	+-
Cupressus sempervirens	Cypress	+		+-
Curcuma longa	Turmeric			
Cymbopogon citratus	Lemongrass	+-	+-	
Cymbopogon martinii	Palmarosa	+-	+-	+
Cymbopogon nardus	Citronella			
Daucus carota	Wild carrot (seeds)			
Elettaria cardamomum	Cardamom		+-	
Eucalyptus citriodora	Lemon-scented gum	++	+-	
Eucalyptus globulus	Tasmanian blue gum	+++^^	+--	
Eucalyptus dives	Broad-leaved peppermint	+	+--	+
Eucalyptus radiata	Narrow-leaved peppermint	+	+--	+-
Eucalyptus smithii	Gully gum	+-		+-
Eucaria spicata	Australian sandalwood	+	+++*	
Evernia prunastri	Oak moss			
Foeniculum vulgare dulce	Fennel	+	+--	
Gaultheria procumbens	Wintergreen			
Helichrysum angustifolium	Curry plant	++		
Hyssopus officinalis	Hyssop	++	+--	+
Illicium verum	Star anise		+--	
Inula heleinium	Elecampane/horse-heal		+	+-
Kunzea ericoides	Kanuka		+-	
Juniperus communis	Common juniper			
Juniperus virginiana	Red cedar			
Laurus nobilis	Bay			+-
Lavandula angustifolia	Lavendar	+++^^^	++*	
Lavandula intermedia super	Lavandin		+--	+-

(Continued)

TABLE 1.1 (CONTINUED)
Antimicrobial Activities of Essential Oils

Binomial Name	Common Name	AB	AM	AV
Lavandula latifolia	Spike lavander	+	+−−	+
Leptospermum scoparium	Manuka	+−	+−	+
Levisticum officinalis	Lovage			++
Lippia citriodora	Verbena			
Litsea cubeba	May Chang			
Matricaria recrutita	German chamomile	+−	+	
Melaleuca alternifolia	Tea tree	+++^	++*	
Melaleuca leucadendron	Cajeput	+++^	++*	++
Melaleuca viridiflora	Broad-leaved paperbark	++	+−−	++
Melissa officinalis	Lemon balm/Melissa		+−−	+
Mentha arvensis	Field mint		+−−	
Mentha piperita	Peppermint	++	!	+
Mentha spicata	Spearmint		+−	
Mentha suaveolens	Apple mint			
Myristica fragrans	Nutmeg	+		
Myrtus communis	Myrtle	+	+−	
Nardostachys jatamansi	Spikenard		+	
Nepeta cataria	Catnip		++*	++°
Ocimum basilicum	Basil	+	+	+
Origanum heracleoticum	Greek oregano		++	
Origanum majorana	Sweet marjoram	+++	+−−	+
Origanum vulgare	Oregano	++		
Ormenis multicaulis	Moroccan chamomile	+		
Pelargonium graveolens	Geranium	++		+−
Pelargonium asperum	Geranium	++	+−−	+−
Petroselinum sativum	Parsley			
Picea abies	Norway spruce			
Pimenta dioica	Allspice			++
Pimenta racemosa	West Indian bay			+
Pimpinella anisum	Aniseed	+−	++*	
Pinus cembra	Swiss stone pine			
Pinus pinaster	Maritime/cluster pine			
Pinus sylvestris	Scots pine			
Piper nigrum	Black pepper	+−		++
Pistacia lentiscus	Mastic			
Pogostemon cablin	Patchouli		+	
Ravensara aromatica	Clove nutmeg	+−		++°°
Rosa damascena	Damask rose	+		
Rosmarinus officinalis	Rosemary	+	+−	+
Rosmarinus officinalis verbenone	Rosemary verbenone	+	+−	++

(Continued)

TABLE 1.1 (CONTINUED)
Antimicrobial Activities of Essential Oils

Binomial Name	Common Name	AB	AM	AV
Salvia officinalis	Sage		+	++
Salvia sclarea	Clary sage			
Santalum album	Indian sandalwood			
Santalum spicatum	Australian sandalwood		+−	
Satureja hortensis	Summer savory	+++^		+−
Satureja montana	Winter savory	+++^	+−−	+−
Syzygium aromaticum	Clove	+++^	++	++°
Tagetes marigold (patula)	Marigold	+	+−	
Tagetes minuta	Southern cone marigold			
Thuya occidentalis	Northern white cedar			
Thymus capitatus	Spanish oregano	+++^	+++*	
Thymus mastichina	Spanish majoram	+	+−	
Thymus serpyllum	Wild thyme	+	+−	+−
Thymus vulgaris	Thyme	+++^	+−	++
Valeriana officinalis	Valerian			
Vetiveria zizanioides	Vetiver			
Zingiber officinalis	Ginger			

Source: Adapted from Price, S., and Price, L., *Aromatherapy for Health Professionals*, Churchill Livingstone Elsevier, London, 2012.

Note: AB: Antibacterial activity; AM: Antimycotic activity; AV: Antiviral activity; ^, Gram-positive and Gram-negative; ^^, *Diplococcus pneumoniae*; ^^^, betahemolytic *Streptococcus*. *, *Candida* species; °, herpes simplex; °°, herpes zoster.

in writing. The tribes of the Amazon have long relied on the antiseptic, fungicidal, and anti-inflammatory properties of Copaiba oil, which is rich in oleic and linoleic acids. Closer to home, the various populations that inhabit the Mediterranean region have an ancient tradition of exploiting the fungicidal and antibacterial properties of coriander oil, and coriander seeds were even found in the tomb of Egyptian pharaoh Ramses the Great. Antibacterial action has also been documented for the essential oils of garlic and Seville orange (obtained by cold-pressing the fresh peel), which is also fungicidal. Other antifungal antibacterial essential oils include sweet orange, lavender, lemon, laurel, rose geranium, and hyssop. The antiseptic properties of cajeput oil have been attributed to a specific antiviral action, and essential oils from the cedar and spotted gum can be used to treat cold sores (herpes simplex). Eucalyptus oil is also effective against the herpes virus, and this, as well as its antiseptic action, makes it useful in the treatment of respiratory infections.

The antimicrobial and antiseptic actions summarily described above are potentiated by the many other benefits of essential oils, such as anti-inflammatory, cicatrizing, stimulant, and fluidificant properties. Little wonder then that, over the centuries, in some parts of the world the cultivation of the source plants for particular essential oils has shaped the geographical surroundings and culture of certain populations, who have wisely preserved and transmitted the relative know-how down through the generations, despite the waxing and waning of the interest in such products.

1.2 BERGAMOT: A REGIONAL TREASURE

The *Citrus bergamia* (bergamot), cultivated for centuries in a certain region of Calabria, southern Italy, produces an essential oil with certain biochemical characteristics that has long been undervalued and used predominantly as a stabilizer for the luxury fragrance market. However, oil of bergamot has recently been proven to possess a powerful antimycotic antimicrobial action [12], and its volatile products are antiseptic, cicatrizing, and psychoactive [13]. Its antimicrobial properties have attracted interest from researchers from all over the globe, and it has been the subject of numerous articles recently published in major scientific journals [14], testament to their scientific rigor. This has thrust bergamot oil from its humble origins as a local product firmly onto the international stage.

There are several varieties of the bergamot plant (*Citrus bergamia*, family Rutaceae) grown in Calabria, namely *"castagnaro"*, *"femminello"*, and *"fantastico"*. Its branches are irregular and its leaves dark green, and it grows best in sunny areas close to the sea. Its flowers, which appear at the end of March in its preferred climate, are highly fragrant and known in the local dialect as *zagara* (from the Arabic *zahara*, "flower"). The fruit, the bergamot orange, is rounded in shape and has a peel (epicarp) that turns from green to yellow as it ripens. The peel is covered with the utricles that contain the essential oil. The endocarp or pulp, which makes up 65%–70% of the fruit, contains juice that is used in medicine to combat high cholesterol, and the spongy mesocarp is rich in pectin (Figure 1.4).

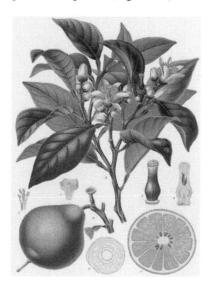

FIGURE 1.4   *Citrus bergamia.*

The fruits are harvested from October to January, as soon as they are ripe enough for the utricles to open and permit the ready extraction of their essential oil. Until the advent of the industrial revolution, bergamot oranges were picked by hand, and their clear greenish yellow oil was extracted with the aid of a sharp knife and collected in natural sponges. In 1844, however, Nicola Barilla invented "the Calabrian machine," which was specifically designed to extract the essence of bergamot. Nowadays, however, this has been superseded, and the process considerably accelerated, by hydraulic peeling machines with rotating rollers or plates.

1.3 BERGAMOT ESSENCE: A HISTORY OF THE RESEARCH

Empirical observations on the antimicrobial, cicatrizing, and balsamic properties of the essence of bergamot were first published in 1800 by Francesco Calabrò, a physician from Reggio Calabria [15]. According to Calabrò, bergamot had been grown commercially in Calabria since before the mid-1700s. This was disputed by several sources, which stated that the first commercial crop was planted in 1750 in the countryside close to Reggio Calabria, but in reality, Gian Paolo Feminis from Santa Maria Maggiore, near Novara, had begun to market his bergamot-based "Admirabilis Aqua" as a painkiller as early as 1660, presumably after the essential oil had become available. Later, in 1676, Feminis relocated to Cologne, and in 1727 he patented this "miraculous" water as "Eau de Cologne," whereupon it was promptly pirated in Italy and elsewhere.

Calabrò, thanks to his medical training, was the first to commission a detailed chemical analysis of bergamot extract [16] in the attempt to provide scientific support for the empirical evidence. Although he did make accurate reference to the possible deposition of gelatin or gluten products that may promote wound healing, the chemist that Calabrò entrusted with this analysis was unable to characterize the volatile products of the essence, to which the latter ascribed its "heroic virtues," leading him to conclude that "given its physical qualities, I would like to believe that, in addition to its excitatory and stimulatory action, it must possess other singular properties in the treatment of wounds, the nature of which we are unaware, whose action depends on its principal components."

Undeterred by the technological limitations of the age, Calabrò widened his research and proposed the use of compresses soaked in a moderate quantity of bergamot essence to heal lacerations, contusions, and knife wounds. He also recommended its use in fever and reported an interesting anecdote regarding its antimalarial properties: "In 1760, Colonel Bernardo Scasanto used the essence as an antimalarial. In fact, having been given 5–6 kilos of essence of bergamot from a nephew from Reggio Calabria, Salvadore Pandari, he used it to treat the soldiers of his regiment affected with tertian or quartan fever."

Calabrò's observations were subsequently published in the *Annales de Thérapeutique* [17], a French medical journal, and commented upon in detail by another Calabrian physician, Francesco Rognetta. Rognetta noted that the workers employed to extract bergamot essence using very sharp knives often cut themselves, but due to the fact that their hands were soaked in bergamot oil, they healed rapidly without medical intervention; he therefore concluded that essence of bergamot promoted cicatrization and prevented suppuration.

Another physician from Reggio Calabria, Vincenzo De Domenico, also studied the medicinal properties of bergamot, describing several cases of malarial fever that he treated with bergamot essential oil, and noted its dynamic hypotensive action [18]. He also used it to bring down fever, with consistently encouraging results, and as a vermicide. Being a liquid, according to De Domenico, bergamot oil could readily be administered using any type of beverage as a vehicle. De Domenico also decided to test this potion in its topical form for its effectiveness against scabies. Once again, he reported very encouraging results, which led him to recommend it to Don Ferdinando Bergamo, surgeon to the 12th regiment, stationed at that time in Reggio Calabria. Bergamo appears to have used this "ointment" to cure many cases of scabies, noting that the essence "heals even the scabs." He also went so far as to state that bergamot essence was a more efficacious treatment than sulfur, as it "acts on the mood of the patient" [19]. To provide experimental proof of his observations, De Domenico conducted a series of trials, first testing the essence of bergamot on dogs, and then, to verify its effect on "healthy men," he decided to self-administer, describing its effects with extreme precision [18].

These initial empirical observations were soon followed by more scientific investigations into the benefits of bergamot essential oil, with specific focus on its antiseptic and antibacterial properties. In 1869, the Scottish chemist Robert Angus Smith, taking up where his predecessor, David MacBride, left off, confirmed the antiseptic efficacy of the volatile oils of various essences, bergamot included [20,21], and Charles Chamberland, celebrated French microbiologist and friend to Louis Pasteur, demonstrated the inhibitory effect of several on the growth of anthrax bacteria (*Bacillus anthracis*) [22]. In 1894, Francesco Maltese, a lecturer in dentistry at the University of Naples, investigated the use of a bergamot-based preparation in his field [23], inspiring Guido Bracchetti to use a 10% solution of bergamot essence to sterilize root canals and fully heal infected periapical and periradicular tissues, demonstrating its superiority with respect to other essences, like oil of cloves and thyme, as well as carbolic acid [24,25].

Giuseppe Sergi, in an article published in Reggio Calabria in 1925, described the properties of bergamot essence as follows: "This essence rapidly moderates and heals wounds, impeding their suppuration; if applied promptly, it impedes phlogosis and cyanosis in surgical lesions, fortifies and vivifies healthy tissue, and, finally, encompasses the virtue of a strongly aromatic analgesic; it is necessary to apply it always to the affected parts by means of a little cotton impregnated with it in the quantities deemed to be sufficient" [26,27].

Around the same time, Arturo Sabatini, military physician, found that in its raw state the essence of bergamot was an excellent antiseptic and rapidly cicatrized the alveolus and gum after dental extraction, as well as sterilizing dental caries and curing various disorders of the scalp. Among its advantages, he highlighted the fact that it did not irritate damaged tissue, even in high doses. Bursting with tables and experimental data, Sabatini's paper also compared the effects of bergamot essence with those of other essences and their vapors, calculating the time to its onset of action on various bacterial species *in vitro*. His paper also contained the results of his *in vivo* experiments, conducted on guinea pigs and frogs, which he used to calculate the lethal dose [28]. Sabatini also repeated research performed by Albert Morel and

Anthelme Rochaix, who, in his series of works on bergamot essence, had obtained very satisfactory results in treating meningitis, diphtheria, typhus, and pustules [29].

In the decade that followed, Prof. Antonino Spinelli, head surgeon at Reggio Calabria hospital, experimented with bergamot essence in his operating theater. He successfully used it for disinfecting small wounds, and in the treatment of contused lacerations and anfractuous lesions, concluding that it possessed evident bactericidal action against both cutaneous and dermal infections. He added that it neither stained the skin nor caused irritation or toxicity upon absorption, and was particularly useful for treating putrid, malodorous wounds, due to its pleasing fragrance. Spinelli confirmed his deductions regarding the efficacy of the preparation via a battery of *in vivo* tests on rabbits, guinea pigs, and rats [30].

In 1933, Fulvio Pulcher, from the University of Genoa, published the results of his research demonstrating the disinfectant action of a bergamot essence soap emulsion, with which he successfully overcame the difficulties in obtaining a stable hydroalcoholic preparation of the essential oil [7], citing studies on its antiseptic action by Robert Koch, C. Cadéac, and A. Meunier (bactericidal effect on the glanders bacillus), C. Guargena, W. Collier, and Y. Nitta, and others. Also in 1933, Prof. Giovanni Carossini, head surgeon at Reggio Calabria hospital, published his observations on a disinfectant called Sabeol, invented and patented by a certain Dr. Usellini of Milan, which was made from bergamot essence "purified and subjected to a particular chemical treatment." Carossini was enthusiastic about its excellent disinfectant properties and its pronounced detersive and anaesthetic effects on wounds and sores, and he also noted that it produced marked keratinization of ulcers [6]. The effectiveness of bergamot as a surgical disinfectant was also confirmed 2 years later by Prof. S. Puglisi-Allegra, who used a 15% alcoholic solution of the essence in surgery and in the treatment of suppurating lesions [31].

One of the milestones in the rich history of publications on the properties of the essence of bergamot is the study by the man considered the father of aromatherapy, Prof. René-Maurice Gattefossé. In his laboratory at the University of Lyon Faculty of Medicine, he tested various formulations of the essence (lotions, irrigations, powders, ointments, tablets, syrups, paints, etc.) in numerous infective processes of the skin and respiratory and urinary systems and on wounds, with excellent results [9,32]. Another luminary, Giuseppe Sanarelli, hygiene lecturer for the Universities of Bologna, Siena, and Rome, also conducted a wide-ranging study on the properties of bergamot. Published in 1936, his memoirs recounted a series of tests conducted on an aqueous solution of the essence called Bergamon, which had been prepared by means of a process developed by another Calabrian son, Dr. F. Romeo. Sanarelli described two preparations, Bergamon-alpha and Bergamon-beta, the latter being more concentrated, and demonstrated the bactericidal action of both on typhus and diphtheria, as well as pyogenic *Staphylococcus* species and *Vibrio cholerae*. He concluded that this bergamot-based disinfectant was of comparable efficacy to better-known, more powerful antiseptics, but did not possess their disadvantages; like the essential oil it was based on, Bergamon had a pleasant smell, did not stain, irritate, or corrode, and above all, was nontoxic, making its field of experimentation and application almost limitless [33]. Citing an article that had appeared in the *Journal of the American Association of Medical Research* in November 1935, Romeo described specific cases in which an aromatic disinfectant like Bergamon would be particularly beneficial to patients, namely childbearing women, neurasthenics, convalescents, and those affected by insomnia and respiratory disorders.

Bergamon was also popular with Antonino Spinelli [34], who, like Dr. Attilio Anedda of the University of Cagliari, used it in surgical settings. In 1940, the latter also reported his observations on its usefulness in the treatment of scabies [35]. The same topic was discussed by Lt. Col. Dr. Dogalino Maimone of Rome's military hospital [36] and many other Italian civilian and military researchers. In ophthalmology, Bergamon was used with excellent results by G. Gandolfi and G. Boari of Parma University [37], as well as Carlo Gandolfi of the same university's eye clinic [38]. Prof. Pompeo Scoto from the University of Cagliari used it in obstetrics [39] and described it as a "powerful antiseptic at various dilutions, and a rapid cicatrizing agent."

REFERENCES

1. Focà A. (a cura di). Sull'azione anti-microbica dell'essenza di bergamotto. Dip. di Scienze Mediche, Università "Magna Graecia," Catanzaro, 2001.
2. Carson, C.F., Hammer, K.A., and Riley, T.V. Broth microdilution method for determining the susceptibility of *Escherichia coli* and *Staphylococcus aureus* to the essential oil of *Melaleuca alternifolia*. *Microbios* 82:181–185, 1995.
3. Carson, C.F., Cookson, B.D., Farrelly, H.D., and Riley, T.V. Susceptibility of methicillin-resistant *Staphylococcus aureus* to the essential oil of *Melaleuca alternifolia*. *J Antimicrob Chemother* 35:421–424, 1995.
4. Lima, E.O., Gompertz, O.F., Giesbrecht, A.M., and Paulo, M.Q. In vitro antifungal activity of essential oils obtained from officinal plants against dermatophytes. *Mycoses* 36:333–336, 1993.
5. Focà, A. *Dell'essenza di bergamotta*. F. Pancallo Ed., Locri, 2005.
6. Carossini, G. Un nuovo antisettico in chirurgia: Il "Sabeol" (a base di essenza di bergamotto). *Rivista Italiana di Terapia*, anno VII, no. 10:1–7, 1933.
7. Pulcher, F. Ricerche sull'azione disinfettante dell'essenza di bergamotto in emulsioni saponose. *L'igiene moderna*, anno XXVI, no. 12:1–21, 1933.
8. Price, S., and Price, L. *Aromatherapy for Health Professionals*. Churchill Livingstone Elsevier, London, 2012.
9. Gattefossé, R.M. *Aromathérapie*. Libreria Girardot, Paris, 1926.
10. Valussi, M. *Il grande Manuale dell'aromaterapia. Fondamentali di scienza degli oli essenziali*. Tecniche Nuove Ed., Milano, 2005.
11. Valnet, J. *The Practice of Aromatherapy*. Healing Arts Press, Rochester, VT, 1990.
12. Aloui, H., Khwaldia, K., Licciardello, F., Mazzaglia, A., Muratore, G., Hamdi, M., and Restuccia, C. Efficacy of the combined application of chitosan and locust bean gum with different citrus essential oils to control postharvest spoilage caused by *Aspergillus flavus* in dates. *Int J Food Microbiol* 170:21–28, 2014.
13. Ni, C.H., Hou, W.H., Kao, C.C., Cang, M.L., Yu, L.F., Wu, C.C., and Chen, C. The anxiolitic effect of aromatherapy on patients awaiting ambulatory surgery: A randomized controlled trial. *Evid Based Complement Alternat Med* 2013:927419, 2013.
14. Werdin Gonzàlez, J.O., Gutierrez, M.M., Ferrero, A.A., and Fernandez Band, B. Essential oils nanoformulations for stored-product pest control: Characterization and biological properties. *Chemosphere* 100:130–138, 2014.
15. Focà, A. *Francesco Calabrò medico, patriota, autore dei primi studi sul bergamot*. Laruffa Ed., Reggio Calabria, 1998.

16. Calabrò, F. Della Balsamica virtù dell'essenza di bergamotta nelle ferrite. Tip. Fiumara e Nobolo, Messina, 1804.
17. Rognetta, F.F. Calabrò. *Annales de Thérapeutique, medicale et chirurgicale et de toxicologie* (Paris) 5:96–97, 1844.
18. De Domenico, V. Sulla efficacia della essenza di bergamotta nel trattamento delle febbri intermittenti, Tip. D. Siclari, Reggio Calabria, 1854 (1930).
19. Bergamo, F. Cenno storico intorno alla cura della scabbia con l'essenza di bergamotto. Tip. L. Ceruso, Reggio Calabria, 1853.
20. Smith, A. *Disinfectants and Disinfection*. Edmoston and Douglas, Edinburgh, 1869.
21. Marino, V. Sull'azione disinfettante dell'essenza di bergamotto. *Annali d'Igiene*, no. 3, 1935.
22. Chamberland, C. Les essences au point de vue de leurs proprietes antiseptique. *Ann Inst Pasteur* 1:153, 1887.
23. Maltese, F. Potere microbicida dell'essenza di bergamotto. Napoli, 1894.
24. Bracchetti, G. *La stomatologia*, p. 833. Ed. Federazione Dentisti d'Italia, Milano, 1923.
25. Bracchetti, G. Risultati di ricerche sperimentali sull'azione dell'essenza di bergamotto. *Rivista di agricoltura subtropicale e tropicale*, 44–45, 1950.
26. Sergi, G. *Il bergamotto ed i suoi derivati*. Ed. Vitalone, Reggio Calabria, 1926.
27. Sergi, G. *Le piante narcotiche nelle voluttà dei popoli*. Tipografia ed. L'Avvenire di M. Borgia, Reggio Calabria, 1925.
28. Sabatini, A. Ricerche farmacologiche sulla essenza di bergamotto—Nota 1 Cenni storici—La chimica della essenza di bergamotto Ricerche tossicologiche. *Annali di Clinica Terapeutica*, anno V, vol. IX, no. 8, Roma, 1927.
29. Morel, A., and Rochaix, A. Action microbicide par contact de quelques essences végétales a l'état liquide. *Compt. Rend. Hobd. Séances Mém. Soc. Biol.* 86:933–934, 1922.
30. Spinelli, A. L'essenza di bergamotto. Nuovo antisettico nella pratica chirurgica. *Policlinico* (Sez. Chir.) 39, 1932.
31. Puglisi, A.S. L'olio essenziale di bergamotto e di limone in chirurgia. *Il Policlinico* (Sez. Prat.) 39, 1935
32. Gattefossé, R.M. *Usi terapeutici dell'essenza di bergamotto*. Officina fotoincisione S. Michele, Roma, 1932.
33. Sanarelli, G. *Il Bergamon e le sue applicazioni*. Quinta edizione. Tip. Imperia, Roma, 1950.
34. Spinelli, A. Il Bergamon nella disinfezione chirurgica. *Il Policlinico* (Sez. Prat.) XLIV, 1937.
35. Anedda, A. *Rassegna Medica Sarda*. Brevi note sulla terapia della scabbia e specialmente sull'uso del Bergamon Alfa puro XLII, no. 3, 1940.
36. Maimone, D. L'Essenza di bergamotto nella cura della scabbia. *Il Dermosifilografo* XV(7), 1940.
37. Gandolfi, G., and Boari, G. Ricerche sperimentali sull'azione disinfettante e terapeutica del Bergamon sulla congiuntiva. *Annali di oftalmologia e Clinica Oculistica* LXVIII, 1940.
38. Gandolfi, G. Il Bergamon nella terapia oculare. *L'Ateneo Parmense* XII:5–6, 1940.
39. Scoto, P. Vantaggi e svantaggi di un nuovo disinfettante nella pratica ostetrica. *L'Ateneo Parmense*, Maggio–Giugno 1939.

2 The Olfactory System
From Odorant Molecules to Perception

Simone Pifferi and Anna Menini

CONTENTS

2.1 INTRODUCTION

The process leading to olfactory perception begins in the nasal cavity, where odorant molecules reaching the olfactory epithelium bind to a large number of different odorant receptors located in the cilia of olfactory sensory neurons. The number of odorant receptors varies between about 300 in humans and 1200 in mice, representing about 1%–4% of proteins encoded by the entire genome. However, each olfactory sensory neuron expresses only one odorant receptor type that can bind different odorant molecules. Vice versa, each odorant molecule can bind to several odorant receptors according to a unique combinatorial code. Axons of olfactory sensory neurons send information to second-order neurons (mitral and tufted cells) in the olfactory bulb, which in turn project to several cortical areas. Sensory coding in the olfactory bulb is based on a high level of convergence of projections from neurons of the olfactory epithelium. Indeed, all olfactory sensory neurons expressing a given odorant receptor project to specific synaptic units, called glomeruli, in the olfactory bulb. Thus, an individual glomerulus represents a single odorant receptor, and each odorant produces the activation of a unique combination of spatially invariant glomeruli in the olfactory bulb.

From the olfactory bulb, mitral and tufted cells transmit signals from glomeruli to cortical neurons in several anatomically distinct areas collectively named the primary olfactory cortex, including the piriform cortex and the cortical amygdala. It is of interest to note that, different from other sensory systems, the olfactory system sends signals directly to the cortex without first connecting to the thalamus. Two different patterns of projections have been found from the olfactory bulb to the piriform cortex and the cortical amygdala. The topographical organization of odorant information of the olfactory bulb is not maintained in the piriform cortex, where axons of mitral and tufted cells from a given glomerulus project diffusely without apparent spatial order. Moreover, individual odorants activate a sparse ensemble of piriform neurons without spatial preference. In the cortical amygdala, projections from different glomeruli are organized in broad but anatomically distinct regions, suggesting that the cortical amygdala may be critical in processing information related to innate behaviors.

Each area of the olfactory cortex sends information to other regions of the brain and also has extensive projections back to the olfactory bulb, allowing top-down modulation of the olfactory bulb activity. Neurons of the primary olfactory cortex directly project to the orbitofrontal cortex and also to the hippocampus, hypothalamus, and mediodorsal nucleus of the thalamus. Moreover, several of these regions are reciprocally connected. This complex neuroanatomical organization is at the basis of olfactory perception, a process that depends not only on the specific odorant molecules binding to odorant receptors, but also on how the brain filters, organizes, and interprets the olfactory information according to several other factors, including learning, experience, expectations, attention, memory, and emotion.

This chapter presents an overview of the current knowledge of the organization and function of the olfactory system in mammals, from the binding of odorant molecules to odorant receptors to human olfactory perception.

2.2 ODORANT MOLECULES

Odorant molecules are small volatile organic compounds with a molecular mass of <300 Da that activate odorant receptors (see Section IV) and the subsequent components of the olfactory system. Odorant molecules include aliphatic and aromatic compounds with various functional groups, such as esters, alkanes, cyanides, imines, thiols, halides, formates, amines, ketones, carboxylic acids, alcohols, and aldehydes, as shown in Figure 2.1a. In general, an olfactory stimulus is composed of a complex mixture of dozens of different types of odorant molecules. For example, it has been estimated that a rose emits more than 200 types of volatile molecules (Ohloff 1994), although not all of them bind to odorant receptors. A recent study investigated the

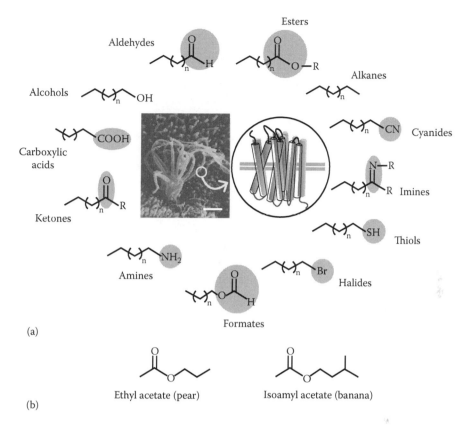

FIGURE 2.1 (a) Chemical structures of several functional groups in some odorant molecules. Center, left: Scanning electron micrograph of the knob of a human olfactory sensory neuron with several cilia. (Modified from Morrison, E.E., and Costanzo, R.M., *J Comp Neurol* 297: 1–13, 1990. With permission.) Center, right: Schematic representation of an odorant receptor showing seven-transmembrane domains typical of GPCRs. (b) Chemical structures of molecules that smell like a pear and a banana.

number of discriminable olfactory stimuli and estimated that humans can discriminate more than 1 trillion olfactory stimuli (Bushdid et al. 2014), whereas previous estimates indicated that humans could discriminate about 10,000 olfactory stimuli. As the human visual system seems to be able to discriminate among 2.3 million and 7.5 million colors and the auditory system can distinguish about 340,000 tones (Nickerson and Newhall 1943; Pointer and Attridge 1998; Stevens and Davis 1983), the human olfactory system outperforms other sensory systems in the number of different stimuli it can discriminate (Bushdid et al. 2014).

The olfactory system has very high detection capabilities; indeed, some odorants have a very low detection threshold. For example, ethyl mercaptan (ethanethiol) can be perceived by humans at a concentration as low as 1 part in 2.5 billion parts of air (Whisman et al. 1978). For this reason, ethyl mercaptan is added to natural gas, which is odorless, as a warning for escaping gas.

The olfactory system also has a high power of discrimination among small changes in the chemical structure of an odorant molecule. For example, ethyl acetate is the main component of the odor of pear, while the structurally similar isoamyl acetate mediates the odor of banana (Figure 2.1b). Moreover, some pairs of enantiomers can elicit different odors. For example, R-carvone smells like spearmint, while its mirror image, S-carvone, smells like caraway (Laska and Teubner 1999).

2.3   NOSE AND OLFACTORY EPITHELIUM

During inspiration through the nostrils, odorant molecules reach the olfactory epithelium, located in the upper part of the nasal cavity (Figure 2.2). The nasal cavity is largely occupied by turbinates that determine the direction of the airflow, and during normal respiration, only 5%–10% of the inhaled air reaches the olfactory epithelium. However, many animals actively explore the presence of odorant molecules in the external environment by sniffing. A sniff consists of taking air into the nose in short breaths to increase the percentage of air reaching the olfactory epithelium, without carrying the air deep into the lung. In humans, a typical sniff lasts on average 1.6 s, with an inhalation velocity of 27 L/min and a volume of 500 cm^3 (for review, see Mainland and Sobel 2006).

Odorant molecules reach the olfactory epithelium not only with the air passing through the nostrils (orthonasal pathway), but also through the nasopharynx

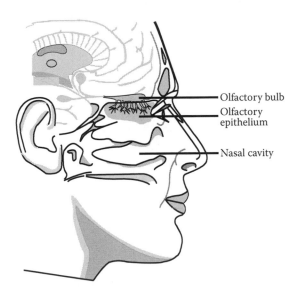

FIGURE 2.2   Anatomical organization of the olfactory system. The olfactory epithelium is located in the upper part of the nasal cavity. Odorant molecules can reach the olfactory epithelium both with the air inspired through the nostrils (orthonasal pathway) and with the air expired through the nasopharynx when food or drinks are ingested (retronasal pathway). Axons of olfactory sensory neurons in the olfactory epithelium directly project to the olfactory bulb passing through the cribriform plate of the ethmoid bone.

(retronasal pathway) during mastication or drinking. The retronasal pathway plays a fundamental role in the generation of food or drink flavor, as volatile molecules released in the mouth during mastication reach the olfactory epithelium through the nasopharynx during expiration (for review, see Shepherd 2006).

The olfactory epithelium is a specialized pseudostratified epithelium mainly composed of three types of cells: olfactory sensory neurons, sustentacular cells, and basal cells (Figure 2.3). In humans, the olfactory epithelium has an average surface of 2–4 cm^2 (Leopold et al. 2000; Moran et al. 1982) and contains about 6 million olfactory sensory neurons in each nasal cavity (Moran et al. 1982; Rowley et al. 1989).

Olfactory sensory neurons are responsible for the detection of odorant molecules and the generation of the electrical response that is transmitted to the brain (Kleene 2008; Pifferi et al. 2010; Schild and Restrepo 1998). They have a bipolar morphology, with a single dendrite that terminates in a knob with several cilia exposing their membrane to the external environment to contact odorant molecules, and a single axon projecting directly to the olfactory bulb of the brain.

In the human olfactory epithelium, the typical diameter of the cell body of an olfactory sensory neuron is about 4–6 μm, while that of the dendritic knob is about 1–2 μm, and the axon has a diameter of 0.1–0.4 μm. Each neuron bears a variable number of cilia, up to about 30, each with a diameter of 0.1–0.3 μm. Cilia have different lengths, varying from 1–5 μm up to 30 μm (Morrison and Costanzo 1990). Cilia of different neurons are tightly intermingled and are embedded in a thick layer of mucus produced by Bowman's glands (Getchell and Getchell 1992). The presence of numerous cilia allows a large increase of the membrane area available for interaction with odorant molecules.

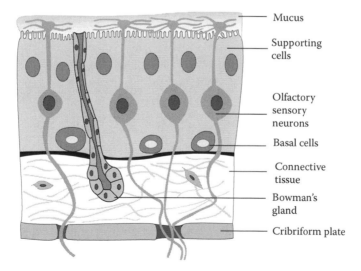

FIGURE 2.3 Organization of the olfactory epithelium. The olfactory epithelium is composed of olfactory sensory neurons, supporting cells, and basal cells. Bowman's glands are responsible for the production of mucus covering the surface of the epithelium.

2.4 ODORANT RECEPTORS

The molecular era of olfactory research began in 1991 with the cloning of odorant receptors by Linda Buck and Richard Axel (1991), who subsequently received
the Nobel Prize in Physiology or Medicine in 2004 for their discoveries of odorant
receptors and the organization of the olfactory system. This breakthrough discovery opened the possibility to understand the mechanisms of olfactory coding at the
molecular level.

Odorant receptors belong to the superfamily of G protein–coupled receptors
(GPCRs) and have a typical general structure comprising seven transmembrane
domains, as shown in Figure 2.1a (Katritch et al. 2013). Mammals have about 1000
odorant receptor genes, but each species has a different number of functional odorant
receptor genes. Primates, including humans, have about 300–400 functional odorant
receptor genes, while mice and rats have about 1000–1200 intact genes (Gilad et al.
2004; Niimura and Nei 2005, 2007; Quignon et al. 2005).

To understand how the olfactory system discriminates among odorants, it is
important to know how many types of odorant receptors are expressed in each olfactory sensory neuron and to determine the ligands of each odorant receptor.

It has been well established that each olfactory sensory neuron expresses only one
odorant receptor gene (for review, see Magklara and Lomvardas 2013; Rodriguez
2013). Moreover, the pattern of expression of odorant receptors in the olfactory epithelium has been extensively studied in rodents (for review, see Malnic et al. 1999).
Recent data have been reported in macaques (Horowitz et al. 2014), while data from
humans are still missing. Based on the expression pattern of odorant receptors, the
olfactory epithelium can be divided into four (mouse and rat) or two (macaque) zones.
Inside a given zone, olfactory sensory neurons expressing a given odorant receptor
are randomly distributed (Horowitz et al. 2014; Mombaerts et al. 1996; Ressler et al.
1993; Vassar et al. 1993; for review, see Mombaerts 2004).

Several studies have attempted to determine the ligands of odorant receptors,
but unfortunately, it has been very difficult to express odorant receptors in heterologous systems suitable for high-throughput screening (Mombaerts 2004; Peterlin et
al. 2014). Thus, at present, our knowledge of the pairing between odorant receptors
and their odorant ligands is very limited, and about 90% of human odorant receptors
are still orphan receptors (for review, see Peterlin et al. 2014).

Despite these limitations, it has been well established that the odorant receptor
family uses a combinatorial code to discriminate among odorant molecules. Each
odorant receptor can be activated by several types of odorant molecules, and a given
type of odorant molecule can activate many odorant receptors (Araneda et al. 2000;
Malnic et al. 1999). However, each odorant is encoded by the activation of a unique
combination of odorant receptors (Figure 2.4). One great advantage of this combinatorial code is the possibility to detect and discriminate a very large number of
odorant molecules.

In addition to the classical odorant receptors described above, a second class of
chemoreceptors has been reported to be expressed in the olfactory epithelium of
mice and macaques (Horowitz et al. 2014; Liberles and Buck 2006). These receptors

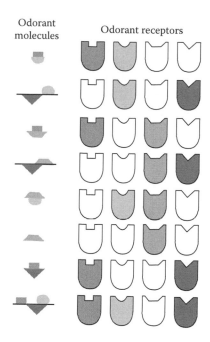

Odorant
molecules   Odorant receptors

FIGURE 2.4 Combinatorial code used by odorant receptors to discriminate different odorant molecules. Four odorant receptors are schematically drawn on the right. The highlighted receptors can be activated by the corresponding odorant molecules depicted in the left column. A given odorant molecule activates a particular combination of odorant receptors. One odorant receptor can be activated by several odorant molecules.

are unrelated to the previously discovered odorant receptors and belong to the trace amine–associated receptor (TAAR) family (for review, see Sotnikova et al. 2009).

The mouse genome has 15 intact genes encoding for TAARs, while macaques and humans have only 6 functional TAAR genes (Liberles and Buck 2006; Niimura and Nei 2007). Horowitz et al. (2014) have recently shown that five TAARs are expressed by olfactory sensory neurons of the macaque, a high primate, and suggested that these receptors may also be expressed in the human olfactory epithelium. Olfactory sensory neurons expressing TAARs do not express the canonical odorant receptors. Moreover, each olfactory sensory neuron is likely to express only a single TAAR gene, in both mice and macaques (Horowitz et al. 2014; Liberles and Buck 2006). Heterologous expression of some human and mouse TAARs showed activation by volatile amines. For example, mouse, macaque, and human TAAR5 are activated by trimethylamine (Horowitz et al. 2014; Wallrabenstein et al. 2013; Zhang et al. 2013). Moreover, human TAAR5 responds to extracts from rotten salmon, whereas it does not respond to extracts from fresh salmon (Horowitz et al. 2014). As trimethylamine is produced by bacteria during spoilage of food and is responsible for the typical unpleasant and repulsive smell of rotten fish (Gram and Dalgaard 2002), it has been suggested that human TAAR5 may be used to elicit innate responses of avoidance toward spoiled foods that may be dangerous if ingested (Horowitz et al. 2014).

2.5 ELECTRICAL RESPONSES OF OLFACTORY SENSORY NEURONS

The binding of odorant molecules to odorant receptors is converted into an electrical signal in olfactory sensory neurons. Electrophysiological recordings from individual sensory neurons have shown that they respond to odorants in different ways (Figure 2.5). Some olfactory sensory neurons can detect several odorants, and a given odorant can activate neurons with various odorant specificities (Firestein et al. 1993; Ma et al. 1999; Reisert et al. 2005).

In many animal models the physiological response of olfactory sensory neurons to odorant stimuli has been well characterized with electrophysiological techniques. The current response of isolated olfactory sensory neurons to odorant stimulation has been recorded with the whole-cell patch-clamp technique in the voltage-clamp mode (Figure 2.5a). At the membrane potential of –55 mV, a brief application of odorants induced a rapid development of an inward current that returned to the basal level after the removal of the stimulus (Figure 2.5b). Different olfactory sensory neurons can have very different patterns of responses to odorants. For example, the

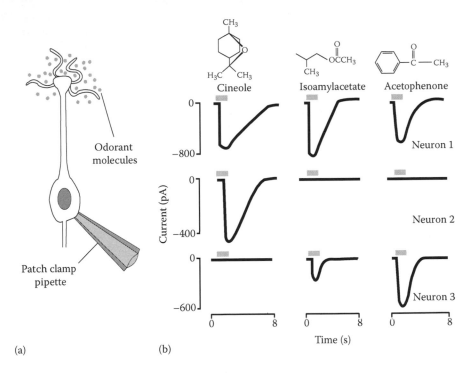

FIGURE 2.5 Electrical responses of olfactory sensory neurons to odorant stimulations. (a) Schematic representation of the experimental approach used to record odorant responses from dissociated olfactory sensory neurons by the whole-cell patch-clamp technique. (b) Responses of three different neurons to three structurally unrelated odorant molecules shown at the top. The holding potential was –55 mV and the odorant was applied for 1.2 s. In the first neuron, each odorant evoked a similar response. Neuron 2 responded to one odorant only, while neuron 3 responded to two of the three odorants with different amplitudes. (Modified from Firestein, S. et al., *J Physiol* 468: 1–10, 1993.)

first neuron in Figure 2.5b was activated by each of three structurally unrelated odorants, while the second neuron was activated by just one odorant, and the third neuron responded to two of the three odorants with responses of different amplitudes (Firestein et al. 1993). This general scheme was confirmed in various animal models using different experimental approaches and reflects the combinatorial code used by odorant receptors illustrated in Figure 2.4 (Araneda et al. 2000; Ma et al. 1999; Reisert and Restrepo 2009; Reisert et al. 2005).

2.5.1 MOLECULAR MECHANISMS OF OLFACTORY TRANSDUCTION

Olfactory transduction is the cellular process that converts the information carried by odorant molecules into a bioelectric signal (Figure 2.6). Transduction takes place in the cilia of olfactory sensory neurons, which, despite expressing different odorant receptors, largely share the same molecular transduction mechanisms (see reviews in Kleene 2008; Pifferi et al. 2010; Tirindelli et al. 2009). The binding of odorant molecules to an odorant receptor causes the activation of a trimeric G protein composed of $G\alpha_{olf}$ and $\beta\gamma$ subunits. In turn, the G protein stimulates the enzymatic activity of a specific adenylyl cyclase (ACIII) causing an increase in the concentration of cyclic AMP (Bakalyar and Reed 1990). The ciliary membrane expresses cyclic-nucleotide gated (CNG) channels that are directly gated by cyclic AMP. CNG channels are nonselective cation channels, and therefore the activation of odorant receptors causes a depolarizing influx of Na^+ and Ca^{2+} (Kaupp and Seifert 2002). The increase of intracellular Ca^{2+} concentration causes the activation of a second type of ion channel, named TMEM16B or anoctamin2, which is selective for Cl^- (Pifferi et al. 2009, 2012; Ponissery Saidu et al. 2013; Stephan et al. 2009). Since olfactory sensory neurons maintain an unusually high intracellular Cl^- concentration, the activation

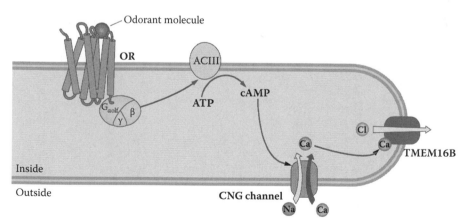

FIGURE 2.6 Molecular mechanisms of olfactory transduction. Schematic representation of olfactory transduction taking place in the cilia. The binding of odorant molecules to an odorant receptor (OR) activates a G protein, which in turn activates adenylyl cyclase (ACIII) producing cyclic AMP (cAMP), which opens cyclic nucleotide-gated (CNG) channels. Ca^{2+} entry causes the activation of TMEM16B generating a depolarizing efflux of Cl^-.

of TMEM16B causes an efflux of Cl^- and the consequent amplification of the odorant response (Kaneko et al. 2004; Reisert et al. 2005). Although the transduction current is composed of up to 90% by the Cl^- current (Boccaccio and Menini 2007; Reisert et al. 2005), the precise role of this current for normal olfaction is unclear. Indeed, the olfactory function of knockout mice for TMEM16B and wild-type mice was not significantly different (Billig et al. 2011). In addition, the olfactory function of human patients having TMEM16B partially deleted was not significantly impaired (Cenedese et al. 2015).

The depolarization generated by the binding of odorants in the cilia is passively transmitted along the dendrite and soma of the neuron and is converted in trains of action potentials that are conducted along the axon to the olfactory bulb (Schild and Restrepo 1998).

Several mechanisms are involved in the termination of the response. The most important are (1) intrinsic GTP-ase activity of $G\alpha_{olf}$ that stops the stimulation of ACIII (Firestein et al. 1991), (2) degradation of cyclic AMP by phosphodiesterase (Cygnar and Zhao 2009; Yan et al. 1995), (3) Ca^{2+}-calmodulin-dependent inhibition of CNG channels (Song et al. 2008), and (4) extrusion of Ca^{2+} through a Na^+/Ca^{2+} exchanger and Ca^{2+}-ATPase (Antolin et al. 2010; Stephan et al. 2012).

2.5.2 ODORANT ADAPTATION

It is a general experience that the continuous or repeated exposure to an odorant causes a reduction in the perception of that odorant. For example, in a recent study in humans, Stuck et al. (2014) found a complete absence of perception after exposure for about 60 s to 4 parts per million of hydrogen sulfide (which smells like rotten eggs), while 10% (v/v) of phenylethyl alcohol (which smells like roses) needed about 160 s to induce a complete adaptation.

The entire olfactory system is involved in adaptation, including olfactory sensory neurons. Indeed, electrophysiological recordings obtained with electro-olfactograms, field recordings of the electrical activity of the olfactory epithelium, showed a reduction of about 20% of the response to repeated odorant stimulations (Hummel et al. 1996). The molecular mechanisms of adaptation in olfactory sensory neurons are still not completely understood. However, experiments in several animal models showed that the main player in this process is the modulation of CNG channels by Ca^{2+}-dependent mechanisms. Indeed, the increase of intracellular Ca^{2+} concentration during odorant stimulation causes a shift of the sensitivity of CNG channels toward higher concentrations of cyclic AMP and therefore increases the detection threshold of olfactory sensory neurons. This mechanism will allow neurons to discriminate higher odorant concentrations without saturating the transduction process (Kurahashi and Menini 1997; Song et al. 2008). Indeed, it is important to note that adaptation is not a mere reduction of response to a continuous or repeated stimulus, but an active process that allows the olfactory system to respond over a broad range of stimuli.

2.6 OLFACTORY BULB

The olfactory bulb is the first part of the encephalon devoted to process the information transmitted by olfactory sensory neurons about odorant molecules present in the external world. Axons of olfactory sensory neurons make synaptic contacts with dendrites of the principal cells of the bulb, mitral and tufted cells, in glomeruli at the superficial layer of the bulb (Figure 2.7).

Genetic and tracing studies in rodents revealed a high level of convergence in the projections of olfactory sensory neurons to the olfactory bulb. Indeed, all olfactory sensory neurons expressing a particular odorant receptor gene send their axons to two glomeruli in each half of the olfactory bulb (Figure 2.7). Moreover, each glomerulus receives only the axons of neurons expressing the same odorant receptor gene (Mombaerts 2004; Mombaerts et al. 1996). Thus, in rodents, the number of glomeruli is approximately twice the number of odorant receptors. A further processing of odorant information occurs through the activity of interneurons that connect different glomeruli.

Recordings from a large population of glomeruli using different experimental approaches showed that, as expected, the activation of glomeruli follows the same combinatorial code observed for odorant receptors. A chemotopic map was observed in the olfactory bulb, where different chemical properties of an odorant molecule, such as the carbon chain length or particular functional groups, activated different populations of glomeruli. Therefore, odorant information is spatially represented in the olfactory bulb, where each odorant molecule is encoded by the activation of a unique combination of glomeruli (for review, see Mori et al. 2006).

It is still unclear if this organization is conserved in humans. Maresh et al. (2008) found an unexpectedly large number of about 5500 glomeruli in the human olfactory bulb. Because humans express only 350 intact odorant receptors, the ratio between the number of glomeruli and functional odorant receptor genes is much higher in humans, 16:1, than in rodents, 2:1 (Maresh et al. 2008; Meisami 1990; Mombaerts 2004; Royet et al. 1988).

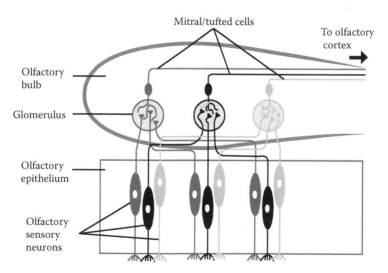

FIGURE 2.7 Functional organization of the olfactory bulb. All olfactory sensory neurons expressing a particular odorant receptor project to the same glomerulus in the olfactory bulb. In turn, each mitral or tufted cell is connected to a single glomerulus and projects to the primary olfactory cortex.

The olfactory bulb in humans is a pair of oval-shaped structures, with a volume of about 30–60 mm³, located under the ventral surface of the frontal lobe of the brain (Figure 2.2). Unfortunately, the position of the olfactory bulb close to the sinus reduces the signal available for functional magnetic resonance imaging (fMRI), and the small size of the bulb precludes the possibility of using positron emission tomography (PET).

2.7 CORTICAL ORGANIZATION OF THE OLFACTORY SYSTEM

Mitral and tufted cells are the projection neurons that transmit signals from glomeruli in the olfactory bulb to cortical neurons in several areas collectively named the primary olfactory cortex (Figure 2.8). Most of the projections are ipsilateral, although a subset of neurons also sends axons from the olfactory bulb to the controlateral cortex. The olfactory cortex is composed of several anatomically distinct areas, including the piriform cortex, olfactory tubercle, anterior olfactory nucleus, cortical amygdala, and lateral entorhinal cortex (Carmichael et al. 1994; Shipley and Ennis 1996). Each of these regions in turn projects to other brain areas. The piriform cortex directly projects

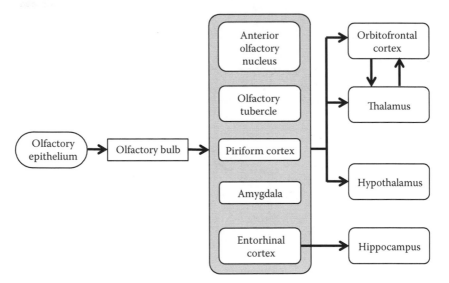

FIGURE 2.8 Organization of the olfactory system. Olfactory information detected in the olfactory epithelium is transmitted to the olfactory bulb, which in turn is connected to the primary olfactory cortex, composed of the anterior olfactory nucleus, olfactory tubercle, piriform cortex, amygdala, and entorhinal cortex. The anterior olfactory nucleus does not project to higher centers, and it is mainly connected to the piriform cortex. The olfactory tubercle projects to the dorsolateral nucleus of the thalamus. The piriform cortex receives the highest number of projections from the olfactory bulb and projects both directly to the orbitofrontal cortex and to the dorsolateral nucleus of the thalamus, connecting again with the orbitofrontal cortex. The entorhinal cortex projects mainly to the hippocampus, while the amygdala is connected to both the hippocampus and the thalamus. Several areas of the primary olfactory cortex are linked by complex intracortical connections and send centrifugal projections to the olfactory bulb.

to the orbitofrontal cortex and to the mediodorsal thalamus, which sends reciprocal projections to the orbitofrontal cortex (Figure 2.8). The entorhinal cortex mainly projects to the hippocampus, while the cortical amygdala is mostly connected to the hypothalamus. The absence of an obligatory thalamic relay to access the neocortical structures is a distinctive feature of the olfactory system organization (see also Section 2.8.2).

Every area of the primary olfactory cortex, with the exception of the olfactory tubercle, sends extensive projections back to the olfactory bulb, and this high number of centrifugal projections is another peculiar feature of the olfactory system (Boyd et al. 2012; Johnson et al. 2000; Kay and Laurent 1999; Luskin and Price 1983; Markopoulos et al. 2012). In rodents, the activation of neurons in the piriform cortex and in the anterior olfactory nucleus can modulate the spike activity of mitral cells in the olfactory bulb, indicating a role of centrifugal connections in the modulation of the response (Boyd et al. 2012; Markopoulos et al. 2012).

2.7.1 Piriform Cortex

The piriform cortex is the largest area of the olfactory cortex, and several studies have investigated its properties. One central question is related to the understanding of how the information elaborated by the olfactory bulb is sent to the piriform cortex. In the olfactory bulb, one type of odorant activates well-defined and spatially invariant glomeruli. In rodents, anatomic studies combined with genetic approaches indicate that the topographical organization of odorant information of the olfactory bulb is not maintained in the piriform cortex. Indeed, some studies used tracing techniques to visualize the projections from individual glomeruli in the bulb to the cortex and found that axons of mitral and tufted cells from a given glomerulus project diffusely to the piriform cortex without apparent spatial preference (Ghosh et al. 2011; Miyamichi et al. 2011; Sosulski et al. 2011). In accordance with this anatomical organization, functional experiments using electrophysiology and optical imaging have shown that each odorant activates a unique combination of neurons that are widely distributed without apparent spatial preference (Illig and Haberly 2003; Poo and Isaacson 2009; Rennaker et al. 2007; Stettler and Axel 2009). Moreover, an individual piriform neuron receives inputs from random collections of olfactory bulb glomeruli, and adjacent neurons respond to structurally different odorants, suggesting a discontinuity in the receptive field profile (Stettler and Axel 2009). Thus, the spatial organization in the olfactory bulb is not maintained in the piriform cortex, in which every neuron receives inputs from several areas of the olfactory bulb.

In humans, studies using fMRI also showed that the piriform cortex responds to different odorant molecules with dispersed and largely overlapping patterns of activation, indicating an evolutionary conserved coding mechanism (Howard et al. 2009).

2.7.2 Cortical Amygdala

Projections from the olfactory bulb to the cortical amygdala have a different organization from projections to the piriform cortex. In mice, axons of mitral and tufted cells from different glomeruli in the olfactory bulb project to broad but anatomically distinct regions of the cortical amygdala. These regions have stereotyped positions in different mice, indicating that the cortical amygdala may be involved in the generation of innate olfactory behaviors (Miyamichi et al. 2011; Sosulski et al. 2011). Moreover, most of the projections to the cortical amygdala originate from the dorsal olfactory bulb, whereas the piriform cortex receives inputs from the entire olfactory bulb (Miyamichi et al. 2011).

The two very different patterns of projections, with inputs that are apparently randomly distributed in the piriform cortex, compared with inputs that have determined and stereotyped positions in different mice in the cortical amygdala, are likely to be the basis for different odorant-evoked olfactory processing. The cortical amygdala is likely to be critical in processing information related to innate behaviors. In mice, a very recent study used a combination of genetic strategies and behavioral assays and demonstrated that a stereotypical neural circuit that transmits information from the olfactory bulb to the cortical amygdala is necessary for the generation of innate responses of aversion or attraction to volatile odorants (Root et al. 2014). The critical role played by the cortical amygdala in the generation of innate odorant-evoked behaviors does not exclude the possibility that the cortical amygdala may also be involved in learned olfactory behaviors (Root et al. 2014).

2.7.3 ORBITOFRONTAL CORTEX

Neurons of the primary olfactory cortex directly project to the orbitofrontal cortex and also to the hippocampus, hypothalamus, and mediodorsal nucleus of the thalamus. The orbitofrontal cortex plays a key role in higher-order olfactory processing; indeed, it is involved in odor discrimination learning, encoding food-based reward, and multisensory integration (Critchley and Rolls 1996; Rolls and Baylis 1994; Schoenbaum and Eichenbaum 1995a, 1995b).

In humans, the role of the orbitofrontal cortex in olfactory information processing was established by early imaging studies showing a robust odorant-induced activation of the right orbitofrontal cortex (Zatorre et al. 1992) and confirmed by fMRI recordings (Boyle et al. 2007; Cerf-Ducastel and Murphy 2006; Gottfried et al. 2002a, 2002b; Howard and Gottfried 2014; O'Doherty et al. 2000; Small et al. 1997). Electrophysiological recordings from primates also showed odorant-induced responses in the orbitofrontal cortex (Critchley and Rolls 1996), and studies on patients with lesions in the orbitofrontal cortex showed that these patients exhibited olfactory deficits (Jones-Gotman and Zatorre 1988, 1993; Li et al. 2010; Potter and Butters 1980; Zatorre and Jones-Gotman 1991).

2.8 OLFACTORY PERCEPTION

The process of olfactory perception depends not only on the specific odorant molecules binding to odorant receptors, but also on how the brain filters, organizes, and interprets the olfactory information received from the external world according to several other factors, including learning, experience, expectations, attention, memory, and emotion.

2.8.1 PERCEPTUAL LEARNING

Olfactory perceptual learning is the improvement through experience in the detection or discrimination of olfactory stimuli. Studies in humans have shown that the repeated exposure to a given odorant could decrease its detection threshold (Dalton et al. 2002; Stevens and O'Connell 1995). Moreover, although many people cannot smell androstenone, they become sensitive to its smell after repeated exposures to this odorant (Mainland et al. 2002; Wysocki et al. 1989).

2.8.2 OLFACTORY OBJECTS

Most odorants in the external environment are composed of a complex mixture of structurally different odorant molecules, but the olfactory system is able to synthesize these signals into a unitary perceptual object. In the natural context, a given odorant stimulus must be perceived in the presence of a variable background of several other odorants; therefore, the olfactory system must be able to selectively filter the information from the background while perceiving the relevant information. Moreover, an olfactory object does not have a constant composition of its odorant components, and the molecules reaching the olfactory epithelium may change for several reasons. For example, a rose may have some odorant components different from those of other roses, the presence of the wind may modify the flux of molecules reaching the olfactory epithelium, or some molecules of the mixture may be degraded with time. However, the olfactory system is often capable of perceiving the overall smell as that of a rose.

The process of adaptation, occurring at several levels of the olfactory system, plays an important role for the identification of an olfactory object in the presence of other odorants, as it produces a decrease of the response to background odorants, allowing the detection of other stimuli.

Several studies have addressed the issue of how the olfactory system may produce the synthetic representation of an olfactory object. Wilson (2003) investigated the activity of the piriform cortex in rats in response to a mixture of two odorants, A + B, or to only one of its components, A, and showed that the piriform cortex (but not the olfactory bulb) was able to encode the mixture (A + B) as an olfactory object distinct from that represented by one of its components (A). Indeed, after 50 s of adaptation to the mixture, neurons of the piriform cortex showed a reduced activity to a second application of the mixture, but not to A alone, indicating that the piriform cortex was able to build a new olfactory object from its components (Wilson 2003). These results were extended by recent data imaging the activity of large ensembles of piriform neurons, confirming that activation of the piriform cortex by an odorant mixture does not correspond to the superimposition of activities of the individual components of the mixture (Stettler and Axel 2009).

Psychophysical data showed that humans responded more rapidly to odorant stimulation when the stimulus was expected, showing that attention can affect olfactory perception (Spence et al. 2001). Moreover, fMRI recordings showed activation of different areas of the piriform cortex depending on the attentional state of the subject (Zelano et al. 2005). Finally, Plailly et al. (2008) showed that the connection between the mediodorsal nucleus of the thalamus and the orbitofrontal cortex is an active modulatory target of olfactory attention, suggesting a role of the thalamus in this process (Plailly et al. 2008).

2.8.3 HEDONIC VALUES OF ODORANTS

Some odorants have a positive hedonic value and are labeled by humans as pleasant, while other odorants have a negative hedonic value and are labeled as unpleasant. It is generally agreed that the hedonic value of an odorant may vary among populations and also among individuals of the same population, and some studies have shown that hedonic responses are often learned on the basis of experience.

The subjective pleasantness of an odorant may be modified by several factors, including emotions, sensory-specific satiety, and cognitive information.

In humans, early studies using positron emission tomography (PET) found that highly aversive unpleasant odorants, such as a mixture of sulfide gases, caused a significant activation of the amygdala (Zald and Pardo 1997). However, intensity and hedonic value are often tightly interconnected; for example, a pleasant odorant at a given concentration may become unpleasant when its concentration is very high. Using different concentrations of pleasant, neutral, and unpleasant odorants, researchers found that the amygdala was primarily activated by the intensity of pleasant or unpleasant odorants, but not by odorants that had a neutral hedonic value (Anderson et al. 2003; Winston et al. 2005). Moreover, the amygdala is involved in emotion-state-dependent olfactory processing. Under anxiety conditions, previously neutral odorants may be perceived as unpleasant, and fMRI recordings revealed an increase of odorant-evoked activity in the amygdala that remained sustained after anxiety adaptation (Krusemark et al. 2013).

The hedonic value of an odorant is represented in different areas of the orbitofrontal cortex, as well as in other cortical regions. Pleasant odorants preferentially activate medial orbitofrontal regions, while unpleasant odorants activate more lateral orbitofrontal regions (Anderson et al. 2003; Gottfried et al. 2002a; Rolls et al. 2003; Zald and Pardo 1997).

Another example of modification of the subjective pleasantness of an odorant is given by the well-known phenomenon of sensory-specific satiety. O'Doherty et al. (2000) investigated the hedonic responses to the odorants of banana and vanilla before and after banana was eaten to satiety, while measuring the activity of the orbitofrontal cortex by fMRI. Before eating, the pleasantness ratings of banana and vanilla were similar and the odorants produced a similar activation of a region of the orbitofrontal cortex, as measured by fMRI. However, after banana was eaten to satiety, its smell became unpleasant and the activation of the same region of the orbitofrontal cortex decreased, whereas there was no similar decrease for the odor of vanilla, a food not eaten in the meal, and the smell of vanilla remained pleasant. These results show that activation of a region of the human orbitofrontal cortex is related to olfactory sensory-specific satiety (O'Doherty et al. 2000).

Howard and Gottfried (2014) investigated sensory-specific satiety to peanut butter and some of the individual types of odorant molecules responsible for its smell.

Interestingly, they found that the decrease of the fMRI response mediating olfactory sensory-specific satiety to peanut butter could be reproduced by stimulation with single components, indicating that the orbitofrontal cortex can extract information from single elements of a complex olfactory object. In contrast, in the amygdala, single components of peanut butter did not change fMRI signals after olfactory sensory-specific satiety (Howard and Gottfried 2014).

Cognitive information influences the representations of odorants' pleasantness in the human brain. de Araujo et al. (2005) conducted experiments presenting an odorant together with the projection on a screen of a word descriptor of the odorant. The test odorant was a combination of isovaleric acid with a small amount of cheddar cheese flavor and was labeled in some trials with the words *cheddar cheese* and in other trials with the words *body odor.* fMRI showed that the medial orbitofrontal cortex was more activated by the same test stimulus when it was described as cheddar cheese than when it was labeled as body odor. Furthermore, the activation of the orbitofrontal cortex was correlated with the rating of pleasantness, with body odor being unpleasant and cheddar cheese close to neutral (de Araujo et al. 2005). These results indicate that cognitive effects can produce a top-down modulation of cortical olfactory information.

2.8.4 Conscious Olfactory Awareness

Conscious olfactory awareness seems to require an intact right orbitofrontal cortex, as indicated by a study on a patient who developed complete anosmia following a traumatic brain injury to the right orbitofrontal cortex (Li et al. 2010). This patient had no history of smell or taste problems before the brain injury, which produced selective damage to the right orbitofrontal cortex, whereas he was not aware of smell perception after the trauma. To test odorant-evoked responses, two unpleasant and neutral odorants were selected. The two strongly unpleasant odorants were trimethylamine, usually perceived as rotten fish, and valeric acid, which has a sweaty and rancid smell, while the two neutral odorants were rose oxide and pinene. Although the patient did not have conscious perceptual awareness of the presence of odorants, physiological responses evoked by odorants could be measured in different ways. For example, the delivery of unpleasant odorants increased skin conductance responses compared to the value measured with neutral odorants. Moreover, fMRI showed activation by odorants of both the left and the right piriform cortex, indicating that the olfactory pathway (of both the left and the right) was functional up to the piriform cortex. On the contrary, fMRI of the orbitofrontal cortex showed that odorant-evoked responses were present in the left and absent in the right orbitofrontal cortex.

Li et al. (2010) suggested that the case of the patient described in their study may also satisfy the criteria for "blind smell," a phenomenon of the olfactory system involving detection of olfactory stimuli in the absence of conscious perception (Sobel et al. 1999). The term *blind smell* originates from a well-known phenomenon of the visual system named blindsight. Some patients with cortical damage in the primary visual cortex have the ability to detect visual stimuli, although they are not aware of their visual ability (Weiskrantz 2002).

These results indicate that the left olfactory pathway is not sufficient for conscious olfaction, whereas the right orbitofrontal cortex is necessary for mediating conscious perception of smell, although it is not known whether the effect is intrinsic to the right orbitofrontal cortex or is caused by other connected brain regions or their network (Li et al. 2010).

ACKNOWLEDGMENTS

This work was supported by a grant from the Italian Ministry of Education, University and Research. S. Pifferi is a recipient of an EU Marie Curie Reintegration Grant (OLF-STOM no. 334404).

REFERENCES

Anderson, A.K., K. Christoff, I. Stappen, D. Panitz, D.G. Ghahremani, G. Glover, J.D.E. Gabrieli, and N. Sobel. 2003. Dissociated neural representations of intensity and valence in human olfaction. *Nat Neurosci* 6: 196–202.
Antolin, S., J. Reisert, and H.R. Matthews. 2010. Olfactory response termination involves Ca^{2+}-ATPase in vertebrate olfactory receptor neuron cilia. *J Gen Physiol* 135: 367–378.
Araneda, R.C., A.D. Kini, and S. Firestein. 2000. The molecular receptive range of an odorant receptor. *Nat Neurosci* 3: 1248–1255.
Bakalyar, H.A., and R.R. Reed. 1990. Identification of a specialized adenylyl cyclase that may mediate odorant detection. *Science* 250: 1403–1406.
Billig, G.M., B. Pál, P. Fidzinski, and T.J. Jentsch. 2011. Ca^{2+}-activated Cl^- currents are dispensable for olfaction. *Nat Neurosci* 14: 763–769.
Boccaccio, A., and A. Menini. 2007. Temporal development of cyclic nucleotide-gated and Ca^{2+}-activated Cl^- currents in isolated mouse olfactory sensory neurons. *J Neurophysiol* 98: 153–160.
Boyd, A.M., J.F. Sturgill, C. Poo, and J.S. Isaacson. 2012. Cortical feedback control of olfactory bulb circuits. *Neuron* 76: 1161–1174.
Boyle, J.A., J. Frasnelli, J. Gerber, M. Heinke, and T. Hummel. 2007. Cross-modal integration of intranasal stimuli: A functional magnetic resonance imaging study. *Neuroscience* 149: 223–231.
Buck, L., and R. Axel. 1991. A novel multigene family may encode odorant receptors: A molecular basis for odor recognition. *Cell* 65: 175–187.
Bushdid, C., M.O. Magnasco, L.B. Vosshall, and A. Keller. 2014. Humans can discriminate more than 1 trillion olfactory stimuli. *Science* 343: 1370–1372.
Carmichael, S.T., M.C. Clugnet, and J.L. Price. 1994. Central olfactory connections in the macaque monkey. *J Comp Neurol* 346: 403–434.
Cenedese, V., M. Mezzavilla, A. Morgan, R. Marino, C.P. Ettorre, M. Margaglione, P. Gasparini, and A. Menini. 2015. Assessment of the olfactory function in Italian patients with type 3 von Willebrand disease caused by a homozygous 253 kb deletion involving VWF and TMEM16B/ANO2. *PloS One* 10: e0116483.
Cerf-Ducastel, B., and C. Murphy. 2006. Neural substrates of cross-modal olfactory recognition memory: An fMRI study. *NeuroImage* 31: 386–396.
Critchley, H.D., and E.T. Rolls. 1996. Olfactory neuronal responses in the primate orbitofrontal cortex: Analysis in an olfactory discrimination task. *J Neurophysiol* 75: 1659–1672.
Cygnar, K.D., and H. Zhao. 2009. Phosphodiesterase 1C is dispensable for rapid response termination of olfactory sensory neurons. *Nat Neurosci* 12: 454–462.
Dalton, P., N. Doolittle, and P.A.S. Breslin. 2002. Gender-specific induction of enhanced sensitivity to odors. *Nat Neurosci* 5: 199–200.

de Araujo, I.E., E.T. Rolls, M.I. Velazco, C. Margot, and I. Cayeux. 2005. Cognitive modulation of olfactory processing. *Neuron* 46: 671–679.

Firestein, S., B. Darrow, and G.M. Shepherd. 1991. Activation of the sensory current in salamander olfactory receptor neurons depends on a G protein-mediated cAMP second messenger system. *Neuron* 6: 825–835.

Firestein, S., C. Picco, and A. Menini. 1993. The relation between stimulus and response in olfactory receptor cells of the tiger salamander. *J Physiol* 468: 1–10.

Getchell, M.L., and T.V. Getchell. 1992. Fine structural aspects of secretion and extrinsic innervation in the olfactory mucosa. *Microsc Res Tech* 23: 111–127.

Ghosh, S., S.D. Larson, H. Hefzi, Z. Marnoy, T. Cutforth, K. Dokka, and K.K. Baldwin. 2011. Sensory maps in the olfactory cortex defined by long-range viral tracing of single neurons. *Nature* 472: 217–220.

Gilad, Y., V. Wiebe, M. Przeworski, D. Lancet, and S. Pääbo. 2004. Loss of olfactory receptor genes coincides with the acquisition of full trichromatic vision in primates. *PLoS Biol* 2: E5.

Gottfried, J.A., J. O'Doherty, and R.J. Dolan. 2002a. Appetitive and aversive olfactory learning in humans studied using event-related functional magnetic resonance imaging. *J Neurosci* 22: 10829–10837.

Gottfried, J.A., R. Deichmann, J.S. Winston, and R.J. Dolan. 2002b. Functional heterogeneity in human olfactory cortex: An event-related functional magnetic resonance imaging study. *J Neurosci* 22: 10819–10828.

Gram, L., and P. Dalgaard. 2002. Fish spoilage bacteria: Problems and solutions. *Curr Opin Biotechnol* 13: 262–266.

Horowitz, L.F., L.R. Saraiva, D. Kuang, K. Yoon, and L.B. Buck. 2014. Olfactory receptor patterning in a higher primate. *J Neurosci* 34: 12241–12252.

Howard, J.D., and J.A. Gottfried. 2014. Configural and elemental coding of natural odor mixture components in the human brain. *Neuron* 84: 857–869.

Howard, J.D., J. Plailly, M. Grueschow, J.-D. Haynes, and J.A. Gottfried. 2009. Odor quality coding and categorization in human posterior piriform cortex. *Nat Neurosci* 12: 932–938.

Hummel, T., M. Knecht, and G. Kobal. 1996. Peripherally obtained electrophysiological responses to olfactory stimulation in man: Electro-olfactograms exhibit a smaller degree of desensitization compared with subjective intensity estimates. *Brain Res* 717: 160–164.

Illig, K.R., and L.B. Haberly. 2003. Odor-evoked activity is spatially distributed in piriform cortex. *J Comp Neurol* 457: 361–373.

Johnson, D.M., K.R. Illig, M. Behan, and L.B. Haberly. 2000. New features of connectivity in piriform cortex visualized by intracellular injection of pyramidal cells suggest that "primary" olfactory cortex functions like "association" cortex in other sensory systems. *J Neurosci* 20: 6974–6982.

Jones-Gotman, M., and R.J. Zatorre. 1988. Olfactory identification deficits in patients with focal cerebral excision. *Neuropsychologia* 26: 387–400.

Jones-Gotman, M., and R.J. Zatorre. 1993. Odor recognition memory in humans: Role of right temporal and orbitofrontal regions. *Brain Cogn* 22: 182–198.

Kaneko, H., I. Putzier, S. Frings, U.B. Kaupp, and T. Gensch. 2004. Chloride accumulation in mammalian olfactory sensory neurons. *J Neurosci Off J Soc Neurosci* 24: 7931–7938.

Katritch, V., V. Cherezov, and R.C. Stevens. 2013. Structure-function of the G protein-coupled receptor superfamily. *Annu Rev Pharmacol Toxicol* 53: 531–556.

Kaupp, U.B., and R. Seifert. 2002. Cyclic nucleotide-gated ion channels. *Physiol Rev* 82: 769–824.

Kay, L.M., and G. Laurent. 1999. Odor- and context-dependent modulation of mitral cell activity in behaving rats. *Nat Neurosci* 2: 1003–1009.

Kleene, S.J. 2008. The electrochemical basis of odor transduction in vertebrate olfactory cilia. *Chem Senses* 33: 839–859.

Krusemark, E.A., L.R. Novak, D.R. Gitelman, and W. Li. 2013. When the sense of smell meets emotion: Anxiety-state-dependent olfactory processing and neural circuitry adaptation. *J Neurosci* 33: 15324–15332.

Kurahashi, T., and A. Menini. 1997. Mechanism of odorant adaptation in the olfactory receptor cell. *Nature* 385: 725–729.

Laska, M., and P. Teubner. 1999. Olfactory discrimination ability of human subjects for ten pairs of enantiomers. *Chem Senses* 24: 161–170.

Leopold, D.A., T. Hummel, J.E. Schwob, S.C. Hong, M. Knecht, and G. Kobal. 2000. Anterior distribution of human olfactory epithelium. *Laryngoscope* 110: 417–421.

Li, W., L. Lopez, J. Osher, J.D. Howard, T.B. Parrish, and J.A. Gottfried. 2010. Right orbitofrontal cortex mediates conscious olfactory perception. *Psychol Sci* 21: 1454–1463.

Liberles, S.D., and L.B. Buck. 2006. A second class of chemosensory receptors in the olfactory epithelium. *Nature* 442: 645–650.

Luskin, M.B., and J.L. Price. 1983. The topographic organization of associational fibers of the olfactory system in the rat, including centrifugal fibers to the olfactory bulb. *J Comp Neurol* 216: 264–291.

Ma, M., W.R. Chen, and G.M. Shepherd. 1999. Electrophysiological characterization of rat and mouse olfactory receptor neurons from an intact epithelial preparation. *J Neurosci Methods* 92: 31–40.

Magklara, A., and S. Lomvardas. 2013. Stochastic gene expression in mammals: Lessons from olfaction. *Trends Cell Biol* 23: 449–456.

Mainland, J., and N. Sobel. 2006. The sniff is part of the olfactory percept. *Chem Senses* 31: 181–196.

Mainland, J.D., E.A. Bremner, N. Young, B.N. Johnson, R.M. Khan, M. Bensafi, and N. Sobel. 2002. Olfactory plasticity: One nostril knows what the other learns. *Nature* 419: 802.

Malnic, B., J. Hirono, T. Sato, and L.B. Buck. 1999. Combinatorial receptor codes for odors. *Cell* 96: 713–723.

Maresh, A., D. Rodriguez Gil, M.C. Whitman, and C.A. Greer. 2008. Principles of glomerular organization in the human olfactory bulb: Implications for odor processing. *PloS One* 3: e2640.

Markopoulos, F., D. Rokni, D.H. Gire, and V.N. Murthy. 2012. Functional properties of cortical feedback projections to the olfactory bulb. *Neuron* 76: 1175–1188.

Meisami, E. 1990. A new morphometric method to estimate the total number of glomeruli in the olfactory bulb. *Chem Senses* 15: 407–418.

Miyamichi, K., F. Amat, F. Moussavi, C. Wang, I. Wickersham, N.R. Wall, H. Taniguchi, B. Tasic, Z.J. Huang, Z. He et al. 2011. Cortical representations of olfactory input by trans-synaptic tracing. *Nature* 472: 191–196.

Mombaerts, P. 2004. Genes and ligands for odorant, vomeronasal and taste receptors. *Nat Rev Neurosci* 5: 263–278.

Mombaerts, P., F. Wang, C. Dulac, S.K. Chao, A. Nemes, M. Mendelsohn, J. Edmondson, and R. Axel. 1996. Visualizing an olfactory sensory map. *Cell* 87: 675–686.

Moran, D.T., J.C. Rowley III, B.W. Jafek, and M.A. Lovell. 1982. The fine structure of the olfactory mucosa in man. *J Neurocytol* 11: 721–746.

Mori, K., Y.K. Takahashi, K.M. Igarashi, and M. Yamaguchi. 2006. Maps of odorant molecular features in the mammalian olfactory bulb. *Physiol Rev* 86: 409–433.

Morrison, E.E., and R.M. Costanzo. 1990. Morphology of the human olfactory epithelium. *J Comp Neurol* 297: 1–13.

Nickerson, D., and S.M. Newhall. 1943. A psychological color solid. *J Opt Soc Am* 33: 419–419.

Niimura, Y., and M. Nei. 2005. Comparative evolutionary analysis of olfactory receptor gene clusters between humans and mice. *Gene* 346: 13–21.

Niimura, Y., and M. Nei. 2007. Extensive gains and losses of olfactory receptor genes in mammalian evolution. *PloS One* 2: e708.

O'Doherty, J., E.T. Rolls, S. Francis, R. Bowtell, F. McGlone, G. Kobal, B. Renner, and G. Ahne. 2000. Sensory-specific satiety-related olfactory activation of the human orbitofrontal cortex. *Neuroreport* 11: 893–897.

Ohloff, G. 1994. *Scent and Fragrances: The Fascination of Odors and Their Chemical Perspectives*. Berlin: Springer-Verlag.

Peterlin, Z., S. Firestein, and M.E. Rogers. 2014. The state of the art of odorant receptor deorphanization: A report from the orphanage. *J Gen Physiol* 143: 527–542.

Pifferi, S., M. Dibattista, and A. Menini. 2009. TMEM16B induces chloride currents activated by calcium in mammalian cells. *Pflüg Arch* 458: 1023–1038.

Pifferi, S., A. Menini, and T. Kurahashi. 2010. Signal transduction in vertebrate olfactory cilia. In *The Neurobiology of Olfaction*, ed. A. Menini. Boca Raton, FL: CRC Press.

Pifferi, S., V. Cenedese, and A. Menini. 2012. Anoctamin 2/TMEM16B: A calcium-activated chloride channel in olfactory transduction. *Exp Physiol* 97: 193–199.

Plailly, J., J.D. Howard, D.R. Gitelman, and J.A. Gottfried. 2008. Attention to odor modulates thalamocortical connectivity in the human brain. *J Neurosci* 28: 5257–5267.

Pointer, M.R., and G.G. Attridge. 1998. The number of discernible colours. *Color Res Appl* 23: 52–54.

Ponissery Saidu, S., A.B. Stephan, A.K. Talaga, H. Zhao, and J. Reisert. 2013. Channel properties of the splicing isoforms of the olfactory calcium-activated chloride channel anoctamin 2. *J Gen Physiol* 141: 691–703.

Poo, C., and J.S. Isaacson. 2009. Odor representations in olfactory cortex: "Sparse" coding, global inhibition, and oscillations. *Neuron* 62: 850–861.

Potter, H., and N. Butters. 1980. An assessment of olfactory deficits in patients with damage to prefrontal cortex. *Neuropsychologia* 18: 621–628.

Quignon, P., M. Giraud, M. Rimbault, P. Lavigne, S. Tacher, E. Morin, E. Retout, A.-S. Valin, K. Lindblad-Toh, J. Nicolas et al. 2005. The dog and rat olfactory receptor repertoires. *Genome Biol* 6: R83.

Reisert, J., and D. Restrepo. 2009. Molecular tuning of odorant receptors and its implication for odor signal processing. *Chem Senses* 34: 535–545.

Reisert, J., J. Lai, K.-W. Yau, and J. Bradley. 2005. Mechanism of the excitatory Cl⁻ response in mouse olfactory receptor neurons. *Neuron* 45: 553–561.

Rennaker, R.L., C.-F.F. Chen, A.M. Ruyle, A.M. Sloan, and D.A. Wilson. 2007. Spatial and temporal distribution of odorant-evoked activity in the piriform cortex. *J Neurosci* 27: 1534–1542.

Ressler, K.J., S.L. Sullivan, and L.B. Buck. 1993. A zonal organization of odorant receptor gene expression in the olfactory epithelium. *Cell* 73: 597–609.

Rodriguez, I. 2013. Singular expression of olfactory receptor genes. *Cell* 155: 274–277.

Rolls, E.T., and L.L. Baylis. 1994. Gustatory, olfactory, and visual convergence within the primate orbitofrontal cortex. *J Neurosci* 14: 5437–5452.

Rolls, E.T., M.L. Kringelbach, and I.E.T. de Araujo. 2003. Different representations of pleasant and unpleasant odours in the human brain. *Eur J Neurosci* 18: 695–703.

Root, C.M., C.A. Denny, R. Hen, and R. Axel. 2014. The participation of cortical amygdala in innate, odour-driven behaviour. *Nature* 515: 269–273.

Rowley III, J.C., D.T. Moran, and B.W. Jafek. 1989. Peroxidase backfills suggest the mammalian olfactory epithelium contains a second morphologically distinct class of bipolar sensory neuron: The microvillar cell. *Brain Res* 502: 387–400.

Royet, J.P., C. Souchier, F. Jourdan, and H. Ploye. 1988. Morphometric study of the glomerular population in the mouse olfactory bulb: Numerical density and size distribution along the rostrocaudal axis. *J Comp Neurol* 270: 559–568.

Schild, D., and D. Restrepo. 1998. Transduction mechanisms in vertebrate olfactory receptor cells. *Physiol Rev* 78: 429–466.

Schoenbaum, G., and H. Eichenbaum. 1995a. Information coding in the rodent prefrontal cortex. II. Ensemble activity in orbitofrontal cortex. *J Neurophysiol* 74: 751–762.

Schoenbaum, G., and H. Eichenbaum. 1995b. Information coding in the rodent prefrontal cortex. I. Single-neuron activity in orbitofrontal cortex compared with that in pyriform cortex. *J Neurophysiol* 74: 733–750.

Shepherd, G.M. 2006. Smell images and the flavour system in the human brain. *Nature* 444: 316–321.

Shipley, M.T., and M. Ennis. 1996. Functional organization of olfactory system. *J Neurobiol* 30: 123–176.

Small, D.M., M. Jones-Gotman, R.J. Zatorre, M. Petrides, and A.C. Evans. 1997. Flavor processing: More than the sum of its parts. *Neuroreport* 8: 3913–3917.

Sobel, N., V. Prabhakaran, C.A. Hartley, J.E. Desmond, G.H. Glover, E.V. Sullivan, and J.D. Gabrieli. 1999. Blind smell: Brain activation induced by an undetected air-borne chemical. *Brain J Neurol* 122 (Pt 2): 209–217.

Song, Y., K.D. Cygnar, B. Sagdullaev, M. Valley, S. Hirsh, A. Stephan, J. Reisert, and H. Zhao. 2008. Olfactory CNG channel desensitization by Ca^{2+}/CaM via the B1b subunit affects response termination but not sensitivity to recurring stimulation. *Neuron* 58: 374–386.

Sosulski, D.L., M.L. Bloom, T. Cutforth, R. Axel, and S.R. Datta. 2011. Distinct representations of olfactory information in different cortical centres. *Nature* 472: 213–216.

Sotnikova, T.D., M.G. Caron, and R.R. Gainetdinov. 2009. Trace amine-associated receptors as emerging therapeutic targets. *Mol Pharmacol* 76: 229–235.

Spence, C., F.P. McGlone, B. Kettenmann, and G. Kobal. 2001. Attention to olfaction. A psychophysical investigation. *Exp Brain Res* 138: 432–437.

Stephan, A.B., E.Y. Shum, S. Hirsh, K.D. Cygnar, J. Reisert, and H. Zhao. 2009. ANO2 is the cilial calcium-activated chloride channel that may mediate olfactory amplification. *Proc Natl Acad Sci USA* 106: 11776–11781.

Stephan, A.B., S. Tobochnik, M. Dibattista, C.M. Wall, J. Reisert, and H. Zhao. 2012. The Na^+/Ca^{2+} exchanger NCKX4 governs termination and adaptation of the mammalian olfactory response. *Nat Neurosci* 15: 131–137.

Stettler, D.D., and R. Axel. 2009. Representations of odor in the piriform cortex. *Neuron* 63: 854–864.

Stevens, S., and H. Davis. 1983. *Hearing: Its Psychology and Physiology*. New York: Acoustical Society of America.

Stevens, D.A., and R.J. O'Connell. 1995. Enhanced sensitivity to androstenone following regular exposure to pemenone. *Chem Senses* 20: 413–419.

Stuck, B.A., V. Fadel, T. Hummel, and J.U. Sommer. 2014. Subjective olfactory desensitization and recovery in humans. *Chem Senses* 39: 151–157.

Tirindelli, R., M. Dibattista, S. Pifferi, and A. Menini. 2009. From pheromones to behavior. *Physiol Rev* 89: 921–956.

Vassar, R., J. Ngai, and R. Axel. 1993. Spatial segregation of odorant receptor expression in the mammalian olfactory epithelium. *Cell* 74: 309–318.

Wallrabenstein, I., J. Kuklan, L. Weber, S. Zborala, M. Werner, J. Altmüller, C. Becker, A. Schmidt, H. Hatt, T. Hummel et al. 2013. Human trace amine-associated receptor TAAR5 can be activated by trimethylamine. *PloS One* 8: e54950.

Weiskrantz, L. 2002. Prime-sight and blindsight. *Conscious Cogn* 11: 568–581.

Whisman, M.L., J.W. Goetzinger, F.O. Cotton, and D.W. Brinkman. 1978. Odorant evaluation: A study of ethanethiol and tetrahydrothiophene as warning agents in propane. *Environ Sci Technol* 12: 1285–1288.

Wilson, D.A. 2003. Rapid, experience-induced enhancement in odorant discrimination by anterior piriform cortex neurons. *J Neurophysiol* 90: 65–72.

Winston, J.S., J.A. Gottfried, J.M. Kilner, and R.J. Dolan. 2005. Integrated neural representations of odor intensity and affective valence in human amygdala. *J Neurosci* 25: 8903–8907.

Wysocki, C.J., K.M. Dorries, and G.K. Beauchamp. 1989. Ability to perceive androstenone can be acquired by ostensibly anosmic people. *Proc Natl Acad Sci USA* 86: 7976–7978.

Yan, C., A.Z. Zhao, J.K. Bentley, K. Loughney, K. Ferguson, and J.A. Beavo. 1995. Molecular cloning and characterization of a calmodulin-dependent phosphodiesterase enriched in olfactory sensory neurons. *Proc Natl Acad Sci USA* 92: 9677–9681.

Zald, D.H., and J.V. Pardo. 1997. Emotion, olfaction, and the human amygdala: Amygdala activation during aversive olfactory stimulation. *Proc Natl Acad Sci USA* 94: 4119–4124.

Zatorre, R.J., and M. Jones-Gotman. 1991. Human olfactory discrimination after unilateral frontal or temporal lobectomy. *Brain J Neurol* 114 (Pt 1A): 71–84.

Zatorre, R.J., M. Jones-Gotman, A.C. Evans, and E. Meyer. 1992. Functional localization and lateralization of human olfactory cortex. *Nature* 360: 339–340.

Zelano, C., M. Bensafi, J. Porter, J. Mainland, B. Johnson, E. Bremner, C. Telles, R. Khan, and N. Sobel. 2005. Attentional modulation in human primary olfactory cortex. *Nat Neurosci* 8: 114–120.

Zhang, J., R. Pacifico, D. Cawley, P. Feinstein, and T. Bozza. 2013. Ultrasensitive detection of amines by a trace amine-associated receptor. *J Neurosci* 33: 3228–3239.

Section I

Botanical, Phytochemical, Analytical, and Technological Issues

3 Physiology, Taxonomy, and Morphology of Aromatic Plants
A Botanical Perspective

Salvatore Ragusa

CONTENTS

3.1 INTRODUCTION

Aromatherapy is a practice that takes advantage of the health properties of therapeutic plants and essential oils. The term *aromatherapy* was coined in 1928 by Frenchman Rene-Maurice Gattefosse; his interest in essential oils and their use in medicine was such that he wrote a book in 1937 on the subject: *Aromathérapie: les huiles essentielles hormones végétales*. Essential oils, essences, or volatile oils are volatile mixtures whose chemical compositions are very complex and present in more than 17,000 plants. Families involving species that are rich in essential oils are Apiaceae, Asteraceae, Cupressaceae, Lamiaceae, Lauraceae, Liliaceae, Magnoliaceae, Myrtaceae, and Rutaceae (Tutin et al., 1993; Capasso, 2011). Essential oils are complexes of volatile substances that are liquid at a relatively low boiling point, present in all plant organs, insoluble or poorly soluble in water, and soluble in alcohol, ether, and fixed oils. Due to their volatile nature, they all have a strong, mostly pleasant, odor. The main chemical constituents of essential oils are represented by hydrocarbons, terpenes, or aromatic and oxygenated derivatives (e.g., alcohols, aldehydes, ketones, and acids).

With regard to the characteristics of the essential oils, the biochemical group of plants that contains them shows the greatest number of chemical breeds, and these include 36 families of bryophyta, gymnosperms, and angiosperms. Reported differences among these species may stem from various external factors other than genetics (Tetenyi, 1975; Lo Presti et al., 2010). There are, for example, three spokes of *Melaleuca bracteata* Muell. (Myrtaceae) that produce essential oils containing mainly methyl eugenol, methyl isoeugenol, and elemicin, respectively. These compounds may be transformed into one another by simple chemical steps, indicating that one of these compounds (e.g., methyl eugenol) is present in all breeds. With the appropriate enzyme, methyl isoeugenol can be formed through the displacement of a double bond and elemicin by the addition of a hydroxyl group and subsequent methylation (Trease and Evans, 1996).

Lamiaceae, Myrtaceae, and Rutaceae are among the families that include species that are rich in essential oils.

3.2 PHYSIOLOGY

Every living organism incorporates from the outside a number of substances used as nutrients and constantly eliminates a number of substances as waste products of the metabolism. For plants, these substances may be the end product of the demolition of more complex substances of an organic nature: the photosynthetic process, for instance, uses light energy, and plants use water and carbon dioxide to synthesize carbohydrates and accumulate energy in the form of chemical bonds. These compounds therefore represent the tanks of chemical energy that the plant, like the animal organism, demolishes at every turn and, with the process of respiration, then oxidizes as end products that are returned to the environment as water and carbon dioxide. However, frequently organic compounds endowed with relatively complex structures are eliminated. This elimination concerns not only products having slag parts, but also very noble substances, or at least ones that are further usable. The elimination of these substances can be definitive or temporary. Cellulose, for example, cannot be regarded as a metabolic waste, and even if under certain circumstances a plant cell ejects it permanently from its protoplast, this is so it can be used as the main constituent of the cell wall. Starch and aleurone grains are substances that are temporarily expelled from the cytoplasm stored in insoluble forms in plastids and vacuoles, outside the whirlwind of metabolic reactions. In this case, the expulsion from the cytoplasm is only temporary since the materials set aside as reserve substances, such as glucose, with which the primary starch is synthesized, are accumulated for a few hours and their excess could disturb the smooth running of further training. Finally, expulsion may relate to minerals; introduced in excess from the outside, these are deleted without even being introduced in the chemistry of life. This is the case, for example, of some soluble salts that, when present in large quantities in the land, plants can introduce and then delete without actually handling small quantities. According to these accounts for plant organisms, in principle, it is possible to envisage a sort of segregation, a term that encompasses the three functional aspects of these phoenomena: excretion, secretion, and *recrezione*. Excretion means elimination of the final products of the demolition or removal of organic substances that also, although not fully exploited, are abandoned as a waste of parts. For secretion, the expulsion of substances that are not waste but rather are reserved for functional tasks is intended. Recrezione is the expelling of substances that are not eligible to participate in the metabolic exchange of the plant cell. However, it should be kept in mind that excreta, namely, products of excretion, only in a few cases are considered useless for the plant that produced or held them without function.

In most cases, they undergo important biological tasks; accordingly, examples are pollinators that offer defense against excessive perspiration, support wound healing, or protect against trauma. Thus, the distinction between excretions and secretions is often conventional and admits several intermediate cases. With regard to plant biology, it is doubtful that the concept of excretion has the same meaning in animal biology. For this reason, today the term *secretion* is preferred (Bruni, 2014); it avoids misinterpretations of the classification of excretions on a quantitative base. In the group of secretory products, also excluded are those compounds that, stored temporarily in different cellular compartments, are also intended to be taken up again and placed in metabolic processes. These are thus considered secretory tissues that give rise to well-defined types of substances (terpenes, essential oils, resins, etc.). From the metabolic point of view, these appear to be more or less abundant. Regardless of the functional significance of the products of vegetable secretion, it is possible to distinguish two types of secretory tissues: (1) those that excrete substances secreted out of the plant or even, in the interior of it, in the intercellular spaces after they had thus been secreted extracellularly and (2) those that eliminate substances secreted in the vacuoles and then store them in the interior of the cells (intracellular secretion). Based solely on morphological criteria, the first group can be indicated by the name *glandular tissues* and the second with the name *secretory tissues*. It must be said that the secretory function is not always exercised by polyplast forming real tissues; it is not rare that it is entrusted to the individually isolated cell in the breast tissue of another type, therefore having the value of idioblast. The latter are known as secretory cells and glandular cells (Svodoba and Svodoba, 2000). The secretion products, contained in the interior of these cells (whether isolated or combined in complexes), may be solids, such as crystals of calcium oxalate, or liquids, such as ethereal oils, mucilage, resins, gums, gum resins, balsams, tannins, alkaloids, latexes, and pigments (e.g., anthocyanins). To the category of secretory tissues, which retains in the lumen the cellular product of their activities, belong the so-called *lactiferous* or *lactiferous tubes*, isolated and elongated cells, or series of elongated cells fused together, featured to contain an emulsion, which is given the name latex. They are typical of certain families that are all among the Magnophyta (Apocinaceae Asclepiadaceae, Asteraceae, Campanulaceae, Convolvulaceae, Euphorbiaceae, Lobeliaceae, Moraceae, Papaveraceae, etc.); these are herbaceous species, trees and shrubs located especially in tropical climates. When present, the lactiferous are located in all parts of the plant, from the roots to the leaves and fruits.

Cells and glandular tissues are cells that, isolated or combined in tissues, pour out the product of their metabolism. These can originate from both apical and sided meristems so that they can be found in both the primary and the secondary body of the plant. However, the rationale for their classification is based on their location, for example, superficial or deep; in fact, cells and glandular tissues of an external source and epidermal cells and glandular tissues of an internal, parenchymatous, source do exist. Cells and glandular tissues are considered the external epidermal formations; the most common examples are given by glandular hairs, the scales by secreting digestive hairs, and stinging hairs from nectaries from glandular emergencies. The products of their secretion, exiting through porosity or laceration of the cuticle, are poured outside, just after they had been secreted. As for the glandular tissues and parenchymatous origin, their position is such that the products that are expelled do not spill out of the plant but will collect in the intercellular spaces (endogenous secretion) that are formed among secretory cells for their mutual distancing and which therefore have schizogene origin. The shape of these intercellular spaces may be that of the cavity, more or less equal in size or highly elongated. In either case, the intercellular space is bordered all around by a layer of glandular cells forming a glandular epithelium. Examples of pocket fragmenting bounded by a glandular epithelium are those that, in the leaves of *Hypericum perforatum* L., have the appearance of tanks of essential oil, but also more frequent are intercellular channels that, branched or not, in many plants through a large part of their body, and communicating between them, often form the true channel system. The secretory product that fills them can be of various natures and be represented by resins, mucilages, gums, and so forth, and named after their nature as resiniferous channels, mucilaginous channels, and so forth. Intercellular spaces, more or less isodiametric, may have an schizolysigenous origin. These spaces are formed following lysis of secretory cells, which, after being filled with the product of their activity, pour into the cavity (pockets or lysigene bags) that has come to form, as in the case of many genera belonging to the Myrtaceae family or even to the Rutaceae. In the case of the genus *Citrus*, however, where the essential oil is found in the peel of hesperidium, localized between the flavedo and albedo, the source is schizolysigenous (Tonzig and Marrè, 1983).

3.3 TAXONOMY

Taxonomy establishes the criteria useful to group and sort hierarchically, in a classification system, an identified unit's diversity. The diversity of plant organisms is studied by systematic botany, characterizing them using all the notions concerning the morphology, the histological and anatomical organization, the physiology of the plant, the playback mode, and ontogenetic cycles. It takes into account the ecological and geographical distribution and investigates the possible evolutionary origin and the phylogenetic relationships existing among organisms (Bayer et al., 2009). Thus, the systematic task is to identify groups of natural diversity and what sort of taxonomy in systems of increasing values. These groupings, of different sizes, are called taxa (Maity, 2012).

In particular, medicinal plants can be categorized in different ways depending on what to pursue: (1) if it is the line, the biological evolutionary criterion is paramount; (2) if it is a phytochemical criterion, the biologically active principles prevail; and (3) if it is a pharmacological criterion, their mode of action is the priority. It can be said that, except for the criterion of evolution, all the criteria are, in fact, artificial or utilitarian (Acquaah, 2012). The classification of objects of study of pharmaceutical biology shall appropriately begin by the criterion of evolution, knowing that in practice you can follow other, opportunistic classification criteria, based on the convenience of grouping plants and drugs for different characteristics (presence of active principles, pharmacological action, plant structure and drugs, etc.). In the field of medicinal plants, most classification systems are, in fact, based on different criteria, and all meet specific needs.

The morphological, phylogenetic classification, which attempts to reconstruct the evolution of plants from ancestral progenitors, does not have a pharmaceutical interest except that it is necessary to classify the plants under study in very precise terms. Its relevance concerns the value of an identification that reduces the margin of error in the recognition of a medicinal species. However, positive identification of a plant includes knowledge of macro- and micromorphological, chemical, and genetic methods (De Pasquale and Ragusa, 1979; Rapisarda et al., 1996; Applequist, 2006; Upton et al., 2011).

Initially, plants were grouped on the basis of their practical use, in particular, as pharmaceuticals and food. To this period belongs the work of Hippocrates, doctor of Kos, born around 460 BCE, who provided lists of medicinal plants and is knowledgeable for having established the fundamental importance of the observation, repudiating previous magical conceptions. The first real scientific organizer of ancient thought was Aristotle (384–322 BCE), who also grouped a classification of the natural world. His disciple Theophrastus (371–285 BCE), who wrote *Historia plantarum* and *De causis plantarum*, was equipped with a wide knowledge of the plant world. He was the author of a remarkable series of both morphological and physiological observations and intuition, and in his classification he divided plants according to their general appearance, but he himself admitted the limits of this transaction, noting that there are intermediate cluster forms identified. For many centuries, however, attention was polarized around the work of Dioscorides, considered a great doctor of the first century CE, who had described and shown about 600 plants, grouping them according to an empirical criterion (food plants, herbs, medicines). He is considered the founding father of pharmacology, having laid the scientific rationale of drug therapy. He gathered all the therapeutic knowledge derived from Egypt, the Middle East, and Roman Greece in a work entitled *De materia medica*—a work of primary importance in the field of medicine that was unmatched by others of his time and known for its clear and detailed descriptions of drugs, based on the rational method and still valid today. From this original work, which was the main, though not exclusive, reference text for more than a millennium, were derived many versions: one of the oldest is *Dioscorides Neapolitanus*, which in 172 cards richly illustrated, with miniaturized drawings, the form of *herbarium* properties and therapeutic uses of 409 plant species (Aboca, 2013). In the second half of the fifteenth century began the classification of plants on the basis of a few morphological characteristics, giving rise to *artificial classifications*. Indeed, they do not gather organisms actually similar to each other, but approachable for one or a few characteristics. This was the period of the great herbals that had significant spread thanks to the advent of printing. Some, like Pierandrea Mattioli (1500–1577), still used the setting given by Dioscorides; others differed sharply. The study of plants for their intrinsic interest, and not in terms of their use, has developed only since the late sixteenth and early seventeenth centuries thanks to the works of A. Cesalpino (1519–1603) and the brothers J. Bauhin (1541–1603) and G. Bauhin (1560–1624), who can be considered the first true taxonomists of the plant world. The beginning of 1700 saw the emergence of fundamental works for the development of botany. Among these is the *Istitutiones herbariae rei*, by J.P. de Tournefort (1656–1708), in which about 9000 species grouped in 698 genera are classified with artificial criteria, and the work of J. Ray (1607–1705), including the second edition of his

Nova methodus plantarum (1703), where plants are classified on the basis of a large number of characteristics, that is, vegetative reproduction. The sexual system of Linnaeus (1707–1778) belongs to the artificial classifications. It is essentially based on the consideration of characteristics related to flowers and fruits; for the flower, the number of stamens is considered, often related to the gynoecium. The importance of Linnaeus, however, is that he adopted the binomial nomenclature still used today (Imbesi, 1964; Index Kewensis, 1997).

3.4   MORPHOLOGY

Among the aromatic plants the Lamiaceae family certainly occupies a leading position in the pharmaceutical, food, and health categories. It belongs to the order of Lamiales, together with other families of pharmacognostic interest, such as the Boraginaceae and Verbenaceae (Capasso, 2011; Senatore, 2012). In a recent subdivision of angiosperms, based on the phylogenetic relationships revealed by molecular studies (Cronk, 2009; Acquaah, 2012), the order of Lamiales was inserted in Asteride, including in the class of eudicots. The asterids are a major group of eudicots that comprise a large percentage of angiosperms in total. The asterids are divided into 14 orders (Simpson, 2010). The species belonging to the family of Lamiaceae are mostly herbaceous or suffruticose (*Lavandula* spp., *Melissa* spp., *Mentha* spp., *Origanum* spp., *Rosmarinus* spp., *Salvia* spp., *Teucrium* spp., *Thymus* spp., etc.) and of pharmaceutical and pharmacognostic interest (Imbesi, 1964; Aqel, 1991; Pignatti, 1997; Iauk et al., 2014); they have simple leaves, are rarely pinnate-compound, and are often opposite, decussate. Their flowers are hermaphrodite, pentamer, and zygomorphic. They are almost always in inflorescences bracteate, among which the most common are the spikelet and verticillaster; calix gamosepalous, sometimes bilabiate; and corolla bilabiate, rarely unilabiate. There are four stamens and two didinami, pistil bicarpellare with an ovary quatrefoil in maturity at the base, and a disk nectar. Fruit dry when ripe is divided into four achenes. The family is cosmopolitan, but is particularly well represented in the Mediterranean region. Almost all species of this family secrete essential oils, processed in the glandular hairs of the leaves and flowers; they also contain abundant di- and triterpenes and phenolic compounds (Lo Presti et al., 2005; Condurso et al., 2013). They are among the numerous genera belonging to the family of Lamiaceae, and that definitely includes aromatic plants of major interest from the genera *Lavandula* and *Rosmarinus*.

The genus *Lavandula* is made up of different species and varieties of pharmaceutical and pharmacognostic interest, such as *Lavandula angustifolia* Miller subsp. *angustifolia* (= *L. officinalis* Chaix, *L. spica* L., *L. fragrans* Jordan, and *L. vera* DC.), *true lavender*; *Lavandula latifolia* Medicus, *lavender aspic*; and hybrids between these two species, the so-called sinks; *Lavandula* × *intermedia* Emeric (= *L. hybrida* Reverchon) and *Lavandula stoechas* L. These species are fragrant shrubs, densely bushy, with woody branches at the base, herbaceous, and quadrangular in the apical part. A genus of 32 species, *Lavandula* is native to the Canary Islands, Cape Verde, Madeira, the Mediterranean area, the Near East, North Africa, northeast tropical Africa, Arabia, and India. Some of the species are grown for their essential oil used in perfumery, the fragrance industry, and aromatherapy. The are cultivated as ornamental plants, for the herb garden, and some as low informal hedges or bee plants. In cooler climates, the Canary Island species and *L. viridis* L. are best treated as cool glasshouse subjects, and *L. multifida* Burm. f. as an annual. With full sun and good drainage, all thrive in most soil types. Propagation is by shoot cutting, best taken in late summer and spring, or seed, except for named clones, may be sown in spring (Chaytor, 1937; De Wolf, 1955; Tucker and Hensen, 1985).

The European Pharmacopoeia contains the essential oil obtained by steam distillation from the flowering tops of *Lavandula angustifolia* Mill. (*Lavandula officinalis* Chaix), a shrub of 50 cm. Leaves (2–5 cm × 3–5 mm) are mainly linear-lanceolate, entire, with gray felt hairs when young, becoming greener with age. The inflorescence stalks are 10–25 cm, unbranched, and usually with compact spikes of 4–5 or 8 cm; some have lower flower clusters distant from the main spike. There are five to seven (sometimes nine) flowered whorls and minute bracteoles present. Bracts are broadly ovate diamond shaped to obovate. Flowers are stalked. The 13-veined calyx has an appendage, cylindric in shape. The corolla is strongly bilaterally symmetric, nearly twice the length of the calyx, with prominent lobes, and is shades of blue-mauve, rarely violet pink in color. Three main subspecies are known: *L. angustifloia* Mill. subsp. *angustifolia* is the source of true lavender oil. There are many cultivars, for example, *Hidecote* (30 cm deep lilac flowers), *Munstead* (45 cm blue-lilac flowers), *Rosea* (45 cm pink flowers), and *Nana Alba* (20 cm dwarf, white). This species is often listed as *L. spica* L., but this name has been questioned as being ambiguous. *L. angustiflolia* Mill. subsp. *pirenaica* (DC.) Guinea is smaller (25–35 cm) with very large bracts; *L. angustifolia* Mill. subsp. *delphinensis* (Jordan) de Bolos et Vigo is larger, more robust (to 50 cm), with longer, more interrupted robust spikes. Seed occasionally distributed as a hardy plant under the name *L. burmanni* Bentham appears to be *L. angustifolia*. *L. bipinnata* Kuntze var. *rothiana* Kuntze (*L. burmannii* Bentham) is a tender Indian species that is not generally cultivated (Cullen et al., 2000).

The genus *Lavandula* has been thoroughly studied mostly for its essential oil from flowers and inflorescences of *Lavandula angustifolia* Mill. obtained, according to pharmacopoeias, by treatment in a current of aqueous vapor; however, other species, varieties, or hybrids are often used in order to improve both quality and yield. Particular attention has thus been turned to the study of exogenous and endogenous factors (genetic, ontogenetic, cultural, climatic, pathological, extraction techniques, etc.) that determine the considerable variability of the composition of the essence itself (De Pasqual et al., 1989; Kokkalou, 1998). The histological studies were initially confined to the commercially better known and more important species. A systematic histological investigation (Bhatnagar and Dunn, 1961, 1962, 1963) was aimed at preparing an analytical key for the microscopic identification of the genus *Lavandula*, grouping them into five sections. However, the morphofunctional aspects of the glandular system of *Lavandula* flowers that produces the essential oil have been little studied.

Using optic and electron microscopy, the distribution and ultrastructure of secretory tissues of the superficial flower *Lavandula* spp. have been studied (Ragusa et al., 1995, 2000). This allowed correlations between the topochemistry of the secretory apparatus and the production of essential oil to be made. Furthermore, laser scanning electron microscopy has allowed a more precise interpretation of the micromorphology and organization of the glandular structures (Figures 3.1 and 3.2) (Ragusa et al., 1997).

The genus *Rosmarinus* L. consists of aromatic evergreen shrubs of three species native to the Mediterranean area, except for the eastern part. They are cultivated as ornamental shrubs, culinary herbs, and for essential oil used in perfumery and aromatherapy. Most soil types are suitable, but plants need full sun and good drainage to thrive. *Rosmarinus officinalis* L. is a bushy, branched evergreen shrub, 1–2 m high, with leaves sessile, opposite, narrow, entire, and strongly reflected in the edges, of leathery texture, dark green on the upper side, whitish and tomentose on the lower side, for the presence of numerous coatings and glandular trichomes. The blue flowers, rarely white, are placed at the apex of the branches' leaf axils. It is a spontaneous species, characteristic of the Mediterranean region, commonly grown in gardens. The drug is made

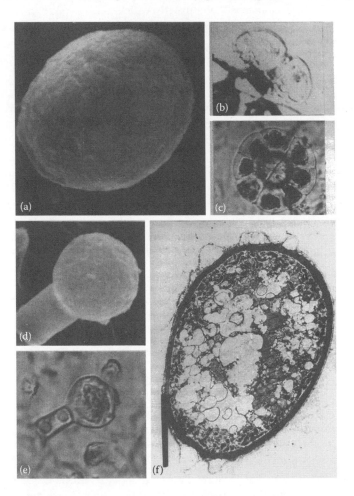

FIGURE 3.1 Light and electron micrographs of glandular hairs (types A and B) of *Lavandula angustifolia* Mill. flowers. Bar = 10 μm. (a) Globular head of type A glandular hair (SEM). (b) Globular head of type A, with short stalk cell (LM). (c) Eight-celled head of type A glandular hair (LM). (d, e) Glandular hair type B, with sub-cylindrical stalk cell (d: SEM; e: LM). (f) Head of type B glandular hair (TEM). (From Ragusa, S. et al., *Riv. It. EPPOS*, 21, 27–33, 1997.)

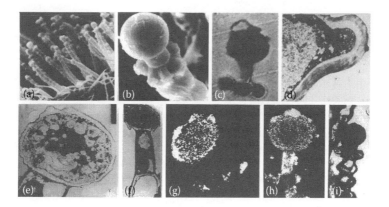

FIGURE 3.2 Light and electron micrographs of glandular hairs (type C) of *Lavandula angustifolia* Mill. flowers. Bar = 10 μm. (a) Globular head of type A glandular hair (SEM). (b) Globular head of type A, with short stalk cell (LM). (c) Eight-celled head of type A glandular hair (LM). (d, e) Glandular hair type B, with sub-cylindrical stalk cell (d: SEM; e: LM). (f) Head of type B glandular hair (TEM). (From Ragusa, S. et al., *Riv. It. EPPOS*, 21, 27–33, 1997.)

from the leaves and flowering tops. Leaves have a lead coating, branched trichomes, and glandular hairs and are peltate. The main constituents of the essential oil are camphor, cineole, α-pinene, and borneol. The composition, however, varies depending on the origin. Two types can be recognized: one of Spanish origin and one of Morocco–Tunisian origin. In the Spanish variety camphor is present in a considerable amount (13%–18%) in the essential oil that also contains 18%–26% of α-pinene and 8%–12% of camphene, although it is poor in cineole. At variance with the latter, the essential oil of the Morocco-Tunisian variety is very rich in cineole (38%–55%), while it is poor in camphor, α-pinene, and camphene (Lo Presti et al., 2005; Maleci Bini et al., 2014).

Many cultivars have been selected, including *Miss Jessopp's Upright, Tuscan Blue*, and *Roseus*. Several varieties are cultivated: *Rosmarinus officinalis* var. *prostratus* Pasquale (*R. lavandulaceus* de Noe, *R. repens* Anon, *R. prostratus* Anon) has a prostrate habit, and *R. officinalis* var. *angustifolius* Gussone (*R. angustifolius* Miller, *R. angustissimum* Fouchard et Mandon) has strongly scented, narrow leaves. The name *form erectus Beguinot* is applied to plants with an erect habit. *Rosmarinus eriocalix* Jordam et Fourreau is a shrub with an upright to sprawling habit, 50–100 cm. Leaves are 5–20 × 1.5–2 mm, gray-green, with margins often rolled under. Bracts are ovate and acuminate, and the calyx is 5–6 mm and densely downy with long simple glandular and nonglandular hairs (Cullen et al., 2000).

The European Pharmacopoeia also contains whole, dried leaves of *Rosmarinus officinalis* L. In particular, the leaves are assile, tough, linear, or linear-lanceolate, 1–4 cm long and 2–4 mm wide, with ricurve edges. The upper surface is dark green, glabrous, and grainy; the lower surface is grayish green and densely tomentose with a preminent midrib, numerous multicellular, extensively branched, covering trichomes of the lower epidermis, and rare conical covering trichomes of the upper epidermis. The glandular trichomes are of two types: the majority have a short, unicellular stalk and radiate head composed of cells, while others, less abundant, have a unicellular stalk and peripherical unicellular or bicellular head (European Pharmacopoeia, 2014).

The family of Rutaceae, along with other pharmaceutical interests such as the Anacardiaceae, Burseraceae, Sapindaceae, and Simarubaceae, is part of Sapindales, an order that is included in the Roside class of eudicots (Simpson, 2010). The Rutaceae in phytochemical terms can be classified into Rutaceae containing essential oils (*Citrus* spp., *Ruta* spp., *Agathosoma* spp., etc.) and Rutaceae containing alkaloids (*Pilocarpus* spp., etc.).

The plants belonging to the family of Rutaceae are generally woody, sometimes thorny, and frequently with pinnate leaves or trifoliate; they rarely have simple, generally available alternates. They are evergreen or deciduous, perennial trees or shrubs, and rarely herbaceous. Leaves are opposite or alternate, simple or compound, usually with stipule and glands and often aromatic. Flowers are in cymes or in terminal or axillary umbels; there are head spikes, panicles, and racemes, which are occasionally unisexual.

A family of 150 genera consisting of about 1600 species is found mainly in Africa, Australia, and America. Some important ornamental plants belong to this family, but it is chiefly of note because of citrus fruits (oranges, grapefruit, etc.). The genus *Citrus* has 20–40 stamens and an ovary with 8–15 cells (Cullen et al., 1997).

Belonging to the genus *Citrus* are species that are commonly indicated by the name *citrus*. They are small trees that originated from the East and naturalized in the Mediterranean region in the antiquity or Middle Ages, depending on the species. Currently, many species are cultivated in warm-temperate regions (California, Australia, South America) for their edible fruits. The fruit is a particular type of berry called hesperidium. It has a pericarp that is thickly sprinkled with schizolysigene pockets containing essential oil, a mesocarp rich in pectin and flavonoids, and an endocarp that looks like a thin film made up of hair-rich juice (cloves) in which are found the seeds. *Citrus aurantium* L. bitter orange is a small tree of 4–5 m with a branched trunk and very thorny branches. The leaves are oval, entire, slightly leathery, and shiny. The foil becomes articulated on a stalk of 1 cm in length and is full of schizolysigene pockets, visible under light microscopy. The flowers are white, very fragrant, and gathered in the axils of leaves. The hesperidium is smaller than that of *Citrus sinensis* (L.) Osbeck (= *Citrus aurantium* var. *dulcis*), sweet orange. It has a wrinkled, orange-red skin coloring (flavedo) when ripe and has numerous large schizolysigene pockets that are clearly visible even to the naked eye. The segments contain a little bitter juice, more fragrant than that of sweet and with many seeds. It is a species native to northern India and is widely cultivated, even in climates that are not too mild.

Being a very robust species and less sensitive to other congeners, especially at low temperature, it is often cultivated and employed as a graft holder for other species of the genus *Citrus*. Of particular interest is the zest (peel), namely, epicarp (flavedo), and part of the mesocarp (albedo). The latter, in addition to forming minerals, pectin, and flavonoid glycosides, produces the essence, which is rich in limonene, myrcene, α-pinene, and so forth. The peel is used to prepare the tincture of bitter orange and syrup of orange peel, bitter tonics, stomachic, and flavoring. These peels are in great demand in liqueur (Curaçao) and the food industry (for pectin jellies and jams). Epicarp and mesocarp are reported in the European Pharmacopoeia. Together with the dye, the presence of a considerable amount of flavonoids (esperoside, neoesperoside, naringoside, eridioctyoside, ericitroside) justifies traditional use in the treatment of fragile capillaries. The flower buds contain an essential oil, reported by the European Pharmacopoeia and called the essence of Néroli, containing linalool, linalyl acetate, limonene, β-pinene, and less acetate and geranyl nerile, trans-nerolidolo, trans-trans-farnesol, and so forth. *Citrus* is used in perfumery and in the pharmaceutical industry to prepare the distilled orange flower officinale, used as a flavoring and endowed with antispasmodic properties. The leaves contain an essential oil consisting of terpene (limonene) carbides and especially alcohols (linalool, nerol); it is reportedly used in infusion as a mild sedative and stomachic, often mixed with other drugs.

Citrus bergamia Risso et Pouiteau (*Citrus aurantium* L. ssp. *bergamia* Engl.), Bergamot, is a species cultivated mainly in Calabria, although there are crops in South America and the Ivory Coast. It is cultivated mainly for its essential oil that contains β-pinene, limonene, γ-terpinene, linalool, linalyl acetate, and geranial. The nonvolatile fraction contains bergaptene (from 0.2% to 0.45%) furanocumarine, known to be responsible for the photosensitizing effect of the essential oil. The essence, preferably deprived of bergaptene, is mainly used in perfumery. *Citrus bergamia* Risso et Poiteau is a tree species that presents an average force with posture ranging from assurgent to expanded. The leaf is large and very similar to that of the lemon in color and shape. The flower of bergamot, and other esperidee, is generally called zagara from the arabic *zahar*, which means *flower*. The flower has beautiful, pure white petals and a pleasant scent that differs from that of many other species of the genus *Citrus* because the style and stigma often persist even after the formation of the fruit. The flowering season begins in March in sunny locations, close to the sea, and in April in the innermost areas. Bergamot of Calabria comprises three cultivars: *Femminello* is a variety of quick but reduced growth that is productive and demanding but short-lived. It has leaves of average development and is lanceolate in shape. The fruit is spherical with a thin peel; fruit picking begins in October. *Castagnaro* is a tree of good development and alternating production; it is rustic and durable. It features large leaves that are lanceolate in shape. The fruit is globose with a moderately thick peel. Fruit picking begins in November. *Fantastico* is a rustic tree of good development with high production. It displays larger leaves than the other cultivars. The fruit is globose. Fruit picking takes place from November to December (Ragusa, 2014).

Pharmacobotanical investigations of the fruits of *Citrus bergamia* Risso et Poiteau and other species of the genus *Citrus* have been performed using scanning electron microscopy (SEM) to highlight details concerned, in particular, with the secretory sacs containing the essential oil. SEM observation showed an epidermis of the flavedo (skin) made up of polygonal cells, almost isodiametric with more or less slightly wavy anticlinal walls, just outside the tangential thickened walls and covered with a thick cuticle topped with a layer of continuous wax and sometimes waxy formations in the form of flakes. Parenchymatous cells of the layers, up to the albedo (mesocarp) in cross section, are irregularly polygonal in shape, have somewhat thickened walls, and become larger as they proceed inwardly. Secretory cavities of ellipsoidal or subspheroidal shape are radially elongated, almost going to epidermal cells, and can be found at both surface depressions and intermediate stages. Dipped into the epicarp, they sink in the outer layers of the mesocarp and are formed by a central cavity, surrounded by five or six layers of secretory cells arranged more or less concentrically; they have more developed tangential walls than radials. From a careful observation of the different stages of the formation of such structures (from the initial round, where they appear as clusters of secretory cells, to the final, in which they already have the formation of the cavity, with the epithelium, tangentially elongated, consisting of flattened cells, filled with essential oil, and with fragments of cell walls in decay), it has been possible to confirm that the cavities are of glandular schizolysigenous origin. These are formed initially for the division of a mother cell and mutual estrangement of the daughter cells, and they increase by successive, tangential divisions of the glandular cells, while in the central secreting cells they undergo a process of dissolution (Figure 3.3). Furthermore, the application of image analysis in the study of other species of the genus *Citrus* has been very useful to obtain important information with an accurate criterion: it is valid and reproducible for calculating the potential yield of essential oil for each species studied. The micromorphometric analysis of cross-sectioned fruit peels of *Citrus bergamia* Risso et Poiteau provided a key factor for differentiation of the cultivars *castagnaro*, *fantastico*, and *femminello*. The glands' number per square centimeter in unripe and ripe fruits is constant, even if the size of oil cavities changes. The ratio between the mean volume of glandular cavities and number of glandular cavities per square centimeter indicates the yield in essential oil of the three cultivars of *C. bergamia* Risso et Poiteau fruits: *Fantastico > Castagnaro* (–13%) > *Femminello* (–21%) (Rapisarda et al., 1992, 1995).

The Myrtaceae family, along with those of Lytraceae, Onagaraceae, Punicaceae, and others of pharmacognostic interest, belonging to the order of Myrtales, is inserted

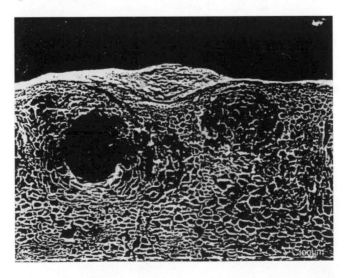

FIGURE 3.3 Electron micrograph of glandular cavities of *Citrus bergamia* Risso et Poiteau fruits. Bar = 100 μm. (From Ragusa, S. et al., *Acta Technol. Legis Medic.*, 6, 377–381, 1995.)

in the Roside class of Eucotiledoni (Conti et al., 1998; Simpson, 2010; Wilson et al., 2005); to this family belong woody plants with simple leaves that are opposite or, less often, alternate and leathery. Tissues containing secretory fragmenting pockets are evident in the leaves. The flowers, solitary or in inflorescences and actinomorphic, are generally tetramers or pentamers; the stamens are usually numerous; the pistil is mostly syncarpous and polycarpel. The fruit is a berry or a capsule and rarely of another type. The Myrtaceae are mainly distributed in subtropical regions, especially in Australia (Maleci Bini et al., 2014). They are trees and shrubs with abundant, scattered secretory cavities containing aromatic oils. Leaves are usually opposite and often leathery; stipules are inconspicuous or absent. Flowers are bisexual and radially symmetric. The fruit is a berry, in capsules or drupes. Seeds range from few to many, and the endosperm is often absent. The family consists of 120 genera and 3850 species from tropical and subtropical areas, mainly America and Australia.

In the Myrtaceae family are *Melaleuca* species (*M. squarrosa* JE Smith, *M. hypercifolia* JE Smith, *M. gibbous* Labill., etc.), which are of Australian origin but grown in different countries. Species of herbal-pharmaceutical interest are *M. linarifolia* Sm. (= *M. alternifolia* Cheel), the wood species from which the distillation of the leaves and the terminal parts of the branches yields an essential oil rich in 1-terpen-4-ol (30%–60%), cineol (5%–15%), terpineol (1.5%–8%), terpinene (15%–25%), and many other terpenes. The smell is reminiscent of eucalyptol. Endowed with antibacterial properties, the essential oil is reportedly useful in disinfecting the oral tract, intestines, genital area, and skin. In susceptible individuals, heartburn is a possible side effect of *M. uncinata* P. Br., whose leaves are chewed popularly against catarrh. However, the *M. leucadendron* L. tree, vegetating in the area between the Malaysian archipelago and Australia, is well known; it has different varieties (cajuputi, viridiflora), and from its fresh twigs and leaves an essential oil is obtained that is yellowish, with the smell of camphor, the said oil, or cajeput (Cajput), and containing mainly 1,8-cineol, pinene, terpinol, and aldehyde compounds. It is used for its antiseptic, antirheumatic, anthelmintic, and carminative, and slightly sedative for outdoor use. *M. viridiflora* Soland ex Gaertn. (= *M. leucadendron* var. *viridiflora*) is an evergreen tree species from Australia and Indonesia. The fruit is a capsule. The leaves provide an essential oil essence, niaouli, and are very rich in 1,8-cineol (50%–65%), along with α-terpineol, limonene, aldehydes, and sulfur compounds. It looks like a mobile, colorless or yellow-citrine liquid, and it smells and tastes like camphor and peppermint. Likewise, to the essence of eucalyptus are ascribed the following properties: antiseptic mucous membranes and respiratory tract, hyperemic, and for the treatment of rheumatism, colds, and acne. In rare cases, as a result of habituation, side effects (i.e., diarrhea, nausea, and vomiting) can occur. Also ascribed to the essence is the property of insect repellent. For external use, it is also recorded in sports for use in invigorating massages. The essence is also known commercially as gomenolo. To obtain the essence, the following additional species are also used: *M. pungens* Brongn. et Gris., *M. gnidiodes* Brogn. et Gris., *M. quinquienervia* (Cav.) S.T. Blake, *M. leucodendron* L., *M. cajeputi* Roxb. and *M. linarifolia* Sm. The essential oils of the leaves are attributed antiseptic properties. The Italian Official Pharmacopoeia (FUI) reports the niaouli essential oil, obtained by steam distillation of fresh leaves of *M. viridiflora* Soland. ex Gaertn. It must contain between 50% and 60% of 1,8-cineole (57.3%), α-terpineol (16.6%), and α-pinene (4.1%) and is to be stored in glass containers (to avoid plastic) and protected from light and temperatures above 15°C (FUI, 2008).

It is a genus of about 15–220 species, mainly cultivated in Australia, New Caledonia, New Guinea, and Malesia for its flowers, overall appearance, and wind resistance. The species require full light and well-drained soil (they are intolerant of chalk soils), preferably without much nitrogen. They propagate by seed in spring or by semiripe cutting in summer (Byrnes, 1984; Cullen et al., 1997).

The species of the genus *Melaleuca* consists of evergreen shrubs or trees. Leaves are opposite, some with three or more pronounced longitudinal veins, stalked or stalkless, entire, flat, concave or semicylindric, and leathery. Inflorescences are terminal or axillary spikes or headlike. Flowers are bisexual or male and stalkless. The fruit is a woody capsule remaining on the stem and sometimes embedded in a thickened stem; seeds are with embryo, with cotyledons equal to or longer than the hypocotyls in length.

REFERENCES

Aboca. *De Materia Medica, il Dioscoride di Napoli.* Aboca Edizioni, Sansepolcro, 2013.

Acquaah, G. *Principles of Plant Genetics and Breeding.* Wiley-Blackwell, Hoboken, 2012.

Applequist, W. *The Identification of Medicinal Plants.* American Botanical Council, Austin, 2006.

Aqel, M.B. Relaxant effect of the volatile oil of *Rosmarinus officinalis* on tracheal smooth muscle. *J. Ethnopharmacol.*, 33 (1991): 57–62.

Bayer, R.J., Mabberley, D.J., Morton, C., Miller, C.H., Sharma, I.K., Pfeil, B.E., Rich, S., Hitchoock, R., and Siskes, S. A molecular phylogeny of orange subfamily (Rutaceae: Aurantioideae) using nine cpDNA sequences. *Am. J. Bot.*, 96 (2009): 668–685.

Bhatnagar, J.K., and Dunn, M.S. Histological studies of the genus Lavandula. IV. Section Spica. Comparative histology of the leaves of Lavandula officinalis Chaix, L. latifolia Vill., and L. lanata Bioss. *Am. J. Pharm. Sci. Support Public Health*, 133 (1961): 327–343.

Bhatnagar, J.K., and Dunn, M.S. Histological studies of genus Lavandula. VIII. Histological key for the identification of some species of the genus Lavandula. *Am. J. Pharm. Sci. Support Public Health*, 134 (1962): 332–333.

Bhatnagar, J.K., and Dunn, M.S. Histological studies of the genus Lavandula. III. Section Stoechas. Lavandula dentata Linn., Lavandula viridis L'Herit. and L. peduncolata Cav. *Am. J. Pharm. Sci. Support Public Heaalth*, 135 (1963): 288–306.

Bruni, A. *Biologia farmaceutica.* Pearson Italia, Milano, 2014.

Byrnes, A. A revision of *Melaleuca* L. (Myrtaceae). In northern and eastern Australia. *Austrobaileya*, 1 (1984): 65–76.

Capasso, F. *Farmacognosia.* Springer-Verlag Italia, Milano, 2011.

Chaytor, D.A. A taxonomic study of the genus *Lavandula. J. Linn. Soc. Bot.*, 51 (1937): 153–204.

Condurso, C., Verzera, A., Ragusa, S., Tripodi, G., and Dima, G. Volatile composition of Italian *Thymus capitatus* (L.) Hoffmanns et Link leaves. *J. Essent. Oil Res.*, 25 (2013): 239–243.

Conti, E., Litt, A., Wilson, P.G., Graham, S.A., Briggs, B.G., Johnson, L.A.S., and Sytsma, K.J. Interfamilial relationship in Myrtales: Molecular phylogeny and patterns of morphological evolution. *Syst. Bot.*, 22 (1998): 629–647.

Cronk, Q.C.B. *The Molecular Organography of Plants.* Oxford University Press, Oxford, 2009.

Cullen, J., Alexander, J.C.M., Brickell, C.D., Edmondson, J.R., Green, P.S., Heywood, V.H., Jorgensen, P.M., Jury, S.L., Knees, S.G., Marxwell, H.S., Miller, D.M., Robson, N.K.B., Walters, S.M., and Yeo, P.F. *The European Garden Flora.* Vol. V. Cambridge University Press, Cambridge, 1997.

Cullen, J., Alexander, J.C.M., Brickell, C.D., Edmondson, J.R., Green, P.S., Heywood, V.H., Jorgensen, P.M., Jury, S.L., Knees, S.G., Marxwell, H.S., Miller, D.M., Robson, N.K.B., Walters, S.M., and Yeo, P.F. *The European Garden Flora.* Vol. VI. Cambridge University Press, Cambridge, 2000.

De Pasqual, J.T., Ovejero, J., Anaya, J., Caballero, E., Hernández, J.M., and Caballero, C. Chemical composition of the Spanish spike oil. *Planta Med.*, 55 (1989): 398–399.

De Pasquale, A., and Ragusa, S. Applications de la microscopie électronique à balayage en pharmacognosie. *Pl. méd. et phytothér.*, 13 (1979): 46–65.

De Wolf, G.P. Notes on cultivated labiates 5, Lavandula. *Baileya*, 3 (1955): 47–57.

European Pharmacopoeia. 8th ed. Council of Europe, Strasbourg, 2014.

Farmocopea Ufficiale della Repubblica Italiana (FUI). 7th ed. Istituto poligrafico e zecca dello stato, Roma, 2008.

Iauk, L., Acquaviva, R., Mastrojeni, S., Amodeo, A., Pugliese, M., Ragusa, M., Loizzo, M.R., Menichini, F., and Tundis, R. Antibacterial, antioxidant and hypoglyceaemic effects of *Thymus capitatus* (L.) Hoffmanns, et Link leaves' fractions. *J. Enzyme Inhib. Med. Chem.*, 30 (2014): 360–365.

Imbesi, A. *Index plantarum quae in omnium populorum Pharmacopoeis sun adhuc receptae.* Scilla Edizioni, Messina, 1964.

Index Kewensis 2.0. Oxford University Press, Oxford, 1997.

Kokkalou, E. The constituents of the essential oil from *Lavandula stoechas* growing wild in Greece. *Planta Med.*, 54 (1998): 59.

Lo Presti, M., Ragusa, S., Trozzi, A., Dugo, P., Visinoni, F., Fazio, A., Dugo, G., and Mondello, L. A comparison between different techniques for the isolation of rosemary essential oil. *J. Sep. Sci.*, 28 (2005): 273–280.

Lo Presti, M., Crupi, M.L., Costa, R., Dugo, G., Mondello, L., Ragusa, S., and Santi, L. Seasonal variations of *Teucrium flavum* L. *J. Essent. Oil Res.*, 22 (2010): 211–216.

Maity, D. *Perspective of Plant Taxonomy, Exploration, Herbarium, Nomenclature and Classification.* NayaUdyog, Kolkat, 2012.

Maleci Bini, E., Maugini, E., and Mariotti Lippi, M. *Botanica farmaceutica.* Piccin Nuova Libreria S.p.A., Padova, 2014.

Pignatti, S. *Flora d'Italia.* Edagricole, Bologna, 1997.

Ragusa, S. Bergamotto: Aspetti farmacobotanici. In *Bergamotto*, 65–69. Iiriti Editore, Reggio Calabria, 2014.

Ragusa, S., Rapisarda, A., and Iauk, L. Caratteri micromorfologici dei fiori di *Lavandula maroccana* Murb. *Acta Technol. Legis Medic.*, 6 (1995): 377–381.

Ragusa, S., Forestieri, A.M., and Rapisarda, A. Glandular tissues of *Lavandula angustifolia* Mill. flowers: Ultrastructural and histochemical survey. *Riv. It. EPPOS*, 21 (1997): 27–33.

Ragusa, S., Iauk, L., and Rapisarda, A. Indagini micromorfologiche sui fiori di *Lavandula stoechas* L. *Essenze Derivati Agrumari*, 70 (2000): 9–13.

Rapisarda, A., Lauk, L., and Ragusa, S. Impiego di una miscela di metil-e idrossipropilmetacrilato nello studio di tessuti vegetali al SEM. *Riv. It. EPPOS*, 3 (7) (1992): 56–58.

Rapisarda, A., Caruso, C., and Ragusa, S. Indagini strutturali sulle sacche secretrici dei frutti di *Citrus bergamia* Risso et Poit. e *Citrus medica* L. *Acta Technol. Legis Medic.*, 6 (1995): 382–387.

Rapisarda, A., Pancaro, R., and Ragusa, S. Image analysis for micromorphometric characterization of vegetable drugs obtained by cogeneric species. *Phytoter. Res.*, 10 (1996): S172–S174.

Senatore, F. *Biologia e Botanica farmaceutica.* Piccin Nuova Libraria S.p.A., Padova, 2012.

Simpson, M.G. *Plant Systematics.* Elsevier Academic Press, Amsterdam, 2000.

Svodoba, K., and Svodoba, T. *Secretory Structures of Aromatic and Medicinal Plants.* Microscopic Publications, Powys, 2010.

Tetenyi, P. Chemical polymorphism and chemical polytypism in essential oil producing plant species. *Planta Med.*, 28 (1975): 244–256.

Tonzig, S., and Marrè, E. *Botanica generale, I.* Casa Editrice Ambrosiana, Milano, 1983.

Trease, G.E., and Evans, W.C. *Pharmacognosy.* WB Saunders, London, 1996.

Tucker, A.O., and Hensen, K.J.W. The cultivars of Lavender and Lavandin. *Balleya*, 22 (1985): 166–177.

Tutin, T.G., Burges, N.A., Chater, A.O., Edmondson, J.R., Heywood, V.H., Moore, D.M., Valentine, D.H., Walters, S.M., and Webb, D.A. *Flora Europaea.* Cambridge University Press, London, 1993.

Upton, R., Graff, A., Jolliffe, G., Langer, R., and Williamson, E. *American Herbal Pharmacopoeia: Botanical Pharmacognosy—Microscopic Characterization of Botanical Medicines.* CRC Press, Boca Raton, FL, 2011.

Wilson, P.G., O'Brien, M.M., Heslewood, M.M., and Quinn, C.J. Relationships within Myrtaceae sensu lato based on a matK phylogeny. *Plant Syst. Evol.*, 251 (2005): 3–19.

4 Phytochemical Components of Aromatic Plants and Factors Influencing Their Variability

Giancarlo Statti

CONTENTS

4.1 INTRODUCTION

Throughout the world, hundreds of species are used as medicinal and aromatic plants. Some of them are among the most popular spices and herbs, like basil, peppermint, and sage. Some of these plants are utilized as a source of phytochemical components (e.g., essential oil) or herbal drugs, especially because in recent times, significant progress in biological and phytochemical investigations has been made.

Most studies, as well as clinically applied experience, have indicated that various essential oils, such as lavender, lemon, and bergamot, can help to relieve stress, anxiety, depression, and other mood disorders. Most notably, inhalation of essential oils can communicate signals to the olfactory system and stimulate the brain to exert neurotransmitters (e.g., serotonin and dopamine), thereby further regulating mood.

The development of techniques for the phytochemical characterization of mixtures of essential oils and the analysis of their variability have allowed us to better define the composition and characteristics of the essences. Essential oils, also called essences (quintessential oils), volatile oils, and ethereal oils, are mixtures of aromatic substances produced by many plants and present in the form of tiny droplets in the leaves, the peel of the fruit, the resin, the branches, and wood. They have a very complex chemical composition, and terpenoids (primarily), shikimates, and polyketides (a few) are the most important secondary metabolites present in essential oils. The analysis of their presence and variability in aromatic plants is therefore the main focus of this chapter.

4.2 BIOSYNTHETIC PATHWAYS

Secondary metabolism is typical of plants and microorganisms, and secondary metabolites are known to derive from the acetate, shikimate, and mevalonate pathways. According to the general scheme[1] of the formation of secondary metabolites (Figure 4.1), compounds from fundamental processes such as glycolysis, photosynthesis, and the Krebs cycle may be employed for the formation of biosynthetic intermediates, instead of being used in processes for the generation of energy.

The biosynthetic pathways that lead to the formation of specific metabolites are dependent on factors affecting the chemical composition of the plants, such as exogenous factors (classified into genetic and nongenetic) and endogenous factors (related to the habitat in which all plants perform their life cycle) (Figure 4.2). Indeed, Franz[2] reported that evaluation of chemical variation in essential oils involves the study of at least three major factors: (1) individual genetic variability, (2) variation among different plant parts and the different developmental stages, and (3) modifications due to the environment the endogenous factors, while exogenous factors.

But, why do so many plants produce essential oils? The adaptation of vegetative habitat is the best answer to this question. Some essential oils may not only act as insect repellents, but also prevent their reproduction. In many cases, it has been shown that plants attract insects that in turn assist in pollinating the plant. It has also been shown that some plants communicate through the agency of their essential oils. Sometimes essential oils are considered to be simply metabolic waste products. This may be so in the case of eucalypts, as the oil cells present in the mature leaves of *Eucalyptus* species are completely isolated and embedded deeply within the leaf structure. In some cases, essential oils act as germination inhibitors, thus reducing competition by other plants.[3]

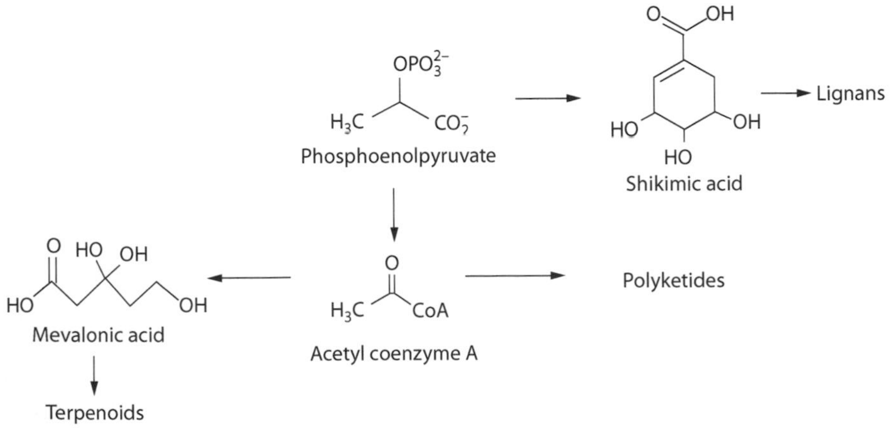

FIGURE 4.1   General scheme of the formation of secondary metabolites.

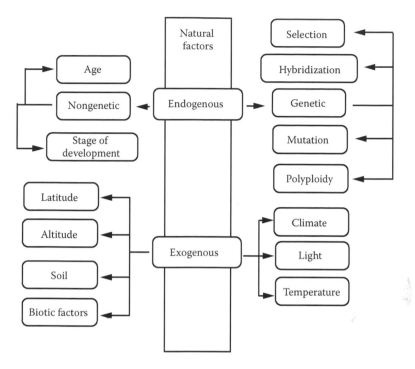

FIGURE 4.2   Factors affecting the chemical composition.

4.3   TERPENOIDS

As written above, the essential oils are mixtures of compounds derived from differ-ent biosynthetic pathways. The terpenoids are, by far, the most important group of natural products as far as essential oils. They are defined as substances composed of isoprene (2-methylbutadiene) units. Isoprene is not found in essential oils, but the 2-methylbutane skeleton is easily discernible in terpenoids. The direction of coupling of isoprene units is almost always in one direction, the so-called head to-tail coupling, which explains the biosynthesis of all terpenoids.[1] The terpenoids are classified according to the number of carbon atoms they contain (multiples of 5). The first group contain molecules with 10 carbon atoms and are called monoter-penes, those that contain molecules with 15 carbon atoms are called sesquiterpenes, those with 20 carbon atoms diterpenoids, and so on. In general, only the monoter-penoids and sesquiterpenoids are sufficiently volatile to be components of essential oils.

The precursor for the monoterpenoids is geranyl pyrophosphate, through which we get coupling of the two isoprene units (dimethyl allyl pyrophosphate [DMPP] and isopentenyl pyrophosphate [IPP]) through the formation of an allyl carbocation (of DMPP) that is added to the double bond of IPP. The chemistry of the reactions of formation takes place under control of the enzymes present in any given plant. In fact, it involves a passage of stereospecific loss of a proton (Figure 4.3). Thus, the essential oil composition can give information about the genetic makeup of the plant.

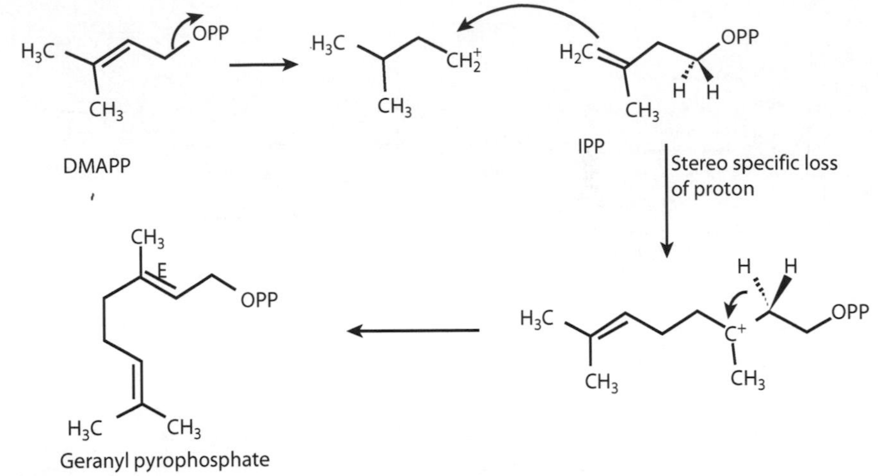

FIGURE 4.3 Geranyl pyrophosphate formation.

Linalyl PP and neryl PP are isomers of geranyl PP, and their formation stems from the formation of the carbocation of geranyl PP (Figure 4.4).[4]

These compounds evolve through simple transformations that pass through the formation of carbocations that are neutralized by nucleophiles (especially water), or through the loss of a proton, or by reaction of intramolecular cyclization or Wagner–Meerwein transpositions. These reactions lead to the formation of simple monoterpenes (hydrocarbons, alcohols, aldehydes, and esters). See Figure 4.5 for the formation of monoterpenes.

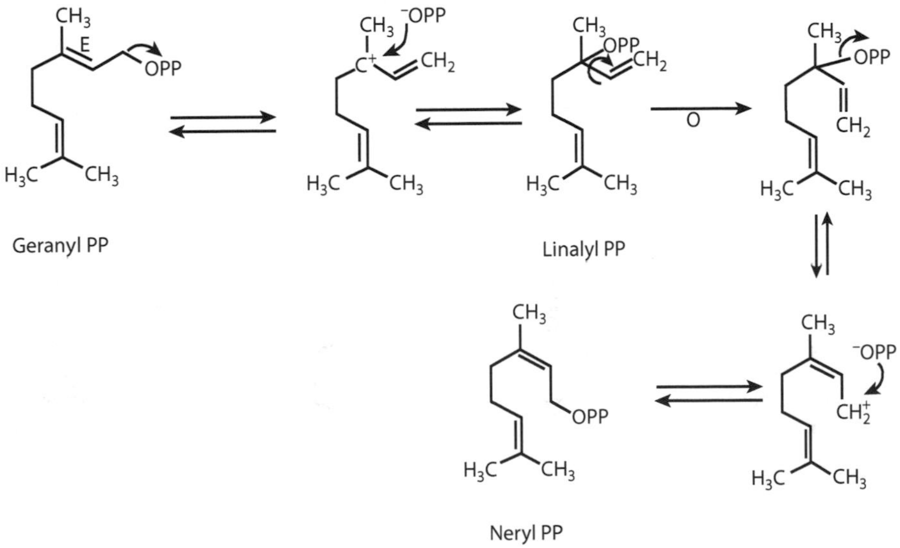

FIGURE 4.4 Isomerization of geranyl PP.

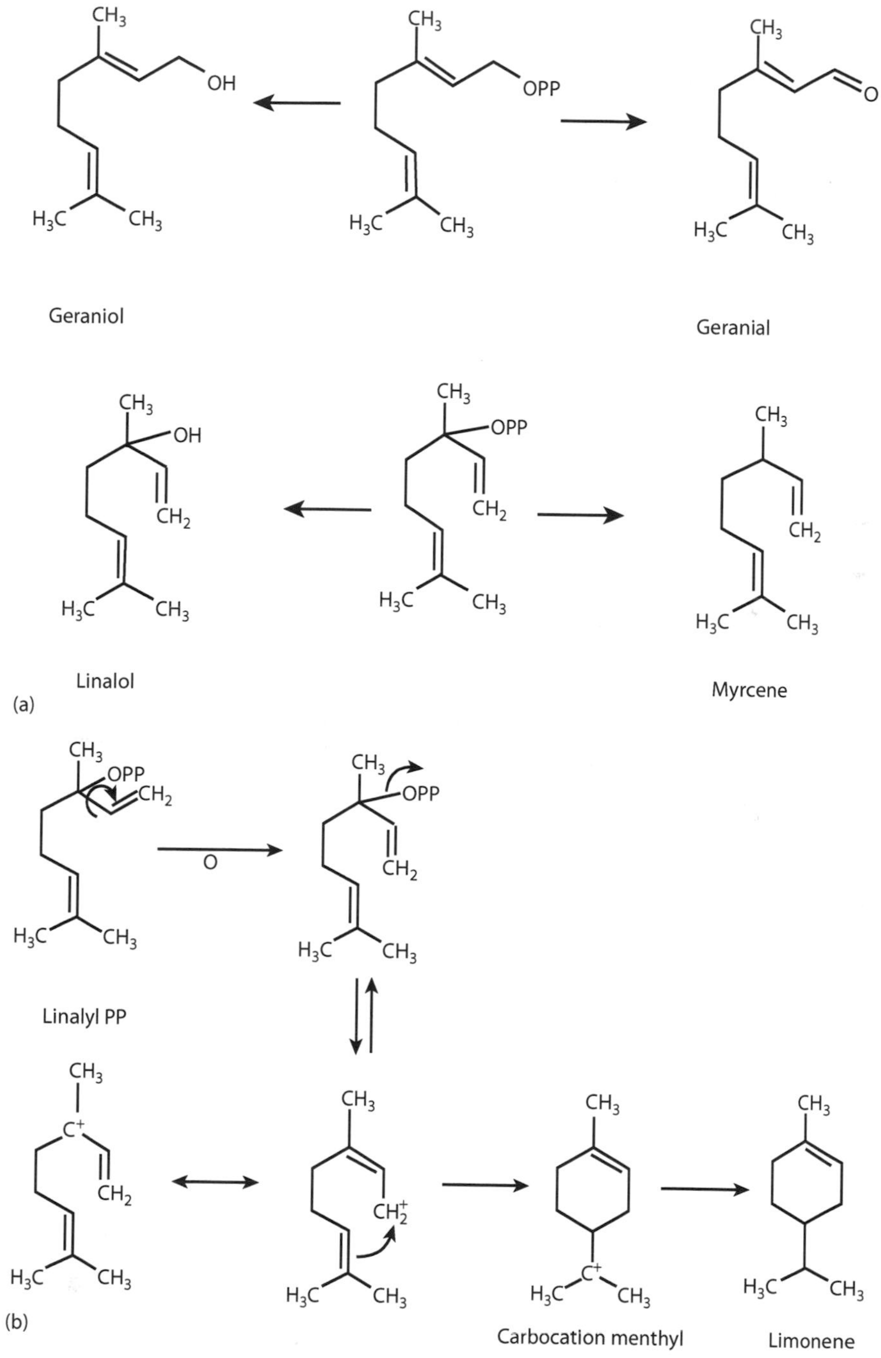

FIGURE 4.5 Formation of cyclic monoterpenes.

These types of reactions often lead to the formation of both alpha and beta forms of simple monoterpenes. However, often one of two forms is most frequently encountered, as in the case of dell'ocimene, whose beta form is more frequently encountered.[5,6]

The reactions of cyclizations take place thanks to the particular stereochemistry of linalyl PP and neryl PP, which are the direct precursors of the system monocyclic carbocation menthyl. This, for loss of a proton, leads to limonene, which is the most abundant monoterpene in many essential oils of the genus *Citrus*. These oils contain the dextrorotatory (R)-enantiomer; its antipode is much less common (Figure 4.6).

A large number of compounds that are commonly present in essential oils are chiral, and consequently, the possible differences existing among the biological activity, metabolism, and toxicology of the enantiomeric pairs occurring in the sample must be carefully assessed. Through applications of enantioselective techniques, it is possible to determine the presence of one or both enantiomers. In the essential oils *Mentha spicata* or *Mentha acquatica*, for example, (R)- and (S)-limonene were found.[7]

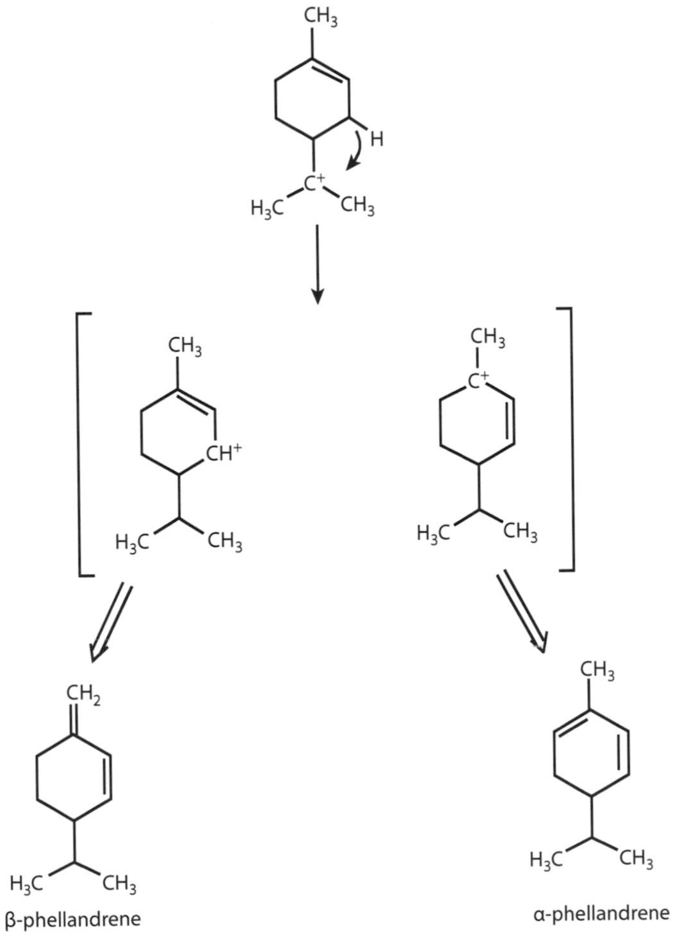

FIGURE 4.6 Formation of phellandrene.

To obtain a more stable carbocation, often occurring migration of carbon atoms or hydride ions. These rearrangements allow the formation of tertiary carbocations or less tense cycles. For example, the cation menthyl undergoes the migration of a hydride ion to form a carbocation allyl stabilized by resonance (Figure 4.6). In this way, for example, phellandreni is obtained for the particular formation reactions and is found in both isoforms. Both α-phellandrene and β-phellandrene occur widely in essential oils. For example, (−)-α-phellandrene is found in *Eucalyptus camaldulensis*[8] and (S)-(−)-β-phellandrene in the lodgepole pine, *Pinus contorta*.[9]

The carbocation menthyl is a key intermediate in the synthesis of monoterpenes that constitute the essential oils. In fact, from it a second intramolecular addition gives the pinyl carbocation (75), which can lose a proton to give either α-pinene or β-pinene (Figure 4.7), which are among the most abundant bicyclic monoterpenes in nature.

The synthesis of acyclic (myrcene), cyclic (limonene), and bicyclic (pinene) compounds is catalyzed by a single enzyme, which facilitates the folding and cyclization of the substrate.[4]

Alcohol monoterpenes are obtained by hydrolysis of the carbocation. Simple hydrolysis of geranyl pyrophosphate gives geraniol, (*E*)-3,7-dimethylocta-2,6-dienol. This is often accompanied in nature by its geometric isomer, nerol, so that the name geraniol is often used to describe a mixture of geraniol and nerol. Both isomers occur in a wide range of essential oils, geraniol being particularly widespread. The oil of *Cymbopogon martini*[10] (palmarosa) contains more than 60% geraniol. The richest natural sources of nerol

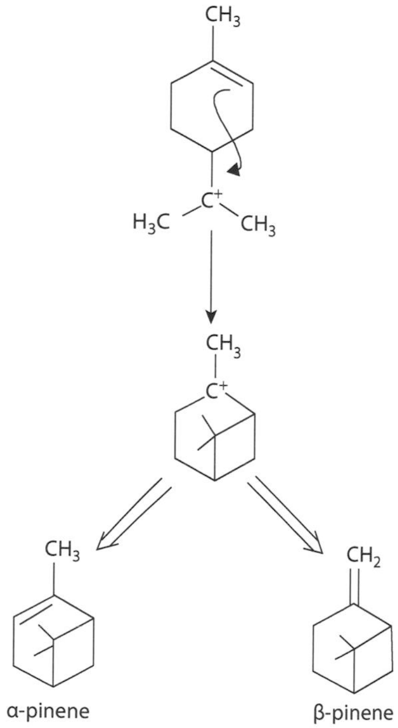

FIGURE 4.7 α-Pinene or β-pinene.

include rose (*Rosa damascena* Mill.),[11] palmarosa,[10] citronella,[12] and davana (*Artemisia pallens* Wall.),[13] although its level in these is usually only in the 10%–15% range.

From geranyl PP you also get citronellol, which is a dehydrogenated form of geraniol. Geraniol, nerol, and citronellol, together with 2-phenylethanol, are known as the rose alcohols because of their occurrence in rose oils.[14]

From geranyl PP linalool is obtained by allylic hydrolysis. Like geraniol, linalool occurs widely in nature. The richest source is jojoba oil (pronounced ho-ho-bah), which is a wax produced from the seeds of jojoba (*Simmondsia chinensis*), containing well over 90% linalool, and coriander oil contains 70%.[15] Linalool is found in all the essential oils from plants of the genus *Citrus*, which is the most abundant component after limonene.[16] Linalool acetate is also frequently encountered and is a significant contributor to the odors of lavender and citrus leaf oils.

Cyclic monoterpene alcohols are also very abundant in nature. α-Terpineol is found in many essential oils, as is its acetate. It is formed by the allylic carbocation resulting from linali PP, neutralized by H_2O (Figure 4.8).

The cation menthyl can undergo migration of a hydride to form the cation terpinen-4-ile, from which is obtained the isomer of α-terpinene, terpinen-4-ol (Figure 4.9).

The isomeric terpinen-4-ol is an important component of ti-tree oil, but its acetate, surprisingly, is more widely occurring, being found in herbs such as oregano (*Origanum vulgare* L.),[17] marjoram (*Origanum majorana*), and rosemary.[18]

Menthol is one of the most common monoterpene alcohols. The main sources are various species of mint. Biosynthesis is complex. From limonene through a two-stage oxidation we get to pulegone, from which all stereoisomers of menthol

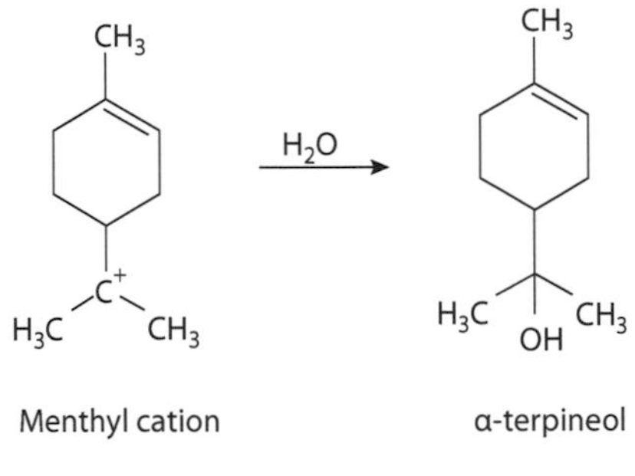

FIGURE 4.8   α-Terpineol.

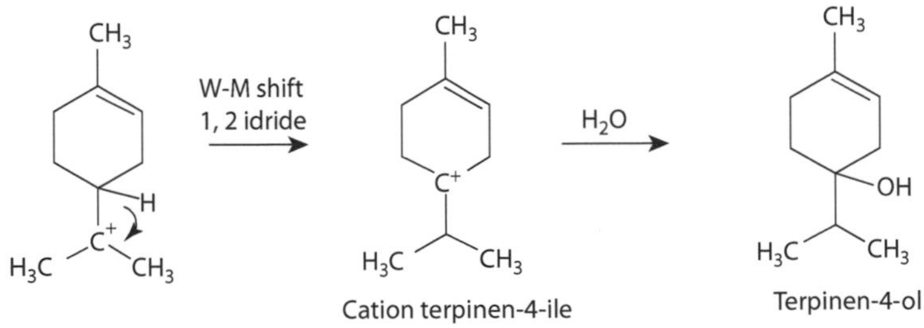

FIGURE 4.9   Terpinen-4-ol.

originate.[19] In this compound there are three asymmetric carbon atoms, and thus it occurs in eight stereoisomers (Figure 4.10a and b) as four pairs of optical isomers, namely, (+)- and (−)-isomenthol, (+)- and (−)-menthol, (+)- and (−)-neomenthol, and (+)- and (−)-neoisomenthol,[20] of which L-menthol is the most common for both distribution and its biological activity.

Menthol is well known for its cooling effect or sensation when it is inhaled, chewed, consumed, or applied to the skin due to its ability to chemically activate the cold-sensitive transient receptor potential cation channel (TRPM8).[21]

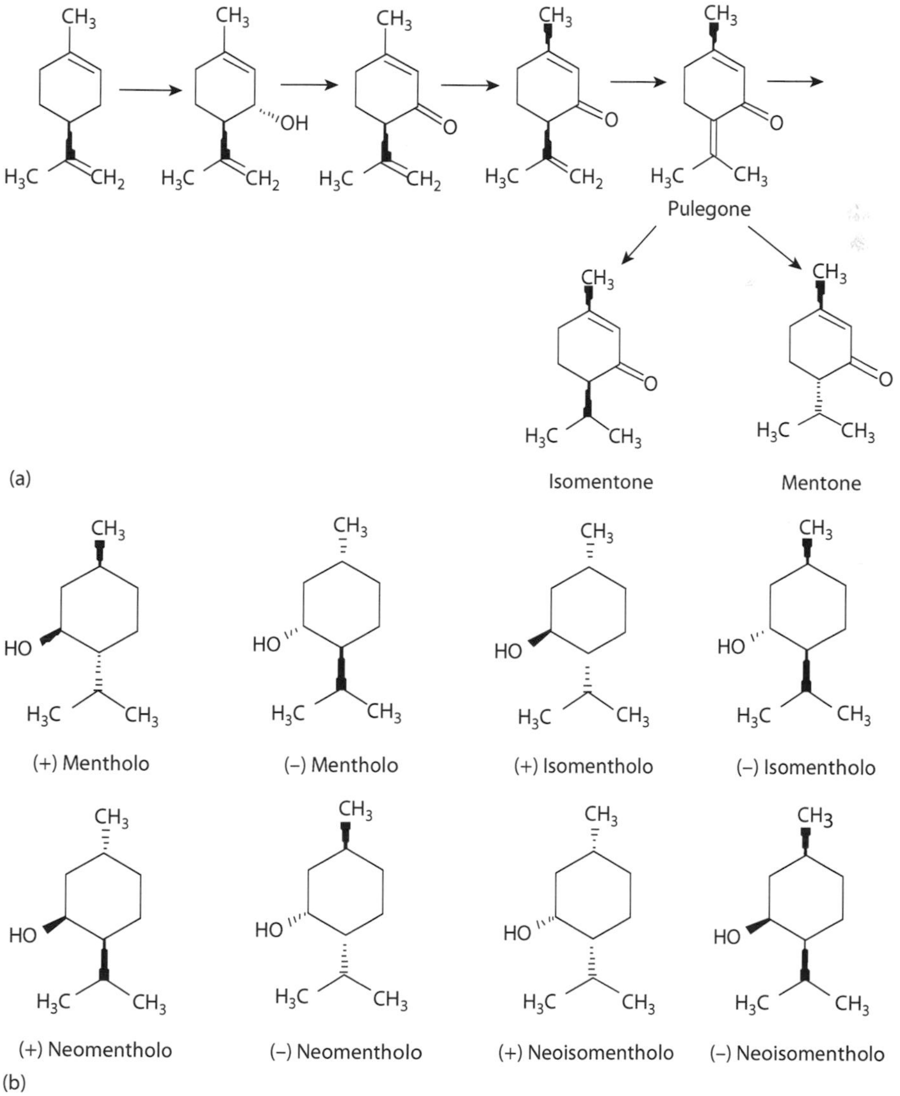

FIGURE 4.10 Biosynthesis of the precursors of menthol. (a and b) Stereoisomers of menthol.

The series of monoterpene alcohols include citronellol, geraniol, linalool,[22] myrcenol, nerol, and nerolidol.[23]

Borneol (endo-1,7,7-trimethylbicyclo[2.2.1]heptan-2-ol) and esters thereof, particularly the acetate, occur in many essential oils: lavender,[24] pinus,[25] and thymus.[26]

Moreover, in this section you need to report the aromatic alcohols thymol and carvacrol (Figure 4.11a), which have the particularity to be produced in nature through the mevalonate pathway rather than from acetate or the shikimic acid pathway. They are present in the thymus,[27] oregano,[28] and lippia.[29] Being phenols, they possess antimicrobial properties, and their oils, such as thyme and basil, are used in herbal remedies.

The presence of a hydroxyl group in the molecules of monoterpenes often induces the formation of ethers. From ethers commonly found in aromatic plants is 1,8-cineole, more commonly referred to simply as cineole (Figure 4.11b).

It is present in 40%–50% of the oil, and *Eucalyptus globulus*,[30] cajeput oil, can also be found in a wide range of other oils and often as an important component. This is very relevant even in myrtle[31] and *Salvia*.[32]

Monoterpenes that have aldehyde and ketone functional groups determine the scent of the plant, giving the characteristic note of an essential oil. The two most significant monoterpene aldehydes are citral and its dihydro analog, citronellal. The word *citral* is used to describe a mixture of the two geometric isomers geranial and neral without specifying their relative proportions. Both isomers are usually present, and the ratio between them is usually in the 40:60 to 60:40 range.

The formation reaction is simple. Derived from the allyl cation geranyl that, neutralized with a molecule of H_2O, forms geranoiolo and nerol, these easily undergo oxidation to the corresponding aldehydes (Figure 4.12).

The citral is responsible for the characteristic smell of lemons, although lemon oil usually contains only a few percent of it. The largest quantities are found in

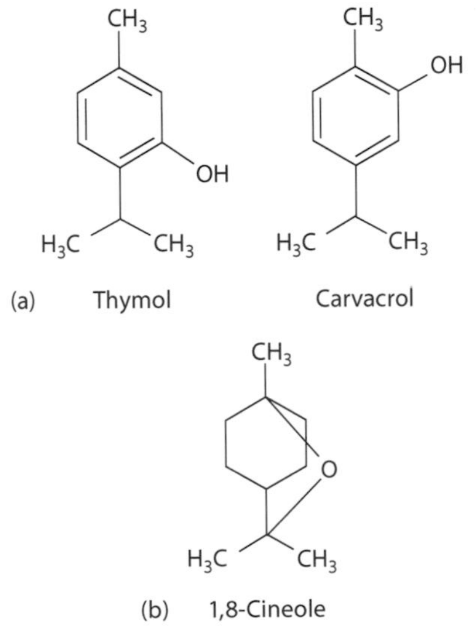

(a)   Thymol   Carvacrol

(b)   1,8-Cineole

FIGURE 4.11   (a) Thymol and carvacrol. (b) Cineole.

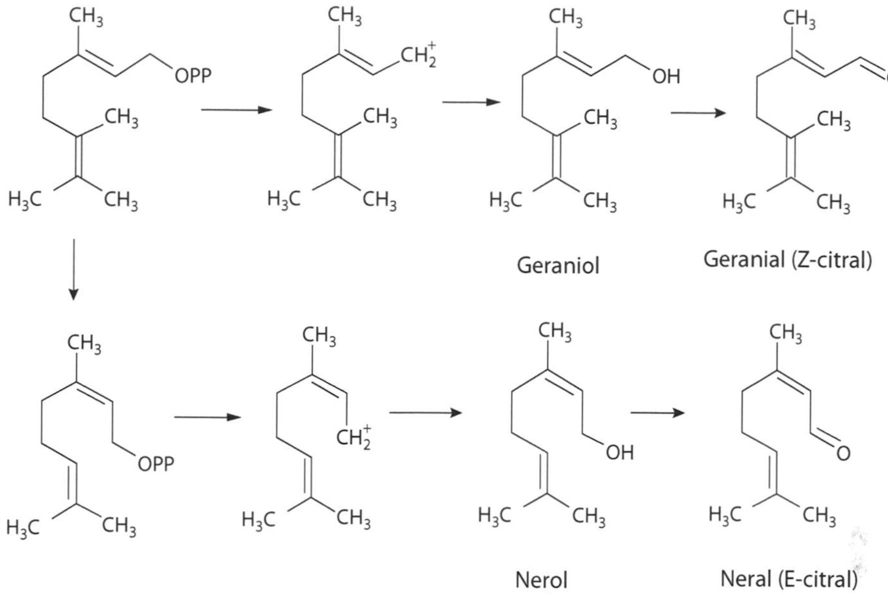

FIGURE 4.12 Citral.

Cymbopogon citratus (DC.) Stapf (Poaceae family), commonly known as lemon-grass, and contain 70%–90% citral.[33] It also occurs in *Eucalyptus*,[34] *Citrus bergamia* Risso,[35] lippia,[36] and verbena.[37]

Along with aldehydes, very important for the organoleptic and biological properties of the essential oils are monoterpene ketones. They are formed through oxidation of monoterpene alcohols. In fact, from limonene are obtained both carveol and isopiperitenol through an oxidative step. Isopiperitenol is oxidized to give isopiperitenone, which is further metabolized to piperitenone (Figure 4.13a).

Isopiperitone is a key intermediate in the biosynthesis of the ketone monoterpene. In fact, piperitenone is obtained by allylic isomerization (Figure 4.13a), while for the oxidation isopulegone is obtained, which isomerizes to pulegone, which, as seen previously (Figure 4.10), leads to menthone and isomentone.

The (R)-(–)- and (S)-(+)-enantiomers of the monoterpene ketone carvone are found in various plants. While (S)-(+)-carvone is the main constituent of the essential oil of caraway (*Carum carvi*), the oil of spearmint leaves (*Mentha spicata* var. *crispa*) contains about 50% of (R)-(–)-carvone besides other terpenes.[38] (R)-(+)-Pulegone is a monoterpene ketone present in essential oils from many mint species. Two mints, *Hedeoma pulegoides* and *Mentha pulegium*, both commonly called pennyroyal, contain essential oils, which are chiefly pulegone.[39] This is also present in plants of the genus *Agastache*. *Agastache* is a small genus of Lamiaceae, comprising 22 species of perennial aromatic medicinal herbs: the strong scent reminiscent of anise, for example, in the case of *Agastache anethiodora*, or mint, in the case of *Agastache mexicana*, or the smell of sour apple in the species. In *Agastache anethiodora* the content of pulegone reaches up to 30%.[40] Also in *Mentha longifolia*, an

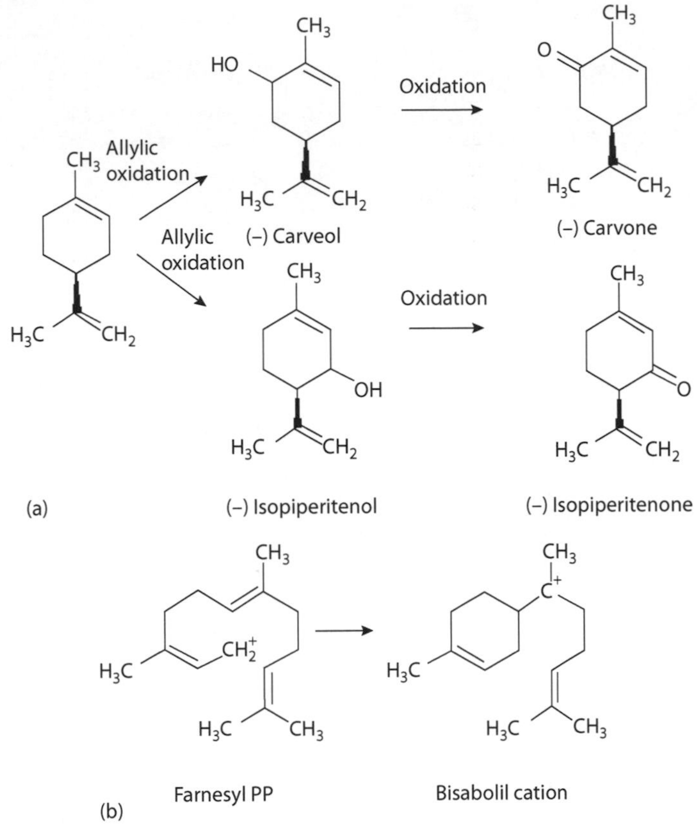

FIGURE 4.13   (a) Formation of ketone monoterpenes. (b) Bisabolil cation.

herb with a wide range of pharmacological properties such as antimicrobial, gastro-intestinal, and nervous system effects, the pulegone is the main compound, followed by menthone, isomenthone, and piperitenone.[41] In *Agastache foeniculum* the content isomentone can reach 40%.[42]

Of the volatile fraction of aromatic plants, essential oils are also part of sesqui-terpenes. By definition, sesquiterpenoids contain 15 carbon atoms and are derived from three isoprene units. It is clear that this results in their having lower volatilities and hence higher boiling points than monoterpenoids. Therefore, fewer of them (in percentage terms) contribute to the odor of essential oils, but those that do often have low-odor thresholds and contribute significantly as endnotes. They are also impor-tant as fixatives for more volatile components.

The precursor of sesquiterpenoids is therefore the farnesyl PP. This is obtained by addition of an isoprene unit to geranyl PP with the intervention of the prenil trans-ferase enzyme.

Starting from farnesyl pyrophosphate, the variety of possible cyclic structures is much greater than that from geranyl pyrophosphate because there are now three double bonds in the molecule.

The formation of sesquiterpenes from farnesyl diphosphate catalyzed by sesquiterpene synthases employs carbocationic-based reaction mechanisms similar to those of monoterpene synthases. As for the monoterpenes, sesquiterpenes, the most common structures, can be attributed to reactions that go through carbocations. For example, the cation bisabolile is similar to the system of monoterpene menthane (Figure 4.13b).

If farnesol is the sesquiterpenoid equivalent of geraniol and nerolidol of linalool, then α-bisabolol is the equivalent of α-terpineol (Figure 4.14).

The richest natural source is *Myoporum crassifolium* Forst.,[43] a shrub from New Caledonia, but α-bisabolol can be found in many other species, including chamomile[44] (of which the bisabolol and its oxide are the main components) and sage,[45] and a less explored source of α-bisabolol is the wood of *Eremanthus erythropappus* (DC.) MacLeish (Asteraceae), known in Brazil by the common name candeia,[46] which may contain up to 85% of α-bisabolol. *Lychnophora ericoides* is a Brazilian medicinal plant used in folk medicine whose essential oil contains more than 50% of α-bisabolol.[47]

Bisabolols are closely related to the structures of bisabolene, zingiberene, and sesquifellandrene (Figure 4.15).

These compounds are found mainly in plants of the genus *Zingiberaceous*, including *Zingiber officinalis*,[48] of which, for example, the bisabolene contributes to the aroma of ginger.

The cyclization to the double bond gives a carbocation with the germacrane skeleton. This is an intermediate in the biosynthesis of odorous sesquiterpenes such as nootkatone and α-vetivone (Figure 4.16).

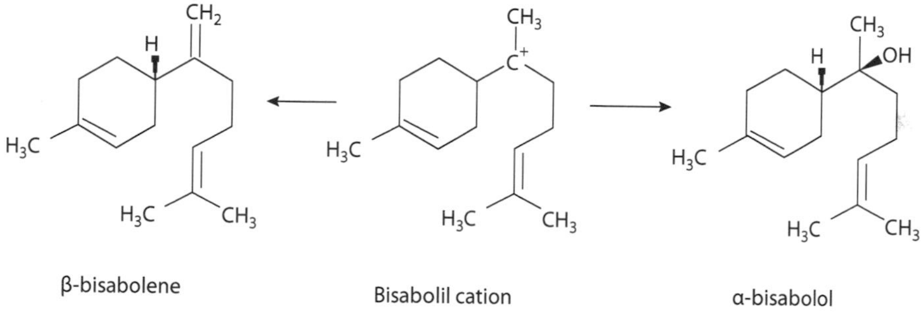

β-bisabolene   Bisabolil cation   α-bisabolol

FIGURE 4.14 Bisabolol.

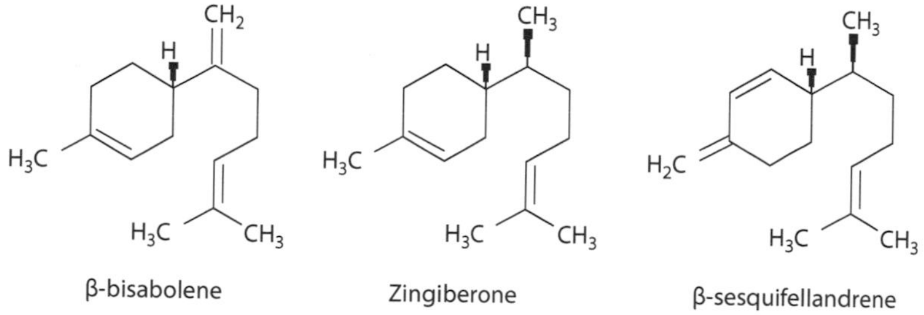

β-bisabolene   Zingiberone   β-sesquifellandrene

FIGURE 4.15 Similar bisabolol sesquiterpenes.

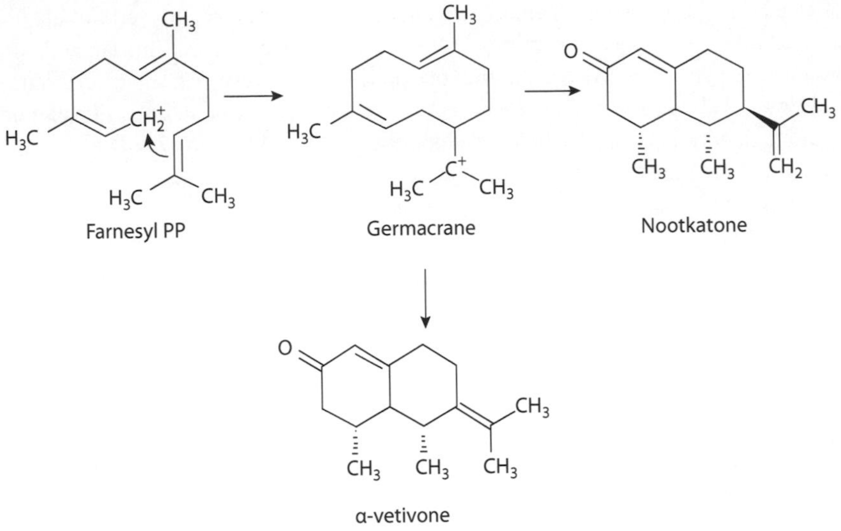

FIGURE 4.16   Nootkatone and α-vetivone.

(+)-Nootkatone is also an important entity for industries that manufacture perfumes.[49] In fact, it is also derived from peels of various fruits like kabusu (*Citrus aurantium* L.), bergamot (*Citrus bergamia* Risso), and pummelo (*Citrus grandis* L. Osbeck).[50] Nootkatone exhibits unique odor characteristics, rendering it a highly sought after flavor and fragrance compound.

Vetiver essential oil is a basic ingredient of the perfume industry, where it is appreciated for its tenacious and long-lasting earthy woody scent. It is obtained by hydrodistillation of the fragrant roots of *Chrysopogon zizanioides* L. (formerly known as *Vetiveria zizanioides* L.), a perennial grass growing wild or cultivated in tropical and subtropical countries such as Haiti, Indonesia, India, Brazil, China, and La Réunion.[51] β-Vetivone (Figure 4.17) is synthesized through a route that also produces various alcohols, and ethers that have the eudesmane skeleton.

Among the odorous components in vetiver oils from different sources, β-vetivone, along with α-vetivone and khusimol, is the major constituent, and its presence is often considered as the fingerprint of the oil.

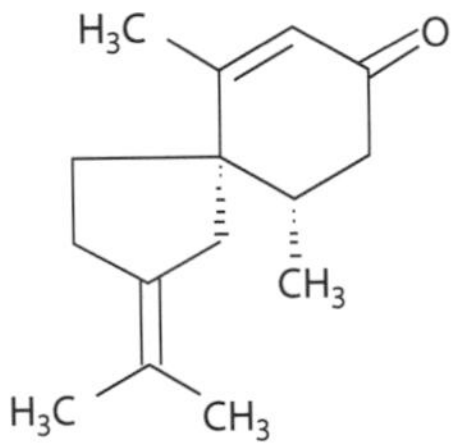

FIGURE 4.17   β-vetivone.

Cedrol (Figure 4.18) has a more complex structure than the sesquiterpenes bisabolol and vetivone. It is the main constituent in a wide range of species, the most significant being trees of the Juniperus,[52] Cupressus,[53] and Thuja[54] families.

Also, santalols are sesquiterpenes with a complex structure (Figure 4.19).

Both α-santalol and β-santalol are major constituents of sandalwood[55] (*Santalum album* L.) and have a distinctive woody scent.

Of particular interest for natural abundance and pharmacological applications are the sesquiterpene lactones, which are prevalent in the Asteraceae (Compositae) plant family. The main families of natural sesquiterpene lactones are germacranolides, eudesmanolides, and guaianolides.

The carbocation farnesyl PP can cyclize to form the carbocation germacryl. Therefore, after oxidative processes, it can have intramolecular cyclization reactions to give sesquiterpene lactones (Figure 4.20).

The parthenolide is an important component of tanacetum,[56] whose essential oil is a traditionally used herbal remedy.

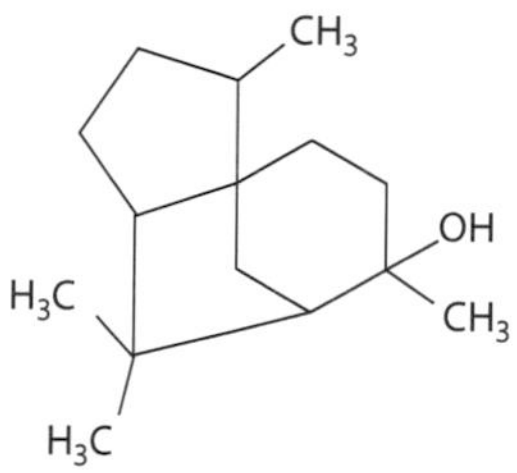

FIGURE 4.18 Cedrol.

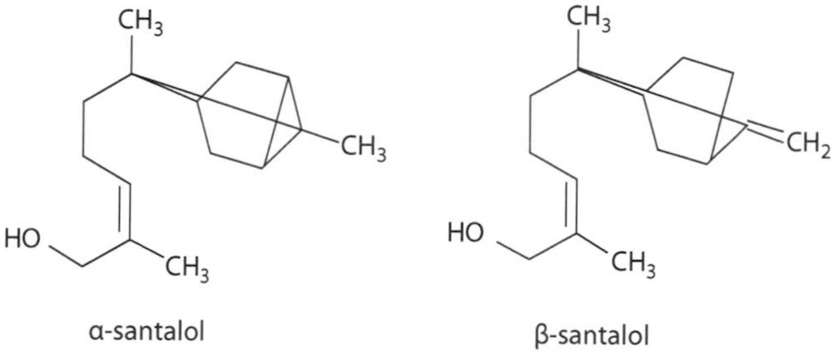

α-santalol   β-santalol

FIGURE 4.19 Santalols.

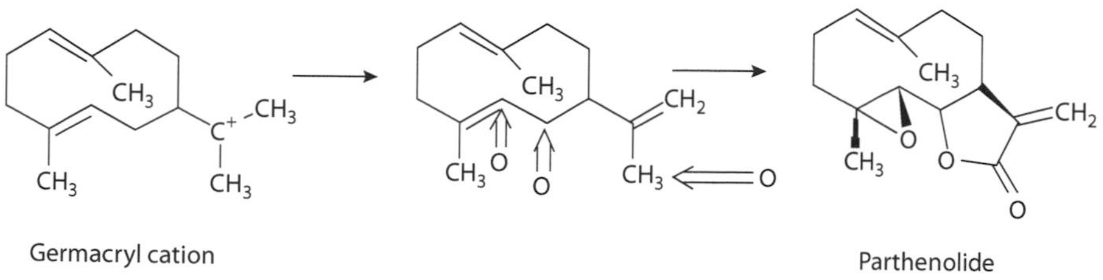

Germacryl cation   Parthenolide

FIGURE 4.20 Lactone sesquiterpenes.

Closely related to the structure of parthenolide are santonin and matricine (as precursor of the artifact chamazulene[57]). Structurally, the most marked difference between santonin and panthenolide regards the presence of the bicyclic ring system of decalin. Despite the similarity, santonine belongs to the family of eudesmanolides. In fact, the basic skeleton is the eudesmanic system, which is formed by the cation germacryl for protonation and cyclization at the eudesmyl cation (Figure 4.21).

Artemisia species possess pharmacological properties that are used for medical purposes worldwide. α-Santonine (Figure 4.22) is the main component of various species of *Artemisia*.[58]

If the protonation of the cation germacrile occurs at the less substituted double bond, anti-Markovnikov addition is obtained by the cation guayl, from which originate guaianolides (Figure 4.23a).

Oxidation and lactonization of Guayl cation leads to the formation of the sesquiterpene lactone matricin (Figure 4.23b).

Structurally related to matricin are the partially labile proazulene substances that, upon heating, will degrade for elimination of acetic acid, water, and subsequent decarboxylation. This group is part of, for example, the chamazulene[59] (Figure 4.24), which is one of the main compounds of the essential oil of camomile for biological activity.

The chamazulene and other bioactive compounds of chamomile (*Matricaria* spp.) are widely used by the pharmaceutical and cosmetic industries for their properties and also as a natural hair dye and fragrance.

An additional opportunity to cyclize the farnesyl PP leads to the formation of the humulyl cation, which finds itself in the humulene (Figure 4.25), or can be modified to give the cariohiillyl cation, which possesses a ring to nine terms fused with a ring to four terms, such as in β-caryophyllene (Figure 4.26).

Germacryl cation   Eudesmyl cation

FIGURE 4.21   Eudesmyl cation.

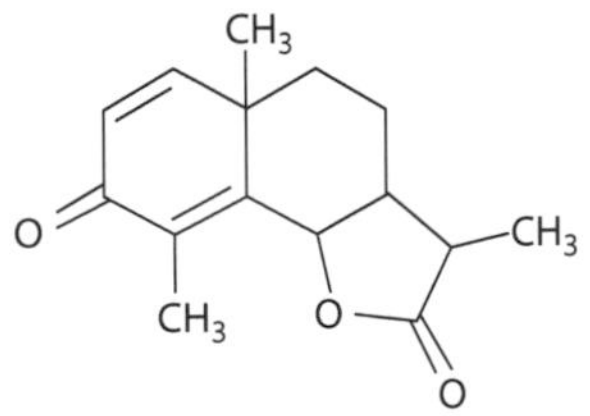

FIGURE 4.22   α-Santonine.

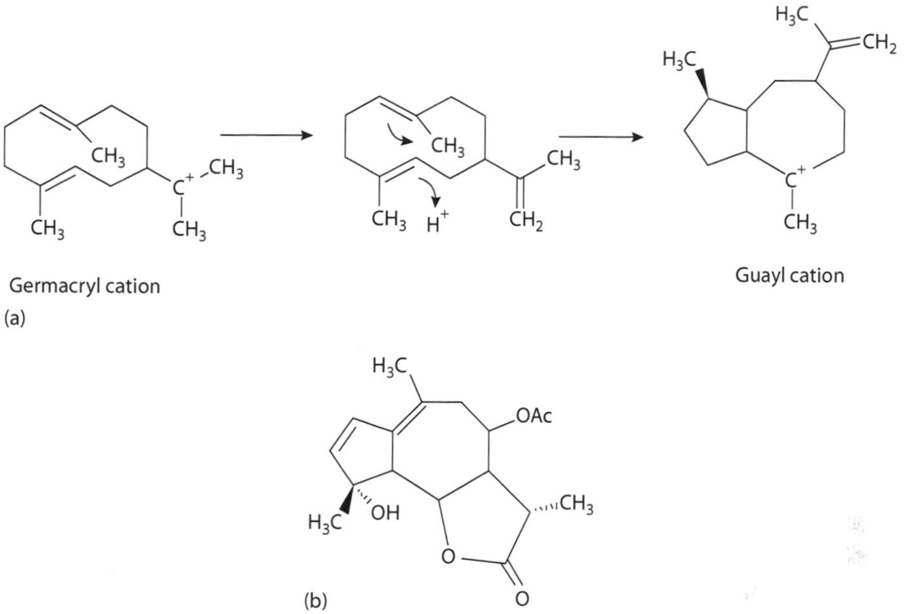

Germacryl cation

Guayl cation

(a)

(b)

FIGURE 4.23 (a) Guayl cation. (b) Matricin.

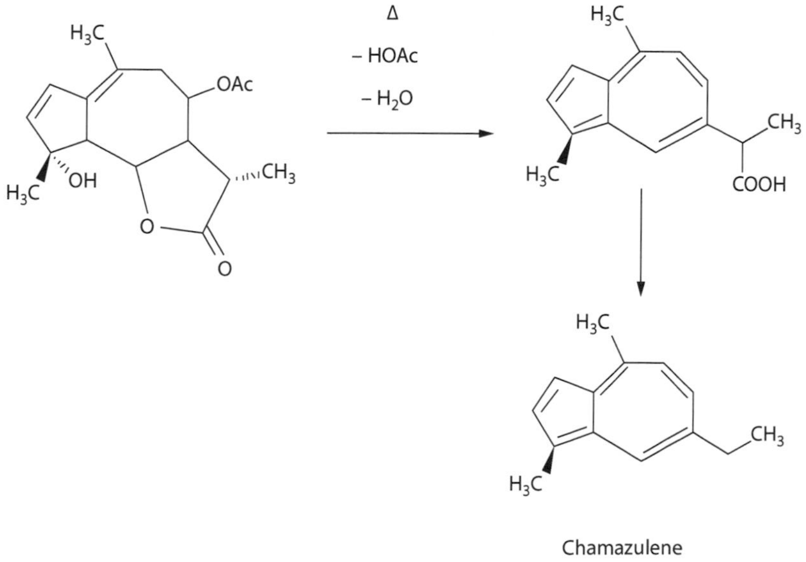

Chamazulene

FIGURE 4.24 Chamazulene: an artifact of the matricin.

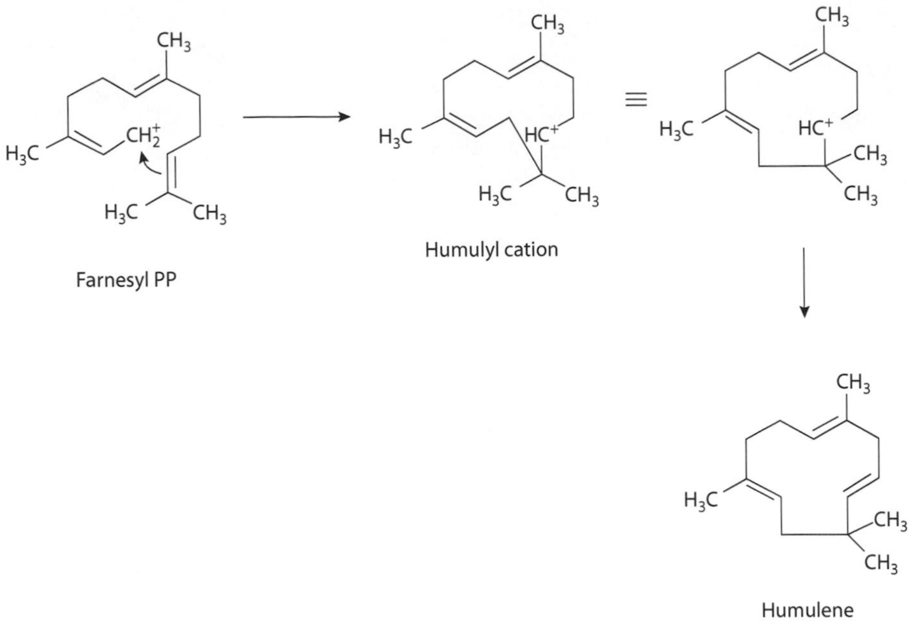

FIGURE 4.25 Humulene.

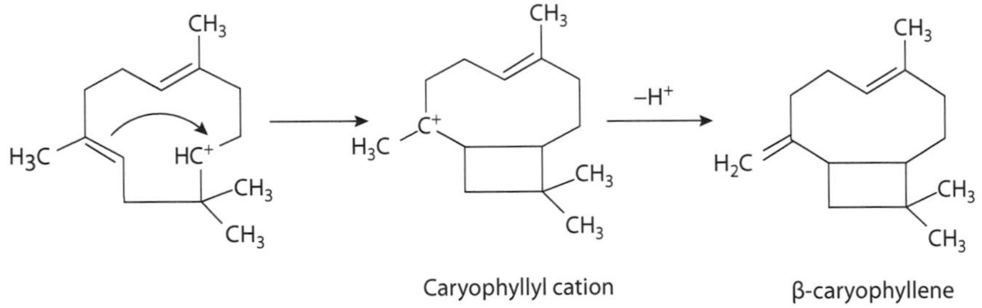

FIGURE 4.26 Cyclization of humulyl cation to β-caryophyllene.

α-Humulene has been found in an ever-increasing number of aromatic plants on all continents, often together with its isomer β-caryophyllene.

Clove (*Syzygium aromaticum*) is one of the most valuable spices; it has been used for centuries as a food preservative and for many medicinal purposes. Clove oil[60] is mostly composed of four compounds: eugenol, β-caryophyllene, α-humulene, and eugenyl acetate.

Lauraceae is an economically important family consisting mostly of trees or tree-like shrubs. Cinnamon leaf and bark are used as spices and in the production of essential oils. Leaves have a hot taste and emit a spicy odor when crushed. Cinnamon offers to the flavor industry a variety of oils with different aroma characteristics and compositions. Among the major compounds identified in the oil of the cinnamon is β-caryophyllene.[61]

4.4 VARIABILITY

The natural abundance of the major compounds present in the essential oils, and their particular biosynthesis, means that they are particularly sensitive to the conditions within which they are produced. For this reason, it is particularly important to take into account all factors that may influence the synthesis. As already mentioned, the evaluation of chemical variation in essential oils involves the study of factors concerning the genetic variability, the variations that depend on the plant (use of different plant parts and the different developmental stages), and factors due to the environment. Population genetics is concerned with the genotypic variation among individuals, but the genotype is not directly observable while it is only the phenotype. Indeed, the term *phenotype* refers to the set of all observable characteristics of a living organism, so its morphology, development, and biochemical properties. The intraspecific variation of characters of vegetable species, including the chemical characters, is the specific item of the chemotaxonomy, which classifies plants based on chemical compounds present and in relation to the possible causes of their variability.[62] Chemical polymorphism consists of the existence of plants from the same species that have modified the production of their secondary metabolites for different reasons. Chemical polymorphism of aromatic plants is a widespread phenomenon described by a number of researchers. Several chemotypes of aromatic plant species have been identified, but have not yet been clearly related to the possible causes.

The genus *Thymus* represents high intraspecific morphological variability and chemical polymorphism caused by environmental factors and genetic variation due to frequent hybridization and sexual dimorphism.[63]

Conifer terpenes have been used as both ecologic and chemotaxonomic markers, beginning at the genus level,[64] and later at the family level.[65] For example, the terpene compositions of essential oil of junipers have shown significant correlation with respect to the geographic distribution.[66]

Also, bergamot (*Citrus bergamia* Risso), while growing and fruiting only in a small area of southern Italy, presents a significant, very high variability, and the composition of the essential oil is reflected in this.[67]

The genus *Lavandula* L. includes 39 species, numerous hybrids, and nearly 400 registered cultivars.[68] Its natural distribution area stretches from the Canary Islands, Cape Verde Islands, and Madeira, across the Mediterranean basin and Arabian Peninsula, all the way to tropical North Africa and, with a disjunction, India. This leads to a very large variability in phytochemistry that can be highlighted through clustering analysis that demonstrates the high degree of polymorphism of the species.[69]

Performing multivariate statistical analysis using variables such as the contents of the main components of essential oil (α-pinene, β-pinene, 1,8-cineole, cis-thujone, camphene, camphor, and borneol) has been shown to also consider intra- and interspecific variability of the genus *Salvia*.[70]

As an explanation of chemical polymorphisms are called exogenous and endogenous factors, such as the possible factors that influence the quality and quantity of secondary metabolites present in a plant species. Essential oil products from aromatic plants are even more sensitive to exogenous factors, in particular, their chemical and physical peculiarities.

4.4.1   EXOGENOUS FACTORS

Generally exogenous factors are related to the environment. Factors such as habitat preference, growth form, vegetative dispersal nature of the soil (pH, constituents), and light precipitation decisively influence the composition of the essential oils of aromatic plants.

In this sense we must consider the cell as a sensitive reaction system that, if it is subject to chemical and physical disturbances, reacts by changing the metabolic final pathways.

A common acclimatization plant response to a variety of environmental stressors is the accumulation of antioxidants and secondary metabolites, including several compounds that are pharmacologically active or nutritionally important, including essential oils.[71] One of the mechanisms that plants possess to help them adapt to enhanced UV-B radiation is the ability to increase the production of secondary metabolites in leaf tissues.[72] Numerous studies have been conducted on the effects of enhanced UV radiation on plant growth, physiology, and secondary metabolites.[73] The studies on the impact of UV-B on aromatic and medicinal plants concern *Ocimum basilicum* L.,[74] *Cymbopogon citratus* (DC.),[75] and *Hypericum perforatum.*[76] In general, these results are in agreement with the observation that many enzymes of the secondary pathways are UV-B dependent.[77]

Also, geographic distance seems to influence the genetic and chemical intraspecific variability, and the altitude plays a key role in the production of volatile compounds in valerian.[78] For some species (*Helichrysum italicum*), however, significant variability among populations present in small areal growth has been highlighted.[79]

Similarly, the latitude plays a significant role in the phytochemical variability of some aromatic species. The positive relationship between latitude and concentration of some terpenes has been demonstrated. The essential oil of *Hyptis suaveolens* L. obtained from low latitudes is richer in sesquiterpenes.[80] Also, in the genus *Savory* (*Satureja* L.), family Lamiaceae, latitude plays an important role in the chemical diversity of the composition of the essential oil,[81] but in vole significant differences can be found in vicinal areal growth. The biovariability of *Citrus bergamia* grown in the wild in Calabria is significant.[82]

This shows that the phytochemical variability is linked to the concomitant presence of ambiantali and the genetic factors mentioned above, and consequently to the definition of chemotypes.

For the aromatic species, analysis of the biochemical pathways that lead to the synthesis of the major compounds of their essential oils (EO) showed a clear fluctuation during the year, but this is important for the purposes of therapeutic applications of essential oils, in order to determine the balsamic time of drug.

In the context of the environmentally regulated factors, the nature of the soil, such as pH and its structure, is sometimes responsible for changes in the chemical composition of the EOs.

4.4.2   ENDOGENOUS FACTORS

Endogenous factors are related to the site of production and accumulation of the EOs in the plant, the age of the plant, and the genetic characteristics that regulate the secondary metabolism. The environment could also affect the DNA of the aromatic plants, leading from chemotypes to different genotypes.

Essential oils are found in all parts of the plant (roots, rhizomes, wood, bark, leaves, flowers, fruits) and also in the secretions of the plants themselves (e.g., in resins). However, the essential oil extracted from an organ of a plant differs from that of other organs of the same plant.

Studies on specific constituents have shown that the methyl eugenol, one of the most common components of the essential oils, is present only in certain plant organs. *Kielmeyera rugosa* (Caryophyllaceae) possesses methyl eugenol only in flowers and not in leaves and fruits.[83] *Valeriana tuberose* (Valerianaceae), a medicinal plant used as a mild sedative, commonly found in Greece, has eugenol and methyl eugenol in similar quantities in inflorescences, but none in roots, stems, or leaves.[84] Also, *Laurus nobilis* (Lauraceae) was reported to contain similar essential oils in all its aerial parts, but in different quantities and quality.[85]

Few studies have reported the influence of the endogenous factor of plant age on the chemical composition of essential oil. Many aromatic plants are annuals and, in any case, along with the age of the plant, should always be considered the vegetative cycle.

The chemical composition of the essential oil from *Thymus vulgaris* L. (Labiatae) and its variation during the life cycle show how the age of the plant represents a further important factor for the variability of the chemical species.[86] Also, in *Eucalyptus camaldulensis*, there is variability concerning the age of the plant and its life cycle.[87] The studies therefore emphasize the importance of choosing the appropriate collection (harvest) period of aromatic plants in order to achieve the highest quality and quantity of the essential oil.

Finally, the exposure of a plant to different exogenous factors for a long time could cause genetic modification. This makes the biosynthetic pathways different and allows variation in the qualitative and quantitative production of volatile secondary products determining chemotypes. Thus, the genotype could be considered the last discrimination after previous identification of ecotypes and chemotypes.

REFERENCES

1. Mann, J., R.S. Davidson, J.B. Hobbs, D.V. Banthorpe, and J.B. Harbourne. 1994. *Natural Products: Their Chemistry and Biological Significance.* London: Longman.
2. Franz, Ch. 1993. Genetics. In *Volatile Oil Crops: Their Biology Biochemistry and Production*, ed. R.K.M. Hay and P.G. Waterman. London: Longman, Harlow, 93–66.
3. Porter, N. 2001. Crop and food research. *Crop and Foodwatch Research*, Christchurch, no. 39, October.
4. Dewic, P.M. 2001. *Medicinal Natural Product: A Biosynthetic Approach.* New York: Wiley.
5. Bakarnga-Via, I. et al. 2014. Composition and cytotoxic activity of essential oils from *Xylopia aethiopica* (Dunal) A. Rich, *Xylopia parviflora* (A. Rich) Benth.) and *Monodora myristica* (Gaertn) growing in Chad and Cameroon. *BMC Complement Altern Med.* 14: 125.
6. Rajendran, M.P. et al. 2014. Chemical composition, antibacterial and antioxidant profile of essential oil from *Murraya koenigii* (L.) leaves. *Avicenna J. Phytomed.* 4(3): 200–14.

7. Barba, C. et al. 2013. Direct enantiomeric analysis of *Mentha* essential oils. *Food Chem.* 141: 542–47.

8. Bayala, B. et al. 2014. Chemical composition, antioxidant, anti-inflammatory and antiproliferative activities of essential oils of plants from Burkina Faso. *PLoS One* 9(3): 1–14.

9. Clark, E.L. et al. 2010. Differences in the constitutive terpene profile of lodgepole pine across a geographical range in British Columbia, and correlation with historical attack by mountain pine beetle. *Can. Entomol.* 142: 557–73.

10. Nirmal, S. et al. 2007. Major constituents and anthelmintic activity of volatile oils from leaves and flowers of *Cymbopogon martini* Roxb. *Nat. Prod. Res.* 21(13): 1217–20.

11. Pellati, F. et al. 2013. Gas chromatography combined with mass spectrometry, flame ionization detection and elemental analyzer/isotope ratio mass spectrometry for characterizing and detecting the authenticity of commercial essential oils of *Rosa damascena* Mill. *Rapid Commun. Mass Spectrom.* 27(5): 591–602.

12. Kpoviessi, S. et al. 2014. Chemical composition, cytotoxicity and in vitro antitrypanosomal and antiplasmodial activity of the essential oils of four *Cymbopogon* species from Benin. *J. Ethnopharmacol.* 151(1): 652–59.

13. Isidorov, V.A. et al. 2001. Gas chromatographic analysis of essential oils with preliminary partition of components. *Phytochem. Anal.* 12(2): 87–90.

14. Sadraei, H. et al. 2013. Inhibitory effect of *Rosa damascena* Mill flower essential oil, geraniol and citronellol on rat ileum contraction. *Res. Pharm. Sci.* 8(1): 17–23.

15. Zheljazkov, V.D. et al. 2014. Hydrodistillation extraction time effect on essential oil yield, composition, and bioactivity of coriander oil. *J. Oleo Sci.* 63(9): 857–65.

16. Oboh, G. et al. 2014. Essential oil from lemon peels inhibit key enzymes linked to neurodegenerative conditions and pro-oxidant induced lipid peroxidation. *J. Oleo Sci.* 63(4): 373–81.

17. Begnini, K.R. et al. 2014. Composition and antiproliferative effect of essential oil of *Origanum vulgare* against tumor. *J. Med Food* 17(10): 1129–33.

18. El-Seedi, H.R. et al. 2012. Chemical composition and repellency of essential oils from four medicinal plants against *Ixodes ricinus* nymphs (Acari: Ixodidae). *J. Med. Entomol.* 49(5): 1067–75.

19. Croteau, R.B. 2005. (–)-Menthol biosynthesis and molecular genetics. *Naturwissens chaften* 92(12): 562–77.

20. Kamatou, G.P. et al. 2013. Menthol: A simple monoterpene with remarkable biological properties. *Phytochemistry* 96: 15–25.

21. Yosipovitch, G. et al. 1996. Effect of topically applied menthol on thermal, pain and itch sensations and biophysical properties of the skin. *Arch. Dermatol. Res.* 288: 245–48.

22. Matsuda, B.M. et al. 1996. Essential oil analysis and field evaluation of the citrosa plant "*Pelargonium citrosum*" as a repellent against populations of Aedes mosquitoes. *J. Am. Mosq. Control Assoc.* 12(1): 69–74.

23. Caissard, J.C. et al. 2006. Chemical and histochemical analysis of 'Quatre Saisons Blanc Mousseux' a moss rose of the Rosa × *damascena* group. *Ann. Bot.* 97(2): 231–38.

24. Nogueira, J.M. et al. 2002. Essential oils from micropropagated plants of *Lavandula viridis*. *Phytochem. Anal.* 13(1): 4–7.

25. Kim, J.H. et al. 2012. Essential oil of *Pinus koraiensis* leaves exerts antihyperlipidemic effects via up-regulation of low-density lipoprotein receptor and inhibition of acylcoenzyme A: Cholesterol acyltransferase. *Phytother. Res.* 26(9): 1314–19.

26. Wu, S. et al. 2013. Chemical composition of essential oil from *Thymus citriodorus* and its toxic effect on liver cancer cells. *Zhong Yao Cai*. 36(5): 756–59.

27. Schmitz, D. et al. 2014. The broadband microwave spectra of the monoterpenoids thymol and carvacrol: Conformational landscape and internal dynamics. *J. Chem. Phys.* 141(3): 034304.

28. Calvo-Irabién, L.M. et al. 2014. Phytochemical diversity of the essential oils of Mexican oregano (*Lippia graveolens* Kunth) populations along an Edapho-climatic gradient. *Chem. Biodivers.* 11(7): 1010–21.

29. Veras, H.N.H. et al. 2013. Topical antiinflammatory activity of essential oil of *Lippia sidoides* cham: Possible mechanism of action. *Phytother. Res.* 27: 179–85.

30. Slimane, B.B. et al. 2014. Essential oils from two eucalyptus from Tunisia and their insecticidal action on *Orgyia trigotephras* (Lepidotera, Lymantriidae). *Biol. Res.* 47: 29.

31. Hsouna, A.B. et al. 2014. *Myrtus communis* essential oil: Chemical composition and antimicrobial activities against food spoilage pathogens. *Chem. Biodivers.* 11: 571–80.

32. Jassbi, A.R. et al. 2012. Chemical classification of the essential oils of the Iranian *Salvia* species in comparison with their botanical taxonomy. *Chem. Biodivers.* 9: 1254–71.

33. Boukhatem, M.N. et al. 2014. Lemon grass (*Cymbopogon citratus*) essential oil as a potent anti-inflammatory and antifungal drugs. *Libyan J. Med.* 9: 25431.

34. Maciel, M.V. et al. 2010. Chemical composition of *Eucalyptus* spp. essential oils and their insecticidal effects on *Lutzomyia longipalpis*. *Vet. Parasitol.* 167: 1–7.

35. Fratini, F. et al. 2014. Antibacterial activity of essential oils, their blends and mixtures of their main constituents against some strains supporting livestock mastitis. *Fitoterapia* 96: 1–7.

36. Gómez, L.A. 2013. Comparative study on in vitro activities of citral, limonene and essential oils from *Lippia citriodora* and *L. alba* on yellow fever virus. *Nat. Prod. Commun.* 8(2): 249–52.

37. De Martino, L. et al. 2009. *Verbena officinalis* essential oil and its component citral as apoptotic-inducing agent in chronic lymphocytic leukemia. *Int. J. Immunopathol. Pharmacol.* 22(4): 1097–104.

38. Wichtel, M. 2002. *Teedrogen und Phytopharmaka*. Stuttgart: Wissenschaftliche Verlagsgesellschaft.

39. Madyastha, K.M. et al. 1992. Metabolic fate of menthofuran in rats. *Drug Metab. Dispos.* 20: 295–301.

40. Bruni, R. et al. 2007. Essential oil composition of *Agastache anethiodora* Britton (Lamiaceae) infected by cucumber mosaic virus (CMV). *Flavour Fragr. J.* 22: 66–70.

41. Mikaili, P. et al. 2013. Pharmacological and therapeutic effects of *Mentha Longifolia* L. and its main constituent, menthol. *Anc. Sci. Life* 33(2): 131–38.

42. Svoboda, K.P. et al. 1995. Analysis of the essential oils of some *Agastache* species grown in Scotland from various seed sources. *Flavour Fragr. J.* 10: 139–45.

43. Menut, C. et al. 2005. Two new furanosesquiterpenes from *Myoporum crassifolium* from New Caledonia. *Flavour Fragr. J.* 20: 621–25.

44. Tomic, M. et al. 2014. Antihyperalgesic and antiedematous activities of bisabolol-oxides-rich matricaria oil in a rat model of inflammation. *Phytother. Res.* 28: 759–66.

45. Viljoen, A.M. et al. 2006. The essential oil composition and chemotaxonomy of *Salvia stenophylla* and its allies *S. repens* and *S. runcinata*. *J Essent. Oil Res.* 18: 37–45.

46. De Souza, A.T. et al. 2008. Supercritical extraction process and phase equilibrium of candeia (*Eremanthus erythropappus*) oil using supercritical carbon dioxide. *J. Supercrit. Fluids* 47: 182–87.

47. Curado, M.A. et al. 2006. Environmental factors influence on chemical polymorphism of the essential oils of *Lychnophora ericoides*. *Phytochemistry* 67(21): 2363–69.

48. Orasa, P. et al. 2000. Phytochemistry of the zingiberaceae. In *Studies in Natural Products Chemistry*, ed. Atta-ur Rahman. Amsterdam: Elsevier Science Publishers, 797–865.

49. Schreier, P. 1997. Enzymes and flavour biotechnology. In *Biotechnology of Aroma Compounds*, ed. R.G. Berger. Berlin: Springer.

50. Wriessnegger, T. et al. 2014. Production of the sesquiterpenoid (+)-nootkatone by metabolic engineering of *Pichia pastoris*. *Metab. Eng.* 24: 18–29.
51. Maffei, M. 2002. *Vetiveria: The Genus Vetiveria*. Medicinal and Aromatic Plants—Industrial Profiles. Boca Raton, FL: CRC Press.
52. Khoury, M. et al. 2014. Chemical composition and antimicrobial activity of the essential oil of *Juniperus excelsa* M.Bieb.: Growing wild in Lebanon. *Chem. Biodivers.* 11: 825–30.
53. El Hamrouni-Aschi, K. et al. 2013. Essential-oil composition of the Tunisian endemic cypress (*Cupressus sempervirens* L. var. *numidica* Trab.). *Chem. Biodivers.* 10: 989–1003.
54. Guleria, S. et al. 2008. Chemical composition and fungitoxic activity of essential oil of *Thuja orientalis* L. grown in the north-western Himalaya. *Z. Naturforsch. C* 63(3–4): 211–14.
55. Zhang, X.H. et al. 2012. Chemical composition of volatile oils from the pericarps of Indian sandalwood (*Santalum album*) by different extraction methods. *Nat. Prod. Commun.* 7(1): 93–96.
56. Salapovic, H. et al. 2013. Quantification of sesquiterpene lactones in Asteraceae plant extracts: Evaluation of their allergenic potential. *Sci. Pharm.* 81(3): 807–18.
57. Vetter, S. et al. 1997. Inheritance of sesquiterpene lactone types within the *Achillea millefolium complex* (Compositae). *Plant Breed.* 116: 79–82.
58. Stappen, I. et al. 2014. Chemical composition and biological effects of *Artemisia maritima* and *Artemisia nilagirica* essential oils from wild plants of western Himalaya. *Planta Med.* 80(13): 1079–87.
59. Tschiggerl, C. et al. 2012. Guaianolides and volatile compounds in chamomile tea. *Plant Foods Hum. Nutr.* 67: 129–35.
60. Yang, Y.-C. et al. 2014. Ultrasound-assisted extraction and quantitation of oils from *Syzygium aromaticum* flower bud (clove) with supercritical carbon dioxide. *J. Chromatogr. A* 1323: 18–27.
61. Jayaprakasha, G.K. et al. 2003. Volatile constituents from *Cinnamomum zeylanicum* fruit stalks and their antioxidant activities. *J. Agric. Food Chem.* 51: 4344–48.
62. Senatore, F. 2000. *Oli essenziali, provenienza estrazione ed analisi chimica*. Rome: Edizioni Mediche Scientifiche Internazionali (EMSI).
63. Maggi, F. et al. 2014. Intra-population chemical polymorphism in *Thymus pannonicus* All. growing in Slovakia. *Nat. Prod. Res.* 28(19): 1557–66.
64. Adams, R.P. et al. 1993. Systematic relationships in *Juniperus* based on amplifed polymorphic DNAs (RAPDs). *Taxon.* 42: 553–71.
65. Otto, A. et al. 2001. Sesqui-, di-, and triterpenoids as chemosystematic markers in extant conifers: A review. *Bot. Rev.* 67: 141–238.
66. Rajčević, N. et al. 2013. Variability of the needle essential oils of *Juniperus deltoides* R.P.Adams from different populations in Serbia and Croatia. *Chem. Biodivers.* 10(1): 144–56.
67. Verzera, A. et al. 1996. The composition of bergamot oil. *Perfum. Flavor.* 21(6): 19–34.
68. Upson, T. et al. 2004. *The Genus Lavandula*. Portland, OR: Timber Press.
69. Benabdelkadera, T. et al. 2011. Essential oils from wild populations of Algerian *Lavandula stoechas* L.: Composition, chemical variability, and in vitro biological properties. *Chem. Biodivers.* 8: 937–53.
70. Hanlidou, E. et al. 2014. Essential-oil diversity of *Salvia tomentosa* Mill. in Greece. *Chem. Biodivers* 11: 1205–15.
71. Jansen, M.A.K. et al. 2008. Plant stress and human health: Do human consumers benefit from UV-B acclimated crops? *Plant Sci.* 175: 449–58.
72. Kakani, V.G. et al. 2003. Field crop response to ultraviolet-B radiation: A review. *Agric. Forest Meteorol.* 120: 191–218.

73. Singh, S.K. et al. 2011. Analysis of phytochemical and antioxidant potential of *Ocimum kilimandscharicum* Linn. *J. Curr. Pharm. Res.* 3: 40–46.

74. Sakalauskaite, J. et al. 2013. The effects of different UV-B radiation intensities on morphological and biochemical characteristics in *Ocimum basilicum* L. *J. Sci. Food Agric.* 93: 1266–71.

75. Kumari, R. et al. 2010. Supplemental UV-B induced changes in leaf morphology, physiology and secondary metabolites of an Indian aromatic plant *Cymbopogon citratus* (D.C.) Staph under natural field conditions. *Int. J. Environ. Stud.* 67: 655–75.

76. Brechner, M.L. et al. 2011. Effect of UV-B on secondary metabolites of St John's wort (*Hypericum perforatum* L.) grown in controlled environments. *Photochem. Photobiol.* 87: 680–84.

77. Kun, D.N. et al. 1984. Induction of phenylalanine ammonia-lyase and 4-coumarate CoA ligase mRNAs in cultured plant cells by UV light or fungal elicitor. *Proc. Natl. Acad. Sci. USA* 81: 1102–6.

78. Sundaresan, V. et al. 2012. Impact of geographic range on genetic and chemical diversity of Indian valerian (*Valeriana jatamansi*) from northwestern Himalaya. *Biochem. Genet.* 50(9–10): 797–808.

79. Leonardi, M. et al. 2013. Essential-oil composition of *Helichrysum italicum* (Roth) G.Don ssp. *italicum* from Elba Island (Tuscany, Italy). *Chem. Biodivers.* 10(3): 343–55.

80. Azavedo, N.R. et al. 2001. Chemical variability in the essential oil of *Hyptis suaveolens*. *Phytochemistry* 57: 733–36.

81. Dunkic, V. et al. 2012. Chemotaxonomic and micromorphological traits of *Satureja montana* L. and *S. subspicata* Vis. (Lamiaceae). *Chem. Biodiver.* 9: 2825–42.

82. Statti, G.A. et al. 2004. Chemical and biological diversity of Bergamot (*Citrus bergamia*) in relation to environmental factors. *Fitoterapia* 75: 212–16.

83. Andrade, M.S. et al. 2007. Volatile compounds of the leaves, flowers and fruits of *Kielmeyera rugosa* Choisy (Clusiaceae). *Flavour Fragr. J.* 22: 49–52.

84. Fokialakis, N. et al. 2002. Essential oil constituents of *Valeriana italic* and *Valeriana tuberosa*: Stereochemical and conformational study of 15-acetoxyvaleranone. *Z. Naturforschung.* 57c: 791–96.

85. Fiorini, C. et al. 1997. Composition of the flower, leaf and stem essential oils from *Laurus nobilis* L. *Flavour Fragr. J.* 12: 91–93.

86. Hudaib, M. et al. 2002. GC/MS evaluation of thyme (*Thymus ulgaris* L.) oil composition and variations during the vegetative cycle. *J. Pharm. Biomed. Anal.* 29: 691–70.

87. Barra, A. et al. 2010. Chemical variability, antifungal and antioxidant activity of *Eucalyptus camaldulensis* essential oil from *Sardinia*. *Nat. Prod. Commun.* 5(2): 329–35.

5 Aromatic Plants
Molecular Biology/ Biotechnology Approach

Candida Vannini and Marcella Bracale

CONTENTS

5.1 INTRODUCTION

Consumer interest in aromatherapy has greatly increased in recent years due to its power to reduce stress, pain, and depression, and to enhance memory, energy, and sleep. As a consequence, aromatherapy is increasingly used in the "emotional design" of environments such as hospitals, spas, retail spaces, restaurants, and hotels.

The essential oils used in aromatherapy are highly concentrated mixtures of odorous volatile organic compounds (VOCs), which are secondary metabolites crucial for the interaction of plants with their surrounding world. VOC mixtures are species specific, with the sites of production and diversity of compounds varying between plant species. Some molecules can be synthesized by all plant tissues, whereas others are produced in a tissue-specific or even in a cell-specific fashion. Synthesis of compounds is usually dependent on environmental conditions, and multistep enzymatic reactions are frequently required. Final VOC levels within plants are low and typically comprise less than 0.1%–5% of the biomass.

Currently, aromatic plants (APs) are mainly harvested from the wild. More than 60% of the world's production derives from developing countries, while the major consumers are the United States, Europe, and Japan.

The intensive collection of plants directly from wild populations has several drawbacks. Such collection often results in unsustainable exploitation of the earth's biological diversity and depletion of natural habitats, and many APs have become extinct in countries such as India (Gantait et al., 2011). Moreover, wild populations often exhibit poor product consistency and quality due to genotypic variation and environmental effects that alter metabolite levels and distribution. Finally, plant supply from wild populations is also limited by changes in political and socioeconomic development in the cultivation regions.

AP agro-cultivation better fulfills market demand in terms of yield, quality standardization, traceability, biodiversity conservation, and socioeconomic development. Agro-technologies also permit the selection of elite varieties that are rich in compounds of interest, free of undesired metabolites, and environmentally tolerant. AP cultivation is based on the selection of suitable plants from the wild population and the use of traditional cultivation methods, such as cuttings, layering, and grafting. The commercial cultivation of different AP species is well developed in several countries. For example, *Lavandula angustifolia* is extensively cultivated in the Mediterranean region; *Pogostemon cabin* is widely grown in China, Indonesia, India, Malaysia, Mauritius, Taiwan, the Philippines, Thailand, Vietnam, and West Africa; and *Vetiveria zizanoides* is farmed in Angola, Argentina, Brazil, China, Haiti, Japan, Java, and the island of Réunion (Bernath, 2014).

Nevertheless, some problems persist for AP cultivation. In many cases, it is difficult to satisfy the environmental requirements of the wild species, such as temperature, soil composition, and pH, in field cultivation. This results in substantial variability in germination rates, yields, and plant concentrations of active compounds. Biotechnological approaches have the potential to complement traditional agriculture in the industrial production of bioactive metabolites from APs.

5.2 PLANT CELL AND TISSUE CULTURE: AN ALTERNATIVE PRODUCTION SYSTEM FOR AROMATICS

In vitro plant culture refers to the growth and multiplication of cells, tissues, and organs of plants on defined media under controlled aseptic conditions. *In vitro* culture allows the efficient achievement of several different objectives: conservation, multiplication, and improvement of diverse plant species; production of high-value compounds as an alternative to whole plant extraction; and dissection of fundamental aspects of physiological and molecular regulation of plant development.

In vitro culture exploits plant cellular totipotency, that is, the ability of fully differentiated somatic cells to regenerate into whole plants. *In vitro* culture techniques are diverse in scope and aim. For APs, the areas of primary concern are micropropagation, cell suspension, and tissue culture.

5.2.1 MICROPROPAGATION

Micropropagation allows the production of a large number of genetically identical plantlets with low production cost (Figure 5.1). Plants are produced *in vitro* under controlled physical and chemical environments and are therefore disease-free and can be obtained year-round, independently of climatic fluctuations. Micropropagation also facilitates the production of plants from species with poor seed yields or low germination rates. Consequently, micropropagation is of particular interest for endangered species. Moreover, this technology requires significantly reduced space compared to field growth. Micropropagation protocols are based on the regeneration of plants from different organs (explants) under sterile conditions.

Explant choice is species specific, and its characteristics (nature, age, size, and phytosanitary conditions) are key factors for micropropagation success rate and efficiency. Basic components of culture media include a carbon source and essential elements such as salts, vitamins, and amino acids, but growth media can be specifically tailored to different plant species. Plant growth regulators such as auxins and cytokinins are critical media components that determine the developmental pathway taken by the explant cells.

Upon appropriate hormonal induction, organized meristems (e.g., shoot tips and node stems) can be induced to develop secondary buds from which several node-leaf cuttings, and ultimately complete plants, can be obtained (Perianez-Rodriguez et al., 2014). Some commercially significant APs have been regenerated from meristem tips, including patchouli, vanilla, and lavender (Sugimura et al., 2007; Gantait et al., 2011; Gonçalves and Romano, 2013).

Alternatively, in several plant species, suitable concentrations of auxin and cytokinin induce the formation of unorganized cell masses called calli (Ikeuchi et al., 2013; Su and Zhang, 2014). Organized structures can be induced from calli via

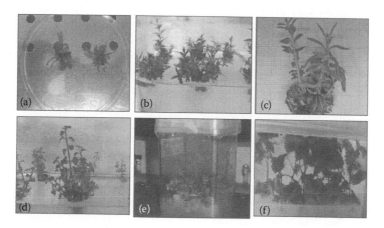

FIGURE 5.1 Micropropagation of some aromatic plants: (a) *Rosmarinus officinalis*, (b) *Myrtus communis*, (c) *Lavandula angustifolia*, (d) *Calamintha nepeta*, (e) *Ocimum basilicum*, and (f) *Melissa officinalis*. (Photos kindly provided by Prof. Luisa Pistelli and Dr. Laura Pistelli, University of Pisa, Italy. With permission.)

either organogenesis (the *de novo* development of shoots and roots) or somatic embryogenesis. The latter refers to the process by which some callus cells recover their embryogenic potential through complete reprogramming of gene expression. Somatic embryos follow the same morphological and developmental pattern as zygotic embryos, through globular, heart, and torpedo stages. A very high multiplication rate is possible with the embryogenic system. Protocols for callus initiation and regeneration have been reported for some *Ocimum* species, *Pelargonium graveolens*, *Cananga odorata*, *Tagetes erecta*, and *Vetiveria zizanoides* (Leupin et al., 2000; Sangduen and Prasertsongskun, 2009; Mathew and Sankar, 2011; Iriawati et al., 2013).

In vitro culture conditions can be mutagenic, and regenerated plantlets sometimes show phenotypic and genotypic variation (somaclonal variation) with respect to the mother plant. Somaclonal variation provides a valuable source for the improvement of crops through the selection of novel elite variants with a desirable natural product composition. Variation in morphology and essential oil production in regenerated plantlets of APs has been investigated (Mathur et al., 1988; Gupta et al., 2001; Tsuro et al., 2001; Ravindra et al., 2012).

Mutations can also be induced using physical and chemical mutagens to allow the production of genetic variants with desirable characteristics. In mutation breeding, the possibility exists to change a single gene or only a few genes without altering the total genetic background of a specific outstanding genotype. For example, Falk et al. (2009) treated lavender calli with ethyl methane-sulfonate (EMS) to induce mutations in regenerating plants. The relative abundance of several mono- and sesquiterpenes in one of these mutants was drastically different from that of wild-type plants. Early flowering and high-yielding mutants in *Ocimum sanctum* were obtained by treatment with gamma irradiation, sodium azide, and EMS (Nasare and Choudhary, 2011). Gamma irradiation treatment of *Pogostemon cabin* produced a mutant with a significantly higher percentage of patchouli alcohol than the wild-type (Rekha et al., 2009). In addition to the development of desirable traits, mutant research provides valuable resources for the investigation of essential oil biosynthetic pathways in plants.

Due to their market importance, *in vitro* culture of some APs has been extensively studied. Patchouli oil is used in aromatherapy to calm nerves and relieve depression and stress. Mass reproduction of patchouli through vegetative cuttings is slow and insufficient for large-scale cultivation. Moreover, natural variations and pathogen infections result in yield fluctuations. The *in vitro* growth and multiplication of shoots is affected by many factors, such as the age of the donor plant and the type of exogenous carbon source added to the medium (Kumara Swamy et al., 2010; Paul et al., 2010). However, rapid plant development, enhanced genetic stability, and high multiplication frequencies were reported from stem tips, axillary buds, leaves, nodal explants, calli, and protoplasts (Padmanabhan et al., 1981; Kukreja et al., 1990; Kageyama et al., 1995; Meena, 1996; Hembrom et al., 2006; Wan Nurul Hidayah et al., 2012).

The regeneration of plants in the *Salvia* genus was also successfully obtained from apical buds, leaves (Figure 5.2), and nodal segments (Arikat et al., 2004; Misic et al., 2006). Specific hormonal requirements for nodal explant growth from *S. officinalis*, *S. fruticosa*, and *S. leucantha* were elucidated (Hosoki and Tahara, 1993;

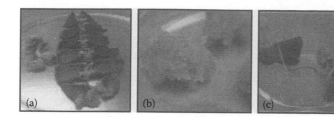

FIGURE 5.2 Plant regeneration from leaves of *Salvia officinalis*. (a) Callus induction from leaf explants. (b) Callus proliferation. (c) Regenerated plantlet. (Photos kindly provided by Prof. Luisa Pistelli and Dr. Laura Pistelli, University of Pisa, Italy. With permission.)

Avato et al., 2005). Several species of lavender were successfully micropropagated from different explants (de Bona et al., 2012; Jahan et al., 2012; Soni et al., 2013).

Essential oil production in micropropagated plants varies with species. Production in a number of species, including *Pogostemon cablin*, *Rosmarinus officinalis* L., *S. officinalis* L., *Satureja hortensis* L., and *Crithmum maritimum* L., was similar to that in the mother plants (Kumara Swamy and Anuradha, 2010; Pistelli et al., 2013). Conversely, addition of selected growth regulators to nutrition media affected essential oil composition and quality in *Melissa officinalis* L. and *Plectranthus ornatus* (Silva et al., 2005; Passinho-Soares et al., 2013).

5.2.2 PLANT CELL CULTURES

Single-cell suspensions can be produced from calli and tissues using enzymatic methods. The homogeneity of cell populations, high rate of cell growth, and good reproducibility make suspension-cultured cells potentially valuable for the production of secondary metabolites of commercial interest. Unfortunately, commercial exploitation of plant cell cultures has had limited success to date and is restricted to a few secondary metabolites. Undifferentiated cells produce secondary metabolites in very low amounts compared with the intact plant, and yields remain unpredictably variable. Strategies for improving the accumulation of desired metabolites in suspension cultures are based on the optimization of media composition, the modulation of physical parameters (aeration and light), and the selection of highly productive cell lines. For example, the production of rosmarinic acid by *Lavandula vera* DC. lines was enhanced by optimizing the medium composition, oxygen, and temperature (Pavlov et al., 2000, 2005).

Synthesis of secondary plant compounds is highly inducible, and it is therefore possible to increase their production in cell culture by the addition of precursors and elicitors. Elicitors are compounds that mimic stress, thereby activating plant biosynthetic pathways and increasing production of secondary metabolites. The positive effects of fungal elicitors, methyl jasmonate, and phenylalanine on the production of rosmarinic acid were reported in cell cultures of *S. officialis* (Nabila et al., 2003), *Ocimum sanctum* (Lukmanul et al., 2011), and *L. vera* (Georgiev et al., 2007). Attempts were also made to increase the yield of patchouli alcohol in cell cultures of *P. cablin* by using precursor feeding in the early part of the stationary phase of growth (Bunrathep et al., 2006).

5.3 GENE DISCOVERY AND FUNCTIONAL GENOMICS

Essential oils consist of a variety of volatile molecules, sometimes comprising more than 100 individual substances. However, two or three compounds are generally present at high proportions (20%–70%), while the remaining components are present in small amounts. Mono- and sesquiterpenes (C_{10} and C_{15} isoprenoids, respectively) are particularly abundant in most essential oils. Although terpenes are extraordinarily diverse, they all derive from the synthesis of two universal precursors, isopentenyl diphosphate (IPP) and its isomer dimethylallyl diphosphate (DMAPP), via two distinct pathways (Figure 5.3). The 2-C-methyl-D-eryhtritol 4-phosphate (MEP) pathway converts IPP/DMAPP to geranyl diphosphate (GPP) and geranylgeranyl diphosphate (GGPP) for the production of mono-, di-, and tetraterpenes in the plastid (Rodríguez-Concepción, 2006; Hasunuma et al., 2010). The MEP pathway begins with the condensation of pyruvate and glyceraldeyde-3-phosphate. The first two steps are catalyzed by 1-deoxy-D-xylulose 5-phosphate synthase (DXS) and 1-deoxy-D-xylulose 5-phosphate reductoisomerase (DXR). The cytosolic mevalonate (MVA)

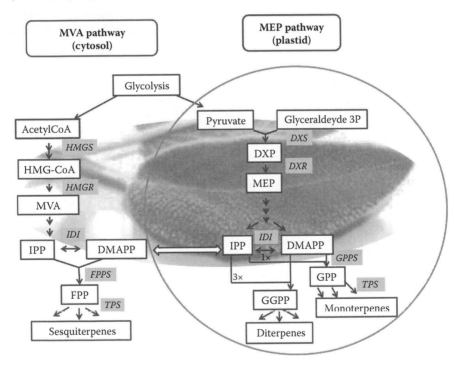

FIGURE 5.3 Synthesis of terpenoid VOCs. Terpenoid VOCs are synthesized by the mevalonic acid (MVA) and methylerythritolphosphate (MEP) pathways. DMAPP, dymethylallyl pyrophosphate; DXP, 1-deoxy-D-xylulose 5-phosphate; *DXR*, DXP reductoisomerase; *DXS*, DXP synthase; FPP, farnesyl pyrophosphate; *FPPS*, FPP synthase; GPP, geranyl pyrophosphate; *GPPS*, GPP synthase; HMG-CoA, hydroxymethylglutaryl-CoA; *HMGR*, HMG-CoA reductase; *HMGS*, HMG-CoA synthase; *IDI*, IPP isomerase; IPP, isopentenyl pyrophosphate; *TPS*, terpene synthase.

pathway is responsible for the conversion of IPP and DMAPP to farnesyl diphos-phate (FPP) for the production of sesqui-, tri-, and polyterpenes (Ganjewala et al., 2009; Rodríguez-Concepción and Boronat, 2002; Rodríguez-Concepción, 2006). The first two steps of this pathway are controlled by 3-hydroxy-3-methylglutaryl-CoA synthase (HMGS) and 3-hydroxy-3-methylglutaryl-CoA reductase (HMGR). Cross talk between the two pathways was reported previously (Hemmerlin et al., 2003; Dudareva et al., 2005).

The late steps of cyclization and oxidation of the precursors of each class of ter-penes are catalyzed by terpene synthases (TPSs). The wide diversity of terpenes results from the large number of different *TPS* genes and the ability of a TPS to pro-duce multiple products from a single substrate (Degenhardt et al., 2009; Dudareva et al., 2013). In addition, several monooxigenases and oxidoreductases are respon-sible for further modifications of the primary terpenes.

There is an increasing interest in improving the quality and yield of essential oils in APs using targeted breeding assisted by molecular markers and metabolic engineering tools.

For biotechnological production of a desired compound at large scale or in a host species, it is necessary to identify the genes participating in its biosynthe-sis. Due to the complexity of terpenoid biosynthesis pathways, many enzyme-encoding genes are still not well defined, particularly the enzymes involved in the last stage of terpenoid biosynthesis. In addition, some key enzymes such as DXS and HMGR are encoded by small gene families whose members are not known in most APs.

The monoterpene biosynthetic pathways in *Mentha* × *piperita* and *Mentha spi-cata* were initially elucidated with time-course studies using labeled precursors (for reviews of the pathway, see Croteau, 1987; Wise and Croteau, 1999). After enzyme identification, peptide sequencing allowed the design of degenerate primers based on conserved domains. These primers were used to clone the enzyme-encoding genes responsible for the synthesis of many monoterpenes and sesquiterpenes in several aromatic species (Bohlmann et al., 1998).

Limonene synthase (LS) was the first TPS identified in *M. spicata* and was elu-cidated by screening a leaf cDNA library with three distinct oligonucleotide probes designed from the amino acid sequence of the purified enzyme from oil glands (Colby et al., 1993). A similarity-based approach was also used to amplify the genes encod-ing enzymes for terpene biosynthesis in *L. angustifolia* (Landmann et al., 2007), *Mentha* (Burke et al., 1999; Lupien et al., 1999), *Abies grandis* (Bohlmann et al., 1997), *S. officinalis* (Wise et al., 1998), *Citrus limon* (Lucker et al., 2002), *P. cablin* (Deguerry et al., 2006), *Valeriana officinalis* (Dong et al., 2013), *Thymus caespiti-tius* (Lima et al., 2013; Mendes et al., 2014), and *Cinnamomum osmophloeum* (Lin et al., 2014).

Genomic sequence databases are not yet available for most APs. However, sequencing of the nuclear and chloroplast genomes of some APs, including *Salvia miltiorrhiza, Mentha spicata, Picea abies, Origanum vulgare, Eucalyptus globulus*, and *Pelargonium*, was recently completed (http://www.genomesonline.org/index; Qian et al., 2013).

Nevertheless, transcriptomic approaches allowed the large-scale sequencing of expressed sequence tags (ESTs) from different tissues, and this facilitated the discovery of new genes involved in the biosynthesis of unique compounds in various species. The rationale of this approach was that the tissue in which a particular metabolite is produced is likely to express the biosynthetic genes at high levels. In APs, mono- and sesquiterpenes are produced and accumulated in highly specialized secretory cells (or oil glands) present on the surfaces of leaves and floral tissues (Wagner, 1991; McCaskill et al., 1992; Lange et al., 2000; Turner et al., 2000). In particular, in Lamiaceae, secretory cells can accumulate metabolites at levels up to 10%–15% of the leaf dry weight (Wagner et al., 2004). These cells can thus be considered biosynthetic factories and therefore constitute attractive targets for metabolic engineering (Schilmiller et al., 2008). The development of methods for the purification of intact glandular cells from different APs (Gershenzon et al., 1992; Crocoll et al., 2010; Olofsson et al., 2012) provided an enriched source of terpene biosynthetic enzymes and allowed identification of their corresponding transcripts.

Lange et al. (2000) generated an EST library by sequencing a pool of 1300 random cDNA sequences from *M. × piperita* oil glands in which at least 18% of sequences were involved in terpene metabolism. An additional 7% of genes were responsible for the biosynthesis of transporters, some of which were likely involved in metabolite trafficking and oil secretion. Screening of this library facilitated the isolation and functional characterization of several genes encoding later menthol pathway enzymes (Bertea et al., 2001; Ringer et al., 2003, 2005; Davis et al., 2005). To further understand the regulation of monoterpene biosynthesis, Bertea et al. (2003) compared cDNA libraries from a control plant and from a Scotch spearmint mutant that had an altered essential oil composition.

The menthol biosynthetic pathway in *M. × piperita* gland cells was thus elucidated, making this plant a good experimental system for metabolic engineering (Figure 5.4) (Croteau et al., 2005).

Two cDNA libraries from flowers and leaves of *L. angustifolia* were constructed and used to obtain 15,000 ESTs (Lane et al., 2010). Moreover, 8000 ESTs were isolated from the glandular trichomes of *Lavandula × intermedia* flowers (Demissie et al., 2012). The screening of *Lavandula* EST databases led to the isolation of cDNAs

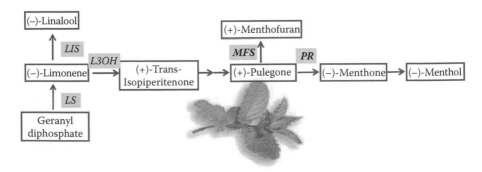

FIGURE 5.4   Menthol pathway scheme. *L3OH*, limonene 3-hydroxylase; *LIS*, linalool synthase; *LS*, (–)-limonene synthase; *MFS*, menthofuran synthase; *PR*, pulegone reductase.

encoding some monoterpene synthases (Lane et al., 2010; Demissie et al., 2011, 2012; Sarker, 2013), a sesquiterpene synthase for the production of caryophyllene (one of the most abundant sesquiterpenes in *Lavandula* essential oil) (Sarker et al., 2013), and a short-chain alcohol dehydrogenase for the conversion of borneol to camphor (Sarker et al., 2012). Moreover, an enzyme was isolated that condensed two DMAPP molecules to generate the monoterpenes lavandulol and lavandulol acetate (Demissie et al., 2013). Gene expression analysis demonstrated that lavender glandular trichomes predominantly utilized the MEP pathway for the production of essential oil constituents.

The glandular trichome-specific EST collections from *Ocimum basilicum* (Gang et al., 2001; Iijima et al., 2004a,b) and *S. fruticosa* (Chatzopoulou et al., 2010) allowed the identification and characterization of genes involved in essential oil biosynthesis in these APs.

The close correlation of absolute terpene synthase expression with essential oil composition in different lines of *O. vulgare* (Crocoll et al., 2010) and *O. basilicum* confirmed that, as reported for other APs, transcriptional regulation was the primary mechanism controlling terpene composition (Dudareva et al., 1996, 2013; Bohlmann et al., 1997; Mahmoud and Croteau, 2003; Boeckelmann, 2008; Lane et al., 2010).

The increasing availability of rapid low-cost sequencing alongside the development of bioinformatic tools for the analysis of sequence data (Collins et al., 2008; Nagalakshmi et al., 2008) has enabled comprehensive analysis of the transcriptome of nonmodel plants. In particular, RNA sequencing (RNA-seq) provides large-scale RNA sequence databases that can be mined for gene discovery, transcript quantification, small RNA discovery, and analysis of regulation. Transcriptome data can be used to investigate the biosynthesis of specialized metabolites of biotechnological interest (Johnson et al., 2012; Xiao et al., 2013; Sangwan, 2014; www.phytometasyn.ca). Using these techniques, transcriptomes from leaves of *O. sanctum* (CIM Ayu—eugenol-rich variety) and *O. basilicum* (CIM Saumya—methylchavicol-rich variety) (Rastogi et al., 2014) were compared. Identified transcripts were 69,117 and 130,043 for *O. sanctum* and *O. basilicum*, respectively. The transcripts were classified into different functional categories and assigned to several functional pathways. Of the discovered transcripts, 501 (*O. sanctum*) and 952 (*O. basilicum*) transcripts were involved in secondary metabolism, with an emphasis on the biosynthesis of terpenoids in *O. sanctum* and phenylpropanoids in *O. basilicum*. Moreover, simple sequence repeat (SSR) markers linked to terpenoid biosynthesis were identified that have potential for use in plant breeding to improve *Ocimum* chemotypes.

Transcriptomes of *Coriandrum sativum* mericarp at three developmental stages, leaves of *Valeriana officinalis*, and leaves and roots of *S. milthiorryza* were sequenced, and relative transcript libraries were produced (Yang et al., 2013; Yeo et al., 2013; Galata et al., 2014).

Transcriptome sequencing offers higher throughput and increased depth than EST sequencing and is a promising tool for the discovery of novel biosynthetic genes.

Recent improvements in high-resolution proteomic and metabolic platforms have allowed large-scale profiling and identification of proteins and metabolites in APs. Proteomic analysis of *M. spicata* peltate trichomes identified 32 proteins involved in terpenoid synthesis and several candidate proteins that might be required for terpenoid transport (Champagne and Boutry, 2013).

The integration of transcriptomic, proteomic, and metabolic profiling data provided a systems-level framework to investigate metabolic pathways in glandular trichomes of different basil lines (Iijima et al., 2004a; Xie et al., 2008).

5.4 METABOLIC ENGINEERING FOR BIOTECHNOLOGICAL PRODUCTION OF ESSENTIAL OILS

Improvement of essential oil yield and quality in aromatic plants through controlling the expression of native-related genes or by the introduction of heterologous genes is another area of research interest. Improvements can be obtained by the overexpression of one or several key genes to increase the flux through the MEP or MVA pathways or by the silencing of specific genes to reduce competing or catabolic branches of the pathways.

To date, the most promising bioengineering results have been obtained in mint, lavender, eucalyptus, and sage (Lange and Ahkami, 2013; Lange and Turner, 2013).

5.4.1 MINT

M. × *piperita* transgenic plants constitutively expressing the *DXR* gene accumulated more essential oil (about 50% yield increase) without changes in monoterpene composition than wild-type plants (Mahmoud and Croteau, 2002). This indicated that the MEP pathway was the sole source of terpenoid precursors in *M.* × *piperita*. Furthermore, the alteration of a committed step improved the flux through the pathway and led to an increase in monoterpene production. An increased essential oil yield was also obtained by the upregulation of the *isopentenyl diphosphate isomerase* (*IDI*) and *geranyl diphosphate synthase* (*GPPS*) genes. In the latter case, the resultant essential oil had a more favorable composition for aromatherapy. Conversely, overexpression of the *DXS* gene did not result in significant increases in oil yield (Lange et al., 2011).

The *LS* gene was the first to be manipulated in *M.* × *piperita* plants with the purpose of essential oil overproduction (Krasnyansky et al., 1999; Diemer et al., 2001; Mahmoud et al., 2004). However, conflicting results were obtained in these studies, and only Diemer et al. (2001) obtained transgenic plants producing higher total concentrations of monoterpenes.

The manipulation of selected downstream biosynthetic steps has been used to improve essential oil composition in mint (Figure 5.4). Limonene-3-hydroxylase (L3-OH) catalyzes the conversion of limonene to trans-isopiperitenol for menthol biosynthesis. Cosuppression resulted in the accumulation of limonene (up to 80% of the essential oil compared to ~2% in wild-type plants) without affecting total oil yield. These results indicate that limonene does not induce feedback inhibition of the synthase enzyme, and that essential oil composition can be significantly altered by pathway engineering without adverse metabolic consequences (Mahmoud et al., 2004).

Transgenic plants of *M.* × *piperita* overexpressing a linalool synthase from *Mentha citrata* produced essential oil containing 0.7% S-linalool compared to 0.4% in control plants.

Menthofuran synthase (MFS) catalyzes the conversion of (+)-pulegone to (+)-menthofuran, an undesirable monoterpenoid component of mint oil. Up- and down-regulation of the *MFS* gene increased or decreased the levels of menthofuran and pulegone, respectively (Mahmoud and Croteau, 2002, 2003). It was subsequently demonstrated that in the absence of menthofuran, the (+)-pulegone reductase (PR) enzyme, responsible for the conversion of (+)-pulegone to menthone, was synthesized readily and produced essential oil with increased menthone and menthol contents. These results suggest that menthofuran yield is regulated at the transcriptional level in peppermint, and *PR* and *MFS* expression are inversely correlated (Rios-Estepa et al., 2008). Moreover, *MFS* antisense plants produced more essential oil. This increase was mainly due to a higher number and higher percentage of mature glandular trichomes on leaves.

The most promising results were obtained by simultaneous downregulation of *MFS* and upregulation of *DXR*. In these transgenic plants, essential oil yield increased by 78% and oil composition was improved compared to control plants (Lange et al., 2011).

5.4.2 LAVENDER

Overexpression of the *DXS* gene in spike lavender plants resulted in a higher essential production and altered monoterpene composition compared to wild-type (Muñoz-Bertomeu et al., 2006). By contrast with *M.* × *piperita*, transgenic spike lavender plants overexpressing the *DXR* gene did not show any increase in essential oil yield (Mendoza-Poudereux et al., 2014). These data indicate that in lavender, the flux of the MEP pathway is controlled by the *DXS* gene. Moreover, lavender plants constitutively overexpressing *HMGR* showed a significant increase in oil yield, suggesting metabolic cross talk between the MEP and MVA pathways (Muñoz-Bertomeu et al., 2007).

Overexpression of the *LS* gene (from *M. spicata*) in spike lavender produced an elevated limonene content (more than 450% increase compared to control) that correlated with elevated transcript accumulation (Muñoz-Bertomeu et al., 2008).

Expression of the *LS* gene in lavandin (*L.* × *intermedia*) under the control of a strong constitutive promoter from *L. angustifolia* resulted in differential expression in leaves and florets. In leaves, *LS* overexpression increased the total essential oil production without alteration of the fragrance. Conversely, in florets, where expression of the endogenous target gene was substantial, the constitutive promoter induced cosuppression of the *LS* gene and led to a reduction in total essential oil production (Tsuro and Asada, 2014).

Transgenic *L. latifolia* plants overexpressing the *linalool synthase* gene from *Clarkia breweri* had significantly higher linalool content than the control (Mendoza-Poudereux et al., 2014).

5.4.3 SAGE

Overexpression of the heterologous *AtDXS* and *AtDXR* genes increased the biosynthesis of diterpenoids in *Salvia sclarea* hairy roots (Vaccaro et al., 2014). Wu et al. (2006) obtained high levels of sesquiterpene production by coexpressing *farnesyl diphosphate synthase* and *sesquiterpene synthase* genes in plastids.

5.4.4 EUCALYPTUS

Eucalyptus camaldulensis was the first woody essential oil plant to be engineered. Transgenic plants overexpressing the *Perilla frutescens LS* gene accumulated limonene, α-pinene, and 1,8-cineole (Ohara et al., 2010).

5.4.5 ENGINEERING CHALLENGES AND PERSPECTIVES IN PLANT ENGINEERING

Plant metabolic engineering can be hampered by unwanted side effects. For example, enzyme catalytic activity can depend on subcellular targeting, and a number of non-specific modifying enzymes can interfere with the production of a desired compound. Moreover, when transgenes are expressed under a strong constitutive promoter, they may have deleterious effects on plant fitness as a result of the interference with other metabolic pathways or toxicity of the resulting compounds (Aharoni et al., 2005; Wu et al., 2006; Tsuro and Asada, 2014). These constraints can be overcome by using inducible promoters or tissue- or organ-specific promoters. The capacity of glandular trichomes to produce and accumulate terpenoids without deleterious effects makes them important targets for metabolic engineering (Schilmiller et al., 2008). Trichome-specific promoters (Tissier, 2012) and transporters could enhance the production of specific terpenoids in trichomes. In addition, essential oil yield is directly proportional to the number of glandular trichomes on leaves, and recent studies identified positive and negative regulators of differentiation and gene expression in trichomes of model plants (Grebe, 2012; Spyropoulou et al., 2014). These data could improve understanding of the formation of glandular trichomes in aromatic plants and potentially allow engineering of new varieties with increased essential oil production.

5.4.6 METABOLIC ENGINEERING IN MICROBES

The improvement of essential oil yield by breeding or genetic engineering of APs is often impossible due to biotechnological or sociopolitical reasons. In recent years, there has been growing interest in using recombinant microbial systems as alternative production platforms for the efficient production of specific bioactive plant compounds. Various research groups described the construction of *Escherichia coli* and yeast strains producing carotenoids, terpenoids, flavonoids, and sesquiterpenes via genetic engineering (Takahashi et al., 2007; Fischer et al., 2011; Misawa et al., 2011; Immethun et al., 2013). For example, Carter et al. (2003) overexpressed *GPPS* from *Abies grandis* and *LS* from *M. spicata* in *E. coli* and achieved an increase in limonene content (>450% with respect to the control). More recently, Alonso-Gutierrez et al. (2013) engineered *E. coli* with a heterologous MEP pathway and *LS* gene to create a limonene synthase platform from simple sugars. The authors also used this platform to produce perillyl alcohol by coexpressing a cytochrome P450 for specific hydroxylation of limonene. This limonene platform could potentially be used to generate any other limonene derivatives.

Selected terpenes such as limonene and α-pinene are widely used to test direct microbial biotransformation. In a recent report, the biotransformation of limonene to α-terpinel, a volatile terpenoid alcohol widely used in aromatherapy, was reported in *E. coli* (Bicas et al., 2009). Vanillin was also produced in high yields through microbial transformation (Daugsch and Pastore, 2005). Ratana Thanasomboon et al. (2012) designed and engineered *E. coli*, using standardized DNA sequences from BioBricks (http://biobricks.org/), to produce linalool. Bacterial cultures overexpressing *GPPS* and *LIS* showed the strongest linalool production after 96 hours of cultivation. Finally, the possibility of introducing large fragments of DNA into bacterial cells suggests that it might be feasible to reconstitute a "trichome cell factory" in a microorganism (Gibson et al., 2009).

5.5 CONCLUSIONS

Recent efforts to manipulate terpenoid production in APs have demonstrated the feasibility of improving the yield and composition of essential oils by metabolic engineering.

However, numerous attempts resulted in disappointing enhancement of terpenoids or unpredicted metabolic consequences due to our insufficient understanding of plant metabolic networks and their regulation. Omic profiling of APs offers promising new avenues for the discovery and characterization of novel biosynthetic genes and for the elucidation of the regulatory mechanisms underlying terpenoid metabolism. In particular, the identification of transcription factors that coordinately regulate gene expression for several endogenous genes can be expected to improve essential oil production in AP cell cultures. Moreover, the characterization of trichome-specific promoters and transporters may allow refinement of metabolic engineering to avoid deleterious effects on plant fitness.

ACKNOWLEDGMENTS

We apologize to colleagues whose studies could not be cited due to space constraints.

REFERENCES

Aharoni, A., Jongsma, M.-A., and Bouwmeester, H.J. Volatile science? Metabolic engineering of terpenoids in plants. *Trends in Plant Science* 10 (2005): 594–602.

Alonso-Gutierrez, J., Chan, R., Batth, T.-S. et al. Metabolic engineering of *Escherichia coli* for limonene and perillyl alcohol production. *Metabolic Engineering* 19 (2013): 33–41.

Arikat, A., Jawad, F., Karam, N. et al. Micropropagation and accumulation of essential oil in wild sage (*Salvia fruticosa* Mill.). *Scientia Horticulturae* 100 (2004): 193–202.

Avato, P., Morone Fortunato, I., Ruta, C. et al. Glandular hairs and essential oils in micropropagated plants of *Salvia officinalis* L. *Plant Science* 169 (2005): 29–36.

Bernath, J. Aromatic plants. Unesco-EOLSS, Paris, 2014. http://www.eolss.net.

Bertea, C.M., Schalk, M., Karp, F. et al. Demonstration that menthofuran synthase of mint (*Mentha*) is a cytochrome P450 monooxygenase: Cloning, functional expression, and characterization of the responsible gene. *Archives of Biochemistry and Biophysics* 390 (2001): 279–286.

Bertea, C., Schalk, M., Mau, C.J.D. et al. Molecular evaluation of a spearmint mutant altered in the expression of limonene hydroxylases that direct essential oil monoterpene biosynthesis. *Phytochemistry* 64 (2003): 1203–1211.

Bicas, J., Dionísio, A.P., and Pastore Gláucia, M. Bio-oxidation of terpenes: An approach for the flavor industry. *Chemical Reviews* 109 (2009): 4518–4531.

Boeckelmann, A. Monoterpene production and regulation in lavenders (*Lavandula angustifolia* and *Lavandula* × *intermedia*). MSc thesis, University of British Columbia–Okanagan, 2008, pp. 70–71.

Bohlmann, J., Steele, C.L., and Croteau, R. Monoterpene synthases from grand fir (*Abies grandis*). cDNA isolation, characterization, and functional expression of myrcene synthase, (–)-(4S)-limonene synthase, and (–)-(1S,5S)-pinene synthase. *Journal of Biological Chemistry* 272 (1997): 21784–21792.

Bohlmann, J., Meyer-Gauen, G., and Croteau, R. Plant terpenoid synthases: Molecular biology and phytogenetic analysis. *Proceedings of the National Academy of Sciences USA* 95 (1998): 4126–4133.

Bunrathep, S., Lockwood, G., Songsakc, T. et al. Chemical constituents from leaves and cell cultures of *Pogostemon cablin* and use of precursor feeding to improve patchouli alcohol level. *Science Asia* 32 (2006): 293–296.

Burke, C.B., Wildung, M., and Croteau, R. Geranyl diphosphate synthase: Cloning, expression, and characterization of this prenyltransferase as a heterodimer. *Proceedings of the National Academy of Sciences USA* 96 (1999): 13062–13067.

Carter, O.A., Peters, R.J., and Croteau, R. Monoterpene biosynthesis pathway construction in *Escherichia coli*. *Phytochemistry* 64 (2003): 425–433.

Champagne, A., and Boutry, M. Proteomic snapshot of spearmint (*Mentha spicata* L.) leaf trichomes: A genuine terpenoid factory. *Proteomics* 13 (2013): 3327–3332.

Chatzopoulou, F.M., Makris, A.M., Argiriou, A. et al. EST analysis and annotation of transcripts derived from a trichome-specific cDNA library from *Salvia fruticosa*. *Plant Cell Reports* 29 (2010): 523–534.

Colby, S.M., Alonso, W.R., Katahira, E.J. et al. 4S-Limonene synthase from the oil glands of spearmint (*Mentha spicata*): cDNA isolation, characterization, and bacterial expression of the catalytically active monoterpene cyclase. *Journal of Biological Chemistry* 268 (1993): 23016–23024.

Collins, L.J., Biggs, P.J., Voelckel, C. et al. An approach to transcriptome analysis of non-model organisms using short-read sequences. *Genome Informatics* 21 (2008): 3–14.

Crocoll, C., Asbach, J., and Gershenzon, J. Terpene synthases of oregano (*Origanum vulgare* L.) and their roles in the pathway and regulation of terpene biosynthesis. *Plant Molecular Biology* 75 (2010): 587–603.

Croteau, R. Biosynthesis and catabolism of monoterpenoids. *Chemical Review* 87 (1987): 929–954.

Croteau, R.B., Davis, E.M., Ringer, K.L. et al. (–)-Menthol biosynthesis and molecular genetics. *Naturwissenschaften* 92 (2005): 562–577.

Daugsch, A., and Pastore, G. Production of vanillin: A biotechnological opportunity. *Química Nova* 28 (2005): 642–645.

Davis, E.M., Ringer, K.L., McConkey, M.E. et al. Monoterpene metabolism: Cloning, expression, and characterization of menthone reductases from peppermint. *Plant Physiology* 137 (2005): 873–881.

de Bona, C.-M., Santos, G.-D., and Biasi, L.-A. *Lavandula* calli induction, growth curve and cell suspension formation. *Revista Brasileira de Ciências Agrárias* 7 (2012): 17–23.

Degenhardt, J., Köllner, T.G., and Gershenzon, J. Monoterpene and sesquiterpene synthases and the origin of terpene skeletal diversity in plants. *Phytochemistry* 70 (2009): 1621–1637.

Deguerry, F., Pastore, L., Wu, S. et al. The diverse sesquiterpene profile of patchouli, *Pogostemon cablin*, is correlated with a limited number of sesquiterpene synthases. *Archives of Biochemistry and Biophysics* 454 (2006): 123–136.

Demissie, Z.-A., Sarker, L.-S., and Mahmoud, S.-S. Cloning and functional characterization of β-phellandrene synthase from *Lavandula angustifolia*. *Planta* 233 (2011): 685–696.

Demissie, Z.-A., Cella, M.-A., Sarker, L.-S. et al. Cloning, functional characterization and genomic organization of 1,8-cineole synthases from *Lavandula*. *Plant Molecular Biology* 79 (2012): 393–411.

Demissie, Z.-A., Erland, L.A.E., Rheault, M.-R. et al. Isolation and biochemical characterization of a novel cis-prenyl diphosphate synthase gene, lavandulyl diphosphate synthase. *Journal of Biological Chemistry* 288 (2013): 6333–6341.

Diemer, F., Caissard, J.C., Moja, S. et al. Altered monoterpene composition in transgenic mint following the introduction of 4S-limonene synthase. *Plant Physiology and Biochemistry* 39 (2001): 603–614.

Dong, L., Miettinen, K., Goedbloed, M. et al. Characterization of two geraniol synthases from *Valeriana officinalis* and *Lippia dulcis*: Similar activity but difference in subcellular localization. *Metabolic Engineering* 20 (2013): 198–211.

Dudareva, N., Cseke, L., Blanc, V.-M. et al. Evolution of floral scent in Clarkia: Novel patterns of S-linalool synthase gene expression in the *C. breweri* flower. *Plant Cell* 8 (1996): 1137–1148.

Dudareva, N., Andersson, S., Orlova, I. et al. The non-mevalonate pathway supports both monoterpene and sesquiterpene formation in snapdragon flowers. *Proceedings of the National Academy of Sciences USA* 102 (2005): 933–938.

Dudareva, N., Klempien, A., Mulhemann J. et al. Biosynthesis, function and metabolic engineering of plant volatile organic compounds. *New Phytologist* 198 (2013): 16–32.

Falk, L., Biswas, K., Boeckelmann, A. et al. An efficient method for the micropropagation of lavenders: Regeneration of a unique mutant. *Journal of Essential Oil Research* 21 (2009): 225–228.

Fischer, M.J., Meyer, S., Claudel, P. et al. Metabolic engineering of monoterpene synthesis in yeast. *Biotechnology and Bioengineering* 108 (2011): 1883–1892.

Galata, M., Sarker, L.S., and Mahmoud, S.S. Transcriptome profiling, and cloning and characterization of the main monoterpene synthases of *Coriandrum sativum* L. *Phytochemistry* 102 (2014): 64–73.

Gang, D.-R., Wang, J., Dudareva, N. et al. An investigation of the storage and biosynthesis of phenylpropenes in sweet basil (*Ocimum basilicum* L.). *Plant Physiology* 125 (2001): 539–555.

Ganjewala, D., Kumar, S., and Luthra, R. An account of cloned genes of methyl-erythritol-4-phosphate pathway of isoprenoid biosynthesis in plants. *Current Issues in Molecular Biology* 11 (2009): 35–45.

Gantait, S., Mandal, N., and Nandy, S. Advances in micropropagation of selected aromatic plants: A review on vanilla and strawberry. *American Journal of Biochemistry and Molecular Biology* 1 (2011): 15–19.

Georgiev, M.I., Kuzeva, S.L., Pavlov, A.I. et al. Elicitation of rosmarinic acid by *Lavandula vera* MM cell suspension culture with abiotic elicitors. *World Journal of Microbiology and Biotechnology* 23 (2007): 301–304.

Gershenzon, J., McCaskill, D., Rajaonarivony, H. et al. Isolation of secretory cells from plant glandular trichomes and their use in biosynthetic studies of monoterpenes and other gland products. *Analytical Biochemistry* 200 (1992): 130–138.

Gibson, D.G., Young, L., Chuang, R.Y. et al. Enzymatic assembly of DNA molecules up to several hundred kilobases. *Natural Methods* 6 (2009): 343–345.

Gonçalves, S., and Romano, A. *In vitro* culture of lavenders (*Lavandula* spp.) and the production of secondary metabolites. *Biotechnology Advances* 31 (2013): 166–174.

Grebe, M. The patterning of epidermal hairs in *Arabidopsis*—updated. *Current Opinion in Plant Biology* 15 (2012): 31–37.

Gupta, R., Mallavarapu, G.-R., Banerjee S. et al. Characteristics of an isomenthone-rich somaclonal mutant isolated in a geraniol-rich rose-scented geranium accession of *Pelargonium graveolens*. *Flavour and Fragrance Journal* 16 (2001): 319–324.

Hasunuma, T., Kondo, A., and Miyake, C. Metabolic engineering by plastid transformation as a strategy to modulate isoprenoid yield in plants. In A.G. Fett-Neto (ed.), *Plant secondary metabolism engineering*, Vol. 643: *Methods in molecular biology*. Humana press, 2010: 213–227.

Hembrom, M.E., Martin, K.P., Patchathundikandi, S.K., and Madassery, J. Rapid *in vitro* production of true-to-type plants of Pogostemon heyneanus through dedifferentiated axillary buds. *In Vitro Cellular & Developmental Biology—Plant* 42 (2006): 283–286.

Hemmerlin, A., Hoeffler, J.F., Meyer, O. et al. Cross-talk between the cytosolic mevalonate and the plastidial methylerythritol phosphate pathways in Tobacco Bright Yellow-2 cells. *Journal of Biological Chemistry* 278 (2003): 26666–26676.

Hosoki, T., and Tahara, Y. *In vitro* propagation of *Salvia leucantha* Cav. *Horticultural Science* 28 (1993): 226–230.

Iijima, Y., Davidovich-Rikanati, R., Fridman, E. et al. The biochemical and molecular basis for the divergent patterns in the biosynthesis of terpenes and phenylpropenes in the peltate glands of three cultivars of basil. *Plant Physiology* 136 (2004a): 3724–3736.

Iijima, Y., Gang, D.-R., Fridman, E. et al. Characterization of geraniol synthase from the peltate glands of sweet basil. *Plant Physiology* 134 (2004b): 370–379.

Ikeuchi, M., Sugimoto, K., and Iwase, A. Plant callus: Mechanisms of induction and repression. *Plant Cell* 25 (2013): 3159–3173.

Immethun, C.M., Hoynes-O'Connor, A.G., Balassy, A. et al. Microbial production of isoprenoids enabled by synthetic biology. *Frontiers in Microbiology* (2013): 4–75.

Iriawati, R., Esyanti, R., Natalia, W. et al. *In vitro* plant regeneration of Java vetiver (*Vetiveria zizanioides*). *International Journal of Biological, Veterinary, Agricultural and Food Engineering* 7 (2013): 532–534.

Jahan, N., Mustafa, R., Zaidi, M.A. et al. Optimization of protocol to enhance the micro propagation of lavender species. *Current Research Journal of Biological Sciences* 4 (2012): 258–260.

Johnson, M.T.J., Carpenter, E.J., Tian, Z. et al. Evaluating methods for isolating total RNA and predicting the success of sequencing phylogenetically diverse plant transcriptomes. *PLoS One* 7 (2012): e50226.

Kageyama, Y., Honda, Y., and Sugimura, Y. Plant regeneration from patchouli protoplasts encapsulated in alginate beads. *Plant Cell Tissue Organ Culture* 41 (1995): 65–70.

Krasnyansky, S., May, R.A., Loskutov, A. et al. Transformation of the limonene synthase gene into peppermint (*Mentha piperita* L.) and preliminary studies on the essential oil profiles of single transgenic plants. *Theoretical Applied Genetics* 99 (1999): 676–682.

Kukreja, A.K., Mathur, A.K., and Zaim, M. Mass production of virus free patchouli plants (*Pogostemon cablin* (Blanco) Benth.) by *in vitro* culture. *Tropical Agriculture* 67 (1990): 101–104.

Kumara Swamy, M., and Anuradha, M. Micropropagation of *Pogostemon cablin* Benth. through direct regeneration for production of true to type plants. *Plant Tissue Culture and Biotechnology* 20 (2010): 81–89.

Kumara Swamy, M., Sudipta, K.-M., Balasubramanya, S. et al. Effect of different carbon sources on *in vitro* morphogenetic response of patchouli (*Pogostemon Cablin* Benth.). *Journal of Phytology* 2 (2010): 11–17.

Landmann, C., Fink, B., Festner, M. et al. Cloning and functional characterization of three terpene synthases from lavender (*Lavandula angustifolia*). *Archives of Biochemistry and Biophysics* 465 (2007): 417–429.

Lane, A., Boecklemann, A., Woronuk, G. et al. A genomics resource for investigating regulation of essential oil production in *Lavandula angustifolia*. *Planta* 231 (2010): 835–845.

Lange, B.-M., and Ahkami, A. Metabolic engineering of plant monoterpenes, sesquiterpenes and diterpenes: Current status and future opportunities. *Plant Biotechnology Journal* 11 (2013): 169–196.

Lange, B.-M., and Turner, G.-W. Terpenoid biosynthesis in trichomes: Current status and future opportunities. *Plant Biotechnology Journal* 11 (2013): 2–22.

Lange, B.-M., Wildung, M.-R., Stauber, E.-J. et al. Probing essential oil biosynthesis and secretion by functional evaluation of expressed sequence tags from mint glandular trichomes. *Proceedings of the National Academy of Sciences USA* 97 (2000): 2934–2939.

Lange, B.M., Mahmoud, S.S., Wildung, M.R. et al. Improving peppermint essential oil yield and composition by metabolic engineering. *Proceedings of the National Academy of Sciences USA* 108 (2011): 16944–16949.

Leupin, R.-E., Leupin, M., Ehret, C. et al. Compact callus induction and plant regeneration of a non-flowering vetiver from Java. *Plant Cell, Tissue and Organ Culture* 62 (2000): 115–123.

Lima, A.S., Schimmel, J., Lukas, B. et al. Genomic characterization, molecular cloning and expression analysis of two terpene synthases from *Thymus caespititius* (Lamiaceae). *Planta* 238 (2013): 191–204.

Lin, Y.-L., Lee, Y.-R., and Huang, W.-K. Characterization of S-(+)-linalool synthase from several provenances of *Cinnamomum osmophloeum*. *Tree Genetics and Genomes* 10 (2014): 75–86.

Lucker, J., El Tamer, M.K., Schwab, W. et al. Monoterpene biosynthesis in lemon (*Citrus limon*): cDNA isolation and functional analysis of four monoterpene synthases. *European Journal of Biochemistry* 269 (2002): 3160–3171.

Lukmanul Hakkim, F., Kalyani, S., Essa, M. et al. Production of rosmarinic in *Ocimum sanctum* (L.) cell suspension cultures by the influence of growth regulators. *International Journal of Biological and Medical Research* 2 (2011): 1158–1161.

Lupien, S., Karp, F., Wildung, M. et al. Regiospecific cytochrome P450 limonene hydroxylases from mint (*Mentha*) species: cDNA isolation, characterization, and functional expression of (–)-4S-limonene-3-hydroxylase and (–)-4S-limonene-6-hydroxylase. *Archives of Biochemistry and Biophysics* 368 (1999): 181–192.

Mahmoud, S.S., and Croteau, R.B. Strategies for transgenic manipulation of monoterpene biosynthesis in plants. *Trends in Plant Science* 7 (2002): 366–373.

Mahmoud, S.S., and Croteau, R.B. Menthofuran regulates essential oil biosynthesis in peppermint by controlling a downstream monoterpene reductase. *Proceedings of the National Academy of Sciences USA* 100 (2003): 14481–14486.

Mahmoud, S.S., Williams, M., and Croteau, R.B. Cosuppression of limonene-3-hydroxylase in peppermint promotes accumulation of limonene in the essential oil. *Phytochemistry* 65 (2004): 547–554.

Mathew, R., and Sankar, D. Comparison of somatic embryo formation in *Ocimum Basilicum* L., *Ocimum Sanctum* L. & *Ocimum Gratissimum* L. *International Journal of Pharma and Biosciences* 2 (2011): 356–367.

Mathur, A.-K., Ahuja, P.-S., Pandey, B. et al. Screening and evaluation of somaclonal variations for quantitative and qualitative traits in an aromatic grass, *Cymbopogon winterianus* Jowitt. *Plant Breeding* 101 (1988): 321–334.

McCaskill, D., Gershenzon, J., and Croteau, R. Morphology and monoterpene biosynthetic capabilities of secretory-cell clusters isolated from glandular trichomes of peppermint (*Mentha-piperita* L.). *Planta* 187 (1992): 445–454.

Meena, M. Regeneration of patchouli (*Pogostemon cablin* Benth.) plants from leaf and node callus, and evaluation after growth in the field. *Plant Cell Reproduction* 15 (1996): 991–994.

Mendes, M.-D., Barroso, J.G., Oliveira, M.M. et al. Identification and characterization of a second isogene encoding γ-terpinene synthase in *Thymus caespititius*. *Journal of Plant Physiology* 171 (2014): 1017–1027.

Mendoza-Poudereux, I., Muñoz-Bertomeu J., Navarro A. et al. Enhanced levels of S-linalool by metabolic engineering of the terpenoid pathway in spike lavender leaves. *Metabolic Engineering* 23 (2014): 136–144.

Misawa, N. Pathway engineering for functional isoprenoids. *Current Opinion in Biotechnology* 22 (2011): 627–633.

Misic, D., Grubisic D., and Konjevic, R. Micropropagation of *Salvia brachyodon* through nodal explants. *Biologia Plantarum* 50 (2006): 473–476.

Muñoz-Bertomeu, J., Arrillaga, I., Ros, R. et al. Up-regulation of 1-deoxy-D-xylulose-5-phosphate synthase enhances production of essential oils in transgenic spike lavender. *Plant Physiology* 142 (2006): 890–900.

Muñoz-Bertomeu, J., Sales, E., Ros, R. et al. Up-regulation of an N-terminal truncated 3-hydroxy-3-methylglutaryl CoA reductase enhances production of essential oils and sterols in transgenic *Lavandula latifolia*. *Journal of Plant Biotechnology* 5 (2007): 746–758.

Muñoz-Bertomeu, J., Ros, R., Arrillaga, I. et al. Expression of spearmint limonene synthase in transgenic spike lavender results in an altered monoterpene composition in developing leaves. *Metabolic Engineering* 10 (2008): 166–177.

Nabila Karam, S., Jawad, M., Arikat, A. et al. Growth and rosmarinic acid accumulation in callus, cell suspension, and root cultures of wild *Salvia fruticosa*. *Plant Cell Tissue Organ Culture* 73 (2003): 117–121.

Nagalakshmi, U., Wang, Z., Waern, K. et al. The transcriptional landscape of the yeast genome defined by RNA sequencing. *Science* 320 (2008): 1344–1349.

Nasare, P.N., and Choudhary, A.D. Early flowering and high yielding mutants in *Ocimum sanctum* linn. *Indian Streams Research Journal* 1 (2011): 202–204.

Ohara, K., Matsunaga, E., Nanto, K. et al. Monoterpene engineering in a woody plant *Eucalyptus camaldulensis* using a limonene synthase cDNA. *Plant Biotechnology Journal* 8 (2010): 28–37.

Olofsson, L., Lundgren, A., and Brodelius, P.E. Trichome isolation with and without fixation using laser microdissection and pressure catapulting followed by RNA amplification: Expression of genes of terpene metabolism in apical and sub-apical trichome cells of *Artemisia annua* L. *Plant Science* 183 (2012): 9–13.

Padmanabhan, C., Sukumar, S., and Sreerangaswamy, S.R. Patchouli plants differentiated *in vitro* from stem tip and callus cultures. *Current Science* 50 (1981): 195–197.

Passinho-Soares, H.-C., Meira, P.R., David, J.-P. et al. Volatile organic compounds obtained by *in vitro* callus cultivation of *Plectranthus ornatus* Codd. (Lamiaceae). *Molecules* 18 (2013): 10320–10333.

Paul, A., Thapa, G., Basu, A. et al. Rapid plant regeneration, analysis of genetic fidelity and essential aromatic oil content of micropropagated plants of patchouli, *Pogostemon cablin* (Blanco) Benth.: An industrially important aromatic plant. *Industrial Crops and Products* 32 (2010): 366–374.

Pavlov, A., Panchev, I., and Ilieva, M. Nutrient medium optimization for rosmarinic acid production by *Lavandula vera* MM cell suspension. *Biotechnology Progress* 16 (2000): 668–670.

Pavlov, A., Georgiev, M., and Ilieva, M. Optimisation of rosmarinic acid production by *Lavandula vera* MM plant cell suspension in a laboratory bioreactor. *Biotechnology Progress* 21 (2005): 394–396.

Perianez-Rodriguez, J., Manzano, C., and Moreno-Risueno, M.-A. Post-embryonic organogenesis and plant regeneration from tissues: Two sides of the same coin? *Frontiers in Plant Science* 5 (2014): 219–225.

Pistelli, L., Noccioli, C., D'Angiolillo, F. et al. Composition of volatile in micropropagated and field grown aromatic plants from Tuscany Islands. *Acta Biochimica Polonica* 60 (2013): 43–50.

Qian, J., Song, J., Gao, H. et al. The complete chloroplast genome sequence of the medicinal plant *Salvia miltiorrhiza*. *PLoS One* 8 (2013): e57607.

Rastogi, S., Meena, S., Bhattacharya, A. et al. *De novo* sequencing and comparative analysis of holy and sweet basil transcriptomes. *BMC Genomics* 15 (2014): 588.

Ravindra, N.S., Ramesh, S.R., Kumar Gupta, M. et al. Evaluation of somaclonal variation for genetic improvement of patchouli (*Pogostemon patchouli*), an exclusively vegetatively propagated aromatic plant. *Journal of Crop Science and Biotechnology* 15 (2012): 1–33.

Rekha, K., Bhan, M.K., and Dhar, A.K. Development of erect plant mutant with improved patchouli alcohol in patchouli (*Pogostemon cablin* [Blanco] Benth). *Journal of Essential Oil Research* 21 (2009): 135–137.

Ringer, K.L., McConkey, M.E., Davis, E.M. et al. Monoterpene double-bond reductases of the (–)-menthol biosynthetic pathway: Isolation and characterization of cDNAs encoding (–)-isopiperitenone reductase and (+)-pulegone reductase of peppermint. *Archives of Biochemistry and Biophysics* 418 (2003): 80–92.

Ringer, K.L., Davis, E.M., and Croteau, R. Monoterpene metabolism: Cloning, expression and characterization of (–)-isopiperitenol/(–)-carveol dehydrogenase of peppermint and spearmint. *Plant Physiology* 137 (2005): 863–872.

Rios-Estepa, R., Turner, G.W., Lee, J.M. et al. A systems biology approach identifies the biochemical mechanisms regulating monoterpenoid essential oil composition in peppermint. *Proceedings of the National Academy of Sciences USA* 105 (2008): 2818–2823.

Rodríguez-Concepción, M. Early steps in isoprenoid biosynthesis: Multilevel regulation of the supply of common precursors in plant cells. *Phytochemical Review* 5 (2006): 1–15.

Rodríguez-Concepción, M., and Boronat, A. Elucidation of the methylerythritol phosphate pathway for isoprenoid biosynthesis in bacteria and plastids: A metabolic milestone achieved through genomics. *Plant Physiology* 130 (2002): 1079–1089.

Sangduen, N., and Prasertsongskun, S. Regeneration and application: From suspension cultured-derived inflorescence of *Vetiveria zizanioides* (L.) Nash. to selection of herbicide resistant cells. *Australian Journal of Technology* 12 (2009): 135–148.

Sangwan, N.S. Transcriptomics in aid to the establishment of secondary metabolic pathways in non-model plants. *Next Generation Sequencing and Application* 1 (2014): e101.

Sarker, L.S. Cloning of *Lavandula* essential oil biosynthetic genes. Dissertation or thesis, University of British Columbia, 2013.

Sarker, L.S., Galata, M., Demissie, Z.-A. et al. Molecular cloning and functional characterization of borneol dehydrogenase from the glandular trichomes of *Lavandula* × *intermedia*. *Archives of Biochemistry and Biophysics* 528 (2012): 163–170.

Sarker, L.-S., Demissie, Z.A., and Mahmoud, S.-S. Cloning of a sesquiterpene synthase from *Lavandula* × *intermedia* glandular trichomes. *Planta* 238 (2013): 983–989.

Schilmiller, A.L., Last, R.L., and Pichersky, E. Harnessing plant trichome biochemistry for the production of useful compounds. *Plant Journal* 54 (2008): 702–711.

Silva, S., Sato, A., Lage, C.L.S. et al. Essential oil composition of *Melissa officinalis* L. *in vitro* produced under the influence of growth regulators. *Journal of the Brazilian Chemical Society* 16 (2005): 1387–1390.

Soni, D.R., Sayyad, F.G., and Sodhi, G.K. Micropropagation studies in *Lavandula aungustifolia*. *Discovery Biotechnology* 4 (2013): 34–37.

Spyropoulou, E.A., Haring, M.-A., and Schuurink, R.C. RNA sequencing on *Solanum lycopersicum* trichomes identifies transcription factors that activate terpene synthase promoters. *BMC Genomics* 15 (2014): 402.

Su, Y.H., and Zhang, X.S. The hormonal control of regeneration in plants. *Current Topics in Developmental Biology* 108 (2014): 35–69.

Sugimura, Y., Padayhag, B.F., Ceniza, M.S. et al. Essential oil production increased by using virus-free patchouli plants derived from meristem-tip culture. *Plant Pathology* 44 (2007): 510–515.

Takahashi, S., Yeo, Y., Greenhagen, B.-T. et al. Metabolic engineering of sesquiterpene metabolism in yeast. *Biotechnology and Bioengineering* 97 (2007): 170–181.

Thanasomboon, R., Warahob, D., Cheevadhanarakc, S. et al. Construction of synthetic *Escherichia coli* producing s-linalool. *Procedia Computer Science* 11 (2012): 88– 95.

Tissier, A. Glandular trichomes: What comes after expressed sequence tags? *Plant Journal* 70 (2012): 51–68.

Tsuro, M., and Asada, S. Differential expression of limonene synthase gene affects production and composition of essential oils in leaf and floret of transgenic lavandin (*Lavandula 3 intermedia Emeric ex Loisel.*). *Plant Biotechnology Reports* 8 (2014): 193–201.

Tsuro, V.M., Inoue, M., and Kameoka, H. Variation in essential oil components in regenerated lavender (*Lavandula vera* DC) plants. *Scientia Horticulturae* 88 (2001): 309–317.

Turner, G.-W., Gershenzon, J., and Croteau, R. Development of peltate glandular trichomes of peppermint. *Plant Physiology* 124 (2000): 665–679.

Vaccaro, M., Malafronte, N., Alfieri, M. et al. Enhanced biosynthesis of bioactive abietane diterpenes by overexpressing *AtDXS* or *AtDXR* genes in *Salvia sclarea* hairy roots. *Plant Cell Tissue Organ Cultures* 119 (2014): 65–77.

Wagner, G.J. Secreting glandular trichomes: More than just hairs. *Plant Physiology* 96 (1991): 675–679.

Wagner, G.J., Wang, E., and Shepherd, R.W. New approaches for studying and exploiting an old protuberance, the plant trichome. *Annals of Botany* 93 (2004): 3–11.

Wan Nurul Hidayah, W.A., Norrizah, J.S., Sharifah Aminah, S.M. et al. Effect of medium strength and hormones concentration on regeneration of *Pogostemon cablin* using nodes explant. *Asian Journal of Biotechnology* 4 (2012): 46–52.

Wise, M.L., and Croteau, R. Biosythesis of monoterpenes. In D.E. Cane (ed.), *Comprehensive Natural Products Chemistry*, Vol. 2: *Isoprenoids Including Carotenoids and Steroids*. Elsevier, Oxford, 1999, pp. 97–153.

Wise, M.-L., Savage, T.-J., Katahira, E. et al. Monoterpene synthases from common sage (*Salvia officinalis*): cDNA isolation, characterization, and functional expression of (+)-sabinene synthase, 1,8-cineole synthase, and (+)-bornyl diphosphate synthase. *Journal of Biological Chemistry* 273 (1998): 14891–14899.

Wu, S., Schalk, M., Clark, A. et al. Redirection of cytosolic or plastidic isoprenoid precursors elevates terpene production in plants. *Nature Biotechnology* 24 (2006): 1441–1447.

Xiao, M., Zhanga, Y., Chenc, X. et al. Transcriptome analysis based on next-generation sequencing of non-model plants producing specialized metabolites of biotechnological interest. *Journal of Biotechnology* 166 (2013): 122–134.

Xie, Z., Kapteyn, J., and Gang, D.R. A systems biology investigation of the MEP/terpenoid and shikimate/phenylpropanoid pathways points to multiple levels of metabolic control in sweet basil glandular trichomes. *Plant Journal* 54 (2008): 349–361.

Yang, L., Ding, G., Lin, H. et al. Transcriptome analysis of medicinal plant *Salvia miltiorrhiza* and identification of genes related to tanshinone biosynthesis. *PLoS One* 8 (11) (2013): e80464.

Yeo, S., Nybo, E., Chittiboyina, A.G. et al. Functional identification of valerena-1,10-diene synthase, a terpene synthase catalyzing a unique chemical cascade in the biosynthesis of biologically active sesquiterpenes in *Valeriana officinalis*. *Journal of Biological Chemistry* 288 (2013): 3163–3173.

6 Extraction, Sample Preparation, and Analytical Methods for Quality Issues of Essential Oils

Paola Montoro, Milena Masullo, Sonia Piacente, and Cosimo Pizza

CONTENTS

Aromatherapy is the therapeutic use of essential oils to cure, mitigate, or prevent diseases, infections, and indispositions mainly by inhalation, but also by the skin (Buchbauer et al., 1993; Lee et al., 2012). In recent years there has been increasing attention to screening plants to study the biological activities of their essential oils from the chemical and pharmacological points of view.

Essential oils are complex mixtures made up of many compounds whose contents can be influenced by several factors. Each of these constituents contributes to the beneficial or adverse effects of these oils. Therefore, a deep knowledge of the essential oil composition is necessary for their therapeutic application (Lahlou, 2004). The presence, yield, and composition of secondary metabolites in plants, and specifically in essential oils, can be affected in a number of ways, from their formation in the plant to their isolation. Several of the factors of influence have been studied, in particular for commercially important crops, to optimize the cultivation conditions and time of harvest and to obtain higher yields of high-quality essential oils.

The factors that determine the chemical variability and yield of essential oils include (1) physiological variations, (2) environmental conditions, (3) geographic variations, (4) genetic factors and evolution, and (5) political and social conditions (Figueiredo et al., 2008). The quality of plant raw materials can also be influenced by human adulterations due to dishonesty or unscrupulous operators. Probable errors could be accidental botanical substitution or intentional botanical substitution. The variability in the content and concentrations of the constituents of plant material, along with the range of extraction techniques and processing steps used by different manufacturers, results in marked variability in the content and quality of commercially available herbal products. Thus, the quality control of essential oils is necessary to ensure the genuineness of the product, the shelf life, and the storage conditions (Bonaccorsi et al., 1999).

In the specific case of essential oils used for aromatherapy, the quality control is an important issue because it guarantees purity, safety, and efficacy. There is a specific term used in this context, *therapeutic grade*, but it is not a label from the Food and Drug Administration (FDA); it is only a market certification.

Recently, European Medicinal Agency published "Reflection Paper on Quality of Essential Oils as Active Substances in Herbal Medicinal Products/Traditional Herbal Medicinal Products," which discusses the importance of and the way to gain quality for essential oils used as active pharmaceutical ingredients or herbal medicinal products. The conclusion, however, is that there is a need for specific guidance, because the current guidance does not fully address the question of essential oils (EMA/HMCP/84789/2013).

Essential oils are complex mixtures that act directly on the gustatory and olfactory receptors in the mouth and nose, leading to taste and aroma responses.

Interacting with the human senses, essential oils have applications in food, preservatives, medicines, symbolic articles in religious and social ceremonies, and remedies to modify behavior. In most cases, essential oils gain widespread acceptance as multifunctional agents due to their strong stimulation of the human gustatory (taste) and olfactory (smell) senses.

Based on histories of use of selected plants and plant products that strongly impact the senses, it is not unexpected that society would bestow powers to heal, cure diseases, and spur desirable emotions in the effort to improve the human condition, often with only a limited understanding or acknowledgment of the toxic effects associated with high doses of these plant products. The *natural* origin of these products and their long history of use by humans have, in part, mitigated concerns as to whether these products work or are safe under conditions of intended use. The adverse effects resulting from the use of these products are often unknown.

In the absence of information concerning efficacy and safety, recommendations for the quantity and quality of natural product to be consumed remain ambiguous. However, when the intended use is as a flavor or fragrance that is subject to governmental regulation, effective and safe levels of use are defined by fundamental biological limits and careful risk assessment.

The safety control of an essential oil is performed in the context of all available data for groups of known constituents and the group of unknown constituents, and any potential interactions that may occur by the essential oil when used in combination with other essential oils, or other natural substances.

Adams and Taylor proposed in 2010 a chemically based approach to the safety evaluation of an essential oil. The approach depends on a quantitative analysis of the chemical constituents in the essential oil. The chemical constituents are assigned to well-defined congeneric groups that are established based on biochemical and toxicologic information, and this is evaluated in the context of intake of the congeneric group resulting from consumption (by olfactory or gustative sense) of the essential oil. The overall objective in safety of essential oils is the knowledge of their chemical composition (Adams and Taylor, 2010).

Sometimes, during the extraction processes, well-known contaminants of synthetic or artificial origin (e.g., plasticizers, chemicals used for solvent stabilization, and butylated hydroxytoluene) are identified as constituents of essential oils and considered to be native plant metabolites. The importance of this problem should be considered since such compounds are still repeatedly being reported as natural products (Radulovic and Blagojevic, 2012). Radulovic investigated some of the most common semivolatile contaminants that could originate from the solvents used during the isolation procedures and analyses of essential oils (Radulovic and Blagojevic, 2012).

6.1 EXTRACTION AND SAMPLE PREPARATION

6.1.1 TREATMENT OF SAMPLE

The first step in the qualitative–quantitative analysis of essential oils is the sample preparation procedure, which has the aim to effectively and rapidly remove the analyte from its matrix. Some harvested plant material may require special treatment of the biomass before oil extraction, for example, grinding or chipping, breaking or cutting up into smaller fragments, and sometimes just drying. In some cases, fermentation of the biomass should precede oil extraction. Drying can be achieved simply by spreading the biomass on the ground where wind movement affects the drying process. Drying can also be carried out by the use of appropriate drying equipment. Drying, too, can affect the quality of the essential oil. Seeds and fruits of the families Apiaceae, Piperaceae, and Myristicaceae usually require grinding up prior to steam distillation. In many cases, the seed has to be dried before comminution takes place. The finer the material is ground, the better will be the oil yield and, owing to shorter distillation times, the quality of the oil. In order to reduce losses of volatiles by evaporation during the comminution of the seed or fruit, the grinding can also be carried out underwater, preferably in a closed apparatus, or cooling the sample. In this respect, several authors have studied the effect of cooling during grinding (Masango, 2005; Meghwal and Goswami, 2013).

Heartwood samples have to be reduced to a very fine powder prior to steam distillation in order to achieve complete recovery of the essential oil. In some cases, coarse chipping of the wood is adequate for efficient essential oil extraction. Plant material containing small branches as well as foliage, which includes pine needles, has to be coarsely chopped up prior to steam distillation. Mechanized harvesting methods automatically affect the chopping up of the biomass. This also reduces the volume of the biomass, thus increasing the quantity of material that can be packed into the still and making the process more economical.

The choice of extraction technique is frequently decided upon consideration of operating costs, simplicity of operation, amount of organic solvent required, and sample throughput. The traditional extraction methods (methods recommended in pharmacopeias, e.g., steam and water distillation, Soxhlet extraction, maceration, percolation, expression, and cold fat extraction) have several shortcomings, including long extraction time and large consumption of solvents, cooling water, and electric energy (Dawidowicz and Wianowska, 2005). It must here again be stressed that only the product obtained by hydrodistillation or steam distillation can be called essential oil (of course, with the exception of cold expression for citrus fruits) (Rubiolo et al., 2010).

6.1.2 EXTRACTION TECHNIQUES

6.1.2.1 Expression

The term *expression* refers to any physical process in which the essential oil glands in the peel are crushed or broken to release the oil. Some volatile oils cannot be distilled without decomposition and thus are usually obtained by expression (lemon oil, orange oil) or by other mechanical means. Among the essential oil extraction methods, expression is probably the oldest. It is used almost exclusively for the production of essential oil from *Citrus* species. Hydrodistillation of *Citrus* fruits yields poor quality oils owing to chemical reactions that can be attributed to heat and acid-initiated degradation of some of the unstable fruit volatiles. Furthermore, some of the terpenic hydrocarbons and esters contained in the peel oils are also sensitive to heat and oxygen. One exception to this exists. Lime oil of commerce can be either cold pressed or steam distilled. The chemical compositions of these two types of oil, as well as their odors, differ significantly from each other. The machines that treat only the peel after removal of juice and pulp are called *sfumatrici*, while those that process the whole fruit are known as *pelatrici*, and both procedures need to obtain the oil from the juice.

6.1.2.2 Enfleurage

Enfleurage, the extraction of elusive floral essential oils with the help of a lipophilic carrier (grease), is widely used in the perfume industry (Eltz et al., 2007). Fat possesses a high power of absorption and, when brought in contact with fragrant flowers, readily absorbs the perfume emitted. This principle, methodically applied on a large scale, constitutes enfleurage. During the entire period of harvest, batches of freshly picked flowers are strewn over the surface of a specially prepared fat base (corps), let there, and then replaced by fresh flowers. Thereafter, the oil is extracted from the fat with alcohol and then isolated.

The long enfleurage time could be reduced by the immersion of petals in molten fat heated at 45°C–60°C for 1 to 2 h, depending on the plant species. It is mainly used for highly delicate flowers whose physiological activities are lost rapidly after their harvest.

6.1.2.3 Hydrodistillation and Steam Distillation

Hydrodistillation (HD), representing the most usual method for the extraction of the essential oil content, is described in pharmacopoeias. In hydrodistillation, the aromatic plant material is packed in a still and water is added and brought to a boil. The laboratory apparatus recommended for hydrodistillations is the Clevenger system. In steam distillation (SD), live steam is injected into the plant charge. Due to hot water and steam, the essential oil is freed from the oil glands in the plant tissue. The vapor mixture of water and oil is condensed by indirect cooling with water. From the condenser, distillate flows into a separator, where oil separates automatically from the distillate water.

The term *hydrodiffusion* refers to the diffusion of essential oils and hot water through plant membranes. In steam distillation, to ease the steam to penetrate the dry cell membranes, the comminution of the plant material is required. To obtain the best quality oil, distillation must be done at low temperatures. The temperature in steam distillation is determined entirely by the operating pressure, whereas in water distillation and in water and steam distillation, the operating pressure is usually atmospheric. Hydrodistillation and steam distillation methods are known to be the most common methods for the extraction of essential oils. It is known that using these conventional methods, the quality of the essential oil extracted should be extremely damaged. Losses of some volatile compounds, low extraction efficiency, degradation of unsaturated or ester compounds through thermal or hydrolytic effects, and toxic solvent residue in the extract may be encountered using these extraction methods (Bayramoglu et al., 2008). Of course, nonvolatile aroma-active compounds are not extracted by hydrodistillation. On the other hand, highly volatile components as well as water-soluble components can get lost during hydrodistillation (Richter and Schellenberg, 2007). Furthermore, hydrodistillation is a very time-consuming method and therefore not useful, especially for the screening of very large quantities of plant samples for their aroma compounds' composition.

Therefore, new technologies have been developed for obtaining essential oils.

6.1.2.4 Soxhlet Extraction

Soxhlet extraction (hot continuous extraction) has been a classical method for decades in the extraction of organic compounds from solid sample. It was developed by von Soxhlet in 1879 (Luque de Castro and Priego-Capote, 2010). Soxhlet extraction is a general and well-established technique that surpasses in performance other conventional extraction techniques, except for the extraction of thermolabile compounds. The contact between the solvent and the substrate in Soxhlet extraction is different from those in hydrodistillation and supercritical fluid extraction. In conventional Soxhlet extraction, the sample is placed in a thimble holder and the solvent is heated to reflux; the vapor passes through a bypass arm to reach the condenser. Then the solvent drips down into the thimble and diffuses into the substrate matrix. The extractable substances then dissolve into the solvent. The mixture of the solvent and extracted substances then diffuses from the substrate matrix back to the bulk solvent. Once the mixture level in the extractor reaches the top of the siphon arm, the solvent and the extract are siphoned back into the lower flask. Thus, Soxhlet extraction is a batch extraction process (Zhao and Zhang, 2014). This operation is repeated more times, and in this way, fresh solvent comes in contact with the plant material a number of times, until the plant material is completely extracted. This performance makes Soxhlet a hybrid continuous–discontinuous technique. In fact, since the extractant acts stepwise, the assembly operates as a batch system; however, extractant is recirculated through the sample, so the system operates in a continuous manner (Luque de Castro and Garcia-Ayuso, 1998; Luque de Castro and Priego-Capote, 2010). The final extract in the distillation still, which is rich in active principle, is concentrated and the solvent is recovered. Worldwide, most of the solvent extraction units are based on the Soxhlet principle with recycling of solvents. Basic equipment for a solvent extraction unit consists of a drug holder–extractor, a solvent storage vessel, a reboiler kettle, a condenser, a breather system (to minimize solvent loss), and supporting structures like a boiler, a refrigerated chilling unit, and a vacuum unit.

Several studies compared the results of the Soxhlet extraction of essential oils with those of other techniques, such as hydrodistillation, steam distillation, super-heated water extraction, and supercritical fluid extraction (Galhiane et al., 2006; Glisic et al., 2010; Kotnik et al., 2007; Ozel and Kaymaz, 2004; Zhao and Zhang, 2014).

The main advantages of conventional Soxhlet lie in the displacement of transfer equilibrium by repeatedly bringing fresh solvent into contact with the solid matrix, in maintaining a relatively high extraction temperature with heat from the distillation flask, and in there being no required filtration of the extract. Moreover, the sample throughput can be increased by simultaneous extraction in parallel, since the basic equipment is inexpensive. It allows us to extract more sample mass than with microwave extraction and supercritical fluid extraction.

The main drawbacks of Soxhlet extraction compared to other techniques for solid sample preparation are the long time required for extraction and the large amount of extractant wasted, the thermal decomposition of thermolabile target species, and the inability of agitation, which is not possible in the conventional Soxhlet device. In addition, the large amounts of extractant require an evaporation–concentration step after extraction. Luque de Castro compared the Soxhlet technique with ultrasound-assisted extraction (UAE), an advisable technique for thermolabile analytes. Better reproducibility and efficiency and less sample manipulation are the advantages of Soxhlet extraction versus UAE, but at the expense of a longer extraction time (Luque de Castro and Garcia-Ayuso, 1998).

Some modifications of conventional Soxhlet extraction have been developed. Soxhlet extraction under high pressure places the extractor in a cylindrical stainless steel autoclave or is performed by the use of supercritical fluid–Soxhlet extractors. The particularity of high-pressure Soxhlet extraction is that the extractants do not reach supercritical conditions.

6.1.2.5 Microwave-Assisted Extraction

Microwave-assisted extraction (MAE) has drawn significant research attention in medicinal plant research, due to its special heating mechanism, moderate capital cost, and good performance under atmospheric conditions (Eskilsson and Bjorklund, 2000).

MAE systems are classified into multimode system and focused-mode system (monomode). The multimode system allows random dispersion of microwave radiation in a cavity by a mode stirrer, while the focused system (monomode) allows focused microwave radiation on a restricted zone in a cavity. Usually, the multimode system is associated with high pressure, while the monomode system is employed under atmospheric operating pressure, but can also run at high pressure. Regarding the pressure, MAE systems are classified as closed systems and open systems, referring to the systems that operate above atmospheric pressure and under atmospheric pressure, respectively (Dean and Xiong, 2000; Luque-Garcia and Luque de Castro, 2003). In a closed MAE system, the extractions are carried out in a sealed vessel with different modes of microwave radiations, under uniform microwave heating. High working pressure and temperature of the system allow fast and efficient extraction. Recent advancements in the closed system have led to the development of high-pressure microwave-assisted extraction (HPMAE). The increase in temperature and pressure accelerates microwave-assisted extraction due to the ability of extraction solvent to absorb microwave energy (Wang et al., 2008). An open MAE system is considered more suitable for extracting thermolabile compounds. This system has higher sample throughput, and more solvent can be added to the system at any time during the process. Basically, an open system operates at more mild conditions, like atmospheric conditions, and only part of the vessel is directly exposed to the propagation of microwave radiation (monomode). The upper part of the vessel is connected to a reflux unit to condense any vaporized solvent. Besides that, multimode radiation can also be employed in an open MAE system with the reflux unit.

The factors that may influence the performance of MAE are solvent nature, solvent-to-feed ratio, extraction time, microwave power, temperature, sample characteristics, and effect of stirring. It is important to understand the effects and interactions of these factors on the MAE processes.

The characteristics of the sample also affect the performance of MAE. The extraction sample is usually dried, powdered, and sieved into fine powder prior to the extraction for optimum extraction yield. Too small particle size would cause difficulty in separating the extract from the residue, and additional cleanup steps may have to be employed. Moreover, if the sample is treated by solvent for 90 min before extraction, this can enhance the heating efficiency of MAE, promote diffusion, and improve mass transfer of active compounds to the solvent (Pan et al., 2003). From the discussion presented, it is clear that particle size, moisture content, and solvent pretreatment have considerable effects on the sample matrix for efficient extraction. Poor extraction yield due to thermal degradation and oxidation of some active compounds has led to the development of more efficient MAE.

6.1.2.6 Ultrasonic Microwave-Assisted Extraction

Enhancement of the mass transfer mechanism in extraction can be achieved by another type of MAE known as ultrasonic microwave-assisted extraction (UMAE). An additional ultrasonic wave emitted by UMAE intensifies the mass transfer mechanism as the combined microwave and ultrasonic waves provide high momentum and energy to rupture the plant cell and elute the active compounds to the extraction solvent (Chen et al., 2010; Yang and Zhang, 2008). As a result, extraction proceeds with shorter extraction time and lower solvent consumption. This technique has been employed in the extraction of essential oil from *Schisandra chinensis* Baill fruits (Cheng et al., 2014).

6.1.2.7 Solvent-Free Microwave Extraction

The solvent-free microwave extraction (SFME) apparatus is an original combination of microwave heating and dry distillation at atmospheric pressure. SFME was conceived for laboratory-scale applications in the extraction of essential oils from different kinds of aromatic plants. Based on a relatively simple principle, this method involves placing plant material in a microwave reactor, without any added solvent or water (Wang et al., 2006). The internal heating of the *in situ* water within the plant material distends the plant cells and leads to rupture of the glands and oleiferous receptacles. This process thus frees essential oil, which is evaporated by the *in situ* water of the plant material. A cooling system outside the microwave oven condenses the distillate continuously. The excess water is refluxed to the extraction vessel in order to restore the *in situ* water to the plant material. SFME significantly reduces extraction time compared to conventional methods, from a few hours to 20–30 min for essential oil extraction (Deng et al., 2006a,b). The SFME technique has been compared with the conventional method, hydrodistillation, in the extraction of essential oils from aerial parts of aromatic herbs, for example, basil (*Ocimum basilicum* L.), garden mint (*Mentha crispa* L.), and thyme (*Thymus vulgaris* L.), belonging to the Labiatae family. Substantially higher amounts of oxygenated compounds and lower amounts of monoterpene hydrocarbons were present in the essential oils of the aromatic plants extracted by SFME in comparison with HD. Results showed that SFME provides more valuable essential oils, offering important advantages, such as shorter extraction times (30 min for the SFME method against 4.5 h for hydro-distillation), substantial energy savings, and a reduced environmental burden (less CO_2 rejected in the atmosphere) (Lucchesi et al., 2004). Moreover, this technique, compared with hydrodistillation, has been employed in the extraction of essential oils of *Calamintha nepeta* (Riela et al., 2008), *Laurus nobilis* (Nehir et al., 2014), and *Rosmarinus officinalis* (Filly et al., 2014) with the same results. SFME can be improved by introducing carbonyl iron powder. Enhanced SFME can extract essential oil from *Cuminum cyminum* and *Zanthoxylum bungeanum* Maxim in 30 min compared to the conventional SFME of 50 min, microwave-assisted hydrodistillation of 90 min, and HD of 180 min (Wang et al., 2006).

6.1.2.8 Microwave-Assisted Hydrodistillation

Microwave-assisted hydrodistillation (MAHD) is an advanced hydrodistillation technique utilizing a microwave oven in the extraction process. It has been developed and used for the extraction of essential oils from *Xylopia aromatica* and *Lippia alba* (Mill.) (Stashenko et al., 2004a,b). MAHD has also been reported for the extraction of essential oils from *Cuminum cyminum* L. and *Zanthoxylum bungeanum* Maxim (Wang et al., 2006).

6.1.2.9 Ultrasound-Assisted Extraction

Ultrasonic vibrations are the source of energy facilitating the release of analytes from the sample matrix (Priego-Capote and Luque de Castro, 2004). Extremely high temperatures and pressures can be produced by the rapid compression of gases and vapors within the numerous tiny bubbles created by the cavitation effect of ultrasound in liquid media and the mechanical rupture of solids. High temperature is conductive to the solubility and diffusivity of analytes, and high pressure can strengthen the penetration of the solvent and the mass transfer of the adsorbed analytes from the sample into aqueous solution (Feng et al., 2014). Ultrasound supplies sufficient energy to disrupt oil-containing glands in order to release essential oil at reduced temperatures. This is beneficial in protecting the essential oil components that are sensitive to heat. Moreover, ultrasound provides an intensified mass transfer between two immiscible phases and facilitates emulsification; hence, it improves liquid–liquid microextraction (Sereshti et al., 2012).

Compared with traditional solvent extraction methods, UAE improves extraction efficiency and rate, reduces extraction temperature, and increases the selection ranges of the solvents. In comparison with supercritical fluid extraction (SFE) and MAE, the equipment is relatively simpler (Kim et al., 2009; Sun et al., 2010) and inexpensive (Sereshti et al., 2012). The other advantages of ultrasound in extraction from plants are mass transfer intensification, cell disruption, improved solvent penetration, and capillary effect (Yang and Zhang, 2008). The type of application of ultrasound depends on the frequency domain. High frequencies (MHz range) lead to product degradation, whereas low frequencies (KHz range) are applied for assisting processes such as emulsification, extraction, filtration, and cell destruction (Sereshti et al., 2012). UAE is used for the extraction of analytes from solid samples, applying ultrasound radiation in a water bath or with other devices, such as probes, sonoreactors, or microplate horns (Tadeo et al., 2010). The most available and cheapest source of ultrasound irradiation is the ultrasonic bath (Tadeo et al., 2010), but at present, a more efficient system using a cylindrical powerful probe for the sonication of samples has been developed (Tadeo et al., 2010). Up to now, this method has been successfully applied in extracting essential oils (Allaf et al., 2013; Clodoveo et al., 2013; Darjazi, 2011; Feng et al., 2014; Liu et al., 2012; Sereshti et al., 2012; Sun et al., 2014; Yang and Zhang, 2008).

6.1.2.10 Supercritical Fluid Extraction

Among innovative process technologies, supercritical fluid extraction (SFE) is indeed the most widely studied application, chiefly because the dissolving power of supercritical fluids can be adjusted by regulating the pressure and temperature conditions. SFE requires less extraction time, does not produce thermal degradation or solvent contamination of samples, and preserves the natural character of the fresh product (Diaz-Maroto et al., 2002). SFE is generally performed using carbon dioxide (CO_2) for several practical reasons: CO_2 has a moderately low critical pressure (74 bar) and temperature (32°C); is nontoxic, nonflammable, and available in high purity at relatively low cost; and is easily removed from the extract. Supercritical CO_2 has a polarity similar to that of liquid pentane and thus is suitable for extraction of lipophilic compounds. Using high CO_2 densities (pressure: 100–300 bar), terpenes and oxygenated terpenes are completely miscible in supercritical CO_2, but other nonvolatile compounds, such as fatty acids, waxes, phytosterols, and paraffins, can appear in the extract (Diaz-Maroto et al., 2002, Reverchon and De Marco, 2006). Several plants, mainly belonging to the Lamiaceae family, such as oregano, thyme, sage, rosemary, mint, basil, and marjoram, have been subject of SFE to produce essential oils (Stamenic et al., 2014). Thus, taking into account the lipophilic characteristic of plant essential oils, it is obvious that SFE using CO_2 emerged as a suitable environmentally benign alternative to the manufacture of essential oil products (Galhiane et al., 2006; Glisic et al., 2010; Kotnik et al., 2007).

The equipment designed for SFE of solid materials implies a semicontinuous procedure. The raw matter (dried and grinded) to be extracted is generally loaded in a basket, located inside the extractor, allowing a fast charge and discharge of the extraction vessel. From the bottom of the extraction vessel the supercritical solvent is continuously loaded; at the exit of the extractor the supercritical solvent with the solutes extracted flows through a depressurization valve to a first separator where, due to the lower pressure, the extracts are separated from the gaseous solvent and collected. Some SFE devices contain two or more separators to fractionate the extract in two or more fractions (on-line fractionation) by setting suitable temperatures and pressures in the separators (Fornari et al., 2012) (Figure 6.1). This distinct fractionation is suitable when different substances, like waxes, are co-extracted with the essential oil compounds. In the last separator of the cascade decompression system the solvent reaches the pressure of the recirculation system (generally around 4–6 MPa), passes through a filter, and then the gaseous solvent is liquefied and stored in a supplier tank. When the solvent is withdrawn from this tank, it is pumped and then heated up to the desired extraction pressure and temperature. Before pumping, precooling of the solvent is generally required in order to avoid pump cavitation. In some cases, an additional pump is employed to pump a cosolvent in the system as a modifier (Fornari et al., 2012). The nature of the modifier depends on the nature of the solute to be extracted, and therefore a modifier represents a good solvent in its liquid state for the target analyte. The addition of large amounts of modifier will change the critical parameters of the mixture. Modifiers can be introduced as mixed fluids in the pumping system with a second pump and mixing chamber, or by simply injecting the modifier as a liquid into the sample before extraction (the latter has the inconvenience of creating concentration gradients within the matrix). An SFE equipment with continuous feeding and discharging of the solid to obtain the continuous process was studied and developed, but design and operation of this alternative are neither cheap nor simple.

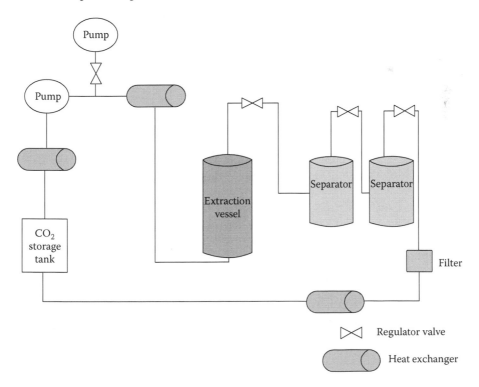

FIGURE 6.1 Supercritical fluid extraction (SFE) system.

6.1.2.10.1   Effect of Matrix Pretreatment and Packing

The particular characteristic of the plant species is a decisive factor in the supercritical extraction kinetics. Recently, Fornari et al. (2012) presented a comparison of the kinetics of the supercritical CO_2 extraction of essential oil from leaves of different plant matrices from the Lamiaceae family: oregano, sage, thyme, rosemary, basil, marjoram, and marigold.

Different factors, such as the particle size, shape, surface area, porosity, moisture, level of extractable solutes, and nature of the matrix, will affect the supercritical fluid extraction results. Regarding the first point, decreasing the particle size of solid matrices leads to a higher surface area, making extraction more efficient (Pourmortazavi and Hajimirsadeghi, 2007). The physical structure of the matrix is of critical importance, as the extraction efficiency is related to the ability of the supercritical fluid to diffuse within the matrix. For that reason, the extraction conditions of the same group of oils may differ from one matrix to another (Pourmortazavi and Hajimirsadeghi, 2007). Essential oil compounds are located inside the vegetable structure in cell organelles. During the extraction process, the surface compounds, such as cuticular waxes, are readily solubilized since they encounter little mass transfer resistance. On the contrary, extraction of essential oil involves a series of complex mass transfer mechanisms (Reverchon et al., 1995).

Many and very different models of mass transfer mechanisms have been used to take into account the various structures of vegetable matter, and the different locations of essential oil can be located (Reverchon and Marrone, 1997). Reverchon, for example, described the fennel essential oil extraction process as a model of desorption from the vegetable matter plus a small mass transfer resistance (Reverchon and Marrone, 1997).

Despite the lipophilic character of essential oil compounds, the water present in the vegetable matrix may interfere in the solute–CO_2 interaction (particularly in the case of terpenoids, which are more polar than terpenes) and produce a decrease of extraction yield. For this reason, drying of the raw material is recommended. Generally, the vegetable matrix should not have water content higher than 12%; the presence of water can cause other undesirable effects, such as the formation of ice in pipelines, due to the rapid depressurization provoked to precipitate the solutes, and hydrolysis of compounds. Moreover, in order to attain an adequate contact with the solvent, a pretreatment to produce cell disruption (comminuting, grinding) is critical. Then, the efficiency of the extraction process is improved by decreasing mass transfer resistance. Indeed, particle size greatly affects process duration, and both variables are interconnected with CO_2 flow rate. The selection of these parameters has the target of producing the exhaustion of the desired compounds in a shorter time.

Particle size plays an important role in SFE processes; if internal mass transfer resistances can be reduced, the extraction is controlled by equilibrium conditions, and thus short extraction times are required. Generally, decreasing particle size improves SFE rate and yield.

6.1.2.10.2   Effect of Extraction Conditions

The extraction pressure is used to tune the selectivity of the supercritical solvent, while the extraction temperature, in the case of thermolabile compounds such as those comprising essential oils, should be set in the range of 35°C–50°C, for example, in the vicinity of the critical point and as low as possible to avoid degradation. Essential oils can be readily extracted using supercritical CO_2 at moderate pressures and temperatures. Higher pressures can also be applied in order to take advantage of the compression effect on the vegetal cell, what enhances mass transfer and liberation of the oil from the cell, but could be determined by the co-extraction of substances other than essential oil. In summary, the higher the pressure, the larger is the solvent power and the smaller is the extraction selectivity. Thus, when high pressures are applied, an on-line fractionation scheme with at least two separators is required to isolate the essential oil from the other co-extracted substances.

6.1.2.10.3   Purification of the Essential Oil Fraction

SFE offers the advantage of fractional extraction or separation (extraction or separation at different pressure and temperature conditions). When substances of several compound families are extracted from the same matrix, it is very useful to improve the selectivity of SFE to produce essential oils. The co-extraction of cuticular waxes represents a further obstacle in the production of essential oils by supercritical extraction. They are located on the surface of the vegetable matter, and the paraffins that typically constitute waxes have low solubilities in supercritical CO_2 if compared to the ones of the odoriferous compounds (Reverchon et al., 1995). Therefore, it is not possible to extract essential oils by supercritical CO_2 using only the data on pure component solubility as a reference. A fractional separation of the supercritical extracts in two or more separators operating at appropriate pressure and temperature conditions is generally necessary (Reverchon et al., 1995).

Fractionation techniques take advantage of the fact that compounds showing different solubilities in supercritical CO_2 and supercritical solvent power can be sensitively varied with pressure and temperature. Applying fractional SFE, natural antioxidants that are soluble in supercritical CO_2 and free of aromatic compounds that could have an impact on organoleptic properties of food can be isolated (Stamenic et al., 2014). Two different fractionation techniques are possible: an extraction accomplished by successive steps (multistep fractionation) and fractionation of the extract in a cascade decompression system (on-line fractionation).

In the multistep fractionation, the conditions applied in the extraction vessel are varied step-by-step, increasing CO_2 density in order to obtain the fractional extraction of the soluble compounds contained in the organic matrix. Thus, the most soluble solutes are recovered in the first fraction, while substances with decreasing solubility in the supercritical solvent are extracted in the successive steps. Essential oils generally constitute the first fraction of a multistep fractionation scheme due to their good solubility in supercritical CO_2.

On-line fractionation is another fractionation alternative that allows operation of the extraction vessel at the same conditions during the whole extraction time, while several separators in series (normally, no more than two or three separators) are set at different temperatures and decreasing pressures. The cascade depressurization is achieved by means of back pressure regulator valves. The scope of this operation is to induce the selective precipitation of different compound families as a function of their different saturation conditions in the supercritical solvent. This procedure has been applied with success in the SFE of essential oils, as it was well established by Reverchon et al. (2006).

6.1.2.11   Pressurized Liquid Extraction or Pressurized Fluid Extraction

Pressurized liquid extraction (PLE) is a technique based on the use of a solvent at elevated pressure and hence at a temperature above its normal boiling point. The application of high pressure in the PLE process facilitates the penetration of the matrix by solvent, leading to the efficient removal of analytes from various matrices. This procedure is also known as accelerated solvent extraction (ASE) and was developed by Richter and collaborators in 1996. The use of liquid solvents at performance compared to extractions at near room temperature and atmospheric pressure promotes higher solubility and mass transfer effects. Indeed, the use of higher temperatures increases the capacity of solvents to solubilize analytes and allows faster diffusion rates. Moreover, increased temperatures can disrupt the strong solute–matrix interactions caused by van der Waals forces, hydrogen bonding, and dipole attractions of the solute molecules and active sites on the matrix. Temperatures above the boiling point are used, exerting sufficient pressure on the solvent during extractions. The use of pressure facilitates the extractions from samples in which the analytes have been trapped in matrix pores. Indeed, the pressure forces the solvent into areas of the matrices that would not normally be contacted by solvents using atmospheric conditions (Richter et al., 1996).

Different techniques based on accelerated solvent extraction have received different names, such as pressurized liquid extraction (PLE), pressurized solvent extraction (PSE), high-pressure solvent extraction (HPSE), pressurized hot solvent extraction (PHSE), high-pressure, high-temperature solvent extraction (HPHTSE), pressurized hot water extraction (PHWE), and subcritical solvent extraction (SSE) (Sun et al., 2012).

The time needed for extraction is significantly shortened (Dawidowicz et al., 2008). In PLE, in comparison with MAE, no additional filtration step is required, since the matrix components that are not dissolved in the extraction solvent may be retained inside the sample extraction cell. In the PLE technique, the sample, placed in the extraction cell, is extracted with an organic solvent at a temperature ranging from ambient to 200°C and at a relatively high pressure (from 4 to 20 MPa). In this approach, the selected solvent is pumped to fill the cell containing the sample, which is kept for a specified time at the selected pressure and temperature. Next, the extracted solvent is transferred to a collection vial. The sample and the connective tubings are then rinsed with a preselected volume of solvent. The inclusion of an additional nitrogen purge guarantees the complete removal of the solvent from the PLE system (Dawidowicz et al., 2012). Extraction time is normally about 15–45 min, although sometimes a longer extraction time is necessary (Nieto et al., 2010). PLE has been employed in the extraction of essential oil components from several plant species, such as mint (*Mentha piperita* L.), sage (*Salvia officinalis* L.), chamomile (*Chamomilla recutita* L.), marjoram (*Origanum majorana* L.), savory (*Satureja hortensis* L.), and oregano (*Origanum vulgare* L.) (Dawidowicz and Rado, 2010; Dawidowicz et al., 2011, 2012).

Several papers have compared the performance of ASE (PLE) with those of other extraction methods, such as Soxhlet extraction, MAE, and SFE. Results have shown that ASE has the advantages of good recoveries, rapidity, adequate precision, and less solvent use, but it has some disadvantages. ASE allows us to reduce the extraction time, but many laboratories will not be able to purchase the equipment because of its high cost. Also, it is difficult to achieve selectivity in the ASE process. Although the extraction time of one sample using the ASE technique is short, the preparation of the extraction cells is time-consuming and uses large volumes of solvents (e.g., for rinsing). Due to low selectivity of the process, the obtained extracts should be cleaned up and reconcentrated before the final analysis (Sun et al., 2012).

The above-cited pressurized hot water extraction (PHWE) is a sample extraction technique based on the use of water as solvent in dynamic mode, at temperatures between 100°C and 374°C (the critical point of water is at 221 bar and 374°C) and a pressure high enough to maintain the liquid state (Deng et al., 2005). Its major advantages are the low cost and environmental friendliness of water. Furthermore, the solvating properties of water are easily altered through change in temperature and pressure. Unfortunately, supercritical water provides a very reactive environment, where oxidation, hydrolysis, and decomposition of compounds can take place (Kamali et al., 2014). This technique has been used for the analyses of essential oils of *Lavandula angustifolia* Mill. and other plants of traditional Chinese medicine (TCM) (Deng et al., 2005; Kamali et al., 2014).

6.1.2.12 Matrix Solid-Phase Dispersion

Matrix solid-phase dispersion (MSPD) is a simple and cheap sample preparation procedure involving simultaneous disruption and extraction of various solid and semi-solid materials, due to the direct mechanical blending of sample with an SPE sorbent (mainly octadecyl-modified silica) (Barker, 2000, 2007; Kristenson et al., 2006). Octadecyl-modified silica used in the classic MSPD process for essential oil analysis (Barker, 2000) acts not only as an abrasive material disrupting the plant sample architecture, but also as a *bound* solvent that accumulates extracted compounds. The sample is dispersed over the surface of the bonded-phase support material, producing a unique mixed-character phase for conducting target analyte isolation. This technique permits complete fractionation of the sample matrix components and has the ability to selectively isolate a single compound or several classes of compounds from the sample. In fact, in this phase apolar components are dispersed in the apolar organic phase on the silica support, while smaller, highly polar molecules are associated with silanols on the surface of the silica support as well as with matrix components able to polarize interactions; large, less polar molecules are accumulated on the surface of the mixed-character phase formed by the bonded octadecyl phase and dispersed matrix. Then, the blended mixture is transferred into an SPE barrel and eluted with an appropriate eluent (Dawidowicz et al., 2011).

The total amount of the essential oil components depends on the type of MSPD dispersing liquid used. A recent report shows that MSPD (Dawidowicz and Rado, 2010; Dawidowicz et al., 2011) efficiency in the essential oil component isolation process from herbs (thyme [*Thymus vulgaris* L.], mint [*Mentha piperita* L.], sage [*Salvia officinalis* L.], chamomile [*Chamomilla recutita* L.], marjoram [*Origanum majorana* L.], savory [*Satureja hortensis* L.], and oregano [*Origanum vulgare* L.]) is better than that of steam distillation (SD), the routine method recommended by pharmacopoeias for the isolation of essential oil in controlling the quality of plant material as its source in the European Pharmacopoeia (Dawidowicz et al., 2011), and equivalent to the efficiency of pressurized liquid extraction (PLE), regarded as one of the most effective techniques of extracting essential oil components (Dawidowicz et al., 2008).

6.1.2.13   Solid-Phase Microextraction

Solid-phase microextraction (SPME) is an evolving technique that reduces the drag of sample preparation and thereby reduces the analysis time. Developed in 1989 by Pawliszyn and coworkers (Arthur and Pawliszyn, 1990), SPME is solvent-free. Extraction and handling of the SPME device is simple (Pawliszyn, 2002) and is similar to handling a syringe. A silica fiber coated with an extracting phase, which can be a liquid (polymer) or a solid (sorbent), is directly injected into the sample (SPME) and analytes are adsorbed to the respective fiber coating. Then the fiber is removed from the sample solution and the analytes are thermally desorbed in the injector of a gas chromatograph (Balasubramanian and Panigrahi, 2011). Hence, sampling, extraction, and preconcentration are accomplished in a single step. This technique is very simple, fast, portable, and inexpensive. SPME has repeatedly been described for the extraction of aroma-active compounds and subsequent gas chromatographic determination. One of the main tasks when developing an SPME method is selecting the most effective fiber and sampling conditions. Several factors influence the choice of fiber and sampling conditions because recovery depends on, among other things, the polarity and volatility of the analytes investigated, the physicochemical characteristics of the polymeric coating and analyte or polymer affinity, and the composition and physical state of the matrix. Yet another important factor is the nature of the fiber coatings, which often consist of two or three components whose recovery capabilities are based on different phenomena (e.g., polydimethylsiloxane [PDMS] on sorption or carboxen [CAR] on adsorption), so as to extend the range of polarities covered and keep good selectivity (Belliardo et al., 2006). Generally, an extraction time of 30 min might be sufficient to obtain desirable results using SPME. However, times as long as 5 h could be necessary to obtain reproducible results in some cases. Since the presence of a high concentration of a "competitive interference compound" might interfere in the adsorption or absorption of the target compound by the fiber and could displace the adsorbed or absorbed target compound from the fiber surface (Pawliszyn, 2002), the extraction time should be selected with reference to the desired analyte to be extracted (Balasubramanian and Panigrahi, 2011). Being a solvent-free technique, it avoids loss of volatiles during the concentration of the extractive solutions. Moreover, the low temperatures normally used during sampling avoid chemical changes in the natural flavor pattern and the formation of artifacts. Finally, the higher concentration capability of this technique allows the identification of many compounds (Maggi et al., 2011). Several factors contribute to the success of SPME, including sampling times that are shorter than those with conventional hydro- or steam distillation; a limited number of parameters to be tuned to maximize analyte recovery, mainly temperature, time, and phase ratio; and the sampling and analysis steps, which are separated for in-the-field or process samplings because the fiber can be stored in its holder, keeping the sample safe over time (Belliardo et al., 2006; Prosen et al., 2010). Solid-phase microextraction has attracted widespread popularity for the analysis of volatile flavor components in various plants and has been employed for determination of essential oils (Adam et al., 2013; Zini et al., 2003). SPME has significant drawbacks, such as its relatively low recommended operating temperature (generally in the range of 240°C–280°C), instability and swelling in organic solvents, fiber breakage, stripping of coatings, and bending of needles and their expense. Moreover, it is very difficult to quantitatively analyze the volatile compounds in plant materials by direct SPME.

6.1.2.14   Liquid-Phase Microextraction and Single-Drop Microextraction

In 1996, liquid-phase microextraction (LPME) was introduced by Jeannot and Cantwell (1996, 1997) in order to overcome the above-cited problem of SPME. LPME is a solvent-minimized sample pretreatment procedure of liquid–liquid extraction (LLE), in which only several microliters of solvent are required to concentrate analytes from various samples, rather than hundreds of milliliters needed in traditional LLE. This relatively new technique is performed by suspending a 1 µl drop of organic solvent on the tip of either a Teflon rod or the needle of a microsyringe immersed in the stirred aqueous solution (Deng et al., 2005). The analytes partition between the bulk aqueous phase and the organic solvent microdrop. It is also compatible with capillary gas chromatography (GC), capillary electrophoresis (CE), and high-performance liquid chromatography (HPLC) (Sarafraz-Yazdi and Amiri, 2010). Single-drop microextraction (SDME), using typically 1–3 µl of an organic solvent at the tip of a microsyringe, has evolved from LPME. After extraction, the microdrop is retracted back into the syringe and transferred for further analysis.

6.1.2.15   Stir Bar Sorptive Extraction

Stir bar sorptive extraction (SBSE) is another sample preconcentration technique, which was developed by Sandra et al. and reported in 1999 (Baltussen et al., 1999; Ng et al., 2012). Stir bars (also known as Twisters) consist of a very thick PDMS film coated on a glass-coated magnetic stir bar, where the analytes are recovered from a liquid or a vapor phase (Sgorbini et al., 2010) (Figure 6.2). The analytes are extracted by stirring the bar in the aqueous sample for a fixed time, recovered by desorbing the stir bar thermally either directly into a GC injector liner or into a glass tube inserted into a thermal desorption system, and then analyzed by GC–capillary flame ionization detector (GC-FID) or capillary GD–mass spectrometry (GC-MS) (Bicchi et al., 2002). Some reviews are reported in the literature, focusing on the general theoretical principles of this technique and the recently developed applications (David and Sandra, 2007; Kawaguchi et al., 2006, 2013). SBSE was applied for the

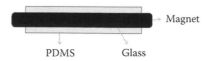

FIGURE 6.2   A PDMS SBSE device made up of a very thick film of PDMS coated onto a glass-coated magnetic stir bar.

enantioselective analysis of chiral monoterpenes in tea tree oil, eucalyptus oil, and thyme oil (Kreck et al., 2002).

6.1.3 Headspace Sampling

In recent years the headspace sampling (HS) technique has been widely employed in the sample preparation of essential oil. The immediate success of HS techniques is due to the fact that they are mainly not time-consuming and solvent-free or solvent-less. They can be combined on-line with analysis, and satisfy the exponential increase in the number of controls required in the essential oil field, which cannot be performed by routine laboratories operating with conventional techniques (Rubiolo et al., 2010).

In HS, the sample is normally placed in a sealed vial and heated in an oven until the volatile compounds reach equilibrium with the gas phase (Belliardo et al., 2006).

Static headspace sampling (S-HS) involves the headspace air not being disturbed by any external means, while diffusion headspace sampling (D-HS) occurs between the fiber and the sample matrix. On the other hand, in dynamic headspace sampling, the headspace air is moved with the help of some air movement devices (Razote et al., 2002). The air velocity is kept constant throughout the sampling process. In some cases, the headspace air is collected in another chamber where the SPME filament or another extraction trap is present (Eisert et al., 1998; Razote et al., 2004) to collect and preconcentrate the headspace gas. In other cases, the SPME fiber is inserted into the same chamber as the sample matrix, and the headspace volatiles are swirled or moved within this chamber at a constant velocity using some device. In the early 1990s, the high-concentration-capacity headspace sampling (HCC-HS) techniques, which act as a bridge between S-HS and D-HS, were developed (Bicchi et al., 2004a, 2008).

The essential oils interact on polymers in sorption or adsorption modes. The recoveries with HCC-HS differ from one component to another, since these techniques are based on the partition between the matrix, headspace, and polymer. The HCC-HS techniques are simple, fast, easy to automate, and as reliable as S-HS, while at the same time showing analyte concentration factors that are very often comparable to those of D-HS (Rubiolo et al., 2010).

Examples of HS sampling techniques are headspace solid-phase microextraction (HS-SPME), headspace sorptive extraction (HSSE), and headspace solvent microextraction (HSME).

6.1.3.1 Headspace Solid-Phase Microextraction

The SPME tecnhique was extended to HS sampling by Zhang and Pawliszyn in 1993. Headspace SPME (HS-SPME) is a technique where fiber used for the SPME is directly injected into the headspace above the sample, and analytes are adsorbed to the respective fiber coating, exposed in the vapor phase above a gaseous, liquid, or solid sample. HS-SPME coupled to GC-MS has been shown to be a simple method, and was widely employed in analyzing essential oil (Deng et al., 2005; Di et al., 2004; Isidorov et al., 2003; Kim and Lee, 2002; Li et al., 2006; Rohloff, 2002; Stashenko et al., 2004a,b). For the extraction of mostly volatile aroma-active components, the extraction from the headspace above the sample is preferred over the direct liquid extraction out of the sample, since many interference problems are eliminated, because the fiber is not in contact with the sample. HS-SPME is especially useful in the case of highly volatile analytes, while for semivolatile compounds, the low volatility and relatively large molecular weight may slow the mass transfer from the matrix to the headspace, resulting in a long extraction time (Florez Menendez et al., 2000). The polydimethylsiloxane 100 μm fiber is most commonly used, since it is well suited for the extraction of essential oil components and is further characterized by a high stability (Richter and Schellenberg, 2007). The choice of fiber and sampling condition is affected not only by the above-cited parameters of SPME, but also by the HS equilibration temperature and time, and analyte diffusion and equilibration time from the vapor phase to the fiber surface (Belliardo et al., 2006).

6.1.3.2 Headspace Sorptive Extraction

As an extension to SBSE, headspace sorptive extraction (HSSE) was developed by Sandra et al. in 2000 (Tienpont et al., 2000) to extract volatiles from the headspace. HSSE was applied to the aromatic and medicinal plants rosemary, sage, thyme, and valerian, and the results were compared to those obtained by SPME (Bicchi et al., 2000). Whereas HSSE and SPME are based on the same extraction principles, the extracting support of the former is a magnetic stir bar coated with a larger volume of sorbent phase than the SPME fibers (up to 110 μl vs. a maximum of 0.5 μl, respectively) (Gallidabino et al., 2014). The concentration capability, evaluated through the relative abundance of some typical components of the plants investigated, in the HSSE was better than that obtained with HS-SPME with different fibers (Bicchi et al., 2005). In the solvent-enhanced HSSE (SE-HSSE) system the PDMS concentration capability is improved with the help of a solvent (Sgorbini et al., 2010). The analytes are concentrated into the solvent stored inside a short piece of PDMS tubing sealed at one end and suspended in the aqueous sample so that they can diffuse through the PDMS, which acts as a selective nonporous membrane and concentrates them into the inner solvent by sorptive extraction. The solvent-impregnated PDMS tubing is suspended using harmonic stainless steel wire in the sample HS for a fixed time (Figure 6.3).

6.1.3.3 Headspace Liquid-Phase Microextraction

Jeannot and Cantwell introduced headspace liquid-phase microextraction (HS-LPME) and demonstrated the feasibility of the application of the microdrop headspace mode to preconcentration of volatile organic compounds (Theis et al., 2001). In the HS-LPME mode, an extraction solvent with a high boiling point and low vapor pressure was required. In order to overcome this limit, Shen and Lee developed a novel HS-LPME mode, where the thin organic solvent film (OSF) formed in a microsyringe barrel through the movement of the plunger was used as an extraction interface (Deng et al., 2005). A review reports the isolation of 27 compounds of the essential oil (e.g., camphor, borneol, and borneol acetate) in a TCM, *Fructus amomi*, and pressurized hot water extraction, followed by extraction and concentration with HS-LPME (Yan et al., 2014), and the determination of the essential oil component of star anise (*Illicium*

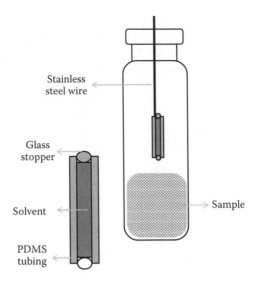

Stainless
steel wire

Glass
stopper

Solvent

PDMS
tubing

Sample

FIGURE 6.3   SE-HSSE system: the solvent-impregnated PDMS tubing is suspended using harmonic stainless steel wire in the sample HS.

verum Hook.f.) was performed using simultaneous hydrodistillation-static headspace liquid-phase microextraction (Gholivand et al., 2009).

6.1.3.4   Headspace Solvent Microextraction

The above-cited techniques with the headspace sampling led to headspace solvent microextraction (HSME), a modern sampling and sample preparation method, used for isolation and preconcentration of volatile compounds from the headspace of the plant matrix. HSME uses a microdrop of organic solvent as an extracting phase. During transport, storage, and manipulation, the microdrop is retracted into the needle of the microsyringe. During extraction and vaporization of the analytes, the microdrop is exposed. The analytes occurring in the headspace of a sample are extracted into the microdrop, depending on its type. The process continues until equilibrium is reached between the extracting solvent and the sample. Once the extraction is finished, the microdrop is retracted back into the needle, and the microsyringe is transferred into the injection port of a gas chromatograph for analyte separation and determination. In comparison with traditional extraction methods, HSME has the advantages of a renewable drop (no sample carryover), good precision, wide selection of available solvents, low cost, simplicity and ease of use, minimal solvent use, short preconcentration time, possibility of automation, and no conditioning required (as is the case with the fiber in solid-phase microextraction) (Besharati-Seidani et al., 2006; Fakhari et al., 2005). This technique has been usefully associated with the hydrodistillation in HD-HSME, a new, rapid, and eco-friendly method used for essential oil analysis of aromatic plants and their seeds (Fakhari et al., 2005; Salehi et al., 2007a,b). HD-HSME is performed by using an apparatus, as shown in Figure 6.4. The flask (Fl) containing the plant material and water is heated at 100°C by a mantle. The needle (Ne) of the syringe (Sy), rinsed and primed with the solvent or

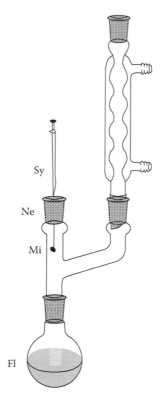

FIGURE 6.4 HSME apparatus. Fl, flask containing the plant material; Mi, microdrop; Ne, needle of the syringe; Sy, syringe.

standard solution, is inserted into the headspace of the plant sample. The extraction starts, and from the syringe a microdrop of extracting solvent is suspended from the needle tip. After an optimized period of time, the microdrop is retracted back into the syringe. The needle is removed from the headspace and its content is injected into the GC system.

6.2 ANALYTICAL METHODS

6.2.1 CLASSICAL METHODS AND THIN-LAYER CHROMATOGRAPHY

The long history of use of essential oils has given rise to a great number of quality control measures. The organoleptic test of smell is probably the oldest method, still used in perfumery, but adulteration cannot be recognized by a too simple method.

Several physicochemical techniques are commonly applied to assess essential oil physical properties (d'Acampora Zellner et al., 2010).

Specific gravity is the measurement of relative density, $[\rho]^{T(^\circ C)}$, defined as the ratio of the density of a given oil and the density of water when both are at the same temperature. The resulting value is characteristic for each essential oil and commonly falls in the range between 0.696 and 1.118 at 15°C. Another physical analysis typical for essential oils is the determination of the refractive index, usually ranging from 1.450 to 1.590. The Abbé-type refractometer, equipped with a monochromatic sodium light source, is recommended for routine essential oil analysis; a similar instrument is generally calibrated through the analysis of distilled water at 20°C, producing a refractive index of 1.3330. If the measurement is performed at a temperature above or below 20°C, a correction factor per degree must be added or subtracted, respectively.

Another recognized technique is the optical rotation, $[\alpha]_{20}^{D}$, that can be determined by using a polarimeter, with the angle of rotation depending on parameters of the oil, such as its nature, and parameters not depending on the oil, such as the length of the column through which the light passes, the temperature, and the applied wavelength. The degree of rotation can give an indication of the purity assessment, since it is related to chiral molecules in the sample.

A procedure that can be applied for the purity assessment of essential oils is based on the water solubility test, which reveals the presence of polar substances, such as alcohols, glycols and their esters, and glycerin acetates: aged or improperly stored oils frequently present decreased solubility.

The evaluation of melting and freezing points, as well as the boiling range of essential oils, is also of great importance for identity and purity assays. Melting point estimation permits us to control essential oil purity, since a large number of molecules generally comprised in essential oils melt within a range of 0.5°C or, in the case of decomposition, over a narrow temperature range. On the other hand, the determination of the congealing point is usually applied when the essential oil consists mainly of one molecule; for these cases, such a test enables the evaluation of the percentage amount of the abundant compound. At congealing point, crystallization occurs, accompanied by heat liberation, leading to a rapid increase in temperature, which is then stabilized at the so-called congealing point.

An additional test, usually performed in essential oil analysis, is the evaporation residue, in which the percentage of the oil that is not released at 100°C is determined.

The use of qualitative information alone is not sufficient to correctly characterize an essential oil, and quantitative data are of extreme importance. Classical methods are generally focused on chemical groups, and the assessment of quantitative information through titration is widely applied.

Essential oils are also often analyzed by means of chromatographic methods. In fact, the most important step in the analysis of secondary plant products was obtained with the introduction of chromatographic methods, of which planar chromatography (thin-layer chromatography [TLC] and paper chromatography [PC]) and gas chromatography (GC) have had the highest impact on essential oil analysis. Planar chromatography may be referred to as a classical method for essential oil analysis, being well represented by TLC and PC. In both techniques, the stationary phase is distributed as a thin layer on a flat support, in PC being the same paper, while in TLC a stationary phase coated on a glass, plastic, or metal surface; the mobile phase is allowed to ascend through the layer by capillary forces. TLC is a fast and inexpensive method for identifying substances and testing the purity of compounds, being widely used for preliminary analyses (Falkenberg, 1999).

TLC is still a valid tool for rapidly obtaining phytochemical fingerprints of complex matrices. In combination with densitometric and spectroscopic methods, the advanced technique related to planar chromatography, (HP)TLC, has actually made a comeback in quality control. TLC combines several attractive features: the equipment is cheap and easy to use, more than a sample can be analyzed in a single run, and several detection methods can be applied to the same analysis (fluorescence, UV detection, chemical methods). Many pharmacopoeias include TLC analysis. There are, however, limits, principally in the poor reproducibility of R_f values.

In recent years several authors have used HPTLC with the aim of characterizing essential oils, or of assessing simple and reproducible methods for quality control (Stan et al., 2014).

6.2.2 Gas Chromatography and Gas Chromatography–Mass Spectrometry

By their nature, essential oils range from volatile through to semivolatile compounds. Being derived from natural flora, they will serve as highly volatile alarm-type compounds, which must rapidly diffuse into the surrounding air, through more waxy leaf compounds that have a smaller vapor pressure and provide part of the structural constituents of a plant.

Gas chromatography (GC) is the most important technique for the analysis of essential oils (Adlard, 2011). Separation of the constituents of a mixture depends on the polarity and volatility of the analytes. GC is based on differential partitioning of solutes between the mobile (gas) and stationary phase (liquid or solid). It is quite simple, fast, reliable, and applicable to the separation of volatile materials that are stable at a temperature up to 350°C. The columns can be packed or capillary and are further classified according to column length material and diameter. One of the most important criteria for good GC separations is to select the most suitable stationary phase and column size.

Since the introduction of capillary columns, especially based on fused silica, gas chromatography is the method of choice if there is necessity of high resolution, sensitivity, and linearity, without too high of a cost. Therefore, based on the state that essential oils are substantially volatile compounds, GC is the ideal method to evaluate complex essential oils or medicinal products derived from them. This is also recognized by modern pharmacopoeias, which include an increasing number of GC assays.

The best accuracy is provided by splitless injection, preferably using a programmed temperature vaporizing (PVT) injector, or by cold on-column injection (Caja and Herraiz, 2009; Zheng et al., 2006).

Headspace analysis, which is very important in food and fragrances, is less suitable in the case of aromatherapy because the composition of odor above the product is different from the product itself. The same is true for the latest development of headspace sampling by solid-phase microextraction (SPME).

The qualitative analysis of essential oils by GC is based on the comparison of the peaks in the chromatogram of the essential oil with those of authentic standards separated in the same chromatographic conditions. Chromatographic data useful for the identification are Kovats indices, linear retention indices, relative retention times, and retention time locking, obtained from a detector or from a spectrometric detection (GC-MS). In addition, spectroscopic data can be used to confirm identification. GC-MS is used for correct identification of each peak (ideally single compound) separated from the essential oil. Spectroscopic information, in some cases, is an unavoidable alternative, together with the use of retention indices and other relative retention parameters. The use of qualitative information alone is not sufficient to correctly characterize an essential oil, and quantitative data are also important. For this reason, selection of the detector is of extreme importance. Apart from the flame ionization detector (FID), each detector has associated with it a compound-specific response factor (Baser and Buchbauer, 2010). FID is considered the more reliable and accurate detector but has low selectivity, while an electron-capture detector (ECD) is used to selectively detect compounds with a high electron affinity. Therefore, GC-MS is preferred for qualitative identification and gives the most accurate quantitative results for individual compounds. In recent years, hyphenated chromatographic and spectroscopic techniques have been used more extensively for the qualitative–quantitative analysis of essential oils. Rarely GC was hyphenated with detection systems, like Fourier transform infrared spectroscopy (FTIR) or UV. Both methods have not gained much importance in the field of essential oil analysis and quality control (Bicchi et al., 2011; Mosandl and Juchelka, 1997; Schipilliti et al., 2010). However, the most important innovation of GC applied to the field of essential oils, in the past years, regards high-speed GC, enantioselective GC, and GC–olfactometry (Smelcerovic et al., 2013).

6.2.2.1   High-Speed GC Separation

High-speed GC separation is based on the reduction of the analysis time, usually used for conventional GC, maintaining the separation, and providing qualitative and quantitative results. Theoretical and practical aspects of high-speed GC methods have been reviewed by Cramers et al. (1999) and Korytar et al. (2002). The method translation approach has been described by Bicchi et al. (2011) and can be seen as an important contribution to fast GC in routine analysis; a further improvement has been introduced by Klee and Blumberg (2002), which makes it possible to find the optimal separation and speed trade-off for a conventional GC method and to derive fast GC conditions from it automatically. Over the years, instruments and methods have been developed to considerably increase the analysis speed of capillary GC, enabling the routine use of fast GC with short narrow-bore columns and the introduction of modern GC instruments provided with automatic injectors, electronic flow control, ovens with high precision temperature and temperature rate controls, and detectors with high sensitivity, electronic stability, and frequency of signal acquisition. To have a high analysis speed in the field of plant volatiles, two approaches are available. The most common is based on the use of a narrow-bore column (Bicchi et al., 2004b; Mondello et al., 2003, 2004). The second one is the short capillary column approach that has been proved to be useful in the rapid analysis of low to medium complexity samples (Bicchi et al., 2001). Rubiolo et al. (2008) investigated the compatibility of fast gas chromatography-quadrupole mass spectrometry (GC-qMS) in essential oil analysis, in a study dealing with the separation, identification, and quantification of components of peppermint essential oils.

6.2.2.2   Enantioselective Gas Chromatography

Enantioselective Gas Chromatography (ES-GC) has allowed detailed study of enantiomeric composition of volatile compounds; its success was linked to the development of stable chiral phases for gas chromatography, mostly based on cyclodextrins (Bicchi et al., 1999). A large number of essential oils have already been investigated by means of ES-GC using distinct chiral stationary phases, but it has appeared that effective separation may not be achieved on a single chiral column. In fact, there are several stationary phases based on different enantiomeric selectivities. Although more than 100 stationary phases with immobilized chiral selectors have been used so far, there is no universal chiral selector with widespread potential for separation of enantiomers (Rubiolo et al., 2010). Chiral recognition of the component of a complex sample often needs a two-dimensional approach (Bicchi et al., 2011).

6.2.2.3   Gas Chromatography–Olfactometry

Gas chromatography–olfactometry (GC-O) is a largely applied GC technique that enables the assessment of odor-active components in complex mixtures, based on the correlation between the chromatographic peaks of the eluted substances revealed simultaneously by two detectors, one of them being the human olfactory system and the other a detector for GC.

GC-O has been frequently employed in essential oil analysis (Benzo et al., 2007; Breme et al., 2009; Costa et al., 2008; Eyres et al., 2007; Ravi et al., 2007); a lot of literature is available on the application of this technique on *Citrus* spp. essential oils (Lin and Rouseff, 2001; Sawamura et al., 2006) by using different assessment methods. Results of GC-O analysis can give information about the presence or absence of odor in a mixture, measure the duration of odor activity, describe the quality of the odor, and quantify the intensity of the specific odorant, which may have an ultimate purpose in the application of such compounds in industry of flavor and fragrances.

6.2.2.4   Mass Spectrometry

Mass spectrometry (MS) can be defined as the study of systems through the formation of gaseous ions, with or without fragmentation, which are then characterized by their mass-to-charge ratios (m/z) and relative abundances (Todd 1995). The analyte may be ionized thermally, by an electric field or by impacting energetic electrons, ions, or photons. Although the sample is destroyed by the mass spectrometer, the technique is very sensitive and only low amounts of material are used in the analysis.

In addition, the potential of combined gas chromatography–mass spectrometry (GC-MS) for determining volatile compounds, contained in very complex flavor and fragrance samples, is well known. The subsequent introduction of powerful data acquisition and processing systems, including automated library search techniques, ensures that the information content of the large quantities of data generated by GC-MS instruments can be fully exploited. The most frequent and simple identification method in GC-MS consists of the comparison of the acquired unknown mass spectra with those contained in a reference MS library. A mass spectrometer produces an enormous amount of data, especially in combination with chromatographic sample inlets (Vekey, 2001). Over the years, many approaches for the analysis of

GC-MS data have been proposed using various algorithms, many of which are quite sophisticated, in efforts to detect, identify, and quantify all the chromatographic peaks. Library search algorithms are commonly provided with mass spectrometer data systems with the purpose of assisting in the identification of unknown compounds (McLafferty et al., 1999).

However, as it is well known, compounds such as isomers, when analyzed by means of GC-MS, can be incorrectly identified, a drawback that is often observed in essential oil analysis. As it is widely known, the composition of essential oils is mainly represented by terpenes, which generate very similar mass spectra; hence, a favorable match factor is not sufficient for identification, and peak assignment becomes difficult and can be gained only by the combination of mass spectral data with chromatographic information: to increase the reliability of the analytical results and to address the qualitative determination of the composition of complex samples by GC-MS, retention indices can be an effective tool. The use of retention indices in conjunction with the structural information provided by GC-MS is widely accepted and used to confirm the identity of compounds (Costa et al., 2007).

According to Joulain and Konig (1998), provided data contained in mass spectrometry libraries have been recorded using authentic samples; thus, the mass spectrum of a given sesquiterpene is usually sufficient to ensure its identification when associated with its retention index obtained on methyl silicone stationary phases. Indeed, for the afore-cited class of compounds, there would be no need to use a polyethylene glycol phase, which could even lead to misinterpretations caused by possible changes in the retention behavior of sesquiterpene hydrocarbons as a result of column aging or deterioration. Three types of libraries are available for essential oil composition identification: commercial libraries, specific libraries, and in-house libraries.

Commercial libraries contain nonspecific collections of spectra mainly taken from the literature. The evaluation of data from commercial libraries needs deep attention since they contain mass spectrometry data taken under different conditions using different instruments. The main drawback of such libraries is the lack of retention data to compare with the retention indices. The National Institute of Standards and Technology (NIST) has recently started providing such a service (Babushok et al., 2007). Among the commercially available GC-MS libraries for essential oil components and aroma chemicals, Wiley, NIST, National Bureau of Standards (NBS), Triskelion volatile compounds in food databank (TNO), Environmental Protection Agency (EPA), National Institutes of Health (NIH), Adams, MassFinder, Flavor and Fragrance Natural and Synthetic Compounds (FFNSC) and Tkachev can be mentioned.

Specific libraries are dedicated to specific applications or compound groups. The Adams, MassFinder, FFNSC, and Joulain and Konig collections are available for these applications. While Adams and MassFinder are general essential oil libraries, the FFNSC and Joulain and Konig collections are prepared for flavors and fragrances of natural and synthetic compounds and sesquiterpene hydrocarbons, respectively. These libraries contain specific information for the compounds of interest, such as retention times, retention indices, and physicochemical information.

Researchers dealing mainly with a certain group of products may develop their own libraries (in-house libraries) with the aim to facilitate and expedite compound characterization. Such libraries are more reliable since they are created using certified compounds under identical conditions and contain retention data. The BASER library of essential oil constituents is an example of an in-house library (Baser and Ozek, 2012).

6.2.3 SUPERCRITICAL FLUID CHROMATOGRAPHY

In 1990 supercritical fluid chromatography (SFC) was introduced as an alternative to capillary GC in aromatic plant analysis (Manninen et al., 1990). Capillary SFC was applied to the analysis of some plant volatile oils. The results were compared with those obtained by capillary GC. For thyme oil, SFC without derivatization gave about the same percentage composition of the main compounds. For a complex mixture of peppermint oil or basil oil, SFC seems to give more reliable quantification than capillary GC, especially for oxygenated compounds. However, the separation efficiency of capillary GC for monoterpene hydrocarbons was, as expected, much better than that of SFC. For this reason, in the last 25 years very few publications appeared using this technique in the field of essential oils, principally on *Citrus* spp. oil, *Thymus* spp. Oil, and *Humulus lupulus* L. oil (Auerbach et al., 2000; Blum et al., 1997; Dugo et al., 1996).

6.2.4 LIQUID CHROMATOGRAPHY AND LC-MS

HPLC-UV is a supplementary method for analysis of volatile oils due to its versatility, sensitivity, and selectivity. HPLC is the method of choice in the analysis of less volatile constituents of essential oils (Lockwood, 2001; Rauber et al., 2005), principally aromatic fraction. This is not a secondary fraction in the essential oils because oxygen heterocyclic compounds can have an important role in the identification of a cold-pressed oil, in the control of both quality and authenticity. The improvement of HPLC detectors and mainly the development of HPLC-MS technologies have afforded a lot of information about the content and nature of the constituents of essential oils.

Atmospheric pressure chemical ionization (APCI) is a choice source system for less polar compounds and of lower molecular weight than electrospray ionization (ESI) (Dugo et al., 2000). However, only a small number of reports on essential oil analyses by HPLC can be found in the literature (Turek and Stintzing, 2011). In most cases, its use has been reserved for the detection of the nonvolatile fraction in citrus oils (Buiarelli et al., 1996; Dugo et al., 2005). The oxygen heterocyclic compounds present in the nonvolatile residue of *Citrus* essential oils have also been extensively investigated by means of high-performance liquid chromatography–atmospheric pressure ionization–mass spectrometry (HPLC-API-MS). The use of normal-phase (NP)– and reversed-phase (RP)–HPLC with microbore columns and UV detection has also been reported for lemon and bergamot bitter orange and grapefruit (Buiarelli et al., 1996) essential oils. Orange and mandarin essential oils have also been analyzed by RP-HPLC, with UV and spectrofluorimetric detection in series (Buiarelli et al., 1991). Apart from *Citrus* spp. oils, other essential oils have also been analyzed by means of LC, such as the blackcurrant bud essential oil (Piry and Pribela, 1994), the volatile compounds in Virgin olive oils (Germek et al., 2013), and *Achillea millefoliun* L. essential oil (Smelcerovic et al., 2010).

Sometimes HPLC in the analysis of essential oils is described as a sample cleaning or fractionating step prior to GC and, in rare cases, for the detection of specific terpenoid volatiles (Rauber et al., 2005).

6.2.5 MULTIDIMENSIONAL TECHNIQUES

Multidimensional chromatographic techniques can be divided into multidimensional GC techniques, multidimensional LC techniques, and multidimensional GC-LC techniques.

6.2.5.1 Multidimensional GC Techniques

Due to the complexity of the essential oil composition, a capillary column is often unable to resolve completely all the components of interest in a short time. The overlapping of the peaks can make difficult the identification of compounds through the MS spectra. Unambiguous identification of minor compounds is extremely difficult when high-concentration constituents mask their presence in the sample. For this reason, in many cases two-dimensional GC (GC-GC) has to be performed. This technique implies coupled columns of different polarities and subject-selected analytes to two independent separation steps, characterized by complementary (or orthogonal) selectivities. The convention wants to use as the first column a low-polarity stationary-phase column, which affects displacement of the sample components along the x-axis of the two-dimensional separation plane, while the second column is a polar stationary-phase column (Figure 6.5).

This conventional system can be changed based on the specific characteristics of each sample. Different compounds undergo different separation mechanisms, and there are no fixed rules to the combination of column phase types as long as they provide orthogonal separation. The unresolved effluent fractions from a first column are transferred onto the second one (Marriott et al., 2003; Namara et al., 2007).

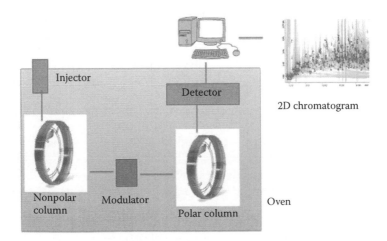

FIGURE 6.5   A GC × GC system used in the analysis of essential oils.

The instrumentation involves a transfer device (modulator), situated between the two dimensions, which presents the key of the system and enables the entire procedure.

In the first multidimensional gas chromatography (MDGC) systems, the transfer of eluted fractions from the first to the second dimension was achieved through mechanical valves. This approach was soon abandoned and replaced by a new interface based on a pressure balance between two columns. Later, the system was improved and largely applied in the studies of enantiomeric volatile components in *Citrus* spp. oils. A different and inexpensive approach for transferring individual GC peaks into a second column has been presented by Kubeczka (Baser and Buchbauer, 2010), using a solid-phase microextraction (SPME) device, while Mondello et al. (1998) developed a six-way rotary mechanical valve as interface.

A detailed study of different aspects in bidimensional gas chromatography for the analysis of essential oils and chiral compounds was given by Shellie (2009).

It is possible to construct a complete two-dimensional chromatogram by continuously taking small-volume heart-cuts from the first column and subjecting each of these to the second-dimension separation. The current knowledge of essential oils is available due to the GC-MS technique, taking into account the number of published manuscripts presenting the composition of essential oils determined by GC-MS. Some authors suggest that GCMS can be considered a two-dimensional analysis system; therefore, hyphenation of GC-GC with mass spectrometry represents tripledimensional analysis. Time-of-flight analyzer mass spectrometry (TOFMS) is the most applied technology.

Among the essential oils previously studied by means of GC × GC are peppermint (Cordero et al., 2006) and Australian sandalwood (Shellie et al., 2004), with the latter also analyzed through GC × GC/TOFMS in the same work. Essential oils derived from *Thymbra spicata* L. (Ozel et al., 2003), *Pistacia vera* L. (Ozel et al., 2004), hop (Roberts, 2004), *Teucrium chamaedrys* L. (Ozel et al., 2006a), *Rosa damascena* Mill. (Ozel et al., 2006b), coriander (Eyres et al., 2007), and *Artemisia annua* L. (Ma et al., 2007), as well as tobacco (Zhu et al., 2007), have also been subjected to GC × GC/TOFMS analyses. The references cited herein represent only a few examples of the studies performed by means of GC × GC on essential oils.

6.2.5.2 Multidimensional LC Techniques

Comprehensive two-dimensional LC is an innovative technique coupling two independent LC separation processes with orthogonal selectivities (Dugo et al., 2008a). This technique was completely described and reviewed by Dugo et al. (2004). If compared to single-dimension chromatography, the separation power of comprehensive two-dimensional chromatography is greatly increased. For the same reasons described in two-dimensional GC, the columns used should have different stationary phases and retention mechanisms. The most used in essential oil analysis is the combination of a normal-phase stationary phase (first dimension) and a reversedphase stationary phase (second dimension). A scheme for an LC × LC instrument is reported in Figure 6.6.

In literature, there are several manuscripts on the application of comprehensive two-dimensional LC for analysis of essential oils (Dugo et al., 2008b,c).

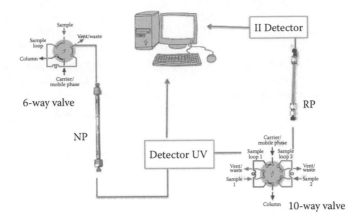

FIGURE 6.6   An LC × LC system used in the analysis of essential oils.

6.2.5.3   Multidimensional GC-LC Techniques

Sample components in essential oil analysis belong to a variety of chemical classes and are present in a wide range of concentrations; this fact makes the analysis complicated. The multidimensional LC-GC approach combines the selectivity of the LC separation with the high efficiency and sensitivity of GC separation, enabling the separation of compounds with similar physicochemical properties in samples characterized by a great number of chemical classes. This technique was first applied to *Citrus* spp. essential oil analysis; later, on-line LC-GC coupled with Fourier transform infrared spectroscopy (FTIR) was used for the determination of some components in bergamot oil sample. The LC-GC technique was applied for the study of single classes of components, mono- and sesquiterpene in citrus oil, aldehyde composition in sweet orange oil, and the enantiomeric distribution of monoterpene

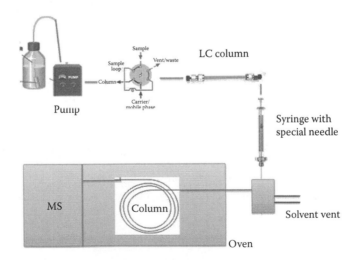

FIGURE 6.7   An LC × GC system used in the analysis of essential oils.

alcohols in lemon, mandarin, sweet orange, and bitter orange oils (Dugo et al., 1994a,b; Mondello et al., 1994, 1995, 1996). The hyphenation of an LC-GC system to a mass spectrometer (LC-GC-MS) increases the potential of the technique, giving the opportunity of spectra collection and identification of the components of the mixture (Figure 6.7).

6.2.6 SPECTROSCOPIC FINGERPRINT: NMR AND NIR

Nuclear magnetic resonance (NMR) is an analytical technique that provides the most information of all spectroscopic methods for the determination of the structure of pure compounds.

Application of NMR in the analysis of complex mixtures such as essential oils is limited due to its low sensitivity, high number of signals and their overlapping, and difficulties in coupling GC to NMR. In general, ^{13}C-NMR is used off-line, while ^{1}H-NMR is applied on-line.

A powerful analytical technique is obtained by on-line coupling of GC and NMR because the excellent separation characteristics of gas chromatography are combined with NMR data about the structure of oil constituents. Commercial available NMR instruments with high magnetic fields and microprobes can record the NMR spectra of a sample in the gaseous phase. Albert and coworkers (Grynbaum et al., 2007; Kuehnle et al., 2008) demonstrated the potential of the hyphenation of capillary GC to solenoidal-type microprobe ^{1}H-NMR detection as a technique for the analysis of volatile compounds.

NMR fingerprint is generally based on ^{1}H-NMR and is applied in combination with other techniques, mainly GC-MS, when used for the characterization of essential oils (Guerrini et al., 2006, 2011).

Near-infrared (NIR) spectroscopy, which is related to the first experiments performed by Herschel in 1800, has been widely used in agricultural and food sectors. A real breakthrough of NIR spectroscopy as a routine analytical technique was first obtained in the early 1980s, when efficient chemometric algorithms were successfully introduced. Generally, the statistical support improved the interpretation of the NIR data dramatically and contributed strongly to this spectroscopy tool, which is today one of the fastest analytical technologies. While numerous NIR spectroscopy methods have been established in the field of agriculture for more than four decades, IR spectroscopy has been primarily used as a structure elucidation technique; only limited applications can be found in the literature for characterization of liquid samples, such as fruit juices or other plant extracts. In the field of natural products, NIR has been used for the rapid determination of active constituents of medicinal plants (Laasonen et al., 2002). Since most of the recent advances in NIR have been concerned with chemometric software (Williams and Norris, 2001), its use in the quantification of essential oil components is a relatively new application. One of the potential applications of this technique is in quality control, since large lots or single samples can rapidly be prescreened in order to identify those samples that might require further testing by more time-consuming and expensive methods (Williams and Norris, 2001).

Applications of NIR to quality control are present in the literature and are focused on the analysis of lavander oil (Tankeu et al., 2014), fennel (Steuer and Schulz, 2003), oregano essential oil (Camps et al., 2014), sandalwood oil (Kuriakose and Joe, 2013), and essential oils from African plants (Juliani et al., 2006).

6.3   MULTIVARIATE DATA ANALYSIS

Over the last 10–15 years the elaboration of analytical data, mainly MS data, has strongly progressed not only because of new powerful softwares and the availability of exhaustive and specialized libraries and collections of spectra, but also because of the introduction into routine work of new tools such as MS spectra deconvolution of co-eluting peaks and the interactive combination of chromatographic linear retention indices and MS data, helpful for producing highly effective identification of components (d'Acampora Zellner et al., 2008; Mondello et al., 1995).

On the other hand, and with the same importance, the recent progress in chemometrics and softwares for statistical elaboration has extended the range of information obtainable from a conventional analysis, making the chromatographic profile (or MS profile, or two-dimensional chromatographic profile), defined by the abundances (better if normalized percentage data) of a selected number of markers, a characteristic of the investigated matrix, a further distinctive parameter to characterize a sample.

The importance of the statistical representation of samples based on the analytical profile to characterize a sample or discriminate it within a set is even higher with two-dimensional chromatographic techniques. New fingerprinting approaches specific to comprehensive gas chromatography have recently shown its potential in sample comparisons and correlations, and its ability to locate compounds whose distribution can be correlated to sensory properties and geographical origin, or to monitor the effect of technological treatments on different classes of compounds (Cordero et al., 2008, 2010a,b).

The range of information that can be obtained from a conventional analysis of a plant essential oil has been extended for statistical elaboration (Bicchi et al., 2011). Samples under investigation are usually statistically pretreated and normalized according to their chromatographic profiles defined by the abundance of a selected number of markers set as variables. When the markers are known compounds, a targeted approach is undertaken; when the variables are relative to unknown compounds able to generate a peak or other response, an untargeted approach is undertaken. The most widely used approach is multivariate analysis, in particular principal component analysis (PCA), a method that can explain the differences within a set of samples characterized by a suitable number of components (variables) through the linear combination of those explaining most of the variability in a set of observations, which generally are samples under investigation.

This method allows the differentiation among groups of samples within a set, pointing at variables (individual components or MS fragments) that have the highest statistical significance in sample discrimination, providing valuable information on the origin or chemotypification (Hiltunen and Laakso, 1995) and differentiation among species at intrageneric levels (Petrakis et al., 2005; Radulovic et al., 2010; Smelcerovic et al., 2007) and among technological treatments (Rubiolo et al., 2006).

REFERENCES

Adam, M., Cizkova, A., Eisner, A., and Ventura, K. Solid-Phase Microextraction Based Method for Determination of Essential Oils Components in Herbal Beverages. *Journal of Separation Science* 36, 4 (2013): 764–72.

Adams, T. B., and Taylor, S. V. Safety Evaluation of Essential Oils: A Constituent-Based Approach. In *Handbook of Essential Oils: Science, Technology, and Applications*, ed. K. H. C. Baser and G. Buchbauer. CRC Press, Boca Raton, FL (2010): 185–208.

Adlard, E. R. Chromatography of Aroma Compounds and Fragrances by Tibor Cserhati. *Chromatographia* 73, 11–12 (2011): 1239–40.

Allaf, T., Tomao, V., Ruiz, K., and Chemat, F. Instant Controlled Pressure Drop Technology and Ultrasound Assisted Extraction for Sequential Extraction of Essential Oil and Antioxidants. *Ultrasonics Sonochemistry* 20, 1 (2013): 239–46.

Arthur, C. L., and Pawliszyn, J. Solid-Phase Microextraction with Thermal-Desorption Using Fused-Silica Optical Fibers. *Analytical Chemistry* 62, 19 (1990): 2145–48.

Auerbach, R. H., Dost, K., and Davidson, G. Characterization of Varietal Differences in Essential Oil Components of Hops (*Humulus lupulus*) by SFC-FTIR Spectroscopy. *Journal of AOAC International* 83, 3 (2000): 621–26.

Babushok, V. I., Linstrom, P. J., Reed, J. J., Zenkevich, I. G., Brown, R. L., Mallard, W. G., and Stein, S. E. Development of a database of gas chromatographic retention properties of organic compounds. *Journal of Chromatography A* 1157, (1–2) (2007): 414–21.

Balasubramanian, S., and Panigrahi, S. Solid-Phase Microextraction (SPME) Techniques for Quality Characterization of Food Products: A Review. *Food and Bioprocess Technology* 4, 1 (2011): 1–26.

Baltussen, E., Sandra, P., David, F., and Cramers, C. Stir Bar Sorptive Extraction (SBSE), a Novel Extraction Technique for Aqueous Samples: Theory and Principles. *Journal of Microcolumn Separations* 11, 10 (1999): 737–47.

Barker, S. A. Applications of matrix solid-phase dispersion in food analysis. *Journal of Chromatography A* 880, 1–2 (2000): 63–8.

Barker, S. A. Matrix solid phase dispersion (MSPD)—A review. *Journal of Biochemical and Biophysical Methods* 70, 2 (2007): 151–62.

Baser, K. H. C., and Buchbauer, G., eds. *Handbook of Essential Oils: Science, Technology, and Applications.* CRC Press, Boca Raton, FL (2010).

Baser, K. C. H., and Ozek, T. Analysis of Essential Oils and Fragrances by Gas Chromatography. In *Gas Chromatography*, ed. C. Poole. Elsevier, Amsterdam, 2012, pp. 519–528.

Bayramoglu, B., Serpil, S., and Sumnu, G. Solvent-Free Microwave Extraction of Essential Oil from Oregano. *Journal of Food Engineering* 88, 4 (2008): 535–40.

Belliardo, F., Bicchi, C., Cordero C., Liberto, E., Rubiolo, P., and Sgorbini, B. Headspace-Solid-Phase Microextraction in the Analysis of the Volatile Fraction of Aromatic and Medicinal Plants. *Journal of Chromatographic Science* 44, 7 (2006): 416–29.

Benzo, M., Gilardoni, G., Gandini, C., Caccialanza, G., Finzi, P. V., Vidari, G., Abdo, S., and Layedra, P. Determination of the Threshold Odor Concentration of Main Odorants in Essential Oils Using Gas Chromatography-Olfactometry Incremental Dilution Technique. *Journal of Chromatography A* 1150, 1–2 (2007): 131–35.

Besharati-Seidani, A., Jabbari, A., Yamini, Y., and Saharkhiz, M. J. Rapid Extraction and Analysis of Volatile Organic Compounds of Iranian Feverfew (*Tanacetum parthenium*) Using Headspace Solvent Gas Chromatography/Mass Microextraction (HSME), and Spectrometry. *Flavour and Fragrance Journal* 21, 3 (2006): 502–9.

Bicchi, C., D'Amato, A., and Rubiolo, P. Cyclodextrin Derivatives as Chiral Selectors for Direct Gas Chromatographic Separation of Enantiomers in the Essential Oil, Aroma and Flavour Fields. *Journal of Chromatography A* 843, 1–2 (1999): 99–121.

Bicchi, C., Cordero, C., Iori, C., Rubiolo, P., and Sandra, P. Headspace Sorptive Extraction (HSSE) in the Headspace Analysis of Aromatic and Medicinal Plants. *HRC—Journal of High Resolution Chromatography* 23, 9 (2000): 539–46.

Bicchi, C., Brunelli, C., Galli, M., and Sironi, A. Conventional Inner Diameter Short Capillary Columns: An Approach to Speeding Up Gas Chromatographic Analysis of Medium Complexity Samples. *Journal of Chromatography A* 931, 1–2 (2001): 129–40.

Bicchi, C., Iori, C., Rubiolo, P., and Sandra, P. Headspace Sorptive Extraction (HSSE), Stir Bar Sorptive Extraction (SBSE), and Solid Phase Microextraction (SPME) Applied to the Analysis of Roasted Arabica Coffee and Coffee Brew. *Journal of Agricultural and Food Chemistry* 50, 3 (2002): 449–59.

Bicchi, C., Brunelli, C., Cordero, C., Rubiolo, P., Galli, M., and Sironi, A. Direct Resistively Heated Column Gas Chromatography (Ultrafast Module-GC) for High-Speed Analysis of Essential Oils of Differing Complexities. *Journal of Chromatography A* 1024, 1–2 (2004a): 195–207.

Bicchi, C., Cordero, C., and Rubiolo, P. A Survey on High-Concentration-Capability Headspace Sampling Techniques in the Analysis of Flavors and Fragrances. *Journal of Chromatographic Science* 42, 8 (2004b): 402–9.

Bicchi, C., Cordero, C., Liberto, E., Rubiolo, P., Sgorbini, B., and Sandra, P. Impact of phase ratio, polydimethylsiloxane volume and size, and sampling temperature and time on headspace sorptive extraction recovery of some volatile compounds in the essential oil field. *Journal of Chromatography A* 1071, 1–2 (2005): 111–118.

Bicchi, C., Cordero, C., Liberto, E., Sgorbini, B., and Rubiolo, P. Headspace Sampling of the Volatile Fraction of Vegetable Matrices. *Journal of Chromatography A* 1184, 1–2 (2008): 220–33.

Bicchi, C., Cagliero, C., and Rubiolo, P. New Trends in the Analysis of the Volatile Fraction of Matrices of Vegetable Origin: A Short Overview. A Review. *Flavour and Fragrance Journal* 26, 5 (2011): 321–25.

Blum, C., Kubeczka, K. H., and Becker, K. Supercritical Fluid Chromatography-Mass Spectrometry of Thyme Extracts (*Thymus Vulgaris* L.). *Journal of Chromatography A* 773, 1–2 (1997): 377–80.

Bonaccorsi, I. L., McNair, H. M., Brunner, L. A., Dugo, P., and Dugo, G. Fast HPLC for the Analysis of Oxygen Heterocyclic Compounds of Citrus Essential Oils. *Journal of Agricultural and Food Chemistry* 47, 10 (1999): 4237–39.

Breme, K., Tournayre, P., Fernandez, X., Meierhenrich, U. J., Brevard, H., Joulain, D., and Berdague, J. L. Identification of Odor Impact Compounds of *Tagetes minuta* L. Essential Oil: Comparison of Two GC-Olfactometry Methods. *Journal of Agricultural and Food Chemistry* 57, 18 (2009): 8572–80.

Buchbauer, G., Jager, W., Jirovetz, L., Ilmberger, J., and Dietrich, H. Therapeutic Properties of Essential Oils and Fragrances. *Bioactive Volatile Compounds from Plants* 525 (1993): 159–65.

Buiarelli, F., Cartoni, G., Coccioli, F., and Ravazzi, E. Analysis of Orange and Mandarine Essential Oils by HPLC. *Chromatographia* 31, 9–10 (1991): 489–92.

Buiarelli, F., Cartoni, G., Coccioli, F., and Leone, T. Analysis of Bitter Essential Oils from Orange and Grapefruit by High-Performance Liquid Chromatography with Microbore Columns. *Journal of Chromatography A* 730, 1–2 (1996): 9–16.

Caja, M., del Mar, and Herraiz, M. Rapid Screening of Volatile Compounds in Edible Plants by Direct Chromatographic Analysis. *Food Chemistry* 117, 3 (2009): 456–60.

Camps, C., Gerard, M., Quennoz, M., Brabant, C., Oberson, C., and Simonnet, X. Prediction of Essential Oil Content of Oregano by Hand-Held and Fourier Transform NIR Spectroscopy. *Journal of the Science of Food and Agriculture* 94, 7 (2014): 1397–402.

Chen, Y., Gu, X., Huang, S.-Q., Li, J., Wang, X., and Tang, J. Optimization of Ultrasonic/ Microwave Assisted Extraction (UMAE) of Polysaccharides from Inonotus Obliquus and Evaluation of Its Anti-Tumor Activities. *International Journal of Biological Macromolecules* 46, 4 (2010): 429–35.

Cheng, Z., Yang, Y., Liu, Y., Liu, Z., Zhou, H., and Hu, H. Two-Steps Extraction of Essential Oil, Polysaccharides and Biphenyl Cyclooctene Lignans from *Schisandra chinensis* Baill Fruits. *Journal of Pharmaceutical and Biomedical Analysis* 96 (2014): 162–69.

Clodoveo, M. L., Durante, V., and La Notte, D. Working Towards the Development of Innovative Ultrasound Equipment for the Extraction of Virgin Olive Oil. *Ultrasonics Sonochemistry* 20, 5 (2013): 1261–70.

Cordero, C., Rubiolo, P., Sgorbini, B., Galli, M., and Bicchi, C. Comprehensive Two-Dimensional Gas Chromatography in the Analysis of Volatile Samples of Natural Origin: A Multidisciplinary Approach to Evaluate the Influence of Second Dimension Column Coated with Mixed Stationary Phases on System Orthogonality. *Journal of Chromatography A* 1132, 1–2 (2006): 268–79.

Cordero, C., Bicchi, C., and Rubiolo, P. Group-Type and Fingerprint Analysis of Roasted Food Matrices (Coffee and Hazelnut Samples) by Comprehensive Two-Dimensional Gas Chromatography. *Journal of Agricultural and Food Chemistry* 56, 17 (2008): 7655–66.

Cordero, C., Liberto, E., Bicchi, C., Rubiolo, P., Reichenbach, S. E., Tian, X., and Tao, Q. Targeted and Non-Targeted Approaches for Complex Natural Sample Profiling by GC × GC-QMS. *Journal of Chromatographic Science* 48, 4 (2010a): 251–61.

Cordero, C., Liberto, E., Bicchi, C., Rubiolo, P., Schieberle, P., Reichenbach, S. E., and Tao, Q. Profiling Food Volatiles by Comprehensive 2-Dimensional Gas Chromatography Coupled with Mass Spectrometry: Advanced Fingerprinting Approaches for Comparative Analysis of the Volatile Fraction of Roasted Hazelnuts (*Corylus avellana* L.) from Different Origins. *Journal of Chromatography A* 1217, 37 (2010b): 5848–58.

Costa, R., De Fina, M. R., Valentino, M. R., Dugo, P., and Mondello, L. Reliable Identification of Terpenoids and Related Compounds by Using Linear Retention Indices Interactively with Mass Spectrometry Search. *Natural Product Communications* 2, 4 (2007): 413–18.

Costa, R., d'Acampora Zellner, B., Crupi, M. L., De Fina, M. R., Valentino, M. R., Dugo, P., Dugo, G., and Mondello, L. GC-MS, GC-O and Enantio-GC Investigation of the Essential Oil of *Tarchonanthus camphoratus* L. *Flavour and Fragrance Journal* 23, 1 (2008): 40–48.

Cramers, C. A., Janssen, H.-G., van Deursen, M. M., and Leclercq, P. A. High-Speed Gas Chromatography: An Overview of Various Concepts. *Journal of Chromatography A* 856, 1–2 (1999): 315–29.

d'Acampora Zellner, B., Bicchi, C., Dugo, P., Rubiolo, P., Dugo, G., and Mondello, L. Linear Retention Indices in Gas Chromatographic Analysis: A Review. *Flavour Fragrance Journal* 23, 5 (2008): 297–314.

d'Acampora Zellner, B., Dugo, P., Dugo, G., and Mondello, L. Analysis of Essential Oils. In *Handbook of Essential Oils: Science, Technology, and Applications*, ed. K. H. C. Baser and G. Buchbauer. CRC Press, Boca Raton, FL (2010): 151–183.

Darjazi, B. B. A Comparison of Volatile Components of Flower of Page Mandarin Obtained by Ultrasound-Assisted Extraction and Hydrodistillation. *Journal of Medicinal Plants Research* 5, 13 (2011): 2839–47.

David, F., and Sandra, P. Stir Bar Sorptive Extraction for Trace Analysis. *Journal of Chromatography A* 1152, 1–2 (2007): 54–69.

Dawidowicz, A. L., and Wianowska, D. PLE in the Analysis of Plant Compounds. Part 1: The Application of PLE for HPLC Analysis of Caffeine in Green Tea Leaves. *Journal of Pharmaceutical and Biomedical Analysis* 37, 5 (2005): 1155–59.

Dawidowicz, A. L., and Rado, E. Matrix Solid-Phase Dispersion (MSPD) in Chromatographic Analysis of Essential Oils in Herbs. *Journal of Pharmaceutical and Biomedical Analysis* 52, 1 (2010): 79–85.

Dawidowicz, A. L., Rado, E., Wianowska, D., Mardarowicz, M., and Gawdzik. J. Application of PLE for the Determination of Essential Oil Components from *Thymus vulgaris* L. *Talanta* 76, 4 (2008): 878–84.

Dawidowicz, A. L., Wianowska, D., and Rado, E. Matrix Solid-Phase Dispersion with Sand in Chromatographic Analysis of Essential Oils in Herbs. *Phytochemical Analysis* 22, 1 (2011): 51–58.

Dawidowicz, A. L., Czapczynska, N. B., and Wianowska, D. The Loss of Essential Oil Components Induced by the Purge Time in the Pressurized Liquid Extraction (PLE) Procedure of *Cupressus sempervirens*. *Talanta* 94 (2012): 140–45.

Dean, J. R., and Xiong, G. H. Extraction of Organic Pollutants from Environmental Matrices: Selection of Extraction Technique. *TrAC—Trends in Analytical Chemistry* 19, 9 (2000): 553–64.

Deng, C., Yao, N., Wang, A., and Zhang, X. Determination of Essential Oil in a Traditional Chinese Medicine, *Fructus amomi* by Pressurized Hot Water Extraction Followed by Liquid-Phase Microextraction and Gas Chromatography-Mass Spectrometry. *Analytica Chimica Acta* 536, 1–2 (2005): 237–44.

Deng, C., Ji, J., Li, N., Yu, Y., Duan, G., and Zhang, X. Fast Determination of Curcumol, Curdione and Germacrone in Three Species of Curcuma Rhizomes by Microwave-Assisted Extraction Followed by Headspace Solid-Phase Microextraction and Gas Chromatography-Mass Spectrometry. *Journal of Chromatography A* 1117, 2 (2006a): 115–20.

Deng, C., Mao, Y., Yao, N., and Zhang, X. Development of Microwave-Assisted Extraction Followed by Headspace Solid-Phase Microextraction and Gas Chromatography-Mass Spectrometry for Quantification of Camphor and Borneol in Flos *Chrysanthemi indici*. *Analytica Chimica Acta* 575, 1 (2006b): 120–25.

Di, X., Shellie, R. A., Marriott, P. J., and Huie, C. W. Application of Headspace Solid-Phase Microextraction (HS-SPME) and Comprehensive Two-Dimensional Gas Chromatography (GC × GC) for the Chemical Profiling of Volatile Oils in Complex Herbal Mixtures. *Journal of Separation Science* 27, 5–6 (2004): 451–58.

Diaz-Maroto, C. M., Perez-Coello, S. M., and Cabezudo, D. M. Supercritical Carbon Dioxide Extraction of Volatiles from Spices: Comparison with Simultaneous Distillation-Extraction. *Journal of Chromatography A* 947, 1 (2002): 23–29.

Dugo, G., Verzera, A., Cotroneo, A., d'Alcontres, I. S., Mondello, L., and Bartle, K. D. Automated HPLC-HRGC: A Powerful Method for Essential Oil Analysis. Part II: Determination of the Enantiomeric Distribution of Linalool in Sweet Orange, Bitter Orange and Mandarin Essential Oils. *Flavour Fragrance Journal* 9, 3 (1994a): 99–104.

Dugo, G., Verzera, A., Trozzi, A., Cotroneo, A., Mondello, L., and Bartle, K. D. Automated HPLC-HRGC: A Powerful Method for Essential Oils Analysis. Part I: Investigation on Enantiomeric Distribution of Monoterpene Alcohols of Lemon and Mandarin Essential Oils. *Essenze, Derivati Agrumari* 64, 1 (1994b): 35–44.

Dugo, P., Mondello, L., Dugo, G., Heaton, D. M., Bartle, K. D., Clifford, A. A., and Myers, P. Rapid Analysis of Polymethoxylated Flavones from Citrus Oils by Supercritical Fluid Chromatography. *Journal of Agricultural and Food Chemistry* 44, 12 (1996): 3900–5.

Dugo, P., Mondello, L., Dugo, L., Stancanelli, R., and Dugo, G. LC-MS for the Identification of Oxygen Heterocyclic Compounds in Citrus Essential Oils. *Journal of Pharmaceutical and Biomedical Analysis* 24, 1 (2000): 147–54.

Dugo, P., Favoino, O., Luppino, R., Dugo, G., and Mondello, L. Comprehensive Two-Dimensional Normal-Phase (Adsorption)–Reversed-Phase Liquid Chromatography. *Analytical Chemistry* 76, 9 (2004): 2525–30.

Dugo, G., Tranchida, P. Q., Cotroneo, A., Dugo, P., Bonaccorsi, I., Marriott, P., Shellie, R., and Mondello, L. Advanced and Innovative Chromatographic Techniques for the Study of Citrus Essential Oils. *Flavour and Fragrance Journal* 20, 3 (2005): 249–64.

Dugo, P., Herrero, M., Giuffrida, D., Kumm, T., Dugo, G., and Mondello, L. Application of Comprehensive Two-Dimensional Liquid Chromatography to Elucidate the Native Carotenoid Composition in Red Orange Essential Oil. *Journal of Agricultural and Food Chemistry* 56, 10 (2008a): 3478–85.

Dugo, P., Herrero, M., Kumm, T., Giuffrida, D., Dugo, G., and Mondello, L. Comprehensive Normal-Phase × Reversed-Phase Liquid Chromatography Coupled to Photodiode Array and Mass Spectrometry Detection for the Analysis of Free Carotenoids and Carotenoid Esters from Mandarin. *Journal of Chromatography A* 1189, 1–2 (2008b): 196–206.

Dugo, P., Cacciola, F., Kumm, T., Dugo, G., and Mondello, L. Comprehensive Multidimensional Liquid Chromatography: Theory and Applications. *Journal of Chromatography A* 1184, 1–2 (2008c): 353–68.

Eisert, R., Pawliszyn, J., Barinshteyn, G., and Chambers, D. Design of an Automated Analysis System for the Determination of Organic Compounds in Continuous Air Stream Using Solid-Phase Microextraction. *Analytical Communications* 35, 6 (1998): 187–89.

Eltz, T., Zimmermann, Y., Haftmann, J., Twele, R., Francke, W., Quezada-Euan, J. J., and Lunau, K. Enfleurage, Lipid Recycling and the Origin of Perfume Collection in Orchid Bees. *Proceedings of the Royal Society B* 274, 1627 (2007): 2843–48.

Eskilsson, C. S., and Bjorklund, E. Analytical-Scale Microwave-Assisted Extraction. *Journal of Chromatography A* 902, 1 (2000): 227–50.

Eyres, G., Marriott, P. J., and Dufour, J.-P. The Combination of Gas Chromatography-Olfactometry and Multidimensional Gas Chromatography for the Characterisation of Essential Oils. *Journal of Chromatography A* 1150, 1–2 (2007): 70–77.

Falkenberg, M. B., Santos, R. I., and Simões, C. M. O. Introdução à Análise Fitoquímica. In Farmacognosia: da planta ao medicamento, Chap. 10, C. M. O. Simões et al. (eds), 1999. Florianópolis: Editora da UFSC and Editora da Universidade/UFRG.

Fakhari, A. R., Salehi, P., Heydari, R., Ebrahimi, S. N., and Haddad, P. R. Hydrodistillation-Headspace Solvent Microextraction, a New Method for Analysis of the Essential Oil Components of *Lavandula angustifolia* Mill. *Journal of Chromatography A* 1098, 1–2 (2005): 14–18.

Feng, X.-F., Jing, N., Li, Z.-G., Wei, D., and Lee, M.-R. Ultrasound-Microwave Hybrid-Assisted Extraction Coupled to Headspace Solid-Phase Microextraction for Fast Analysis of Essential Oil in Dry Traditional Chinese Medicine by GC-MS. *Chromatographia* 77, 7–8 (2014): 619–28.

Figueiredo, A. C., Barroso, J. G., Pedro, L. G., and Scheffer, J. J. C. Factors Affecting Secondary Metabolite Production in Plants: Volatile Components and Essential Oils. *Flavour and Fragrance Journal* 23, 4 (2008): 213–26.

Filly, A., Fernandez, X., Minuti, M., Visinoni, F., Cravotto, G., and Chemat, F. Solvent-Free Microwave Extraction of Essential Oil from Aromatic Herbs: From Laboratory to Pilot and Industrial Scale. *Food Chemistry,* 150 (2014): 193–98.

Florez Menendez, J. C., Fernandez Sanchez, M. L., Sanchez Uria, J. E., Fernandez Martinez, E., and Sanz-Medel, A. Static headspace, solid-phase microextraction and headspace solid-phase microextraction for BTEX determination in aqueous samples by gas chromatography. *Analytica Chimica Acta* 415, 1–2 (2000): 9–20.

Fornari, T., Vicente, G., Vazquez, E., Garcia-Risco, M. R., and Reglero, G. Isolation of Essential Oil from Different Plants and Herbs by Supercritical Fluid Extraction. *Journal of Chromatography A* 1250 (2012): 34–48.

Galhiane, M. S., Rissato, S. R., Chierice, G. O., Almeida, M. V., and Silva, L. C. Influence of Different Extraction Methods on the Yield and Linalool Content of the Extracts of *Eugenia uniflora* L. *Talanta* 70, 2 (2006): 286–92.

Gallidabino, M., Romolo, F. S., Bylenga, K., and Weyermann, C. Development of a Novel Headspace Sorptive Extraction Method to Study the Aging of Volatile Compounds in Spent Handgun Cartridges. *Analytical Chemistry* 86, 9 (2014): 4471–78.

Germek, V. M., Koprivnjak, O., Butinar, B., Pizzale, L., Bucar-Miklavcic, M., and Conte, L. S. Influence of Phenols Mass Fraction in Olive (*Olea europaea* L.) Paste on Volatile Compounds in Buza Cultivar Virgin Olive Oil. *Journal of Agricultural and Food Chemistry* 61, 25 (2013): 5921–27.

Gholivand, M. B., Rahimi-Nasrabadi, M., and Chalabi, H. Determination of Essential Oil Components of Star Anise (*Illicium verum*) Using Simultaneous Hydrodistillation-Static Headspace Liquid-Phase Microextraction-Gas Chromatography Mass Spectrometry. *Analytical Letters* 42, 10 (2009): 1382–97.

Glisic, S., Ivanovic, J., Ristic, M., and Skala, D. Extraction of Sage (*Salvia officinalis* L.) by Supercritical CO2: Kinetic Data, Chemical Composition and Selectivity of Diterpenes. *Journal of Supercritical Fluids* 52, 1 (2010): 62–70.

Grynbaum, M. D., Kreidler, D., Rehbein, J., Purea, A., Schuler, P., Schaal, W., Czesla, H., Webb, A., Schurig, V., and Albert, K. Hyphenation of Gas Chromatography to Microcoil H-1 Nuclear Magnetic Resonance Spectroscopy. *Analytical Chemistry* 79, 7 (2007): 2708–13.

Guerrini, A., Sacchetti, G., Muzzoli, M., Rueda, G. M., Medici, A., Besco, E., and Bruni, R. Composition of the Volatile Fraction of *Ocotea bofo* Kunth (Lauraceae) Calyces by GC-MS and NMR Fingerprinting and Its Antimicrobial and Antioxidant Activity. *Journal of Agricultural and Food Chemistry* 54, 20 (2006): 7778–88.

Guerrini, A., Rossi, D., Paganetto, G., Tognolini, M., Muzzoli, M., Romagnoli, C., Antognoni, F., Vertuani, S., Medici, A., Bruni, A., Useli, C., Tamburini, E., Bruni, R., and Sacchetti, G. Chemical Characterization (GC/MS and NMR Fingerprinting) and Bioactivities of South-African *Pelargonium capitatum* (L.) L'Her. (Geraniaceae) Essential Oil. *Chemistry and Biodiversity* 8, 4 (2011): 624–42.

Hiltunen, R., and Laakso, I. Gas Chromatographic Analysis and Biogenetic Relationships of Monoterpene Enantiomers in Scots Pine and Juniper Needle Oils. *Flavour and Fragrance Journal* 10, 3 (1995): 203–10.

Isidorov, V. A., Vinogorova, V. T., and Rafalowski, K. HS-SPME Analysis of Volatile Organic Compounds of Coniferous Needle Litter. *Atmospheric Environment* 37, 33 (2003): 4645–50.

Jeannot, M. A., and Cantwell, F. F. Solvent Microextraction into a Single Drop. *Analytical Chemistry* 68, 13 (1996): 2236–40.

Jeannot, M. A., and Cantwell, F. F. Mass Transfer Characteristics of Solvent Extraction into a Single Drop at the Tip of a Syringe Needle. *Analytical Chemistry* 69, 2 (1997): 235–39.

Joulain, D., and Konig, W. *The Atlas of Spectral Data of Sesquiterpene Hydrocarbons*. E.B.-Verlag, Hamburg, Germany (1998).

Juliani, H. R., Kapteyn, J., Jones, D., Koroch, A. R., Wang, M., Charles, D., and Simon, J. E. Application of Near-Infrared Spectroscopy in Quality Control and Determination of Adulteration of African Essential Oils. *Phytochemical Analysis* 17, 2 (2006): 121–28.

Kamali, H., Aminimoghadamfarouj, N., and Nematollahi, A. Optimization of Process Variables for Essential Oil from *Lavandula angustifolia* by PHWE Using Central Composite Design. *International Journal of ChemTech Research* 6, 2 (2014): 1151–61.

Kawaguchi, M., Ito, R., Saito, K., and Nakazawa, H. Novel Stir Bar Sorptive Extraction Methods for Environmental and Biomedical Analysis. *Journal of Pharmaceutical and Biomedical Analysis* 40, 3 (2006): 500–8.

Kawaguchi, M., Ito, R., Nakazawa, H., and Takatsu, A. Applications of Stir-Bar Sorptive Extraction to Food Analysis. *TrAC—Trends in Analytical Chemistry* 45 (2013): 280–93.

Kim, N. S., and Lee, D. S. Comparison of Different Extraction Methods for the Analysis of Fragrances from *Lavandula* Species by Gas Chromatography-Mass Spectrometry. *Journal of Chromatography A* 982, 1 (2002): 31–47.

Kim, H.-J., Chi, M.-H., and Hong, I.-K. Effect of Ultrasound Irradiation on Solvent Extraction Process. *Journal of Industrial and Engineering Chemistry* 15, 6 (2009): 919–28.

Klee, M. S., and Blumberg, L. M. Theoretical and Practical Aspects of Fast Gas Chromatography and Method Translation. *Journal of Chromatographic Science* 40, 5 (2002): 234–47.

Korytar, P., Janssen, H.-G., Matisova, E., and Brinkman, U. A. Th. Practical Fast Gas Chromatography: Methods, Instrumentation and Applications. *TrAC—Trends Analytical Chemistry* 21, 9–10 (2002): 558–72.

Kotnik, P., Skerget, M., and Knez, Z. Supercritical Fluid Extraction of Chamomile Flower Heads: Comparison with Conventional Extraction, Kinetics and Scale-Up. *Journal of Supercritical Fluids* 43, 2 (2007): 192–98.

Kreck, M., Scharrer, A., Bilke, S., and Mosandl, A. Enantioselective Analysis of Monoterpene Compounds in Essential Oils by Stir Bar Sorptive Extraction (SBSE)-Enantio-MDGC-MS. *Flavour and Fragrance Journal* 17, 1 (2002): 32–40.

Kristenson, M. E., Ramos, L., and Brinkman, U. A. Th. Recent Advances in Matrix Solid-Phase Dispersion. *TrAC—Trends in Analytical Chemistry* 25, 2 (2006): 96–111.

Kuehnle, M., Kreidler, D., Holtin, K., Czesla, H., Schuler, P., Schaal, W., Schurig, V., and Albert, K. Online Coupling of Gas Chromatography to Nuclear Magnetic Resonance Spectroscopy: Method for the Analysis of Volatile Stereoisomers. *Analytical Chemistry* 80, 14 (2008): 5481–86.

Kuriakose, S., and Joe, I. H. Feasibility of Using Near Infrared Spectroscopy to Detect and Quantify an Adulterant in High Quality Sandalwood Oil. *Spectrochimica Acta A* 115 (2013): 568–73.

Laasonen, M., Harmia-Pulkkinen, T., Simard, C. L., Michiels, E., Raesaenen, M., and Vuorela, H. Fast Identification of *Echinacea purpurea* Dried Roots Using Near-Infrared Spectroscopy. *Analytical Chemistry* 74, 11 (2002): 2493–99.

Lahlou, M. Methods to Study the Phytochemistry and Bioactivity of Essential Oils. *Phytotherapy Research* 18, 6 (2004): 435–48.

Lee, M. S., Choi, J., Posadzki, P., and Ernst, E. Aromatherapy for Health Care: An Overview of Systematic Reviews. *Maturitas* 71, 3 (2012): 257–60.

Li, N., Deng, C., Li, Y., Ye, H., and Zhang, X. Gas Chromatography-Mass Spectrometry Following Microwave Distillation and Headspace Solid-Phase Microextraction for Fast Analysis of Essential Oil in Dry Traditional Chinese Medicine. *Journal of Chromatography A* 1133, 1–2 (2006): 29–34.

Lin, J., and Rouseff, R. L. Characterization of Aroma-Impact Compounds in Cold-Pressed Grapefruit Oil Using Time-Intensity GC-Olfactometry and GC-MS. *Flavour Fragrance Journal* 16, 6 (2001): 457–63.

Liu, Y., Wang, H., and Zhang, J. Comparison of MAHD with UAE and Hydrodistillation for the Analysis of Volatile Oil from Four Parts of *Perilla frutescens* Cultivated in Southern China. *Analytical Letters* 45, 13 (2012): 1894–909.

Lockwood, G. B. Techniques for Gas Chromatography of Volatile Terpenoids from a Range of Matrices. *Journal of Chromatography A* 936, 1–2 (2001): 23–31.

Lucchesi, M. E., Chemat, F., and Smadja, J. Solvent-Free Microwave Extraction of Essential Oil from Aromatic Herbs: Comparison with Conventional Hydro-Distillation. *Journal of Chromatography A* 1043, 2 (2004): 323–27.

Luque de Castro, M. D., and Garcia-Ayuso, L. E. Soxhlet Extraction of Solid Materials: An Outdated Technique with a Promising Innovative Future. *Analytica Chimica Acta* 369, 1–2 (1998): 1–10.

Luque de Castro, M. D., and Priego-Capote, F. Soxhlet Extraction: Past and Present Panacea. *Journal of Chromatography A* 1217, 16 (2010): 2383–89.

Luque-Garcia, J. L., and Luque de Castro, M. D. Where Is Microwave-Based Analytical Equipment for Solid Sample Pre-Treatment Going? *TrAC—Trends in Analytical Chemistry* 22, 2 (2003): 90–98.

Ma, C., Wang, H., Lu, X., Li, H., Liu, B., and Xu, G. Analysis of *Artemisia annua* L. Volatile Oil by Comprehensive Two-Dimensional Gas Chromatography Time-of-Flight Mass Spectrometry. *Journal of Chromatography A* 1150, 1–2 (2007): 50–53.

Maggi, F., Conti, F., Cristalli, G., Giuliani, C., Papa, F., Sagratini, G., and Vittori, S. Chemical Differences in Volatiles between *Melittis melissophyllum* L. subsp *melissophyllum* and subsp *albida* (Guss) P. W. Ball (Lamiaceae) Determined by Solid-Phase Microextraction (SPME) Coupled with GC/FID and GC/MS. *Chemistry and Biodiversity* 8, 2 (2011): 325–43.

Manninen, P., Riekkola, M.-L., Holm, Y., and Hiltunen, R. SFC in Analysis of Aromatic Plants. *HRC—Journal of High Resolution Chromatography* 13, 3 (1990): 167–69.

Marriott, P. J., Haglund, P., and Ong, R. C. Y. A Review of Environmental Toxicant Analysis by Using Multidimensional Gas Chromatography and Comprehensive GC. *Clinica Chimica Acta* 328, 1–2 (2003): 1–19.

Masango, P. Cleaner Production of Essential Oils by Steam Distillation. *Journal of Cleaner Production* 13, 8 (2005): 833–39.

McLafferty, F. W., Stauffer, D. A., Loh, S. Y., and Wesdemiotis, C. Unknown Identification Using Reference Mass Spectra: Quality Evaluation of Databases. *Journal of the American Society for Mass Spectrometry* 10, 12 (1999): 1229–40.

Meghwal, M., and Goswami, T. K. *Piper nigrum* and Piperine: An Update. *Phytotherapy Research* 27, 8 (2013): 1121–30.

Mondello, L., Dugo, P., Bartle, K. D., Frere, B., and Dugo, G. Online High-Performance Liquid-Chromatography Coupled with High-Resolution Gas-Chromatography and Mass-Spectrometry (HPLC-HRGC-MS) for the Analysis of Complex-Mixtures Containing Highly Volatile Compounds. *Chromatographia* 39, 9–10 (1994): 529–38.

Mondello, L., Dugo, P., Basile, A., Dugo, G., and Bartle, K. D. Interactive Use of Linear Retention Indices, on Polar and Apolar Columns, with a MS-Library for Reliable Identification of Complex Mixtures. *Journal of Microcolumn Separations* 7, 6 (1995): 581–91.

Mondello, L., Dugo, P., Dugo, G., and Bartle, K. D. On-Line HPLC-HRGC-MS for the Analysis of Natural Complex Mixtures. *Journal of Chromatographic Science* 34, 4 (1996): 174–81.

Mondello, L., Catalfamo, M., Dugo, G., and Dugo, P. Multidimensional Tandem Capillary Gas Chromatography System for the Analysis of Real Complex Samples. Part I: Development of a Fully Automated Tandem Gas Chromatography System. *Journal of Chromatographic Science* 36, 4 (1998): 201–9.

Mondello, L., Casilli, A., Tranchida, P. Q., Cicero, L., Dugo, P., and Dugo, G. Comparison of Fast and Conventional GC Analysis for Citrus Essential Oils. *Journal of Agricultural and Food Chemistry* 51, 19 (2003): 5602–6.

Mondello, L., Shellie, R., Casilli, A., Tranchida, P. Q., Marriott, P., and Dugo, G. Ultra-Fast Essential Oil Characterization by Capillary GC on a 50 μm ID Column. *Journal of Separation Science* 27, 9 (2004): 699–702.

Mosandl, A., and Juchelka, D. Advances in the Authenticity Assessment of Citrus Oils. *Journal of Essential Oil Research* 9, 1 (1997): 5–12.

Namara, K. M., Howell, J., Huang, Y., and Robbat, A., Jr. Analysis of Gin Essential Oil Mixtures by Multidimensional and One-Dimensional Gas Chromatography/Mass Spectrometry with Spectral Deconvolution. *Journal of Chromatography A* 1164, 1–2 (2007): 281–90.

Nehır, S. E., Karagozlu, N., Karakaya, S., and Sahin, S. Antioxidant and Antimicrobial Activities of Essential Oils Extracted from *Laurus nobilis* L. Leaves by Using Solvent-Free Microwave and Hydrodistillation. *Food and Nutrition Sciences* 5, 2 (2014): 97–106.

Ng, K. H., Heng, A., Osborne, M. Quantitative analysis of perfumes in talcum powder by using headspace sorptive extraction. *Journal of Separation Science* 35, 5–6 (2012): 758–762.

Nieto, A., Borrull, F., Pocurull, E., and Marce, R. M. Pressurized Liquid Extraction: A Useful Technique to Extract Pharmaceuticals and Personal-Care Products from Sewage Sludge. *TrAC—Trends in Analytical Chemistry* 29, 7 (2010): 752–64.

Ozel, M. Z., and Kaymaz, H. Superheated Water Extraction, Steam Distillation and Soxhlet Extraction of Essential Oils of *Origanum onites*. *Analytical and Bioanalytical Chemistry* 379, 7–8 (2004): 1127–33.

Ozel, M. Z., Gogus, F., and Lewis, A. C. Subcritical Water Extraction of Essential Oils from *Thymbra spicata*. *Food Chemistry* 82, 3 (2003): 381–86.

Ozel, M. Z., Gogus, F., Hamilton, J. F., and Lewis, A. C. The Essential Oil of *Pistacia vera* L. at Various Temperatures of Direct Thermal Desorption Using Comprehensive Gas Chromatography Coupled with Time-of-Flight Mass Spectrometry. *Chromatographia* 60, 1–2 (2004): 79–83.

Ozel, M. Z., Gogus, F., and Lewis, A. C. Determination of *Teucrium chamaedrys* Volatiles by Using Direct Thermal Desorption-Comprehensive Two-Dimensional Gas Chromatography-Time-of-Flight Mass Spectrometry. *Journal of Chromatography A* 1114, 1 (2006a): 164–69.

Ozel, M. Z., Gogus, F., and Lewis, A. C. Comparison of Direct Thermal Desorption with Water Distillation and Superheated Water Extraction for the Analysis of Volatile Components of *Rosa damascena* Mill. Using GCxGC-TOF/MS. *Analytica Chimica Acta* 566, 2 (2006b): 172–77.

Pan, X., Niu, G., and Liu, H. Microwave-Assisted Extraction of Tea Polyphenols and Tea Caffeine from Green Tea Leaves. *Chemical Engineering and Processing* 42, 2 (2003): 129–33.

Pawliszyn, J. (ed). Solid phase microextraction. In *Comprehensive Analytical Chemistry*, Volume 37. (Sampling and Sample Preparation for Field and Laboratory: Fundamentals and New Directions in Sample Preparation.) ed.; Elsevier: Amsterdam, 2002, pp. 389–477.

Petrakis, P. V., Couladis, M., and Roussis, V. A Method for Detecting the Biosystematic Significance of the Essential Oil Composition: The Case of Five Hellenic *Hypericum* L. Species. *Biochemical Systematics and Ecology* 33, 9 (2005): 873–98.

Piry, J., and Pribela, A. Application of High-Performance Liquid-Chromatography to the Analysis of the Complex Volatile Mixture of Black-Currant Buds (*Ribes nigrum* L). *Journal of Chromatography A* 665, 1 (1994): 105–9.

Pourmortazavi, S. M., and Hajimirsadeghi, S. S. Supercritical Fluid Extraction in Plant Essential and Volatile Oil Analysis. *Journal of Chromatography A* 1163, 1–2 (2007): 2–24.

Priego-Capote, F., and Luque de Castro, M. D. Analytical Uses of Ultrasound. I. Sample Preparation. *TrAC—Trends in Analytical Chemistry* 23, 9 (2004): 644–53.

Prosen, H., Kokalj, M., Janes, D., and Kreft, S. Comparison of Isolation Methods for the Determination of Buckwheat Volatile Compounds. *Food Chemistry* 121, 1 (2010): 298–306.

Radulovic, N. S., and Blagojevic, P. D. The Most Frequently Encountered Volatile Contaminants of Essential Oils and Plant Extracts Introduced during the Isolation Procedure: Fast and Easy Profiling. *Phytochemical Analysis* 23, 2 (2012): 131–42.

Radulovic, N. S., Dordevic, A. S., and Palic, R. M. The Intrasectional Chemotaxonomic Placement of *Hypericum elegans* Stephan Ex Willd. Inferred from the Essential-Oil Chemical Composition. *Chemistry and Biodiversity* 7, 4 (2010): 943–52.

Rauber, C. da S., Guterres, S. S., and Schapoval, E. E. S. LC Determination of Citral in *Cymbopogon citratus* Volatile Oil. *Journal of Pharmaceutical and Biomedical Analysis* 37, 3 (2005): 597–601.

Ravi, R., Prakash, M., and Bhat, K. K. Aroma Characterization of Coriander (*Coriandrum sativum* L.) Oil Samples. *European Food Research and Technology* 225, 3–4 (2007): 367–74.

Razote, E. B., Jeon, I. J., Maghirang, R. G., and Chobpattana, W. Dynamic Air Sampling of Volatile Organic Compounds Using Solid Phase Microextraction. *Journal of Environmental Science and Health B* 37, 4 (2002): 365–78.

Razote, E. B., Maghirang, R. G., Seitz, L. M., and Jeon, I. J. Characterization of Volatile Organic Compounds on Airborne Dust in a Swine Finishing Barn. *Transactions of the ASAE* 47, 4 (2004): 1231–38.

Reverchon, E., and Marrone, C. Supercritical Extraction of Clove Bud Essential Oil: Isolation and Mathematical Modeling. *Chemical Engineering Science* 52, 20 (1997): 3421–28.

Reverchon, E., and De Marco, I. Supercritical Fluid Extraction and Fractionation of Natural Matter. *Journal of Supercritical Fluids* 38, 2 (2006): 146–66.

Reverchon, E., Taddeo, R., and Della Porta, G. Extraction of Sage Oil by Supercritical CO2: Influence of Some Process Parameters. *Journal of Supercritical Fluids* 8, 4 (1995): 302–9.

Richter, J., and Schellenberg, I. Comparison of Different Extraction Methods for the Determination of Essential Oils and Related Compounds from Aromatic Plants and Optimization of Solid-Phase Microextraction/Gas Chromatography. *Analytical and Bioanalytical Chemistry* 387, 6 (2007): 2207–17.

Richter, B. E., Jones, B. A., Ezzell, J. L., Porter, N. L., Avdalovic, N., and Pohl, C. Accelerated Solvent Extraction: A Technique for Sample Preparation. *Analytical Chemistry* 68, 6 (1996): 1033–39.

Riela, S., Bruno, M., Formisano, C., Rigano, D., Rosselli, S., Saladino, M. L., and Senatore, F. Effects of Solvent-Free Microwave Extraction on the Chemical Composition of Essential Oil of *Calamintha nepeta* (L.) Savi Compared with the Conventional Production Method. *Journal of Separation Science* 31, 6–7 (2008): 1110–17.

Roberts, M. T., Dufour, J. P., and Lewis, A. C. Application of comprehensive multidimensional gas chromatography combined with time-of-flight mass spectrometry (GC x GC-TOFMS) for high resolution analysis of hop essential oil. *Journal of Separation Science* 27, 5–6 (2004): 473–8.

Rohloff, J. Volatiles from Rhizomes of *Rhodiola rosea* L. *Phytochemistry* 59, 6 (2002): 655–61.

Rubiolo, P., Belliardo, F., Cordero, C., Liberto, E., Sgorbini, B., and Bicchi, C. Headspace-Solid-Phase Microextraction Fast GC in Combination with Principal Component Analysis as a Tool to Classify Different Chemotypes of Chamomile Flower-Heads (*Matricaria recutita* L.). *Phytochemical Analysis* 17, 4 (2006): 217–25.

Rubiolo, P., Liberto, E., Sgorbini, B., Russo, R., Veuthey, J.-L., and Bicchi, C. Fast-GC-Conventional Quadrupole Mass Spectrometry in Essential Oil Analysis. *Journal of Separation Science* 31, 6–7 (2008): 1074–84.

Rubiolo, P., Sgorbini, B., Liberto, E., Cordero, C., and Bicchi, C. Essential Oils and Volatiles: Sample Preparation and Analysis. A Review. *Flavour and Fragrance Journal* 25, 5 (2010): 282–90.

Salehi, P., Asghari, B., and Mohammadi, F. Hydrodistillation-Headspace Solvent Microextraction: An Efficient Method for Analysis of the Essential Oil from the Seeds of *Foeniculum vulgare* Mill. *Chromatographia* 65, 1–2 (2007a): 119–22.

Salehi, P., Fakhari, A. R., Ebrahimi, S. N., and Heydari, R. Rapid Essential Oil Screening of *Rosmarinus officinalis* L. By Hydrodistillation-Headspace Solvent Microextraction. *Flavour and Fragrance Journal* 22, 4 (2007b): 280–85.

Sarafraz-Yazdi, A., and Amiri, A. Liquid-Phase Microextraction. *TrAC—Trends in Analytical Chemistry* 29, 1 (2010): 1–14.

Sawamura, M., Onishi, Y., Ikemoto, J., Tu, N. T. M., and Phi, N. T. L. Characteristic Odour Components of Bergamot (*Citrus bergamia* Risso) Essential Oil. *Flavour and Fragrance Journal* 21, 4 (2006): 609–15.

Schipilliti, L., Tranchida, P. Q., Sciarrone, D., Russo, M., Dugo, P., Dugo, G., and Mondello, L. Genuineness Assessment of Mandarin Essential Oils Employing Gas Chromatography-Combustion-Isotope Ratio MS (GC-C-IRMS). *Journal of Separation Science* 33, 4–5 (2010): 617–25.

Sereshti, H., Rohanifar, A., Bakhtiari, S., and Samadi, S. Bifunctional Ultrasound Assisted Extraction and Determination of *Elettaria cardamomum* Maton Essential Oil. *Journal of Chromatography A* 1238 (2012): 46–53.

Sgorbini, B., Budziak, D., Cordero, C., Liberto, E., Rubiolo, P., Sandra, P., and Bicchi, C. Solvent-Enhanced Headspace Sorptive Extraction in the Analysis of the Volatile Fraction of Matrices of Vegetable Origin. *Journal of Separation Science* 33, 14 (2010): 2191–99.

Shellie, R. A. Volatile Components of Plants, Essential Oils, and Fragrances. In *Wilson and Wilson's Comprehensive Analytical Chemistry*, ed. L. Ramos. Vol. 55. Elsevier, Amsterdam, 2009, pp. 189–213.

Shellie, R., Marriott, P., and Morrison, P. Comprehensive Two-Dimensional Gas Chromatography with Flame Ionization and Time-of-Flight Mass Spectrometry Detection: Qualitative and Quantitative Analysis of West Australian Sandalwood Oil. *Journal of Chromatographic Science* 42, 8 (2004): 417–22.

Smelcerovic, A., Spiteller, M., Ligon, A. P., Smelcerovic, Z., and Raabe, N. Essential Oil Composition of *Hypericum* L. Species from Southeastern Serbia and Their Chemotaxonomy. *Biochemical Systematics and Ecology* 35, 2 (2007): 99–113.

Smelcerovic, A., Lamshoeft, M., Radulovic, N., Ilic, D., and Palic, R. LC-MS Analysis of the Essential Oils of *Achillea millefolium* and *Achillea crithmifolia*. *Chromatographia* 71, 1–2 (2010): 113–16.

Smelcerovic, A., Djordjevic, A., Lazarevic, J., and Stojanovic, G. Recent Advances in Analysis of Essential Oils. *Current Analytical Chemistry* 9, 1 (2013): 61–70.

Stamenic, M., Vulic, J., Djilas, S., Misic, D., Tadic, V., Petrovic, S., and Zizovic, I. Free-Radical Scavenging Activity and Antibacterial Impact of Greek Oregano Isolates Obtained by SFE. *Food Chemistry* 165 (2014): 307–15.

Stan, M., Lung, I., Opris, O., and Soran, M.-L. High-Performance Thin-Layer Chromatographic Quantification of Some Essential Oils from Anethum Graveolens Extracts. *JPC—Journal of Planar Chromatography—Modern TLC* 27, 1 (2014): 33–37.

Stashenko, E. E., Jaramillo, B. E., and Martinez, J. R. Analysis of Volatile Secondary Metabolites from Colombian *Xylopia aromatica* (Lamarck) by Different Extraction and Headspace Methods and Gas Chromatography. *Journal of Chromatography A* 1025, 1 (2004a): 105–13.

Stashenko, E. E., Jaramillo, B. E., and Martinez, J. R. Comparison of Different Extraction Methods for the Analysis of Volatile Secondary Metabolites of *Lippia alba* (Mill.) N.E. Brown, Grown in Colombia, and Evaluation of Its *In Vitro* Antioxidant Activity. *Journal of Chromatography A* 1025, 1 (2004b): 93–103.

Steuer, B., and Schulz, H. Near-Infrared Analysis of Fennel (*Foeniculum vulgare* Miller) on Different Spectrometers: Basic Considerations for a Reliable Network. *Phytochemical Analysis* 14, 5 (2003): 285–89.

Sun, Y., Liu, D., Chen, J., Ye, X., and Yu, D. Effects of Different Factors of Ultrasound Treatment on the Extraction Yield of the All-Trans-B-Carotene from *Citrus* Peels. *Ultrasonics Sonochemistry* 18, 1 (2010): 243–49.

Sun, H., Ge, X., Lv, Y., and Wang, A. Application of Accelerated Solvent Extraction in the Analysis of Organic Contaminants, Bioactive and Nutritional Compounds in Food and Feed. *Journal of Chromatography A* 1237 (2012): 1–23.

Sun, H., Ni, H., Yang, Y., Chen, F., Cai, H., and Xiao, A. Sensory Evaluation and Gas Chromatography-Mass Spectrometry (GC-MS) Analysis of the Volatile Extracts of Pummelo (*Citrus maxima*) Peel. *Flavour and Fragrance Journal* 29, 5 (2014): 305–12.

Tadeo, J. L., Sanchez-Brunete, C., Albero, B., and Garcia-Valcarcel, A. I. Application of Ultrasound-Assisted Extraction to the Determination of Contaminants in Food and Soil Samples. *Journal of Chromatography A* 1217, 16 (2010): 2415–40.

Tankeu, S. Y., Vermaak, I., Kamatou, G. P. P., and Viljoen, A. M. Vibrational Spectroscopy and Chemometric Modeling: An Economical and Robust Quality Control Method for Lavender Oil. *Industrial Crops and Products* 59 (2014): 234–40.

Theis, A. L., Waldack, A. J., Hansen, S. M., and Jeannot, M. A. Headspace Solvent Microextraction. *Analytical Chemistry* 73, 23 (2001): 5651–54.

Tienpont, B., David, F., Bicchi, C., and Sandra, P. High Capacity Headspace Sorptive Extraction. *Journal of Microcolumn Separations* 12, 11 (2000): 577–84.

Todd, J. F. J. Recommendations for Nomenclature and Symbolism for Mass Spectroscopy (Including an Appendix of Terms Used in Vacuum Technology) (IUPAC Recommendations 1991). *International Journal of Mass Spectrometry Ion Processes* 142, 3 (1995): 211–40.

Turek, C., and Stintzing, F. C. Application of High-Performance Liquid Chromatography Diode Array Detection and Mass Spectrometry to the Analysis of Characteristic Compounds in Various Essential Oils. *Analytical and Bioanalytical Chemistry* 400, 9 (2011): 3109–23.

Vekey, K. Mass Spectrometry and Mass-Selective Detection in Chromatography. *Journal of Chromatography A* 921, 2 (2001): 227–36.

Wang, Z., Ding, L., Li, T., Zhou, X., Wang, L., Zhang, H., Liu, L., Li, Y., Liu, Z., Wang, H., Zeng, H., and He, H. Improved Solvent-Free Microwave Extraction of Essential Oil from Dried *Cuminum cyminum* L. And *Zanthoxylum bungeanum* Maxim. *Journal of Chromatography A* 1102, 1–2 (2006): 11–17.

Wang, Y., You, J., Yu, Y., Qu, C., Zhang, H., Ding, L., Zhang, H., and Li, X. Analysis of Ginsenosides in *Panax ginseng* in High Pressure Microwave-Assisted Extraction. *Food Chemistry* 110, 1 (2008): 161–67.

Williams, P., and Norris, K., eds. *Near-Infrared Technology in the Agricultural and Food Industries*, 2nd ed. AACC (2001).

Yan, Y., Chen, X., Hu, S., and Bai, X. Applications of Liquid-Phase Microextraction Techniques in Natural Product Analysis: A Review. *Journal of Chromatography A* 1368 (2014): 1–17.

Yang, Y., and Zhang, F. Ultrasound-Assisted Extraction of Rutin and Quercetin from *Euonymus alatus* (Thunb.) Sieb. *Ultrasonics Sonochemistry* 15, 4 (2008): 308–13.

Zhang, Z., and Pawliszyn, J. Headspace Solid-Phase Microextraction. *Analytical Chemistry* 65, 14 (1993): 1843–52.

Zhao, S., and Zhang, D. Supercritical CO2 Extraction of Eucalyptus Leaves Oil and Comparison with Soxhlet Extraction and Hydro-Distillation Methods. *Separation and Purification Technology* 133 (2014): 443–51.

Zheng, P., Sheng, X., Ding, Y., and Hu, Y. Study of Organosulfur Compounds in Fresh Garlic by Gas Chromatography/Mass Spectrometry Incorporated with Temperature-Programmable Cold On-Column Injection. *Se Pu* (*Chinese Journal of Chromatography/ Zhongguo Hua Xue Hui*) 24, 4 (2006): 351–53.

Zhu, S., Lu, X., Qiu, Y., Pang, T., Kong, H., Wu, C., and Xu, G. Determination of Retention Indices in Constant Inlet Pressure Mode and Conversion among Different Column Temperature Conditions in Comprehensive Two-Dimensional Gas Chromatography. *Journal of Chromatography A* 1150, 1–2 (2007): 28–36.

Zini, C. A., Zanin, K. D., Christensen, E., Caramao, E. B., and Pawliszyn, J. Solid-Phase Microextraction of Volatile Compounds from the Chopped Leaves of Three Species of Eucalyptus. *Journal of Agricultural and Food Chemistry* 51, 9 (2003): 2679–86.

7 Technological Aspects of Essential Oils

Maria Chiara Cristiano, Donato Cosco, and Donatella Paolino

CONTENTS

7.1 INTRODUCTION

The essential oils are natural products derived from aromatic plants, traditionally used all over the world for disinfection, as anti-inflammatory remedies, and as substances that relax or stimulate; they are full of potential for modern exploitation in clinical medicine. They can be used as natural alternatives to synthetic preparations in the prevention and treatment of diseases. These compounds are promising in the medical, pharmacological, alimentary, and cosmetic fields, to name a few.

Nevertheless, today the use of essential oils is very limited by their low levels of stability and water solubility, their great volatility, and their possible toxic effects when used in direct contact with the skin.

This chapter explores the experimental strategies that research groups all over the world have undertaken toward solving these problems. The lion's share of the attention is focused on technological approaches or, better yet, on the nanotechnological approach. Several works describe nanocarriers as systems able to encapsulate essential oils, modifying their undesirable features. Very interesting results were obtained in the study carried out by Celia and coworkers (2013), in which liposomes were used to deliver bergamot essential oil (BEO), thus overcoming the problem of its notably poor solubility, or the studies of Sinico et al. (2005) and Lai et al. (2007) carried out on *Artemisia arborescens*, which was encapsulated into liposomes and

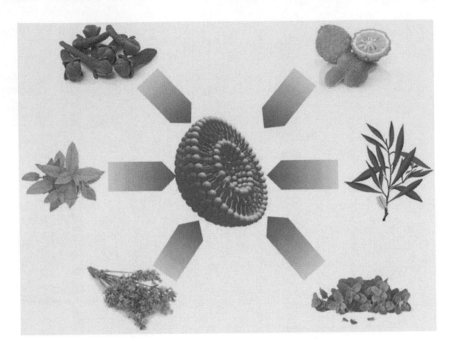

solid lipid nanoparticles so as to enhance its antiviral activity. But these are just some of the possible delivery systems for use with essential oils; other important systems are examined in this chapter, namely, the polymeric and lipidic nanocarriers, cyclodextrins, and nanoemulsions.

7.2   ESSENTIAL OILS: USES AND LIMITATIONS

The International Organization for Standardization (ISO) defines essential oils as products obtained from raw vegetable material, either by distillation with water or steam, from the epicarp of citrus fruit through a mechanical process, or by dry distillation (ISO 9235, 1997). But generally, essential oils (EOs) are complex mixtures of natural, aromatic, volatile, oily liquids that can be obtained from several parts of plants, especially the aerial parts, such as leaves and flowers.

The natural functions of essential oils are to protect plants from pathogenic microorganisms, to repel insects as potential plague vectors, and to limit their consumption by herbivores by conferring an unpleasant taste to the plant. Moreover, EOs facilitate plant reproduction by attracting specific insects that favor the dispersion of pollen and seeds. These aromatic and *attractive* features have been exploited for the production of perfumed products for personal hygiene, such as soaps, perfumes, and toiletries. D-Limonene, geranyl acetate, and D-carvone are examples of essential oils used as fragrances in household cleaning products and as industrial solvents (Bakkali et al., 2008).

In addition to these properties, promising approaches have been reported using essential oils or their components in medicinal products for human or veterinary use (Franz, 2010). In fact, evidence of the wide spectrum of the bioactivity of EOs has been confirmed by several studies and includes antibacterial, antiviral, anti-inflammatory, antifungal, antimutagenic, anticancer, and antioxidant effects, as well as others (Shaaban et al., 2012).

In particular, several studies have demonstrated that some essential oils or their components are able to reduce local tumor volume or tumor cell proliferation through pro-oxidant activity. Several research groups have demonstrated that *Myrica gale* and geraniol exhibit anticancer activity when used on lung and colon cancer cell lines (Carnesecchi et al., 2004; Sylvestre et al., 2005); *Ocimun sanctum*, *Citrus citratus*, *Piper nigrum*, *Lavandula angustifolia* (Manosroi et al., 2006), and others are able to inhibit the proliferation of murine leukemia and the human mouth epidermal carcinoma cell line, and again, the essential oil of a variety of lemongrass (*Cymbopogon flexuosus*) has shown an *in vitro* cytotoxicity against several human cancer cell lines (Parduman et al., 2009).

Antimicrobial activity is another important feature of essential oils. In fact, EOs from various origins seem to have a clear-cut inhibitory profile against pathogenic bacteria and fungi. For example, lemongrass, oregano, peppermint, rosemary, thyme, and clove oil contain essential oils characterized by an ample antimicrobial spectrum (Cava et al., 2007; Choi et al., 2012; Sienkiewicz et al., 2012). This activity is a consequence of their ability to interact with the lipidic cell membranes of microorganisms; due to their hydrophobicity and their short carbon chains, the components of EOs affect the fluidity of external and mitochondrial membranes, leading to their disruption and so to the death of the pathogen (Solórzano-Santos and Miranda-Novales, 2012).

With the increase in antibiotic-resistant bacteria and the lack of new antibiotics appearing on the market, alternative strategies need to be found in order to cope with infections resulting from drug-resistant bacteria. A possible solution may be to combine existing antibiotics with phytochemicals, such as essential oils, to enhance the efficacy of antibiotics (Langevedel et al., 2014); in fact, several works have shown the significant increase that occurs in antibiotic activity against drug-resistant microorganism strains when this strategy is used, a strategy that would make it possible to administer a smaller dose of antibiotics and avoid undesirable side effects (Palaniappan and Holley, 2010). In this scenario, some studies become important, such as those of Yap et al. (2013). The authors demonstrated the pronounced synergistic relationship that exists between piperacillin and several essential oils (such as lavender oil and peppermint oil) against bacteria containing plasmids codifying beta-lactamases. Moreover, the study of de Sousa et al. (2012) highlighted the antibacterial activity of the essential oil of *Lantana montevidensis* and its potential in modifying the resistance of the aminoglycosides analyzed during the study.

The multiple positive effects of essential oils are amply documented in literature, but their nature presents several limitations to their use. The most effective ways to administer most EOs is by topical application, mouthwashes, and gargles or through inhalation therapy. Oral administration is possible, although rarely used, and in these cases the EO is diluted in milk or olive oil. Topical applications are the most frequently used because they are generally safer; here the oil is diluted in a particular formulation or coupled with another oil, such as massage oil. Problems arise with topical application when skin reactions occur due to the direct application of the EO or UV alteration of the oil, both of which can irritate or darken the skin. Moreover, some oils, such as bergamot oil, can cause photosensitization and even induce malignant changes in the skin. Applying excessive amounts of strong oils to a large surface of the skin can also result in significant systemic adsorption and increase the chance of serious side effects (Bilia et al., 2014).

Besides dilution, EOs are also tailored by dispersing them in semisolid media. In this case, the oil-in-water (O/W) types of emulsions are preferred because they are easier to apply to the skin and do not leave an unpleasant, oily residue. Moreover, taking into account the natural antimicrobial profile of many EOs, their use can reduce the necessity for synthetic preservative excipients such as parabens, which are potential allergens.

There are many serious limitations to the use of EOs. They are very volatile essences and are highly sensitive to temperature, light, and oxygen, the exposure to which can lead to a loss of integrity (Turek and Stintzing, 2014). Considering that the main constituents of EOs contain unsaturated carbon chains, their susceptibility to oxidation mediated by light or heat is well known (Neumann and Garcia, 1992). In addition to oxidation, the constituents of EOs may also undergo isomerization, cyclization, or dehydrogenation, triggered either enzymatically or chemically (Scott, 2007). The products of these processes have been demonstrated to have highly allergenic, skin-sensitizing capacities, both of which constitute potent contact reactions.

The great volatility of EO components limits their free use; moreover, their scarce solubility in water further limits possible administration routes. All these factors condition the use of EOs. In this scenario, nanotechnology has become a promising solution for overcoming these problems.

7.3   ESSENTIAL OIL–BASED NANOTECHNOLOGY

Scientific research is focusing more and more on the encapsulation of bioactive compounds as a feasible and efficient approach to modulating drug release, increasing the physical stability of the active substances, protecting them from environmental effects, decreasing their volatility, enhancing their bioactivity, reducing their toxicity, and improving patient compliance and convenience. This type of approach—namely, nanotechnology—is a promising field for interdisciplinary research. It opens up a wide array of opportunities in many sectors, the foremost of which are medical, pharmaceutical, electronic, and agricultural, because it involves not only the delivery of anticancer drugs and anti-inflammatory, chemical, and natural compounds, but also the encapsulation of pesticides and probiotics (Rai and Ingle, 2012).

The encapsulation of EOs in nanometric-sized systems is desirable for the protection of their active compounds against environmental factors (possible thermal or photodegradation or other types of destabilization induced by oxygen, light, moisture, or pH), to decrease their volatility, thus facilitating use, and for transforming the EOs into powder form. Moreover, the design of drug-loaded nanosystems may permit the potentiation of the cellular absorption mechanism and bioefficacy, due to the exploitation of their subcellular sizes (Bilia et al., 2014).

Considering these features, nanosystems could actually overcome the limitations of essential oils. This chapter aims to describe the principal nanocarrier systems that are suitable for EO encapsulation.

7.3.1 Polymeric Nanosystems

Nanoparticles are solid colloidal suspensions, the mean particle size of which is less than 1 μm. They can be morphologically classified as spheres and capsules. In the first case, the particles are made up of a porous and dense matrix in which the drug can be adsorbed or entrapped, while capsule systems are formed by an aqueous or lipophilic core containing drugs enclosed in a shell (Cosco et al., 2008). A wide range of polymers exists that may be of synthetic (such as poly[DL-lactide-co-glycolide] [PLGA]) or natural origin (such as chitosan). If the nanosystem is designed for the pharmaceutical or medical fields, any selected polymer must necessarily be biocompatible, stable, safe, nontoxic, and biodegradable. These features are present especially in natural biomaterials, such as polysaccharides. The ample category of polysaccharides includes compounds of vegetable origin (pectin, cellulose, starch, arabic gum, carrageenan, and alginate) and compounds from microbial or animal origin (xanthan gum and chitosan). Due to their unique properties, nanoparticles made of polysaccharides are promising carriers for delivering and protecting the physiological properties of drugs (Liu et al., 2008). In addition, polysaccharides are abundantly available and their processing costs are low.

The mechanisms that cause the release of the encapsulated drug from nanoparticle colloidal suspensions depend on the characteristics of the colloidal suspension as well as on the physicochemical properties of the drug. In particular, the release of a drug may occur by one of the following mechanisms or by a combination of more than one: (1) drug desorption from the colloidal surface (for both nanospheres and nanocapsules), (2) drug diffusion through the polymeric network of the nanospheres or through the polymeric shell of the nanocapsules, and (3) polymeric matrix erosion of the nanoparticles (Paolino et al., 2006). Different particle structures give origin to different types of drug release. In particular, the compounds loaded into spheres will be released by a zero-order kinetic, while the drugs entrapped in the cores of the capsules will be released by a first-order kinetic (Cosco et al., 2008).

In literature, several types of EO-loaded nanoparticles are described, and in function of the selected polymer, different characteristics and functions of nanosystems can be obtained.

The encapsulation of essential oils into nanoparticles permits the improvement of the problem of their scarce water solubility, as demonstrated by Wu and collaborators (2012). The authors prepared zein nanoparticles containing carvacrol or thymol, and they demonstrated that EO-loaded nanocapsules increased the solubility of the EOs under all tested pH conditions (pH 4, 6.5, and 10) and that different pH conditions influenced the degree of solubility enhancement. Wu et al. demonstrated that encapsulation of EOs in zein nanoparticles allows their dispersion in water, which greatly enhances their potential for use in food preservation and the control of human pathogenic bacteria. In particular, this study demonstrated that encapsulating EOs in zein nanoparticles can enhance their solubility up to 14-fold without hindering their ability to scavenge free radicals or control *Escherichia coli* growth.

Eugenol is the main constituent of diverse EOs, and it is characterized by a high level of volatility and instability, besides being sensitive to oxygen, light, and heat. The encapsulation of this EO into nanocarriers such as polycaprolactone nanoparticles (Choi et al., 2009) or chitosan nanoparticles permits the protection of the compound against light oxidation and thermal stress. In particular, the eugenol-loaded chitosan nanoparticles could be useful as antioxidants for various thermal processing applications (Woranuch and Yoksan, 2013).

Another system that loads eugenol is polylactic glycolic acid nanocapsules. In Gomes et al.'s work (2011), these nanocapsules were shown to be characterized by a two-phase EO release: the first phase was rapid and about 20% of the EO was released after 30 min, which may have been due to the fact that the molecules were adsorbed to the polymeric wall; the second phase was more prolonged, and after 72 h, 64% of the eugenol had been released. The EO released in the second phase corresponded to the total amount of essential oil present in the core of the nanocapsules. Considering that PLGA has a slow degradation rate, it was hypothesized that its release is probably governed by diffusion, with possible additional elements of polymer swelling and bulk erosion.

The same trend of release was shown by carvacrol-loaded PLGA nanocapsules (Iannitelli et al., 2011). The *in vitro* release profile was characterized by an initial *burst*, followed by a slowing down, due to the concentration gradient. In fact, the nanoparticles showed 60% release after 3 h and 95% after 24 h.

Formulation	Essential Oil	Activity	References
Zein-sodium caseinate (SC) nanoparticles	Thymol	Presented efficient antimicrobial activity and two-phase release	Li et al. (2012)
Chitosan nanoparticles	Carvacrol	Enhanced antimicrobial activity	Keawchaoon and Yoksan (2011)
Chitosan nanoparticles	Oregano essential oil	Controlled release	Hosseini et al. (2013)
Chitosan nanoparticles	Eugenol and carvacrol	Decreased cytotoxicity toward mouse cells at MIC in comparison to free EOs	Chen (2012)
Methyl and ethylcellulose nanoparticles	Thymol	Presented efficient antimicrobial activity and is an effective preventive for cosmetic lotions creams and gels	Wattanasatcha et al. (2012)

Tea tree oil was encapsulated into nanocapsules to decrease its tendency to volatilize. The nanostructures presented a mean size of 160–220 nm with a polydispersity index below 0.25 and a negative zeta potential. The pH value was 5.98 ± 0.00 for nanocapsules. The oil content after preparation was 96%. The incorporation of the tea tree oil into the nanocapsules protected it from evaporation, improving its stability and decreasing its pronounced odor. The analysis of mean size and polydispersity index of the experimental formulations presented no significant alteration during storage time (Flores et al., 2011).

7.3.2 LIPID NANOSYSTEMS

Lipid nanosystems include micro- and nanometric-scaled emulsions and lipid nanoparticles, roughly divided into liposomes, micelles, niosomes, solid lipid nanoparticles (SLNs), and nanostructured lipid carriers (NLCs). The association of EOs with lipid nanosystems has different objectives, but the main aims are the enhancement of their stability and solubility in aqueous media, maintenance or even enhancement of their biological activity, and drug targeting (Bilia et al., 2014).

7.3.2.1 Nanoemulsions

Nanoemulsions are submicron-sized emulsions that are currently under extensive investigation as drug carriers for improving the delivery of therapeutic agents. They are by far the most advanced nanoparticle systems for the systemic delivery of biologically active agents for controlled drug delivery and targeting. Nanoemulsions are thermodynamically stable isotropic systems in which two immiscible liquids (water and oil) are put into emulsion to form a single phase by means of an appropriate surfactant or mix with a droplet diameter approximately in the range of 0.5–100 µm. Nanoemulsion droplet sizes fall typically in the range of 20–500 nm and show narrow size distribution (Shah et al., 2010).

Many different applications of nanoemulsions have been reported, including using them as preservatives in foods, for delivering pesticides in the agrochemical sector, and as antimicrobial agents in disinfectant formulas (Buranasuksombat et al., 2011). The antimicrobial property of a nanoemulsion seems to be due to the small size of the oil particles it contains; these particles are characterized by a high surface tension, which can interact with and subsequently disrupt the membranes of isolated microorganisms, so the already-present antimicrobial activity can be enhanced by including substances that possess antimicrobial properties in the nanoemulsions. In this way, the amount of active substances and detergents can be reduced, which would also reduce side effects.

The encapsulation of terpenes extracted from *Melaleuca alternifolia* and D-limonene into a nanoemulsion was investigated by Donsì and coworkers (2011) as a method for improving the safety and quality of foods through the addition of natural preservatives. The most promising formulations were tested in fruit juices, in order to evaluate the preservation of the juice from the activity of spoilage microorganisms (*Lactobacillus delbrueckii, Saccharomyces cerevisiae, E. coli*) inoculated into it. Results showed that the minimum inhibitory concentration (MIC) and minimum bactericidal concentration (MBC) values of the antimicrobial agents encapsulated in nanoemulsions were always lower than or equal to those of the pure compounds, suggesting that the enhancement of transport mechanisms through the cell membranes of the target microorganisms occurs.

Selected cooking oils such as sunflower, castor, coconut, groundnut, and sesame oils were screened for use in the development of a surfactin-based nanoemulsion formulation by Chen et al. (2009). Among the different resulting emulsions, the nanosystems obtained using sunflower oil were of the smallest recorded size (almost 70 nm). And it is noteworthy that the sunflower oil–based nanoemulsion showed the greatest antimicrobial activity against *Salmonella typhi*, *Listeria moosytogenes*, and *Staphylococcus aureus*.

Saranya and collaborators formulated nanoemulsions using eucalyptus oil, Tween 20, and ethanol, obtaining droplets with a mean size of 20 nm. The nanoemulsions were highly stable, transparent, and found to carry on greater bactericidal activity against *Proteus mirabilis* than eucalyptus alone; in fact, growth inhibition was found to be 100% when treated with the nanoemulsion (Sugumar et al., 2013).

The delivery of essential oils in nanoemulsions is important not only in the alimentary sector, but also for the production of insect repellents and products for the prevention of insect-induced diseases. For this reason, Nuchuchua et al. (2009) proposed EO-loaded nanoemulsions characterized by mosquito-repellent activity (*Aedes aegypti*). Nanoemulsions composed of citronella, hairy basil, and vetiver oils were prepared, and the results indicated that those with the smallest droplet size (around 150 nm) have better physical stability, a higher oil release rate, and more prolonged mosquito-repellent activity. The authors found that the longest mosquito protection time (4.7 h) against *A. aegypti* can be obtained with a composition of 10% (w/w) citronella oil, 5% (w/w) hairy basil oil, and 5% (w/w) vetiver oil in a nanoemulsion.

7.3.2.2 Liposomes

Among all the possible types of nanocarriers, the liposomes are certainly the most widely known, and since 1960 they have represented an innovative approach in the field of drug delivery systems. Liposomes are mostly made up of phospholipids, and are therefore highly biocompatible and biodegradable, but they can also be made to contain other components (i.e., steroid molecules, gangliosides, and polymeric materials), which can modify their biodistribution, drug-release profile, and clearance. These carriers have the ability to deliver macromolecules with different physico-chemical characteristics, thus permitting a selective therapeutic effect (Cosco et al., 2008).

Liposomes may be characterized by (1) one bilayer forming unilamellar vesicles (ULVs), (2) several concentric bilayers forming multilamellar vesicles, or (3) non-concentric bilayers forming multivesicular vesicles (MVVs) (Bilia et al., 2014). The importance of liposomal carriers is due to their ability to protect the compartmentalized bioactive compounds against degradation and also, in the case of lipophilic compounds, to increase solubilization (Musthaba et al., 2009).

In literature, the delivery of essential oils in liposomes is amply described. Liposomes are generally able to improve the delivery of the active compounds, releasing them inside the cells; in this way, the EO can carry on its antimicrobial, antifungal, and antiviral activities (Shoji and Nakashima, 2004) to the maximum potential.

For example, Liolios and coworkers (2009) prepared phosphatidylcholine-based liposomes as carriers for cavacrol and thymol isolated from the essential oil of *Origanum dictamnus*. After preparation, the researchers performed tests against four Gram-positive bacteria and four Gram-negative bacteria and three human pathogenic fungi, as well as the food-borne pathogen *Listeria monocytogenes*. Following encapsulation, enhanced antimicrobial activities were observed, in which the above-mentioned natural compounds acted as potent preservative and conservation agents, not only in food, but also in cosmetics and medical preparations.

The effect of liposomal inclusion on the *in vitro* antiherpetic activity of *A. arborescens* L. essential oil was investigated by Sinico et al. (2005). The authors prepared several formulations: multilamellar (MLV) and unilamellar (SUV) positively charged liposomes, using hydrogenated (P90H) or nonhydrogenated (P90) soy phosphatidylcholine. The results showed that the tested EO can be incorporated successfully into the liposomal system. The antiviral assay demonstrated that the system enhanced the *in vitro* antiherpetic activity of the EO against herpes simplex virus type 1 (HSV-1), especially in the case of the MLV made with P90H. Here, the essential oil seems to have been able to render the virus inactive, especially when it was delivered by nanosystems, since these carriers acted as target systems and delivered the EO directly to the action site. Moreover, the authors demonstrated that their innovative systems loading *A. arborescens* are very stable for at least 6 months with no oil leakage or alteration of the vesicle size (Sinico et al., 2005).

A similar study, but with a different trend, was performed by Valenti, who investigated the effect of liposomal inclusion on the stability and *in vitro* antiherpetic activity of *Santolina insularis* EO. This EO is effective in rendering HSV-1 inactive, which is principally due to its direct virucidal effects. In this case, the liposomes were also prepared using hydrogenated soya phosphatidylcholine and cholesterol. Analysis demonstrated that *Santolina insularis* EO-loaded liposomes remained stable for at least 1 year and that the systems are able to prevent EO degradation. Antiviral activity assays gave particular results: when this EO was loaded into liposomes, a certain antiviral activity was still present, though diminished (Valenti et al., 2001). Since viruses possess different types of organization, it is probable that the activity of the EO was hampered by the virus capsule.

The scientific study carried out by Celia et al. (2013) was particularly interesting. The authors investigated the possibility of incorporating bergamot essential oil (BEO) into liposomal carriers. It had been demonstrated that BEO carries on anti-cancer activity against neuroblastoma cells, but the poor solubility of this compound limited its use as a therapeutic agent. In this study, the encapsulation of BEO within liposomes eliminated the need for toxic solubilizing agents and allowed increased anticancer efficacy *in vitro*. Both liposomal BEO and bergapten-free BEO (BEO-BF) were able to reduce the viability of SH-SY5Y cells at far lower concentrations than their free-drug counterparts, highlighting the importance of a liposomal drug delivery system for the future development of BEO as an anticancer agent.

7.3.2.3 Solid Lipid Nanoparticles

Solid lipid nanoparticles (SLNs) were developed in the early 1990s as an alternative carrier system to emulsions, liposomes, and polymeric nanoparticles. These are nanoparticles with a solid lipid matrix presenting an average diameter in the nanometer range, which protects the incorporated active compounds against chemical degradation and modulates their release (drug mobility is much slower in a solid lipid than in a liquid oil). Normally, SLNs are made up of solid lipids (triglycerides, partial glycerides, fatty acids, steroids, and waxes), emulsifiers (poloxamer 188, polysorbate 80, polyvinyl alcohol, sorbitane monopalmitate), and water, all of which are generally recognized as safe substances (Cosco et al., 2008).

Frankincense and myrrh are gum resins obtained from the genera *Boswellia* and *Commiphora*, respectively. As with other essential oils, the instability and poor water solubility of frankincense and myrrh essential oils (FMOs) result in poor bioavailability, which limits their clinical application (Pillmoor et al., 1993); moreover, the components of FMOs are sensitive to light, air, and high temperatures. In order to overcome these limits, Shi et al. (2012) prepared and characterized solid lipid nanoparticles loaded with FMOs. For the preparation, Compritol 888 ATO was used as the solid lipid, showing a reasonable capacity for FMO solubilization. The scarcely water-soluble drug FMOs were efficiently encapsulated into SLNs, presenting a mean diameter of <220 nm. The drug evaporation release study showed that SLN incorporation could prevent the evaporation of FMO components to an interesting degree. Moreover, FMO-SLNs possess significantly greater antitumor efficacy. Therefore, the developed SLNs can be used to increase the stability or improve the *in vivo* antitumor efficacy of FMOs.

The use of SLNs for the topical delivery of active compounds is widely described. The topical application of SLNs favors skin hydration, an effect that is due to their spatial disposition. In particular, the reduced mean sizes of the nanoparticles and the extremely small spaces between the nanoparticles result in a uniform, poreless film that is more effective at preventing water evaporation than the microparticles (Müller et al., 2002). Moreover, a great advantage of SLNs is their protective action on the natural lipid element of the skin induced by their reflective properties, a characteristic that is missing in the other formulations (Cosco et al., 2008).

Considering the promise of SLN for efficient topical delivery, Lai and collaborators (2007) investigated the effect of SLN incorporation on the transdermal delivery and *in vitro* antiherpetic activity of *A. arborescens* essential oil. The prepared formulations were able to entrap EO in high yields, and their mean particle size increased only slightly after 2 years of storage, indicating a great degree of physical stability. The *in vitro* antiviral assay showed that the incorporation of the essential oil into SLNs did not affect its anti-HSV activity. Moreover, the *in vitro* skin permeation experiments demonstrated the capability of SLNs to greatly improve the accumulation of the EO in the skin, while permeation of the oil occurred only when it was delivered by the control solution.

In the same period, the same research team wanted to evaluate the potentiality of *A. arborescens* L. essential oil–loaded SLNs as a fitting delivery system for ecological pesticides. Also in this case, the SLNs showed themselves to be highly stable for 2 months at various storage temperatures. Regarding *in vitro* testing, the release experiments showed that SLNs were able to reduce the rapid evaporation of the EO when compared with the reference emulsions (Lai et al., 2006).

Alhaj and coworkers developed a formulation based on the *Nigella sativa* essential oil in SLNs. The aqueous and oily extracts of the seeds have been shown to possess antioxidant, anti-inflammatory, anticancer, analgesic, and antimicrobial properties, which renders them promising for future use in medicinal and cosmetic applications, and also in the sanitary, cosmetic, agricultural, and food industries. The analysis carried out on the EO-loaded SLNs showed a high degree of physical stability at various storage temperatures during 3 months of storage. In particular, the average diameter of the *N. sativa* EO-loaded SLN did not vary during storage and increased only slightly after freeze-drying of the SLN dispersions. Therefore, results showed that the studied SLN formulations are carriers suitable for use in the pharmaceutical and cosmetic fields (Alhaj et al., 2010).

7.3.2.4 Cyclodextrins

The cyclodextrins (CDs) are an important group of molecular carriers and are already amply present on the market for the delivery of various types of drugs. The CDs are characterized by a lipophilic central cavity and a hydrophilic outer surface. The glucopyranose units present themselves in the form of a chair, and for this reason, the CDs may be represented as a truncated cone. The OH groups are oriented with the primary hydroxyl groups of the various units of glucose on the narrow side of the cone and the secondary OH groups at the larger edge (Paolino et al., 2006).

The most important characteristic of CDs is their ability to form inclusion complexes (ICs) both in solution and in the solid state, in which the guest molecule places itself in the hydrophobic cavity in subtraction from the aqueous environment. This leads to a modification of the physical, chemical, and biological properties of the guest molecules. Moreover, the formation of the inclusion complex increases the guest's *in vivo* stability against hydrolysis, oxidation, decomposition, and dehydration, consequently increasing its bioavailability and bioefficacy. Natural CDs (α-CD, β-CD, γ-CD, in particular β-CD) possess a much lower degree of aqueous solubility with respect to comparable linear or branched dextrins. This is probably due to the relatively strong binding of the CD molecules in the crystal state (i.e., relatively high crystal lattice energy). Moreover, β-CD forms intramolecular hydrogen bonds between the secondary hydroxyl groups, a fact that reduces the number of hydroxyl groups capable of forming hydrogen bonds with the surrounding water molecules (Table 7.1) (Paolino et al., 2006).

Most relative publications are concerned with the encapsulation of essential oils in β-CD and its derivatives, which include randomly methylated-β-cyclodextrin, hydroxypropyl-β-cyclodextrin, and low methylated-β-cyclodextrin.

Starting with the importance of the capacity of cyclodextrins to form inclusion complexes, Ponce Cevallos et al. (2010) wanted to investigate the influence of water adsorption on the ICs of thymol and cinnamaldehyde in β-CD. Thymol is a monoterpene present in Lamiaceae plants, especially oreganos and thymes. Cinnamaldehyde represents 65%–75% of the cinnamon EO. As natural and

TABLE 7.1

Principal Physical-Chemical Characteristics of Natural CDs

	α-CDs	β-CDs	γ-CDs
Molecular weight	972	1135	1297
Units of glucopyranose	6	7	8
Internal diameter, Å	5	6	8
Solubility, mg · 100 ml^{-1}, 25°C	14.2	1.85	23.2
Melting point, °C	250–255	250–265	240–245

Source: Paolino, D. et al., Drug delivery systems, in J.G. Webster (ed.), *The Encyclopedia of Medical Devices and Instrumentations*, 2nd ed, John Wiley & Sons Ltd., Oxford, UK, 2006, pp. 437–495.

artificial flavors, they are very sensitive to the effects of light, oxygen, humidity, and high temperatures.

The results of Ponce Cevallos et al.'s study showed that β-CD efficiently encapsulates both of them, in a 1:1 molar ratio. After preparation, the samples were stored at a constant relative humidity, ranging from 22% to 97%, at 25°C. Water sorption isotherms for β-CD and the complexes showed that constant, low water sorption occurred at relative humidity (RH) < 80%, after which the uptake of water increased abruptly. Concerning the release of essential oils, no thymol or cinnamaldehyde release was detected at RH < 84%, though it did increase abruptly after 84% RH. The stability studies showed that the thymol-β-CD and cinnamaldehyde-β-CD inclusion complexes remain stable up to 75% RH during long storage periods. In fact, the guests released from the β-CD complexes were detectable in the region of the water adsorption isotherm, at which a sharp increase of water content was present (84% RH) (Ponce Cevallos et al., 2010).

B-Caryophyllene (BCP) is a natural sesquiterpene existing in the EOs of many plants that has antimicrobial, anticarcinogenic, anti-inflammatory, anti-oxidant, anxiolytic-like, and local anesthetic effects (Liu et al., 2013). Unfortunately, it is highly volatile and is poorly water soluble; these characteristics limit its application in the pharmaceutical field. For this reason, Liu and coworkers wanted to investigate and compare the oral bioavailability and the pharmacokinetics of the free form of BCP and the BCP/β-CD inclusion complex following a single dose of 50 mg/kg on rats. Through a gas chromatography–mass spectrometry method in selected ion monitoring (GC-MS/SIM) mode, the authors evaluated the free BCP in rat plasma. The *in vivo* data showed that the BCP/β-CD inclusion complex leads to earlier T_{MAX} and higher C_{MAX}, and the AUC_{0-12h} was greater with respect to free BCP. Thanks to these results, the authors demonstrated that the BCP/β-CD inclusion complex significantly increases the oral bioavailability of the drug in rats, compared to the free essential oil (Liu et al., 2013).

Similar to BCP, garlic oil (GO) is also characterized by high volatility and low physicochemical stability, which limits its application as a food-functional ingredient. GO, rich in organosulfuric compounds, has a variety of antimicrobial and antioxidant properties. The study of Wang et al. (2011) was focused on the formation of the GO/β-CD inclusion complex. The complex was obtained by the coprecipitation method in a molar ratio of 1:1; and the formation of the IC was demonstrated through different analytical techniques, including Fourier transform infrared spectroscopy, differential scanning calorimetry, and x-ray diffractometry. The aqueous solubility and stability of GO were significantly increased by inclusion in β-CD.

7.4   CONCLUSION

Scientific research in the medical, cosmetic, pharmacological, and alimentary fields is continuously evolving, as is the need to find solutions to problems related to the use of natural compounds. Essential oils are promising substances that present interesting antimicrobial, anti-inflammatory, and anticancer properties. In particular, the antimicrobial activity of EOs can be exploited in the fields of agriculture, food storage, and the preparation of pharmacological products.

Up to now, the general negative EO characteristics of low water solubility and low stability, together with their great volatility and the side effects associated with their use, have limited their application.

Pharmaceutical technology, above all nanotechnology, is able to solve these major inconveniences. As demonstrated in literature, the encapsulation of essential oils into nanosystems such as liposomes, SLNs, and cyclodextrins is an innovative approach that could lead to the employment of essential oils in major sectors.

REFERENCES

Alhaj, N.A., Shamsudin, M.N., Alipiah, N.M., Zamri, H.F., Abdul, A.B., Ibrahim, S., Abdullah, R. 2010. Characterization of *Nigella sativa* L. essential oil-loaded solid lipid nanoparticles. *American Journal of Pharmacology and Toxicology*, 5, 52–57.

Bakkali, F., Averbeck, S., Averbeck, D., Idaomar, M. 2008. Biological effects of essential oils: A review. *Food and Chemical Toxicology*, 46, 446–475.

Bilia, A.R., Guccione, C., Isacchi, B., Righeschi, C., Firenzuoli, F., Bergonzi, M.C. 2014. Essential oils loaded in nanosystems: A developing strategy for a successful therapeutic approach. *Evidence-Based Complementary and Alternative Medicine*, 2014, 1–14.

Buranasuksombat, U., Kwon, Y., Turner, M., Bhandari, B. 2011. Influence of emulsion droplet size on antimicrobial properties. *Food Science and Biotechnology*, 20, 793–800.

Carnesecchi, S., Bras-Gonçalves, R., Bradaia, A., Zeisel, M., Gossé, F., Poupon, M.F., Raul, F. 2004. Geraniol, a component of plant essential oils, modulates DNA synthesis and potentiates 5-fluorouracil efficacy on human colon tumor xenografts. *Cancer Letters*, 215, 53–59.

Cava, R., Nowak, E., Taboada, A., Marin-Iniesta, F. 2007. Antimicrobial activity of clove and cinnamon essential oils against *Listeria monocytogenes* in pasteurized milk. *Journal of Food Protection*, 70, 2757–2763.

Celia, C., Trapasso, E., Locatelli, M., Navarra, M., Ventura, C.A., Wolfram, J., Carafa, M. et al. 2013. Anticancer activity of liposomal bergamot essential oil (BEO) on human neuroblastoma cells. *Colloids and Surface B*, 112, 548–553.

Chen, F., Shi, Z., Neoh, K.G., Kang, E.T. 2009. Antioxidant and antibacterial activities of euge-nol and carvacrol-grafted chitosan nanoparticles. *Biotechnology and Bioengineering*, 104, 30–39.

Choi, M.J., Soottitantawat, A., Nuchuchua, O., Min, S.G., Ruktanonchai, U. 2009. Physical and light oxidative properties of eugenol encapsulated by molecular inclusion and emulsion diffusion method. *Food Research International*, 42, 148–156.

Choi, J.Y., Damte, D., Lee, S.J., Kim, J.C., Park, S.C. 2012. Antimicrobial activity of lem-ongrass and oregano essential oil against standard antibiotic resistant *Staphylococcus aureus* and field isolates from chronic mastitis cow. *International Journal of Phyto-medicine*, 4, 134–139.

Cosco, D., Celia, C., Cilurzo, F., Trapasso E., Paolino, D. 2008. Colloidal carriers for the enhanced delivery through the skin. *Expert Opinion*, 5, 737–755.

de Sousa, E.O., Rodrigues, F.F.G., Campos, A.R., Lima, S.G., da Costa, J.G.M. 2012. Chemical composition and synergistic interaction between aminoglycosides antibiotics and essen-tial oil of *Lantana montevidensis* Briq. *Natural Product Research*, 27, 942–945.

Donsì, F., Annunziata, M., Sessa, M., Ferrari, G. 2011. Nanoencapsulation of essential oils to enhance their antimicrobial activity in foods. *LWT—Food Science and Technology*, 44, 1908–1914.

Flores, F.C., Ribeiro, R.F., Ourique, A.F., Rolim, C.M.B., Silva, C.B., Pohlmann, A.R., Beck, R.C.R., Guterres, S.S. 2011. Nanostructured systems containing an essential oil: Protection against volatilization. *Quìmica—SciELO Barsil*, 34, 968–972.

Franz, C.M. 2010. Essential oil research: Past, present and future. *Flavour and Fragrance Journal*, 25 (3), 112–113.

Gomes, C., Moreira, R.G., Castell-Perez, E. 2011. Poly(DL-lactide-co-glycolide) (PLGA) nanoparticles with entrapped trans-cinnamaldehyde and eugenol for antimicrobial delivery applications. *Journal of Food Science*, 76, 16–24.

Hosseini, S.F., Zandi, M., Rezaei, M., Farahmandghavi, F. 2013. Two-step method for encap-sulation of oregano essential oil in chitosan nanoparticles: Preparation, characteriza-tion and in vitro release study. *Carbohydrate Polymers*, 95, 50–56.

Iannitelli, A., Grande, R., Di Stefano, A., Di Giulio, M., Sozio, P., Bessa, L.J., Laserra, S., Paolini, C., Protasi, F., Cellini, L. 2011. Potential antibacterial activity of carvacrol-loaded poly(DL-lactide-co-glycolide) (PLGA) nanoparticles against microbial biofilm. *International Journal of Molecular Sciences*, 12, 5039–5051.

Keawchaoon, L., Yoksan, R. 2011. Preparation, characterization and in vitro release study of carvacrol-loaded chitosan nanoparticles. *Colloids and Surfaces B* 84, 163–171.

Lai, F., Wissing, S.A., Muller, R.H., Fadda, A.M. 2006. *Artemisia arborescens* L essential oil-loaded solid lipid nanoparticles for potential agricultural application: Preparation and characterization. *AAPS PharmSciTech*, 7, E1–E9.

Lai, F., Sinico, C., De Logu, A., Zaru, M., Muller, R.H., Fadda, A.M. 2007. SLN as a topical delivery system for *Artemisia arborescens* essential oil: *In vitro* antiviral activity and skin permeation study. *International Journal of Nanomedicine*, 2, 419–425.

Langevedel, W.T., Veldhuizen, E.J.A., Burt, S.A. 2014. Synergy between essential oil compo-nents and antibiotics: A review. *Critical Review in Microbiology*, 40, 76–94.

Li, K.K., Yin, S.W., Yang, X.Q., Tang, C.H., Wei, Z.H. 2012. Fabrication and characterization of novel antimicrobial films derived from thymol-loaded zein–sodium caseinate (SC) nanoparticles. *Journal of Agricultural and Food Chemistry*, 60, 11592–11600.

Liolios, C.C., Gortzi, O., Lalas, S., Tsaknis, J., Chinou, I. 2009. Liposomal incorporation of carvacrol and thymol isolated from the essential oil of *Origanum dictamnus* L. and *in vitro* antimicrobial activity.

Liu, Z., Jiao, Y., Wang, Y., Zhou, C., Zhang, Z. 2008. Polysaccharides-based nanoparticles as drug delivery systems. *Advanced Drug Delivery Reviews*, 60, 1650–1662.

Liu, H., Yang, G., Tang, Y., Cao, D., Qi, T., Qi, Y., Fan, G. 2013. Physicochemical character-ization and pharmacokinetics evaluation of β-caryophyllene/β-cyclodextrin inclusion complex. *International Journal of Pharmaceutics*, 450, 304–310.

Manosroi, J., Dhumtanom, P., Manosroi, A. 2006. Anti-proliferative activity of essential oil extracted from Thai medicinal plants on KB and P388 cell lines. *Cancer Letters*, 235, 114–120.

Müller, R.H., Radtke, M., Wissing, S.A. 2002. Solid lipid nanoparticles (SLN) and nano-structured lipid carriers (NLC) in cosmetic and dermatological preparations. *Advanced Drug Delivery Reviews*, 54, 131–155.

Musthaba, S.M., Baboota, S., Ahmed, S., Ahuja, A., Ali, J. 2009. Status of novel drug delivery technology for phytotherapeutics. *Expert Opinion on Drug Delivery*, 6, 625–637.

Neumann, M., Garcia, N. 1992. Kinetics and mechanism of the light-induced deterioration of lemon oil. *Journal of Agricultural and Food Chemistry*, 40, 957–960.

Nuchuchua, O., Sakulku, U., Uawongyart, N., Puttipipatkhachorn, S., Soottitantawat, A., Ruktanonchai, U. 2009. *In vitro* characterization and mosquito (*Aedes aegypti*) repellent activity of essential-oils-loaded nanoemulsions. *AAPS PharmSciTech*, 10, 1234–1242.

Palaniappan, K., Holley, R.A. 2010. Use of natural antimicrobials to increase antibiotic sus-ceptibility of drug resistant bacteria. *International Journal of Food Microbiology*, 140, 164–168.

Paolino, D., Sinha, P., Fresta, M., Ferrari, M. 2006. Drug delivery systems. In J.G. Webster (ed.), *The Encyclopedia of Medical Devices and Instrumentations*. 2nd ed. Wiley-Interscience, pp. 437–495.

Parduman, R. et al. 2009. Anticancer activity of an essential oil form from *Cymbopogon flexuosus*. *Chemio-Biological Interactions*, 179, 160–168.

Pillmoor, J.B., Wright, K., Terry, A.S. 1993. Natural products as a source of agrochemicals and leads for chemical synthesis. *Pesticide Science*, 39, 131–140.

Ponce Cevallos, P.A., Buera, M.P., Elizalde, B.E. 2010. Encapsulation of cinnamon and thyme essential oils components (cinnamaldehyde and thymol) in β-cyclodextrin: Effect of interactions with water on complex stability. *Journal of Food Engineering*, 99, 70–75.

Rai, M., Ingle, A. 2012. Role of nanotechnology in agriculture with special reference to man-agement of insect pests. *Applied Microbiology and Biotechnology*, 94, 287–293.

Saraya, S., Chandrasekaran, N., Mukherjee, A. 2012. Antibacterial activity of eucalyptus oil nanoemulsion against *Proteus mirabilis*. *International Journal of Pharmacy and Pharmaceutical Sciences*, 4, 668–671.

Scott, R.P.W. 2007. Essential oils. *Encyclopedia of Analytical Science*, 554–561.

Shaaban, H.A.E., El-Ghorab, A.H., Shibamoto, T. 2012. Bioactivity of essential oils and their volatile aroma components: Review. *Journal of Essential Oil Research*, 24, 203–212.

Shah, P., Bhalodia, D., Shelat, P. 2010. Nanoemulsion: A pharmaceutical review. *Systematic Reviews in Pharmacy*, 1, 24–32.

Shi, F., Zhao, J.-H, Liu, Y., Wang, Z., Zhang, Y.-T., Feng, N.-P. 2012. Preparation and char-acterization of solid lipid nanoparticles loaded with frankincense and myrrh oil. *International Journal of Nanomedicine*, 7, 2033–2043.

Shoji, Y., Nakashima, H. 2004. Nutraceutics and delivery systems. *Journal of Drug Targeting*, 12, 385–391.

Sienkiewicz, M., Lysakowska, M., Denys, P., Kowalczyk, E. 2012. The antimicrobial activity of thyme essential oil against multidrug resistant clinical bacterial strains. *Microbial Drug Resistance*, 18, 137–148.

Sinico, C., De Logu, A., Lai, F., Valenti, D., Manconi, M., Loy, G., Bonsignore, L., Fadda, A.M. 2005. Liposomal incorporation of *Artemisia arborescens* L. essential oil and *in vitro* antiviral activity. *European Journal of Pharmaceutics and Biopharmaceutics*, 59, 161–168.

Solórzano-Santos, F., Miranda-Novales, M.G. 2012. Essential oils from aromatic herbs as antimicrobial agents. *Current Opinion in Biotechnology*, 23, 136–141.

Sugumar, S., Nirmala, J., Ghosh, V., Anjali, H., Mukherjee, A., Chandrasekaran, N. 2013. Bio-based nanoemulsion formulation, characterization and antibacterial activity against food-borne pathogens. *Journal of Basic Microbiology*, 53, 677–685.

Sylvestre, M., Legault, J., Dufour, D., Pichette, A. 2005. Chemical composition and anticancer activity of leaf essential oil of *Myrica gale* L. *Phytomedicine*, 12, 299–304.

Turek, C., Stintzing, F.C. 2014. Stability of essential oils: A review. *Comprehensive Reviews in Food Science and Food Safety*, 12, 40–53.

Valenti, D., De Logu, A., Loy, G., Sinico, C., Bonsignore, L., Cottiglia, F., Garau, D., Fadda, A.M. 2001. Liposome-incorporated *Sanolina insularis* essential oil: Preparation, characterization and *in vitro* antiviral activity. *Journal of Liposome Research*, 11, 73–90.

Wattanasatcha, A., Rengpipat, S., Wanichwecharungruang, S. 2012. Thymol nanospheres as an effective anti-bacterial agent. *International Journal of Pharmaceutics*, 434, 360–365.

Woranuch, S., Yoksan, R. 2013. Eugenol-loaded chitosan nanoparticles. I. Thermal stability improvement of eugenol through encapsulation. *Carbohydrate Polymers*, 96, 578–585.

Wu, Y., Luo, Y., Wang, Q. 2012. Antioxidant and antimicrobial properties of essential oils encapsulated in zein nanoparticles prepared by liquid–liquid dispersion method. *LWT—Food Science and Technology*, 48, 283–290.

Yap, P.S.X., Lim, S.H.E., Huc, C.P., Yiap, B.C. 2013. Combination of essential oils and antibiotics reduce antibiotic resistance in plasmid-conferred multidrug resistant bacteria. *Phytomedicine*, 20, 710–713.

Section II

Cell Biological Effects
and Underlying Mechanisms

8 Essential Oils Exploited in Cytotoxicity Studies for Translation into Safer and More Effective Cancer Therapeutics

*Rossella Russo, Maria Tiziana Corasaniti,
Giacinto Bagetta, and Luigi Antonio Morrone*

CONTENTS

8.1   INTRODUCTION

Cancer is one of the leading causes of morbidity and the second leading cause of mortality worldwide, accounting for about 8.2 million deaths in 2012 (Gulland, 2014). Although great advances have been made in cancer prevention, detection, diagnosis, and treatment, the number of people dying of cancer is expected to increase up to 14.6 million in 2035. Limits of the current therapies include development of multidrug resistance, important side effects, and high cost, underscoring the unmet need for more efficacious and less toxic interventions. Plants have always represented an attractive source for drug discovery and development of cancer chemoprevention, and several examples do exist for natural products being included in current protocols to tackle the limits of chemotherapy. Accordingly, vincristine, vinblastine, colchicine, taxol, paclitaxel, and others are plant-derived anticancer drugs used in the clinic (Efferth et al., 2007; Mukherjee et al., 2001; Turrini et al., 2014).

Among phytochemicals, essential oils have been considered attractive for their wide variety of bioactivities. Traditionally, essential oils have been used for their antiseptic (i.e., bactericidal, virulicidal, fungicidal), analgesic, sedative, anti-inflammatory, spasmolytic, and locally anesthetic properties (Bakkali et al., 2008). Moreover, they are used in aromatherapy for health improvement due to their sedative or stimulant properties (Edris, 2007; Yim et al., 2009).

More recently, growing attention has been focused on the potential of essential oils as anticancer treatment, and several studies are now available in the literature (Table 8.1). A MEDLINE survey on PubMed for "essential oil and cancer" (January 2015) retrieved 699 results, with a remarkable surge in publications over the last 15 years (471 out of 699 studies), while a search for "essential oil and cytotoxicity" reported only 282 results, with 243 published in the last 10 years. These numbers suggest that, despite the fact that essential oils have been known since ancient times, the studies in this field have been initiated rather lately.

8.2   CHEMICAL COMPLEXITY OF ESSENTIAL OILS

Essential oils (also called volatile or ethereal oils) are aromatic, highly volatile, hydrophobic liquids produced by aromatic plants as secondary metabolites. To date, about 3000 essential oils are known and about 300 are relevant for the pharmaceutical, agronomic, food, cosmetic, and perfume industries. Aromatic plant sources of essential oils mainly grow in temperate and warm areas, like the Mediterranean and tropical countries. Geographical areas of growing are often restricted, limiting the relevance of some essential oils to the local traditional pharmacopoeia.

Essential oils are a very complex mixture of molecules containing between 20 and 90 components with low molecular weight. Most molecules are present in traces, while two or three are often the most representative components, accounting for 20%–70% of the whole oil, and therefore mainly determining the biological activities of the essential oil (Bakkali et al., 2008).

The constituents of essential oils are classified by their chemical structures as terpene hydrocarbons, distinct in monoterpenes (C10), sesquiterpenes (C15), and diterpenes (C20); terpenes containing oxygen (terpenoids), such as alcohols, ketones,

TABLE 8.1
List of Essential Oils Showing Cytotoxic Properties

Plant Name	Cell Line/Animal	Effects	References
Artemisia annua	Hepatocarcinoma	Apoptosis	Li et al., 2004
Artemisia capillaris	Human oral epidermoid carcinoma	Apoptosis	Cha et al., 2009
Artemisia vulgaris	Human acute myelogenous leukemia Human acute T lymphocytic leukemia Human chronic myelogenous leukemia Breast adenocarcinoma Prostate adenocarcinoma Hepatocellular carcinoma Cervical carcinoma	Growth inhibition apoptosis	Saleh et al., 2014
Cedronella canariensis	Human melanoma Human breast adenocarcinoma Human colon carcinoma	Cytotoxicity	Zorzetto et al., 2015
Citrus bergamia	Human neuroblastoma	Necrosis and apoptosis Cytoskeletal alterations Autophagy induction	Berliocchi et al., 2011; R. Russo et al., 2013, 2014
	Human breast cancer	Autophagy induction	Russo et al., 2014
Citrus sinensis	Colon cancer	Apoptosis inhibition of cell migration Reduced VEGF expression	Chidambara Murthy et al., 2012
Cymbopogon flexuosus	Neuroblastoma Colon Liver Cervix	Cytotoxicity	Sharma et al., 2009
	Solid and ascitic Erlich and Sarcoma-180 tumor models in mice	Tumor growth inhibition Decreased ascitic volume	
Eucalyptus benthamii	Cervical cancer Murine macrophage tumor Human T leukemia	Cytotoxicity	Doll-Boscardin et al., 2012
Eucalyptus sideroxylon	Human breast adenocarcinoma	Cytotoxicity	Ashour, 2008
Eucalyptus torquata	Human breast adenocarcinoma	Cytotoxicity	Ashour, 2008
Laurus nobilis	Amelanotic melanoma	Cytotoxicity	Loizzo et al., 2007

(Continued)

TABLE 8.1 (CONTINUED)
List of Essential Oils Showing Cytotoxic Properties

Plant Name	Cell Line/Animal	Effects	References
Malaleuca alternifolia	Cervical cancer Acute lymphoblastic leukemia Erythromyeloblastoid leukemia Acute myeloid leukemia	Antiproliferative	Hayes et al., 1997; Mikus et al., 2000; Schnitzler et al., 2001; Soderberg et al., 1996
	Human melanoma	Antiproliferative apoptosis	Calcabrini et al., 2004; Soderberg et al., 1996
	Murine mesotelioma Murine melanoma	Cytotoxicity	Greay et al., 2010b
	Melanoma	Reduced migration and invasion	Bozzuto et al., 2011
	Subcutaneous tumor established in mice	Necrosis Slower growth Temporary regression Activation of local immune response	Greay et al., 2010a; Ireland et al., 2012
Melissa officinalis	Human lung, colon, breast cancer leukemias Mouse melanoma	Cytotoxicity	de Sousa et al., 2004
	Human glioblastoma multiforme	Apoptosis	Queiroz et al., 2014
Nigella sativa	Solid tumor-bearing mice	Inhibition of tumor development Reduced liver metastasis	Ait M'barek et al., 2007a
	Erlich ascites carcinoma developed in mice	Improved survival Growth inhibition	Salomi et al., 1991
Rosmarinus officinalis	Human breast cancer Hormone-dependent prostate carcinoma	Antiproliferative	Hussain et al., 2010
	Human ovarian cancer Human hepatocellular liver carcinoma	Cytotoxicity	Wang et al., 2012
Salvia bracteata	Human melanoma	Apoptosis	Cardile et al., 2009
Salvia libanotica	Human colon cancer	Cell cycle arrest and apoptosis	Itani et al., 2008
	Mouse papilloma	Antiproliferative	Gali-Muhtasib and Affara, 2000
	Mouse fibrosarcoma Metastatic human breast carcinoma	Antiproliferative	Kaileh et al., 2007

(Continued)

TABLE 8.1 (CONTINUED)
List of Essential Oils Showing Cytotoxic Properties

Plant Name	Cell Line/Animal	Effects	References
Salvia miltiorrhiza	Human hepatoma	Apoptosis	Liu et al., 2000
Salvia officinalis	Amelanotic melanoma Renal adenocarcinoma	Cytotoxicity	Loizzo et al., 2007
	Human melanoma	Apoptosis	Russo et al., 2013a
	Squamous human carcinoma of the oral cavity	Cytotoxicity	Sertel et al., 2011a
Salvia rubifolia	Human melanoma	Apoptosis	Cardile et al., 2009
Thymus brousonnettii	Human ovarian adenocarcinoma	Cytotoxicity	Ait M'barek et al., 2007a
	Tumor-bearing DBA-2 $\left(H_2^d\right)$ mice	Inhibition of tumor proliferation Reduced tumor volume Delayed mortality	Ait M'barek et al., 2007a
Thymus vulgaris	Human head and neck squamous carcinoma	Cytotoxicity	Sertel et al., 2011b
	Human prostate carcinoma Human lung carcinoma Human breast cancer	Cytotoxicity	Zu et al., 2010
Vepris macrophylla	Human breast adenocarcinoma Human colon carcinoma	Growth inhibition	Maggie et al., 2013
Xilopia frutescens	Human ovarian adenocarcinoma Human bronchoalveolar carcinoma Human metastatic prostate carcinoma	Cytotoxicity	Ferraz et al., 2013
	Mice subcutaneously transplanted with sarcoma cells	Tumor growth inhibition	Ferraz et al., 2013

aldehydes, esters, lactones, and coumarins; and phenylpropanoids, aromatic compounds derived from phenylpropane, that occur less frequently. Monoterpenes are the most abundant constituents, and they have often been identified as the components responsible for the antitumor activity of the phytocomplex (Sobral et al., 2014).

There is an overall high variation in the chemical profile of essential oils depending on the extraction methods, organ used, age and vegetative stage of the plant, time of the harvest, and soil composition (Angioni et al., 2006; Masotti et al., 2003).

Based on the above considerations two important concepts must be stressed when studying or reporting on the biological effects of essential oils: (1) characterization of their chemical composition, together with a good quality of the phytocomplexes

(as reported in analytical monographs of the European Pharmacopeia), is fundamental for their appropriate use, data interpretation, and reproducibility; (2) the
chemical complexity of the phytocomplex contributes to its biological effects,
since each constituent takes part in the overall outcome and may modulate the
effects of the others.

   Therefore, in most cases, it is not possible to ascribe the effects of an essential oil
to a single component, and studies on individual ingredients might report results that
do not recapitulate the effect of treatment with the phytocomplex as a whole. In view
of the latter, in the present chapter we discuss the cytotoxicity and potential anticancer activities of whole essential oils rather than their single constituents.

8.3 MECHANISMS UNDERLYING
THE CYTOTOXICITY OF ESSENTIAL OILS

Cancer is a complex disease in which cells are no longer responsive to the signals
related to proliferation, differentiation, and death. Indeed, hallmarks of cancer cells
include sustaining proliferation signaling, evading growth suppressors, resisting
cell death, inducing angiogenesis, and activating invasion and metastasis (Hanahan
and Weinberg, 2000). Therefore, chemotherapy often relies on the characteristics
of drugs to reduce the ability of cancer cells to grow and divide and to induce cell
damage and death.

   With the aim of testing their possible use as alternative or complementary cancer treatments, several essential oils are under investigation for their cytotoxic and
antiproliferative actions in cancer cell lines or tumor-bearing animals (Edris, 2007;
Lesgards et al., 2014) (Table 8.1). Different mechanisms may account for the reported
effects of essential oils or their constituents on cancer cells. These include induction
of cell death by apoptosis or necrosis, cell cycle arrest, and loss of key organelle
function. Some of these effects are ascribable to the lipophilic nature and low molecular weights of the constituents of essential oils that allow them to cross cell membranes, altering the phospholipid layers, increasing membrane fluidity, and leading
to leakage of ions and cytoplasmic content. Reduced ATP production, alteration of
pH gradient, and loss of mitochondrial potential are just few of the consequences
of disturbed cellular membranes. Furthermore, essential oils can also act as pro- or
antioxidants, affecting the cellular redox state (Azmi et al., 2006; Tuttolomondo et
al., 2013; Wei and Shibamoto, 2010).

8.4 ESSENTIAL OILS FROM LAMIACEAE SPECIES

8.4.1 SAGE

Salvia (commonly called sage) is probably the largest genus among the Lamiaceae
family, consisting of about 900 species widely distributed throughout the world.
The plant mainly grows in temperate, subtropical, and tropical regions, with the
Mediterranean, Central Asia, Mexico, Central and South America, and southern
Africa being the major centers.

As suggested by its Latin name, meaning "to save or to cure," *Salvia*, and in particular the species *S. officinalis*, has been known and utilized for hundreds of years in traditional medicine to treat fever, rheumatisms, perspiration, sexual debility, infection and inflammation of the throat and mouth, chronic bronchitis, and mental diseases (Kamatou et al., 2008). Furthermore, sage leaves and its essential oil have carminative, antiseptic, antispasmodic, astringent, and antihidrotic properties (Raal et al., 2007).

The content profile of *Salvia* essential oil defined by the ISO 9909 standard (ISO, 1997) is the following: α-thujone (18%–43%), β-thujone (3%–8.5%), camphor (4.5%–24.5%), 1,8-cineole (5.5%–13%), humulene (0%–12%), α-pinene (1%–6.5%), camphene (1.5%–7%), limonene (0.5%–3%), linalool (free and esterified [1% maximum]), and bornyl acetate (2.5% maximum).

However, the essential oil does not always match the profile. This is due to several species-specific differences as well as the influence of genetic and environmental factors, climate conditions, time of sample harvesting, and culture site (Ben Farhat et al., 2009).

Cytotoxic and antiproliferative activities have been reported for essential oils from the aerial parts of several *Salvia* species. *S. officinalis* essential oil exerted cytotoxic activity on C32 amelanotic melanoma and renal adenocarcinoma human cell lines, with 50% growth inhibition (IC_{50}) values of 367 and 108 μg/ml, respectively. Conversely, no effects were reported when the essential oil was tested on MCF-7 human breast cancer and LNCaP hormone-dependent prostate carcinoma cell lines (Loizzo et al., 2007). The study did not find significant correlation between the activity of the essential oil and its main component 1,8-cineole, underlying the concept that different constituents might act together to enhance the observed effect. Accordingly, a study on *S. libanotica*, a different species of sage, reported that three bioactive components of the oil—lynalil acetate, α-terpineol, and camphor—synergize, inducing cell cycle arrest and apoptosis in the human colon cancer HCT-116 p53$^{+/+}$ and p53$^{-/-}$ cell lines (Itani et al., 2008). However, the IC_{50} observed upon combining the three components (10^{-3} M) was lower than the effect of the whole oil in SP-1 mouse papilloma cell lines (50 μg/ml) (Gali-Muhtasib and Affara, 2000), L929sA mouse fibrosarcoma cells (180 μg/ml), and MDA-MB 231 metastatic human breast carcinoma cells (290 μg/ml) (Kaileh et al., 2007). In this case a differential sensitivity of various cancer cell lines to the essential oil must also be taken into account. Interestingly, the study by Itani and colleagues (2008) showed that cancer cells have higher sensitivity to the oil, since the growth suppression following exposure to the combined components had only minimal effects on normal human intestinal cells.

The cytotoxicity of *S. bracteata* and *S. rubifolia* essential oils was reported in M14 human melanoma cells; apoptotic induction in tumor cells was observed at concentrations nontoxic in normal cells (Cardile et al., 2009). Similar results were obtained in A375, M14, and A2058 human melanoma cells exposed for 72 h to 18 *S. officinalis* essential oils obtained from different sites located in south-central Italy (A. Russo et al., 2013). *S. miltiorrhiza*, a common species in traditional Chinese medicine, was shown to have cytotoxic effects in a human hepatoma cell line, inducing depletion of glutathione, reduction of mitochondrial potential, and in turn, apoptotic cell death (Liu et al., 2000).

Cell viability of a squamous human carcinoma cell line of the oral cavity (UMSCC1) was significantly reduced following treatment with *S. officinalis* essential oil, and this was associated with changes in the expression of genes involved in aryl hydrocarbon receptor signaling, cell cycle regulation, and p53 signaling (Sertel et al., 2011a).

8.4.2 ROSEMARY

Rosemary (*Rosmarinus officinalis* L.) is a perennial evergreen herb belonging to the Lamiaceae family. Rosemary is widely used as food flavoring, and in addition, it is also known in traditional medicine for its antibacterial, antimutagenic, antioxidant, and chemopreventive properties (Ngo et al., 2011; Oluwatuyi et al., 2004; Pintore et al., 2009). *R. officinalis* essential oil mainly consists of oxygenated monoterpenes and monoterpene hydrocarbons, with 1,8-cineol, α-pinene, camphor, limonene, camphene, and linalool being the major constituents (Hussain et al., 2010). The antiproliferative effect of *R. officinalis* essential oil was studied by 3-(4,5-dimethylthiazol-2-yl)-2,5-diphenyltetrazolium bromide (MTT) assay in human breast cancer (MCF7) and hormone-dependent prostate carcinoma (LNCaP) cell lines; the study reported IC_{50} values of 190.1 and 180.9 μg/ml, respectively (Hussain et al., 2010). A dose-dependent cytotoxicity was also reported following exposure to the essential oil of human ovarian cancer (SK-OV-3 and HO-8910) and human hepatocellular liver carcinoma (Bel-7402) cell lines; the essential oil showed higher cytotoxicity than its main components, with an order of toxicity of essential oil > α-pinene > β-pinene > 1,8-cineole (Wang et al., 2012).

8.4.3 MELISSA

Melissa officinalis L. (Lemon balb) is a medicinal plant widely diffused in Europe and the Mediterranean region. Aqueous and alcoholic extracts are traditionally used for their digestive and antispasmodic (Chakurski et al., 1981), sedative (Lopez et al., 2009), antiviral (Dimitrova et al., 1993; Kucera and Herrmann, 1967) and antioxidant (de Sousa et al., 2004) properties. *M. officinalis* essential oil has been shown to possess antibacterial, antifungal, and spasmolytic activities (Larrondo et al., 1995; Mimica-Dukic et al., 2004; Sadraei et al., 2003), while an antitumoral effect has only recently been reported.

In 2004, de Sousa and colleagues investigated, by MTT assay, the cytotoxic activity of *M. officinalis* essential oil in lung (A549), colon (Caco-2), breast (MCF-7), and leukemia (HL-60 and K562) human cancer cell lines and in a mouse melanoma cell line (B16F10). In this study, dilutions of the essential oil ranging from 1:50,000 to 1:2000 induced a dose-dependent inhibition of cell viability in all tested tumor cell lines, although each culture showed a different sensitivity (de Sousa et al., 2004). The antitumoral effect of *M. officinalis* was later studied in human glioblastoma multiforme cell lines; in U87 and A172 cultures, treatment with the essential oil for 48 h decreased the cell number in a dose-dependent manner, and this was associated with induction of apoptosis, as demonstrated by the presence of DNA fragmentation and activation of caspase-9 and caspase-3 (Queiroz et al., 2014). Glioblastoma multiforme

(GBM) is the most common and aggressive form of glioma, and tumor cell drug resistance limits a successful treatment, worsening the prognosis. Expression of members of the multidrug resistance–related proteins (MRPs), which belong to the ATP binding cassette (ABC) transporter superfamily, is one of the mechanisms contributing to the GBM chemoresistance. Interestingly, treatment with the monoterpene citral, which represents more than 85% of the *M. officinalis* essential oil and reproduces the cytotoxic features of the essential oil, reduces the activity and downregulates the expression of MRP1 in GBM cell cultures that express an active form of the transporter (Queiroz et al., 2014).

The ability of *M. officinalis* essential oil and citral to induce apoptosis in resistant cells that express MRP1 suggests their potential for tumor treatment.

8.4.4 THYME

Thyme belongs to the Lamiaceae family; due to its wide spectrum of pharmacological properties, it has been used in traditional medicine for thousands of years in countries of the Mediterranean basin. Essential oil of the most studied species, *Thyme vulgaris*, and its principal component, thymol, has been shown to have antifungal, antibacterial (Cosentino et al., 1999; Kalemba and Kunicka, 2003), and antioxidant (Miura et al., 2002) activities. Therefore, thyme is usually employed as an expectorant in upper respiratory tract infections, and thymol is often the main antiseptic ingredient in mouth rinses against gingivitis.

In 2007, Ait M'barek and colleagues tested the cytotoxic effect of Moroccan endemic thyme (*Thymus brousonnettii*) essential oil in the human ovarian adenocarcinoma cell line (IGR-OV1) and its parental cell line resistant to three chemotherapeutic drugs currently used to treat the ovarian adenocarcinoma (adriamycin, vincristine, and cisplatinum). In this study all cell lines were sensitive to the cytotoxic effects of the essential oil, although they had different degrees of sensitivity reporting an IC_{50} ranging between 0.39% and 0.94%; importantly, the authors also showed that administration of the essential oil at the tumor site for 30 days in tumor-bearing DBA-2 $\left(H_2^d\right)$ mice inhibited tumor proliferation, reduced tumor volume, and delayed mouse mortality (Ait M'barek et al., 2007a).

In human UMSCC1 head and neck squamous cell carcinoma (HNSCC), subtoxic concentrations of *Thymus vulgaris* essential oil stimulated proliferation and viability, while at higher concentrations, dose-dependent cytotoxic effects were observed (Sertel et al., 2011b); under this experimental setting, the cytotoxicity induced by the essential oil was associated, as shown by microarray-based mRNA expression profiling and pathway analysis, with the regulation of three pathways, namely, interferon signaling, N-glycan biosynthesis, and ERK5 signaling, which could be all involved in the effect of thyme essential oils on cancer cell growth and survival (Sertel et al., 2011b). Interestingly, a recent study testing the cytotoxicity of 10 essential oils (mint, ginger, lemon, grapefruit, jasmine, lavender, chamomile, thyme, rose, and cinnamon) identified thyme as the most effective on human prostate carcinoma (PC3), human lung carcinoma (A549), and human breast cancer (MCF7) cell lines (Zu et al., 2010).

8.4.5 CEDRONELLA CANARIENSIS

Cedronella canariensis (L.) Webb & Berthel is a monotypic species of the Lamiaceae family endemic to the Macaronesian region. Its uses in traditional medicine include as a anticatarrhal, antimicrobic, analgesic, carminative, diuretic, hypotensive, anti-inflammatory, and decongestant of the respiratory tract. The var. *canariensis*, one of the two chemotypes of the essential oil extracted from the aerial parts (i.e., var. *canariensis* and var. *anisata*), presents as major constituents pinocarvone and β-pinene (Lopez-Garcia et al., 1992). The cytotoxicity of *C. canariensis* essential oil was recently evaluated on A375 human malignant melanoma, MDA-MB231 human breast adenocarcinoma, and HCT116 human colon carcinoma. Essential oil showed cytotoxicity in all the cell lines tested, with human melanoma cell lines being more sensitive (IC_{50} 4.33 μg/ml). Lower activity was observed in human colon carcinoma (IC_{50} 11.43 μg/ml) (Zorzetto et al., 2015).

8.5 ESSENTIAL OILS FROM MYRTACEAE SPECIES

8.5.1 EUCALYPTUS

The genus *Eucalyptus*, belonging to the Myrtaceae family, includes about 900 species and subspecies. This evergreen tree is native to Australia and has a worldwide distribution. Traditional uses of *Eucalyptus* leaves are for wound healing and fungal infection, while plant infusions has been indicated for treating cold, influenza, and sinus congestion. In Chinese folk medicine, leaves of *E. globulus* and *E. robusta* are used for the treatment of articular pain, dysentery, and tonsillitis. Those traditional uses are now supported by several studies reporting the anti-inflammatory, antimicrobial, and analgesic properties of *Eucalyptus* spp. Although extracts and components isolated from *Eucalyptus* species have been shown to be endowed with cytotoxic activities, only few reports have been published regarding the anticancer activity of the whole oil.

Ashour showed the cytotoxic activity of the essential oils extracted from *E. torquata* stems and leaves and *E. sideroxylon* leaves on the MCF7 human breast adenocarcinoma cell line, reporting IC_{50} values of 1.34, 5.22, and 6.76 μg/ml, respectively; conversely, oils from both species did not exert cytotoxicity on the HEPG2 human hepatocellular carcinoma cell line (Ashour, 2008). A recent paper reported the cytotoxic effect of the essential oils from young and adult leaves of *E. benthamii* on T leukemia cells (Jurkat) and murine macrophage tumor (J774A.1) and cervical cancer (HeLa) cell lines (Doll-Boscardin et al., 2012). In all cell lines tested, the essential oils of *E. benthamii* showed stronger cytotoxicity than the related terpene compounds, α-pinene and γ-terpinene, suggesting that the effects exerted by the whole oil are the consequence of a synergic effect of monoterpenes and sesquiterpenes (Doll-Boscardin et al., 2012). Conversely, in a study comparing the antiproliferative activity of seven essential oils extracted from plants from Burkina Faso, essential oil from leaves of *E. camaldulensis* did not present any cytotoxic effects on LNCaP and PC-3 prostate cancer cell lines or on SF-763 and SF-767 glioblastoma cell lines at concentrations up to 8 mg/ml (Bayala et al., 2014). Similarly, eucalyptol

(1,8-cineol), the major compound of essential oil of *E. camaldulensis*, had no effects on prostate cancer and glioblastoma cell lines at the maximum tested concentration (1 mg/ml) (Bayala et al., 2014).

8.5.2 MELALEUCA ALTERNIFOLIA

Tea tree oil (TTO) is the essential oil steam distilled from *Melaleuca alternifolia* of the Myrtaceae family, a plant native to Australia. Traditionally, the oil was used by aboriginal Australians for insect bites and skin infections and was rediscovered in the 1920s for its topical antiseptic effects. Today the oil is present in several products for skin treatment and wound care, and its safety and toxicity for topical use have been rigorously examined (Hammer et al., 2006). TTO consists largely of monoterpenes; about half are oxygenated and the rest are hydrocarbons (Brophy et al., 2006). Of the more than 100 components of the oil, terpinen-4-ol, γ-terpinene, α-terpinene, 1,8-cineole, and ρ-cymene are the most represented. Currently, the composition of TTO must adhere to an international standard for oil of the *Melaleuca* terpinen-4-ol type, which sets the upper and lower limits for 14 components of the oil, although it does not indicate the species of *Melaleuca* that must be the source of the oil (Hammer et al., 2006; ISO, 1996). Being that terpinen-4-ol is the most abundant component, it is also thought to be the main active constituent responsible for the several *in vitro* and *in vivo* activities reported for TTO (Mondello et al., 2006). TTO is known for its antibacterial (Carson et al., 2002, 2006), antifungal (Hammer et al., 2003), antiviral (Schnitzler et al., 2001), and anti-inflammatory (Hart et al., 2000) properties, while only recently the phytocomplex and some of its components have been screened for anticancer activities (Bozzuto et al., 2011; Calcabrini et al., 2004; Hayes et al., 1997).

Studies evaluating the cytotoxicity of TTO on cultured cells were initially performed to determine its potential toxic effects. TTO toxicity was tested on a wide panel of human cell cultures, including cervical cancer (HeLa), acute lymphoblastic leukemia (MOLT-4), erythromyeloblastoid leukemia (K562), B cells derived from the bone marrow of a patient with acute myeloid leukemia (CTVR-1), and fibroblast and epithelial cells. In these studies TTO showed an IC_{50} on cell growth ranging from 20 to 2700 μg/ml (Hayes et al., 1997; Mikus et al., 2000; Schnitzler et al., 2001; Soderberg et al., 1996).

The potential antitumoral activity of TTO was reported in a study by Calcabrini and colleagues (2004) in human melanoma M14 wild-type cells and their drug-resistant counterparts, M14 adriamicin-resistant (ADR) cells. TTO, at the higher used concentrations (0.02% and 0.03%), as well as terpinen-4-ol, was able to inhibit the growth and induce caspase-dependent apoptotic cell death in both wild-type and drug-resistant melanoma cells, with the latter being more susceptible to the cytotoxic effect (Calcabrini et al., 2004). The authors suggested that the greater sensitivity to the TTO treatment displayed by the drug-resistant cells could be ascribed to the different lipid composition of the plasma membrane since there is evidence indicating that the multidrug resistance phenotype is also associated with changes in membrane lipid composition (Lavie et al., 1999; Santini et al., 2001). This would suggest that, as claimed for the antimicrobial effect, the cytotoxicity of TTO might be due to the interaction of the lipophilic components of the oil with the phospholipid bilayer of cell membranes, with consequent alteration of cell growth and activity. It is worth noting that an earlier study testing the cytotoxic effect of TTO on "normal" epithelial and fibroblast cells, having susceptibilities to topical agents similar to those of basal keratinocytes (Teepe et al., 1993), did not report toxic effects at concentrations that were shown to affect melanoma cell survival (Soderberg et al., 1996), thus confirming a higher sensitivity of tumor cells than normal cells.

A cytotoxic effect of TTO has been reported in murine mesothelioma (AE17) and melanoma (B16) cell lines, though slightly different IC_{50} values were reported, probably due to the different cell types (Greay et al., 2010b). In this case, TTO and terpinen-4-ol induce time-dependent cancer cell cycle arrest and cell death by primary necrosis and low levels of apoptosis; a differential dose–response between tumor and nontumor fibroblast cells was shown, suggesting that TTO might elicit its effect by inhibiting rapidly dividing cells more readily than slower-growing noncancerous cells (Greay et al., 2010b). More recently, the ability of tea tree oil and its major component, terpinen-4-ol, to interfere with the migration and invasion processes of drug-sensitive and drug-resistant melanoma cells has also been reported (Bozzuto et al., 2011).

Two recent studies investigated the efficacy of topical TTO on aggressive, subcutaneous, chemoresistant tumors in fully immune-competent mice (Greay et al., 2010a; Ireland et al., 2012). The studies showed that topical treatment with 10% TTO, given once a day for 4 consecutive days, induced a significant, though temporary, regression of established subcutaneous AE17 tumors and slowed the growth of B16-F10 tumors. However, the use of dimethyl sulfoxide (DMSO) as carrier was needed to induce the antitumor effect, while no effects were evident when using neat TTO or solvents other than DMSO (i.e., isopropanol or acetone). Similar effects on tumor growth were obtained using a combination of the five major components of TTO (terpinen-4-ol, γ-terpinene, α-terpinene, 1,8-cineole, and ρ-cymene) at doses equivalent to those found in 10% TTO, but not with the single components (Greay et al., 2010b). The antitumor effect of topical TTO was accompanied by skin irritation that, unlike other topical chemotherapeutic agents, resolved quickly and completely.

A follow-up study investigated the mechanism of action underlying the antitumor activity of topical TTO, reporting that topically applied 10% TTO induced a direct cytotoxicity on subcutaneous AE17 tumor cells, which was associated with nontumor-specific activation of locale immune response (i.e., neutrophils, dendritic and T cells) (Ireland et al., 2012). In particular, transmission electron microscopy analysis of AE17 tumor sections from mice treated topically with TTO revealed loss of cellular organization with increased intercellular spaces and accumulation of cell debris, nuclear shrinkage, chromatin condensation, mitochondria swelling and loss of cristae and membranes, significant alteration of endoplasmic reticulum, and less defined cellular membranes. These findings would suggest that, following *in vivo* TTO treatment, tumor cells undergo primary necrosis as previously suggested *in vitro* (Calcabrini et al., 2004; Greay et al., 2010a). Interestingly the topical treatment does not seem to affect the fibroblast adjacent to damaged tumor cells, nor lymphocytes within tumor sections and skeletal muscle fibers adjacent to tumor, suggesting that normal cells might have higher tolerance to TTO cytotoxicity than tumor cells.

8.6 ESSENTIAL OILS FROM CITRUS FRUITS

8.6.1 BLOOD ORANGE

The antiproliferative effects of volatile oil from fresh peels of blood orange (*Citrus sinensis* L. Osbeck) have been recently shown in two colon cancer cell lines, SW480 and HT-29; the cytotoxic effect of citrus oil was associated with the induction of apoptosis, an increased expression ratio of pro-apoptotic markers (Bax/Bcl-2), and a decrease of VEGF expression (Chidambara Murthy et al., 2012). In the same study, a dose-dependent inhibition of cell migration with a concurrent decrease of MMP-9 was shown, suggesting the great potential of the citrus oil for treatment and prevention of colon cancer.

8.6.2 BERGAMOT ESSENTIAL OIL

Bergamot essential oil (BEO) is a well-known plant extract, obtained by cold pressing of the epicarp and, partly, of the mesocarp of the fresh fruit of bergamot (*Citrus bergamia* Risso et Poiteau). The fruit belongs to the genus *Citrus* of the Rutacee family and grows, almost exclusively, in a restricted area along the coast of southern Italy.

BEO comprises a volatile fraction (93%–96% of total) containing monoterpene and sesquiterpene hydrocarbons and oxygenated derivatives, and a nonvolatile fraction (4%–7% of total) characterized by coumarins and furocoumarins (Dugo et al., 2000; Mondello et al., 1993). The most abundant components of the essential oil are the monoterpene hydrocarbon d-limonene and the monoterpene ester linalyl acetate, with d-limonene accounting for about 40% of the whole oil (Verzera et al., 1996, 2003).

BEO has been used by folk medicine as an antiseptic and antihelmintic to facilitate wound healing, and these uses are now supported by experimental data reporting the antifungal (Romano et al., 2005) and antimicrobial (Laird et al., 2012) activities of the phytocomplex, as well as its ability to increase oxidative metabolism in human polimorphonuclear leukocytes (Cosentino et al., 2014). Recent studies attributed to bergamot essential oil analgesic (Bagetta et al., 2010; Sakurada et al., 2009, 2011), anxiolytic (Saiyudthong and Marsden, 2011), and neuroprotective (Amantea et al., 2009; Corasaniti et al., 2007) effects, and these are consistent with the use of the oil in aromatherapy for the relief of pain and symptoms associated with stress-induced anxiety and depression. Furthermore, it has been shown in rodents that BEO affects synaptic transmission by modulating the release of specific amino acid neurotransmitters (Morrone et al., 2007), and it produces a dose-related sequence of sedative and stimulatory behavioral effects in freely moving, normal rats (Rombola et al., 2009).

Despite the number of studies on the effects of bergamot essential oil under pathological or normal conditions, data regarding its potential activity on tumor cells have only recently been gained. Accordingly, a recent study reported that exposure of human SH-SY5Y neuroblastoma cells to 0.02% and 0.03% bergamot essential oils significantly reduced cell viability, inducing necrotic and apoptotic cell death; cytotoxicity induced by the phytocomplex was accompanied by cytoskeletal alteration, mitochondrial dysfunction, caspase-3 activation, DNA fragmentation, plasma membrane damage, and cleavage of pro-survival proteins (Berliocchi et al., 2011). The mixed features of necrotic and apoptotic cell death induced by bergamot essential oil might be related to its complex phytochemical composition, suggesting that different components might activate different pathways to execute cell death. A follow-up study engaged to identify the components responsible for cell death induced by the phytocomplex showed that, at concentrations comparable to the cytotoxic concentrations of the oil, none of the tested constituents (d-limonene, linalyl acetate, linalool, γ-terpinene, β-pinene, bergapten) reduced SH-SY5Y cell viability, while only the combination of limonene and linalyl acetate was able to induce cell death (R. Russo et al., 2013). Accordingly, the bergapten-free fraction of bergamot essential oil was shown to be more effective than the complete phytocomplex, suggesting that bergapten is not the main component responsible for the observed cytotoxicity (Celia et al., 2013).

Interestingly, it was recently shown that bergamot essential oil and its main component, limonene, activate autophagy in SH-SY5Y human neuroblastoma and MCF7 human breast cancer cell lines (Russo et al., 2014). This effect was concentration dependent, unrelated to the effects elicited by the essential oil on cell survival, and occurred with an mTOR-independent mechanism (Russo et al., 2014). In view of the role of autophagy in limiting cancer development while facilitating advanced tumor progression (Kenific and Debnath, 2014), the finding that an essential oil is able to activate this pathway can be extremely relevant for its potential application as a chemotherapeutic, and therefore it stimulates further studies.

As for other essential oils, the hydrophobic nature of bergamot essential oil requires the use of solvents endowed with toxic effects (i.e., DMSO and ethanol) that can limit the therapeutic use of the phytocomplex. Celia and colleagues (2013) recently showed that this limitation could be overcome by loading the essential oil in pegylated liposomes; in addition, the liposomal formulation of bergamot essential oil showed an enhanced cytotoxic effect in neuroblastoma cells compared to the free phytocomplex. Similarly, encapsulation of other essential oils in nanocarriers (i.e., polymeric nanoparticulate formations and lipid carriers such as liposomes) might represent a good strategy for improving water solubility and stability of essential oils while lowering their effective dose and limiting potential side effects (Bilia et al., 2014).

8.7 OTHER ESSENTIAL OILS

Artemisia is a small herbal plant with a worldwide distribution, consisting of several species belonging to the Asteraceae family. Members of the *Artemisia* genus have been widely used as food additives and in folk medicine for the treatment of viral or bacterial infection, inflammation, hepatitis, and malaria (Gilani et al., 2005; Kordali et al., 2005). The essential oil of *Artemisia annua* L. (commonly known as sweet wormwood) induced apoptosis in SMMC-7721 hepatocarcinoma cells (Li et al., 2004), while treatment of the KB human oral epidermoid carcinoma cell line with the essential oil of *Artemisia capillaris* was associated with the induction of apoptosis through mitochondrial- and caspase-dependent mechanisms, as well as the mitogen-activated protein kinase (MAPK)–mediated pathway (Cha et al., 2009).

A recent study by Saleh and colleagues (2014) showed the cytotoxicity of *Artemisia vulgaris* L. essential oil in the HL-60 leukemic cell line. In this study, low concentrations (0.25–2.0 μg/ml) of the essential oil isolated from the aerial part (leaves and buds) of *A. vulgaris* L. inhibited the growth of the human acute myelogenous leukemia cell line (HL-60) in a dose- and time-dependent manner and induced apoptosis by a mitochondria-dependent mechanism; similar effects were reported in various other human cancer cell lines, including acute T lymphocytic (Jurkat) and chonic myelogenous (K-562) leukemia, breast adenocarcinoma (MCF7), prostate adenocarcinoma (PC-3), and hepatocellular (HepG2) and cervical (HeLa) carcinoma (Saleh et al., 2014). Interestingly, the same study also reported, at comparable concentrations, the absence of substantial toxicity for normal nonmalignant mammalian cells, such as human skin fibroblast (BJ) and kidney epithelial (HEK-293) cells (Saleh et al., 2014), suggesting the potential use of the oil for cancer treatment with a low risk of side effects due to unspecific cytotoxicity.

A number of human cancer cell lines, including melanoma, breast, and ovarian cancer, showed hallmarks of apoptosis when treated with the essential oil of the conifer tree *Tetraclinis articulate* (Buhagiar et al., 1999).

The essential oil of *Cymbopogon flexuosus* (eastern lemongrass) showed dose-dependent cytotoxicity in colon (502713), neuroblastoma (IMR-32), liver (Hep-g-2), and cervix (SiHa) cell lines with IC_{50} values ranging from 4.2 to 6.5 μg/ml. The same oil induced dose-dependent growth inhibition and a decrease in the ascitic fluid volume and total ascites cell count in solid and ascitic Ehrlich and S-180 tumor models in mice (Sharma et al., 2009).

A study conducted by Loizzo and colleagues (2007) compared the cytotoxic activities of five essential oils from the Labiatae and Lauraceae families (*Sideritis perfoliata*, *Satureia thymbra*, *Salvia officinalis*, *Laurus nobilis*, and *Pistacia palestina*) on a panel of cancer cell lines; all the tested oils inhibited tumor cell growth, with *L. nobilis* exerting the highest activity on C32 amelanotic melanoma and renal cell adenocarcinoma.

Maggi and colleagues (2013) reported the cytotoxic effect of the essential oil extracted from the leaves of *Vepris macrophylla*, a high evergreen tree endemic of Madagascar. The results showed that the essential oil exhibited strong inhibitory effects on MDA-MB 231 human breast adenocarcinoma and HCT116 human colon carcinoma tumor cell lines, with inhibition values comparable to those of the anticancer drug cisplatin (Maggi et al., 2013).

In vitro and *in vivo* anticancer effects of the leaf essential oil of *Xilopia frutescens*, a medicinal plant found in Central and South America, Africa, and Asia, were recently reported (Ferraz et al., 2013). MTT assay was used to assess essential oil cytotoxicity in ovarian adenocarcinoma (OVCAR-8), bronchoalveolar lung carcinoma (NCI-H358M), and metastatic prostate carcinoma (PC-3M) human tumor cell lines. Interestingly, in the same study, a 7-day intraperitoneal treatment with the tested essential oil dose-dependently inhibited tumor growth in mice subcutaneously transplanted with Sarcoma-180 cells without reporting evident signs of toxicity (Ferraz et al., 2013).

Essential oil of *Nigella sativa* L. (Ranunculaceae family) seeds, known as black seeds or black cumin, and its ethyl acetate fractions possess strong, although differential, cytotoxic effects against tumor cells, while butanol extract has limited effects; the reported differential effects for these extracts seem to be related not only to their chemical composition, but also to the nature of the tumor cell line tested. Interestingly, minimal cytotoxicity was observed for all the extracts toward normal human peripheral blood mononuclear cells (Ait M'barek et al., 2007b). Furthermore, *N. sativa* L. essential oil, when injected at the tumor site of solid tumor-bearing mice, significantly inhibited the tumor development, reduced the incidence of liver metastasis, and improved mouse survival (Ait M'barek et al., 2007b). Consistently, previous findings have shown that *Nigella sativa* methanol extract inhibits the growth of Erlich ascites carcinoma in mice (Salomi et al., 1991).

8.8   CONCLUSIONS

Essential oils have been used in traditional medicine since ancient times; however, research in this area is still in its growing state, and a systematic and rigorous approach to the study of biological activities of potential phytotherapeutics is an achievement of the last few decades. This is particularly true for the cytotoxic effects of phytocomplexes. From the available literature, essential oils seem to have great potential as anticancer therapeutic agents; however, information regarding their mechanisms of action, as well as their toxicities, is still lacking and far from being deciphered.

Indeed, their complex chemical composition makes it difficult to envisage a single mechanism underlying the entirety of the biological effect, with the final outcome conceivably being the sum or synergy of the biological activity of each component. For the same reason, data obtained from single components may not necessarily be, in turn, applied to the whole essential oil.

On the other hand, the presence in the phytocomplex of numerous constituents that simultaneously interfere with multiple signaling pathways might be the key for overcoming the current limit of chemotherapeutic agents, and in particular the development of multidrug resistance.

From the data reviewed in this article, the use of essential oils in cancer therapy is very promising, and therefore, it appears to be of great importance that agencies for research funding (1) continue to support worldwide basic research in the field and (2) stimulate clinical trials for those phytocomplexes where a reasonable wealth of preclinical data is available to limit attrition in late phases of trials. The guidance for effective research and development of essential oils in cancer therapy is based on the available European legislation in the field of herbal medicines (Directive 2004/24/EC [Nisticò and Roth-Behrendt, 2012]) and clinical trials (Regulation No. 536/2014) and the National Institutes of Health (NIH) guidelines for the definition of anticancer activity of any natural or synthetic substance.

REFERENCES

Ait M'barek, L., Ait Mouse, H., Jaafari, A., Aboufatima, R., Benharref, A., Kamal, M., Benard, J., El Abbadi, N., Bensalah, M., Gamouh, A., Chait, A., Dalal, A., Zyad, A. 2007a. Cytotoxic effect of essential oil of thyme (*Thymus broussonettii*) on the IGR-OV1 tumor cells resistant to chemotherapy. *Braz J Med Biol Res* 40, 1537–44.

Ait M'barek, L., Ait Mouse, H., Elabbadi, N., Bensalah, M., Gamouh, A., Aboufatima, R., Benharref, A., Chait, A., Kamal, M., Dalal, A., Zyad, A. 2007. Anti-tumor properties of blackseed (*Nigella sativa* L.) extracts. *Braz J Med Biol Res* 40, 839–47.

Amantea, D., Fratto, V., Maida, S., Rotiroti, D., Ragusa, S., Nappi, G., Bagetta, G., Corasaniti, M.T. 2009. Prevention of glutamate accumulation and upregulation of phospho-Akt may account for neuroprotection afforded by bergamot essential oil against brain injury induced by focal cerebral ischemia in rat. *Int Rev Neurobiol* 85, 389–405.

Angioni, A., Barra, A., Coroneo, V., Dessi, S., Cabras, P. 2006. Chemical composition, seasonal variability, and antifungal activity of *Lavandula stoechas* L. ssp. *stoechas* essential oils from stem/leaves and flowers. *J Agric Food Chem* 54, 4364–70.

Ashour, H.M. 2008. Antibacterial, antifungal, and anticancer activities of volatile oils and extracts from stems, leaves, and flowers of *Eucalyptus sideroxylon* and *Eucalyptus torquata*. *Cancer Biol Ther* 7, 399–403.

Azmi, A.S., Bhat, S.H., Hanif, S., Hadi, S.M. 2006. Plant polyphenols mobilize endogenous copper in human peripheral lymphocytes leading to oxidative DNA breakage: A putative mechanism for anticancer properties. *FEBS Lett* 580, 533–38.

Bagetta, G., Morrone, L.A., Rombola, L., Amantea, D., Russo, R., Berliocchi, L., Sakurada, S., Sakurada, T., Rotiroti, D., Corasaniti, M.T. 2010. Neuropharmacology of the essential oil of bergamot. *Fitoterapia* 81, 453–61.

Bakkali, F., Averbeck, S., Averbeck, D., Idaomar, M. 2008. Biological effects of essential oils: A review. *Food Chem Toxicol* 46, 446–75.

Bayala, B., Bassole, I.H., Gnoula, C., Nebie, R., Yonli, A., Morel, L., Figueredo, G., Nikiema, J.B., Lobaccaro, J.M., Simpore, J. 2014. Chemical composition, antioxidant, anti-inflammatory and anti-proliferative activities of essential oils of plants from Burkina Faso. *PLoS One* 9, e92122.

Ben Farhat, M., Jordan, M.J., Chaouech-Hamada, R., Landoulsi, A., Sotomayor, J.A. 2009. Variations in essential oil, phenolic compounds, and antioxidant activity of tunisian cultivated *Salvia officinalis* L. *J Agric Food Chem* 57, 10349–56.

Berliocchi, L., Ciociaro, A., Russo, R., Cassiano, M.G., Blandini, F., Rotiroti, D., Morrone, L.A., Corasaniti, M.T. 2011. Toxic profile of bergamot essential oil on survival and proliferation of SH-SY5Y neuroblastoma cells. *Food Chem Toxicol* 49, 2780–92.

Bilia, A.R., Guccione, C., Isacchi, B., Righeschi, C., Firenzuoli, F., Bergonzi, M.C. 2014. Essential oils loaded in nanosystems: A developing strategy for a successful therapeutic approach. *Evid Based Complement Alternat Med* 2014, 651593.

Bozzuto, G., Colone, M., Toccacieli, L., Stringaro, A., Molinari, A. 2011. Tea tree oil might combat melanoma. *Planta Med* 77, 54–56.

Brophy, J.J., Craig, D.C., Goldsack, R.J., Fookes, C.J., Leach, D.N., Waterman, P.G. 2006. Triumphalone, a diketone from the volatile oil of the leaves of *Melaleuca triumphalis*, and its spontaneous conversion into isotriumphalone. *Phytochemistry* 67, 2085–89.

Buhagiar, J.A., Podesta, M.T., Wilson, A.P., Micallef, M.J., Ali, S. 1999. The induction of apoptosis in human melanoma, breast and ovarian cancer cell lines using an essential oil extract from the conifer *Tetraclinis articulata*. *Anticancer Res* 19, 5435–43.

Calcabrini, A., Stringaro, A., Toccacieli, L., Meschini, S., Marra, M., Colone, M., Salvatore, G., Mondello, F., Arancia, G., Molinari, A. 2004. Terpinen-4-ol, the main component of *Melaleuca alternifolia* (tea tree) oil inhibits the in vitro growth of human melanoma cells. *J Invest Dermatol* 122, 349–60.

Cardile, V., Russo, A., Formisano, C., Rigano, D., Senatore, F., Arnold, N.A., Piozzi, F. 2009. Essential oils of *Salvia bracteata* and *Salvia rubifolia* from Lebanon: Chemical composition, antimicrobial activity and inhibitory effect on human melanoma cells. *J Ethnopharmacol* 126, 265–72.

Carson, C.F., Mee, B.J., Riley, T.V. 2002. Mechanism of action of *Melaleuca alternifolia* (tea tree) oil on *Staphylococcus aureus* determined by time-kill, lysis, leakage, and salt tolerance assays and electron microscopy. *Antimicrob Agents Chemother* 46, 1914–20.

Carson, C.F., Hammer, K.A., Riley, T.V. 2006. *Melaleuca alternifolia* (tea tree) oil: A review of antimicrobial and other medicinal properties. *Clin Microbiol Rev* 19, 50–62.

Celia, C., Trapasso, E., Locatelli, M., Navarra, M., Ventura, C.A., Wolfram, J., Carafa, M., Morittu, V.M., Britti, D., Di Marzio, L., Paolino, D. 2013. Anticancer activity of liposomal bergamot essential oil (BEO) on human neuroblastoma cells. *Colloids Surf B Biointerfaces* 112, 548–53.

Cha, J.D., Moon, S.E., Kim, H.Y., Cha, I.H., Lee, K.Y. 2009. Essential oil of *Artemisia capillaris* induces apoptosis in KB cells via mitochondrial stress and caspase activation mediated by MAPK-stimulated signaling pathway. *J Food Sci* 74, T75–81.

Chakurski, I., Matev, M., Koichev, A., Angelova, I., Stefanov, G. 1981. (Treatment of chronic colitis with an herbal combination of *Taraxacum officinale, Hipericum perforatum, Melissa officinaliss, Calendula officinalis* and *Foeniculum vulgare*). *Vutr Boles* 20, 51–54.

Chidambara Murthy, K.N., Jayaprakasha, G.K., Patil, B.S. 2012. D-Limonene rich volatile oil from blood oranges inhibits angiogenesis, metastasis and cell death in human colon cancer cells. *Life Sci* 91, 429–39.

Corasaniti, M.T., Maiuolo, J., Maida, S., Fratto, V., Navarra, M., Russo, R., Amantea, D., Morrone, L.A., Bagetta, G. 2007. Cell signaling pathways in the mechanisms of neuroprotection afforded by bergamot essential oil against NMDA-induced cell death in vitro. *Br J Pharmacol* 151, 518–29.

Cosentino, S., Tuberoso, C.I., Pisano, B., Satta, M., Mascia, V., Arzedi, E., Palmas, F. 1999. In-vitro antimicrobial activity and chemical composition of Sardinian thymus essential oils. *Lett Appl Microbiol* 29, 130–35.

Cosentino, M., Luini, A., Bombelli, R., Corasaniti, M.T., Bagetta, G., Marino, F. 2014. The essential oil of bergamot stimulates reactive oxygen species production in human polymorphonuclear leukocytes. *Phytother Res* 28, 1232–39.

de Sousa, A.C., Alviano, D.S., Blank, A.F., Alves, P.B., Alviano, C.S., Gattass, C.R. 2004. *Melissa officinalis* L. essential oil: Antitumoral and antioxidant activities. *J Pharm Pharmacol* 56, 677–81.

Dimitrova, Z., Dimov, B., Manolova, N., Pancheva, S., Ilieva, D., Shishkov, S. 1993. Antiherpes effect of *Melissa officinalis* L. extracts. *Acta Microbiol Bulg* 29, 65–72.

Doll-Boscardin, P.M., Sartoratto, A., Sales Maia, B.H., Padilha de Paula, J., Nakashima, T., Farago, P.V., Kanunfre, C.C. 2012. In vitro cytotoxic potential of essential oils of *Eucalyptus benthamii* and its related terpenes on tumor cell lines. *Evid Based Complement Alternat Med* 2012, 342652.

Dugo, P., Mondello, L., Dugo, L., Stancanelli, R., Dugo, G. 2000. LC-MS for the identification of oxygen heterocyclic compounds in citrus essential oils. *J Pharm Biomed Anal* 24, 147–54.

Edris, A.E. 2007. Pharmaceutical and therapeutic potentials of essential oils and their individual volatile constituents: A review. *Phytother Res* 21, 308–23.

Efferth, T., Li, P.C., Konkimalla, V.S., Kaina, B. 2007. From traditional Chinese medicine to rational cancer therapy. *Trends Mol Med* 13, 353–61.

Ferraz, R.P., Cardoso, G.M., da Silva, T.B., Fontes, J.E., Prata, A.P., Carvalho, A.A., Moraes, M.O., Pessoa, C., Costa, E.V., Bezerra, D.P. 2013. Antitumour properties of the leaf essential oil of *Xylopia frutescens* Aubl. (Annonaceae). *Food Chem* 141, 196–200.

Gali-Muhtasib, H.U., Affara, N.I. 2000. Chemopreventive effects of sage oil on skin papillomas in mice. *Phytomedicine* 7, 129–36.

Gilani, A.H., Yaeesh, S., Jamal, Q., Ghayur, M.N. 2005. Hepatoprotective activity of aqueousmethanol extract of *Artemisia vulgaris*. *Phytother Res* 19, 170–72.

Greay, S.J., Ireland, D.J., Kissick, H.T., Heenan, P.J., Carson, C.F., Riley, T.V., Beilharz, M.W. 2010a. Inhibition of established subcutaneous murine tumour growth with topical *Melaleuca alternifolia* (tea tree) oil. *Cancer Chemother Pharmacol* 66, 1095–102.

Greay, S.J., Ireland, D.J., Kissick, H.T., Levy, A., Beilharz, M.W., Riley, T.V., Carson, C.F. 2010b. Induction of necrosis and cell cycle arrest in murine cancer cell lines by *Melaleuca alternifolia* (tea tree) oil and terpinen-4-ol. *Cancer Chemother Pharmacol* 65, 877–88.

Gulland, A. 2014. Global cancer prevalence is growing at "alarming pace," says WHO. *BMJ* 348, g1338.

Hammer, K.A., Carson, C.F., Riley, T.V. 2003. Antifungal activity of the components of *Melaleuca alternifolia* (tea tree) oil. *J Appl Microbiol* 95, 853–60.

Hammer, K.A., Carson, C.F., Riley, T.V., Nielsen, J.B. 2006. A review of the toxicity of *Melaleuca alternifolia* (tea tree) oil. *Food Chem Toxicol* 44, 616–25.

Hanahan, D., Weinberg, R.A. 2000. The hallmarks of cancer. *Cell* 100, 57–70.

Hart, P.H., Brand, C., Carson, C.F., Riley, T.V., Prager, R.H., Finlay-Jones, J.J. 2000. Terpinen-4-ol, the main component of the essential oil of *Melaleuca alternifolia* (tea tree oil), suppresses inflammatory mediator production by activated human monocytes. *Inflamm Res* 49, 619–26.

Hayes, A.J., Leach, D.N., Markham, J.L. 1997. In vitro cytotoxicity of Australian tea tree oil using human cell lines. *J Essent Oil Res* 9, 15–16.

Hussain, A.I., Anwar, F., Chatha, S.A., Jabbar, A., Mahboob, S., Nigam, P.S. 2010. *Rosmarinus officinalis* essential oil: Antiproliferative, antioxidant and antibacterial activities. *Braz J Microbiol* 41, 1070–78.

International Organization for Standardization (ISO). 1996. ISO 4730: Oil of Melaleuca, terpinen-4-ol type (Tea Tree oil). American National Standards Institute (ANSI), New York.

International Organization for Standardization (ISO). 1997. ISO 9909: Oil of dalmatian sage (*Salvia officinalis* L.). American National Standards Institute (ANSI), New York.

Ireland, D.J., Greay, S.J., Hooper, C.M., Kissick, H.T., Filion, P., Riley, T.V., Beilharz, M.W. 2012. Topically applied *Melaleuca alternifolia* (tea tree) oil causes direct anti-cancer cytotoxicity in subcutaneous tumour bearing mice. *J Dermatol Sci* 67, 120–29.

Itani, W.S., El-Banna, S.H., Hassan, S.B., Larsson, R.L., Bazarbachi, A., Gali-Muhtasib, H.U. 2008. Anti colon cancer components from Lebanese sage (*Salvia libanotica*) essential oil: Mechanistic basis. *Cancer Biol Ther* 7, 1765–73.

Kaileh, M., Vanden Berghe, W., Boone, E., Essawi, T., Haegeman, G. 2007. Screening of indigenous Palestinian medicinal plants for potential anti-inflammatory and cytotoxic activity. *J Ethnopharmacol* 113, 510–16.

Kalemba, D., Kunicka, A. 2003. Antibacterial and antifungal properties of essential oils. *Curr Med Chem* 10, 813–29.

Kamatou, G.P., Makunga, N.P., Ramogola, W.P., Viljoen, A.M. 2008. South African *Salvia* species: A review of biological activities and phytochemistry. *J Ethnopharmacol* 119, 664–72.

Kenific, C.M., Debnath, J. 2014. Cellular and metabolic functions for autophagy in cancer cells. *Trends Cell Biol* 25, 37–45.

Kordali, S., Cakir, A., Mavi, A., Kilic, H., Yildirim, A. 2005. Screening of chemical composition and antifungal and antioxidant activities of the essential oils from three Turkish artemisia species. *J Agric Food Chem* 53, 1408–16.

Kucera, L.S., Herrmann, E.C., Jr. 1967. Antiviral substances in plants of the mint family (labiatae). I. Tannin of *Melissa officinalis*. *Proc Soc Exp Biol Med* 124, 865–69.

Laird, K., Armitage, D., Phillips, C. 2012. Reduction of surface contamination and biofilms of *Enterococcus* sp. and *Staphylococcus aureus* using a citrus-based vapour. *J Hosp Infect* 80, 61–66.

Larrondo, J.V., Agut, M., Calvo-Torras, M.A. 1995. Antimicrobial activity of essences from labiates. *Microbios* 82, 171–72.

Lavie, Y., Fiucci, G., Czarny, M., Liscovitch, M. 1999. Changes in membrane microdomains and caveolae constituents in multidrug-resistant cancer cells. *Lipids* 34 (Suppl), S57–63.

Lesgards, J.F., Baldovini, N., Vidal, N., Pietri, S. 2014. Anticancer activities of essential oils constituents and synergy with conventional therapies: A review. *Phytother Res* 28, 1423–46.

Li, Y., Li, M.Y., Wang, L., Jiang, Z.H., Li, W.Y., Li, H. 2004. (Induction of apoptosis of cultured hepatocarcinoma cell by essential oil of *Artemisia annua* L). *Sichuan Da Xue Xue Bao Yi Xue Ban* 35, 337–39.

Liu, J., Shen, H.M., Ong, C.N. 2000. *Salvia miltiorrhiza* inhibits cell growth and induces apoptosis in human hepatoma HepG(2) cells. *Cancer Lett* 153, 85–93.

Loizzo, M.R., Tundis, R., Menichini, F., Saab, A.M., Statti, G.A., Menichini, F. 2007. Cytotoxic activity of essential oils from Labiatae and Lauraceae families against in vitro human tumor models. *Anticancer Res* 27, 3293–99.

Lopez, V., Martin, S., Gomez-Serranillos, M.P., Carretero, M.E., Jager, A.K., Calvo, M.I. 2009. Neuroprotective and neurological properties of *Melissa officinalis*. *Neurochem Res* 34, 1955–61.

Lopez-Garcia, R.E., Hernandez-Perez, M., Rabanal, R.M., Darias, V., Martin-Herrera, D., Arias, A., Sanz, J. 1992. Essential oils and antimicrobial activity of two varieties of *Cedronella canariensis* (L.) W. et B. *J Ethnopharmacol* 36, 207–11.

Maggi, F., Fortune Randriana, R., Rasoanaivo, P., Nicoletti, M., Quassinti, L., Bramucci, M., Lupidi, G., Petrelli, D., Vitali, L.A., Papa, F., Vittori, S. 2013. Chemical composition and in vitro biological activities of the essential oil of *Vepris macrophylla* (BAKER) I.VERD. endemic to Madagascar. *Chem Biodivers* 10, 356–66.

Masotti, V., Juteau, F., Bessiere, J.M., Viano, J. 2003. Seasonal and phenological variations of the essential oil from the narrow endemic species *Artemisia molinieri* and its biological activities. *J Agric Food Chem* 51, 7115–21.

Mikus, J., Harkenthal, M., Steverding, D., Reichling, J. 2000. In vitro effect of essential oils and isolated mono- and sesquiterpenes on *Leishmania major* and *Trypanosoma brucei*. *Planta Med* 66, 366–68.

Mimica-Dukic, N., Bozin, B., Sokovic, M., Simin, N. 2004. Antimicrobial and antioxidant activities of *Melissa officinalis* L. (Lamiaceae) essential oil. *J Agric Food Chem* 52, 2485–89.

Miura, K., Kikuzaki, H., Nakatani, N. 2002. Antioxidant activity of chemical components from sage (*Salvia officinalis* L.) and thyme (*Thymus vulgaris* L.) measured by the oil stability index method. *J Agric Food Chem* 50, 1845–51.

Mondello, L., Stagno d'Alcontres, I., Del Duce, R., Crispo, F. 1993. On the genuineness of citrus essential oils. XL. The composition of the coumarins and psoralens of Calabrian bergamot essential oil (*Citrus bergamia* Risso). *Flavour Fragr J* 8, 17–24.

Mondello, F., De Bernardis, F., Girolamo, A., Cassone, A., Salvatore, G. 2006. In vivo activity of terpinen-4-ol, the main bioactive component of *Melaleuca alternifolia* Cheel (tea tree) oil against azole-susceptible and -resistant human pathogenic *Candida* species. *BMC Infect Dis* 6, 158.

Morrone, L.A., Rombola, L., Pelle, C., Corasaniti, M.T., Zappettini, S., Paudice, P., Bonanno, G., Bagetta, G. 2007. The essential oil of bergamot enhances the levels of amino acid neurotransmitters in the hippocampus of rat: Implication of monoterpene hydrocarbons. *Pharmacol Res* 55, 255–62.

Mukherjee, A.K., Basu, S., Sarkar, N., Ghosh, A.C. 2001. Advances in cancer therapy with plant based natural products. *Curr Med Chem* 8, 1467–86.

Ngo, S.N., Williams, D.B., Head, R.J. 2011. Rosemary and cancer prevention: Preclinical perspectives. *Crit Rev Food Sci Nutr* 51, 946–54.

Nisticò, G., Roth-Behrendt, D. 2012. The European legislation (Directive 2004/24/EC) brings clarification and recognition to herbal medicinal products. In G. Bagetta, M. Cosentino, M.T. Corasaniti, S. Sakurada (eds.), *Herbal Medicines: Development and Validation of Plant-Derived Medicines for Human Health*, 1–5. CRC Press, Taylor & Francis Group, Boca Raton, FL.

Oluwatuyi, M., Kaatz, G.W., Gibbons, S. 2004. Antibacterial and resistance modifying activity of *Rosmarinus officinalis*. *Phytochemistry* 65, 3249–54.

Pintore, G., Marchetti, M., Chessa, M., Sechi, B., Scanu, N., Mangano, G., Tirillini, B. 2009. *Rosmarinus officinalis* L.: Chemical modifications of the essential oil and evaluation of antioxidant and antimicrobial activity. *Nat Prod Commun* 4, 1685–90.

Queiroz, R.M., Takiya, C.M., Guimaraes, L.P., Rocha Gda, G., Alviano, D.S., Blank, A.F., Alviano, C.S., Gattass, C.R. 2014. Apoptosis-inducing effects of *Melissa officinalis* L. essential oil in glioblastoma multiforme cells. *Cancer Invest* 32, 226–35.

Raal, A., Orav, A., Arak, E. 2007. Composition of the essential oil of *Salvia officinalis* L. from various European countries. *Nat Prod Res* 21, 406–11.

Romano, L., Battaglia, F., Masucci, L., Sanguinetti, M., Posteraro, B., Plotti, G., Zanetti, S., Fadda, G. 2005. In vitro activity of bergamot natural essence and furocoumarin-free and distilled extracts, and their associations with boric acid, against clinical yeast isolates. *J Antimicrob Chemother* 55, 110–4.

Rombola, L., Corasaniti, M.T., Rotiroti, D., Tassorelli, C., Sakurada, S., Bagetta, G., Morrone, L.A. 2009. Effects of systemic administration of the essential oil of bergamot (BEO) on gross behaviour and EEG power spectra recorded from the rat hippocampus and cerebral cortex. *Funct Neurol* 24, 107–12.

Russo, A., Formisano, C., Rigano, D., Senatore, F., Delfine, S., Cardile, V., Rosselli, S., Bruno, M. 2013. Chemical composition and anticancer activity of essential oils of Mediterranean sage (*Salvia officinalis* L.) grown in different environmental conditions. *Food Chem Toxicol* 55, 42–47.

Russo, R., Ciociaro, A., Berliocchi, L., Cassiano, M.G., Rombola, L., Ragusa, S., Bagetta, G., Blandini, F., Corasaniti, M.T. 2013. Implication of limonene and linalyl acetate in cytotoxicity induced by bergamot essential oil in human neuroblastoma cells. *Fitoterapia* 89, 48–57.

Russo, R., Cassiano, M.G., Ciociaro, A., Adornetto, A., Varano, G.P., Chiappini, C., Berliocchi, L., Tassorelli, C., Bagetta, G., Corasaniti, M.T. 2014. Role of D-limonene in autophagy induced by bergamot essential oil in SH-SY5Y neuroblastoma cells. *PLoS One* 9, e113682.

Sadraei, H., Asghari, G., Naddafi, A. 2003. Relaxant effect of essential oil and hydro-alcoholic extract of *Pycnocycla spinosa* Decne. ex Boiss. on ileum contractions. *Phytother Res* 17, 645–49.

Saiyudthong, S., Marsden, C.A. 2011. Acute effects of bergamot oil on anxiety-related behaviour and corticosterone level in rats. *Phytother Res* 25, 858–62.

Sakurada, T., Kuwahata, H., Katsuyama, S., Komatsu, T., Morrone, L.A., Corasaniti, M.T., Bagetta, G., Sakurada, S. 2009. Intraplantar injection of bergamot essential oil into the mouse hindpaw: Effects on capsaicin-induced nociceptive behaviors. *Int Rev Neurobiol* 85, 237–48.

Sakurada, T., Mizoguchi, H., Kuwahata, H., Katsuyama, S., Komatsu, T., Morrone, L.A., Corasaniti, M.T., Bagetta, G., Sakurada, S. 2011. Intraplantar injection of bergamot essential oil induces peripheral antinociception mediated by opioid mechanism. *Pharmacol Biochem Behav* 97, 436–43.

Saleh, A.M., Aljada, A., Rizvi, S.A., Nasr, A., Alaskar, A.S., Williams, J.D. 2014. In vitro cytotoxicity of *Artemisia vulgaris* L. essential oil is mediated by a mitochondria-dependent apoptosis in HL-60 leukemic cell line. *BMC Complement Altern Med* 14, 226.

Salomi, M.J., Nair, S.C., Panikkar, K.R. 1991. Inhibitory effects of *Nigella sativa* and saffron (*Crocus sativus*) on chemical carcinogenesis in mice. *Nutr Cancer* 16, 67–72.

Santini, M.T., Romano, R., Rainaldi, G., Filippini, P., Bravo, E., Porcu, L., Motta, A., Calcabrini, A., Meschini, S., Indovina, P.L., Arancia, G. 2001. The relationship between 1H-NMR mobile lipid intensity and cholesterol in two human tumor multidrug resistant cell lines (MCF-7 and LoVo). *Biochim Biophys Acta* 1531, 111–31.

Schnitzler, P., Schon, K., Reichling, J. 2001. Antiviral activity of Australian tea tree oil and eucalyptus oil against herpes simplex virus in cell culture. *Pharmazie* 56, 343–47.

Sertel, S., Eichhorn, T., Plinkert, P.K., Efferth, T. 2011a. Chemical composition and antiproliferative activity of essential oil from the leaves of a medicinal herb, *Levisticum officinale*, against UMSCC1 head and neck squamous carcinoma cells. *Anticancer Res* 31, 185–91.

Sertel, S., Eichhorn, T., Plinkert, P.K., Efferth, T. 2011b. Cytotoxicity of *Thymus vulgaris* essential oil towards human oral cavity squamous cell carcinoma. *Anticancer Res* 31, 81–87.

Sharma, P.R., Mondhe, D.M., Muthiah, S., Pal, H.C., Shahi, A.K., Saxena, A.K., Qazi, G.N. 2009. Anticancer activity of an essential oil from *Cymbopogon flexuosus*. *Chem Biol Interact* 179, 160–68.

Sobral, M.V., Xavier, A.L., Lima, T.C., de Sousa, D.P. 2014. Antitumor activity of monoterpenes found in essential oils. *ScientificWorldJournal* 2014, 953451.

Soderberg, T.A., Johansson, A., Gref, R. 1996. Toxic effects of some conifer resin acids and tea tree oil on human epithelial and fibroblast cells. *Toxicology* 107, 99–109.

Teepe, R.G., Koebrugge, E.J., Lowik, C.W., Petit, P.L., Bosboom, R.W., Twiss, I.M., Boxma, H., Vermeer, B.J., Ponec, M. 1993. Cytotoxic effects of topical antimicrobial and antiseptic agents on human keratinocytes in vitro. *J Trauma* 35, 8–19.

Turrini, E., Ferruzzi, L., Fimognari, C. 2014. Natural compounds to overcome cancer chemoresistance: Toxicological and clinical issues. *Expert Opin Drug Metab Toxicol* 10, 1677–90.

Tuttolomondo, T., La Bella, S., Licata, M., Virga, G., Leto, C., Saija, A., Trombetta, D., Tomaino, A., Speciale, A., Napoli, E.M., Siracusa, L., Pasquale, A., Curcuruto, G., Ruberto, G. 2013. Biomolecular characterization of wild sicilian oregano: Phytochemical screening of essential oils and extracts, and evaluation of their antioxidant activities. *Chem Biodivers* 10, 411–33.

Verzera, A., Lamonica, G., Mondello, L., Trozzi, A., Dugo, G. 1996. The composition of bergamot oil. *Perfumer Flavorist* 21, 19–34.

Verzera, A., Trozzi, A., Gazea, F., Cicciarello, G., Cotroneo, A. 2003. Effects of rootstock on the composition of bergamot (*Citrus bergamia* Risso et Poiteau) essential oil. *J Agric Food Chem* 51, 206–10.

Wang, W., Li, N., Luo, M., Zu, Y., Efferth, T. 2012. Antibacterial activity and anticancer activity of *Rosmarinus officinalis* L. essential oil compared to that of its main components. *Molecules* 17, 2704–13.

Wei, A., Shibamoto, T. 2010. Antioxidant/lipoxygenase inhibitory activities and chemical compositions of selected essential oils. *J Agric Food Chem* 58, 7218–25.

Yim, V.W., Ng, A.K., Tsang, H.W., Leung, A.Y. 2009. A review on the effects of aromatherapy for patients with depressive symptoms. *J Altern Complement Med* 15, 187–95.

Zorzetto, C., Sanchez-Mateo, C.C., Rabanal, R.M., Lupidi, G., Bramucci, M., Quassinti, L., Iannarelli, R., Papa, F., Maggi, F. 2015. Antioxidant activity and cytotoxicity on tumour cells of the essential oil from *Cedronella canariensis* var. *canariensis* (L.) Webb & Berthel. (Lamiaceae). *Nat Prod Res* 1–9.

Zu, Y., Yu, H., Liang, L., Fu, Y., Efferth, T., Liu, X., Wu, N. 2010. Activities of ten essential oils towards *Propionibacterium acnes* and PC-3, A-549 and MCF-7 cancer cells. *Molecules* 15, 3200–10.

9 Phototoxicity of Essential Oils

*Michele Navarra, Marco Miroddi,
and Gioacchino Calapai*

CONTENTS

9.1 INTRODUCTION

Certain essential oils contain chemical substances that increase the possibility to experience a toxic response to sunlight. This kind of adverse reaction is known as phototoxicity, a particular form of photosensitivity. The phototoxic potential of compounds in essential oils represents a concern regarding their use and production. For this reason, research is focused on identifying what photoreactive agents could be found in these products and how to prevent or manage photosensitivity disorders.

9.2 HISTORY

Photosensitive properties of herbal substances have been recognized for thousands of years. It has been reported that in ancient Egypt, India, and Greece, plant extracts containing psoralen (a photosensitizer chemical compound) were exposed to sunlight to treat skin diseases. In 1897, cases of dermatitis following contact with parsnips or angelica were reported in scientific literature in both the United States and England

(Hann, 1991). Around a century ago, it was observed that the application of eau de cologne containing bergamot oil could produce typical hyperpigmented lesions at sunlight. In 1916, for the first time, it was noticed that the cutaneous application of bergamot essential oil and concurrent exposure to an ultraviolet lamp could lead to a phototoxic reaction consisting of skin reddening, blistering, and residual hyperpigmentation. This reaction was called Berloque dermatitis, but other names have also been used, such as phytodermatitis and bergapten dermatitis (Oppenheim, 1947). In 1938, plant furocoumarins were identified as molecules causing photosensitization (Dubakiene and Kupriene, 2006).

9.3 DEFINITION

Photosensitivity induced by chemical substances is called photodermatosis, a particular pathological condition of the skin determined by exogenous agents, used topically or systemically, that occurs in the presence of ultraviolet (UV) light within the visible range—wavelengths within the UVA (320–400 nm) (Zammit, 2010). UVA penetrates the skin more deeply, and particularly for systemic chromophores, this is certainly the most important spectrum for inducing photodermatosis (Hawk, 1999). Photosensitivity can be more specifically classified into two groups: phototoxicity and photoallergy. Phototoxicity is a direct tissue injury, caused by a phototoxic agent and radiation, which can be seen in every individual, without a specific predisposition. Phototoxic reactions can appear on first exposure to the agent with no cross-sensitivity to chemically related agents. Phototoxic reactions are dose dependent and will occur in almost any one who ingests or applies an adequate amount of the potential toxic agent and is exposed to UV radiation, but the dose necessary to induce such a reaction varies among individuals. They are invariably not dependent on an antigen–antibody relationship or a cell-mediated hypersensitivity reaction. In contrast, photoallergy is a delayed-type hypersensitivity reaction. It is caused by chemicals that are modified by absorbing photon energy. It does not occur during the first exposure, and there is a sensitization phase where the immune system plays a pivotal role. The incidence of photosensitivity is rather low, and phototoxic reactions are far more common than photoallergic reactions (Lehman and Schwarz 2011).

9.4 PATHOPHYSIOLOGY

The pathophysiology of phototoxicity is based on various mechanisms. A potential phototoxic chemical substance absorbs UVA radiation energy. Before this irradiation, the substance, being at its ground state, rises to an excited-state molecule, in consequence of the action of UV energy. This excited chemical state is involved in reactions causing cytotoxic effects. Phototoxic reactions may be photodynamic or nonphotodynamic in nature, the primary difference being that photodynamic reactions require oxygen. These different pathways of chemical reactions can be divided into two major classes: type 1 and type 2 reactions. During type 1 reactions, an electron is transferred to the excited-state photosensitizer, and this reaction is a source of free radical formation. The formation of free radicals results in various oxidation–reduction reactions, leading to cell damage due to peroxide toxicity. Type 2 reactions are energy transfer processes. Again, transfer of energy to ground-state oxygen causes oxygen radical formation. These radicals interact with unsaturated fatty acids, and in the end, hydroperoxides are formed. These substances eventually lead to oxidation of lipids and proteins (Kutlubay et al., 2014).

Biologically active products of complement activation, mast cell–derived mediators, eicosanoids, proteases, and polymorphonuclear leukocytes may also take part in the process of phototoxicity. The epidermal cells are damaged, causing the release of mediators of inflammation with erythema, edema, inhibition of DNA synthesis, inhibition of cell proliferation, and stimulation of melanin production. Interestingly, photosensitizers plus light irradiation are currently used in medical practice in the cure of skin disorders. Furthermore, photosensitizers plus electromagnetic radiation can stimulate apoptosis, cytotoxicity processes useful in the treatment of premalignant and malignant skin lesions (Dubakiene and Kupriene, 2006).

9.5 CLINICAL ASPECTS

Phototoxic reactions are significantly more common than photoallergic reactions and mostly resemble an exaggerated sunburn. In phototoxicity, the damage of skin at the cellular level induces erythema, edema, and stimulation of melanin production (Lugovic et al., 2007). In the acute phase, phototoxic dermatitis shows its effects minutes to hours after exposure to the sunlight. Patients can experience a wide range of clinical manifestations, such as erythematous patches, plaques, vesicles, and bullae. A burning and stinging sensation may be reported, especially on areas of the body that have been exposed to sun irradiation, such as the forehead, nose, V area of the neck, ears, and dorsa of the hands. Severity of symptoms can vary from mild or even asymptomatic phase to severe sunburn. Postinflammatory evolution of photoxic lesions may help physicians in differential diagnosis with common sunburn. The occurrence of dark skin lesions with different degrees of hyperpigmentation typically lasts for weeks or months. All the symptoms are dose dependent, depending on both the dose of the chemical compound used and the dose of the UV radiation to which the individual is exposed. In differential diagnoses, it is important to notice the sparing of areas where UV radiation has not reached, such as the postauricular areas, the submental area, the nasolabial folds, and under clothing. Usually in phototoxic reactions the latency of symptom onset is short, while in Berloque dermatitis acute response first appears after 24 hours and peaks at 48 to 72 hours (Dubertret et al., 1990). The resultant hyperpigmentation may appear atypical, thus leading to an error in diagnosis. Additionally, the condition can sometimes induce or aggravate melasma and may be responsible for other pigmentary disorders of the face and neck of questionable etiology, such as poikiloderma of Civatte, Riehl's melanosis and pigmented peribuccal erythema of Brocq (Zaynoun, 2006). Photo-onycholysis can also be observed as a manifestation of acute phototoxicity (Chandran and Aw, 2013). Chemical compounds derived from plants, such as furocoumarins, are reported to be responsible for this damage (Dubakiene and Kupriene, 2006; Zala et al., 1977). The clinical course of phototoxicity in most patients is usually self-limiting. The symptoms reduce after discontinuation of the responsible agent. In some cases, even after the patient is no longer exposed to the phototoxic chemical, the symptoms persist, sometimes for years. Treatment of phototoxic dermatitis induced by essential oils as other toxic phytophotodermatitis depends on the extent of the lesion. In mild cases, conservative management with application of a moist dressing is sufficient. In severe cases or in those involving more than 30% of the total body surface area, it is highly desirable to admit the patient to a hospital burn unit. Cooling the acute lesions and topical corticosteroid administration may help to alleviate symptoms, and in the case of risk to a bacterial superinfection, the use of antibiotics is indicated (Lugovic et al., 2007). In the case of serious skin inflammation with necrotic lesions, a therapeutic approach is necessary based on systemic corticosteroid administration (Solis et al., 2000; Abali et al., 2012). Avoidance of furocoumarin-containing products as essential oils in direct sunlight can prevent recurrences (Moreau et al., 2014), but it appears mandatory to use photoprotection. Photoprotection is an integral part of the clinical management of phototoxicity; it includes seeking shade, wearing photoprotective clothing, a wide-brimmed hat, and sunglasses, and applying broad-spectrum sunscreens with a sun protection factor (SPF) (Medeiros and Lim, 2010). It is suggested that sunscreens with UVA protection should be used. SPF is not a reliable indicator of protection against drug-induced photoxic reactions and refers to the degree of protection against primarily the UVB range of irradiation (Lugovic et al., 2007). Several studies have reported that clothing, depending on textiles, provides only limited UV protection. Various textile parameters, such as fabric porosity, type, color, weight, and thickness, have an impact on the sun-protective properties against UVA irradiation (Gambichler et al., 2002).

9.6   HISTOLOGY

Histopathologic evaluation of phototoxic lesions revealed epidermal spongiosis and dermal edema, with a mixed infiltrate of lymphocytes, macrophages, and neutrophils. In acute phototoxic reactions, necrotic keratinocytes are present (Lugovic et al., 2007).

9.6.1   Essential Oils That Can Induce Phototoxicity

Rutaceae, Apiaceae, Asteraceae, and Moraceae are the families of plants that most likely contain chemical substances that potentially induce phototoxic reactions. They are rich in a class of substances, including coumarins and in particular furocoumarins (also called furanocoumarins), that are most extensively studied as photoreactive compounds.

9.6.2   Substances Inducing Phototoxicity

Coumarins are compounds that belong to a large class of phenolic substances found in plants and are made of fused benzene and alpha-pyrone rings. Coumarins are contained in about 150 different species distributed over nearly 30 different families (Venugopala et al., 2013). Although distributed throughout all parts of the plant, coumarins occur at the highest levels in fruits; their incidence can be influenced by environmental conditions and seasonal changes. In addition, on the basis of the procedure adopted to produce essential oils, the concentrations of these chemical compounds vary. They are commonly found in cold-pressed citrus oil, for example, but in distilled oils they are scarce. The condition of stockage of raw material can influence the level of furocoumarins. Plants are considered to synthesize these compounds as part of their chemical defense strategy in order to protect, for example, roots or fruits against microbial infections, but actually their function is not fully understood. Some authors suggest that they could be plant growth regulators and even waste products (Ostertag et al., 2002). Furanocoumarins (or furocoumarins) represent one particular type of natural coumarin characterized by flat polycyclic molecules. Furocoumarins are present in a large variety of plants, including a number of species used as food and flavorings and to produce essential oils (Santana et al., 2004). Upon UVA irradiation, furocoumarins can undergo photoactivation, which makes them highly reactive toward cellular target molecules such as proteins or nucleic acids forming complexes by intercalating in the base pairs; thus, they cause toxicity in human skin cells (Gasparro et al., 1997). In plants, the most commonly detected linear furocoumarins are psoralen, 8-methoxypsoralen (8-MOP, xanthotoxin), and 5-methoxypsoralen (5-MOP, bergapten). Angular furocoumarins include angelicin (isopsoralen) and its derivatives. The phototoxic potential of furanocoumarins such as 8-MOP and 5-MOP has been extensively studied. Psoralens are able to produce photomodifications of various biomolecules (Balato et al., 1984; Bordin, 1999; Bylaite et al., 2009). Unlike most other photosensitizing compounds, psoralens mediate their phototoxic effect for the most part through a non-oxygen-dependent photoreaction, although photodynamic reactions may additionally contribute. As opposed to other phototoxic agents, psoralens primarily target DNA. The interaction between psoralens and DNA occurs in two separate steps. In the first step, the nonirradiated ground state of psoralen intercalates inside the nucleic acid duplex. In combination with UVA radiation, the excited psoralen molecules then form monofunctional and bifunctional psoralen–DNA photoadducts (cross-links) with pyrimidine bases—mainly thymine, but also cytosine and uracil. This mechanism may explain the antiproliferative effects of psoralens. Psoralen-induced DNA damage is responsible for adverse effects such as increased mutagenicity and skin cancer (Dall'Acqua et al., 1979). Besides the most prominent and studied psoralen and angelicin, less is known about the phototoxic potential of the numerous other furocoumarins produced by plants and eventually found in their derivative products (Messer et al., 2012). Furocoumarins may not be the only photosensitizer molecules in essential oils. Target herb contains alpha-terthienyl, which is a pontential source of phototoxicity (Opdyke, 1979). However, knowledge of phototoxic and photogenotoxic properties is limited to less than a dozen congeners, while more than 90 congeners have been described to occur in plants (Raquet and Schrenk, 2014).

Notably, as recognized by ancient traditional medicine, phototoxic chemical substances present in plants can be used in the treatment of skin disorders. Phototoxic reactions induced by psoralens constitute the major therapeutic principle of psoralen plus UVA radiation (PUVA) therapy. For PUVA therapy, linear psoralens such as 8-methoxypsoralen, 5-methoxypsoralen, and trimethylpsoralen are mostly used in combination with UVA radiation (Laskin et al., 1986). PUVA is a particular therapy often administered to treat psoriasis, vitiligo, cutaneous T-cell lymphoma (CTCL), eczema, and many other skin diseases (Stern et al., 1999). It has been shown, for example, that psoralen–fatty acid adducts can activate a signaling transduction cascade of reaction stimulating the melanosynthesis in melanocytes. This effect may explain the beneficial effects of PUVA therapy in vitiligo patients (Anthony et al., 1997).

PUVA was especially used in the treatment of severe psoriasis. Although PUVA is generally considered effective, it is also more toxic and more expensive. For this reason, there is criticism regarding its use. It may be accompanied by various adverse effects, such as nausea, vomiting, headache, generalized photosensitization lasting for about 24 hours (Schiener et al., 2007), and the risk of potential photocarcinogenesis, as shown by U.S. and European studies (Archier et al., 2012).

9.6.3 ESSENTIAL OILS INDUCING PHOTOTOXICITY

Phototoxicity of the essential oils is dependent on the content of photoactive components and the solvent used (Kejlova, 2010).

The presence of furocoumarins in essential oils is a potential risk for the development of phototoxic reactions. Furocoumarins are present in different amount in various plants and fruit. Bergapten and psoralens in general are contained not only in expressed bergamot oil (*Citrus bergamia*), but also in other plants, such as figs (*Ficus carica* L.), angelica (*Angelica archangelica* L.), celery (*Apium graveolens* L.), and various citrus fruits (Zammit, 2010).

Herein, we report a list of phototoxic essential oils: *Amni visnaga* oil (*Amni visnaga*), angelica root oil (*Angelica archangelica*), cumin oil (*Cuminum cyminum*), fig leaf absolute (*Ficus carica*), expressed grapefruit oil (*Citrus paradisi*), Saint-John's-wort (*Hypericum perforatum*), cold-pressed lemon oil (*Citrus medica limonum*), expressed lime oil (*Citrus aurantifolia*), cold-pressed mandarin oil (*Citrus reticulata*), absolute, resinoid opoponax oil (*Commiphora erythrea*), bitter orange oil (*Citrus aurantium amara*), parsley leaf oil (*Petroselinum crispum*), petitgrain mandarin oil (*Citrus reticulata* var. *mandarin*), rue oil (*Ruta graveolens*), tagetes oil and absolute (*Tagetes minuta*), cold-pressed tangerine oil (*Citrus reticulata*), and verbena oil (*Lippia citriodora*).

9.7   BERGAMOT (*CITRUS BERGAMIA*) ESSENTIAL OIL

Bergamot essential oil (BEO) is a widely used aromatic (fragrance) ingredient of cosmetics that may be applied on sun-exposed skin areas. BEO is naturally reach in photoactive furocoumarins, such as bergapten and 5- and 8-methoxypsoralen, which are well-known photosensitizers (Costa et al., 2010). The name Berloque dermatitis, or dermatitis in Berloque form, was coined by Rosenthal in 1924 to indicate the phototoxic reaction caused by BEO (Marzulli and Maibach, 1970). The correlation between topical use of bergamot oil–containing products and the occurrence of phototoxic reactive lesions led regulatory agencies to ban it from cosmetic and medicinal products for topical use (see Herbal Medicinal Products Committee of European Medicines Agency, 2011; Navarra et al., 2015). In order to guarantee safety, it has been suggested to remove bergapten and other phototoxic components by distillation; the resulting essential oil is known as furocoumarin-free (FCF) or bergapten-free (BF) bergamot and hydrocarbon fraction–free/bergapten-free bergamot (BEO-HF/BF) (Kejlova et al., 2010; Corasaniti et al., 2007; Navarra et al., 2015).

The International Fragrance Association (Franceschi et al., 2004) recommended a maximum of 0.4% of BEO in the final leave-on products for skin application and potential exposure to sunlight (Franceschi et al., 2004). Despite bergapten-free oils or, better, furocoumarin-free oils being safer and currently present in various products (Dubertret et al., 1990), milder cases occur for the presence of relatively small amounts of bergapten in cosmetic products (Kaddu et al., 2001). Despite the decline in the incidence of phototoxic dermatitis due to BEO during the past decades, phototoxicity induced by BEO is still a health hazard related to the use of psoralen-containing aromatherapy oils. In aromatherapy the exposure to aerosolized (evaporated) essential oil and subsequent UVA radiation results in Berloque dermatitis, with development of dark lesions in 48 to 72 hours (Kaddu et al., 2001).

To identify phototoxic effects, several fragrances (including BEO) were evaluated *in vitro* with a photohemolysis test using suspensions of human erythrocytes exposed to radiation sources rich in UVA or UVB in the presence of the test compounds. Hemolysis was measured by reading the absorbance values, and photohemolysis was calculated as a percentage of the total hemolysis. Moderate phototoxic effects were induced by UVA in the presence of seven fragrances (benzyl alcohol, bergamot oil, costus root oil, alpha-amyl cinnamic aldehyde, laurel leaf oil, lime oil, and orange oil) and by UVB due to incubation with five fragrances (alpha-amyl cinnamic aldehyde, hydroxy-citronellal, cinnamic alcohol, cinnamic aldehyde, and laurel leaf oil). The authors concluded that BEO, as well as lime oil, orange oil, and lemon oil, caused moderate UVA-induced photohemolysis (Placzek et al., 2007).

9.8 ANGELICA (*ANGELICA ARCHANGELICA* L.) ESSENTIAL OIL

In *Angelica archangelica* preparations, essential oils as well the phototoxic furocoumarins 5- and 8-methoxypsoralen are present. For this reason, there is a potential risk to develop phytophotodermatitis after application or assumption of angelica derivative essential oil. To date, it is not available a comprehensive chemical characterization of every single furocoumarin contained in angelica herbal preparation. Though such lack of data, a study tried to develop a procedure for phototoxic risk assessment of angelica products (Herbal Medicinal Products Committee of European Medicines Agency, 2006).

9.9 SAINT-JOHN'S-WORT (*HYPERICUM PERFORATUM*)

Hypericum perforatum L. (Saint-John's-wort), a plant member of the Hypericaceae family, has been used in folk medicine for a long time for a range of indications, including depressive disorders (Linde et al., 2008). This plant material is used for the production of *Oleum hyperici*, which is also used as a carrier oil in aromatherapy and for the distillation of the essential oil. The essential oil is applied topically in a pure form or diffused in a carrier oil (Crockett, 2010). Because of the presence of naphthodianthrone hypericin (a red edanthraquinone derivative), a substance that evidence indicates is a photosensitizer, these products have potential phototoxic action; consequently, its presence in topical formulations has to be carefully evaluated (Cosmetic Ingredient Review Expert Panel, 2001).

9.10   LEMON (*CITRUS LIMON*)

In lemon oil furocoumarin derivatives are present that potentially cause phototoxicity. In a study, lemon oil was fractionated and its phototoxic activity was measured by means of a biological assay. High-performance liquid chromatography identified oxypeucedanin and bergapten as photoxic substances, but the phototoxic potency of oxypeucedanin was only one-quarter of that of bergapten. The concentration of these furocoumarins may vary on the basis of the geographical area where the plants have been cultivated, influencing phototoxic activity. It has been observed that oxypeucedanin may elicit photopigmentation on colored guinea pig skin without preceding visible erythema (Naganuma et al., 1985).

9.11   LIME (*CITRUS AURANTIFOLIA*)

Citrus aurantifolia essential oil has been proven to cause a photodynamic action with a clinical manifestation similar to that of Berloque dermatitis (Sams, 1941). Coumarins with phototoxic potential are present in variable concentrations in the rind and pulp of Persian and key limes, hybrids derived from *C. aurantifolia*. They contain limettin, bergapten, isopimpinellin, xanthotoxin, and psoralen (Nigg et al., 1993).

9.12   PRECLINICAL TESTS ASSESSING PHOTOXICITY

The determination of phototoxicity can be conducted with different preclinical tests. An adverse cutaneous response induced by phototoxic agents can be reproduced *in vitro* using different models (Dijoux et al., 2006). A collaboration involving several laboratories from the European Cosmetic Industry Association (COLIPA) conducted various experiments to indentify *in vitro* models considered suitable to be incorporated into international guidelines for acute phototoxicity testing. This research concluded that the 3T3 mouse fibroblast neutral red uptake phototoxicity test (3T3 NRU PT) could be adopted as designated protocol for evaluation of phototoxicity of chemical substances. The 3T3 NRU PT is designed to detect the phototoxicity induced by the combined action of a test article and light by using an *in vitro* cytotoxicity assay with the Balb/c 3T3 mouse fibroblast cell line. The test permits us to identify aqueous-soluble compounds (or formulations) having the potential to exhibit *in vivo* phototoxicity after systemic application (Spielmann et al., 1998; Yanga et al., 2007). Currently the 3T3 NRU phototoxicity test is used within the context of EU test guidelines (Commission Directive 2000/33/EC, 2000; Council Directive 67/548/ EEC, 2004) and the Organisation for Economic Co-operation and Development (OECD) chemical testing guideline (OECD, 2014). In addition, complementary *in vitro* methods can also be set up using human primary keratinocyte-based tissue models. These experimental protocols have been shown to be useful to identify the phototoxic potential of both soluble and insoluble agents. This type of model allows application of test materials to the air-exposed surface and modification of usage concentrations and formulations, offering a simulation of the human *in vivo* situation (Dijoux et al., 2006). However, the highest nonphototoxic concentrations obtained by the skin model assay can offer a useful starting point that, in certain cases, needs to be confirmed with a subsequent human photopatch test aimed to identify safe concentrations for human use (Kejlova, 2010).

REFERENCES

Abali, A.E., Aka, M., Aydogan, C., Haberal, M. Burns or phytophotodermatitis, abuse or neglect: Confusing aspects of skin lesions caused by the superstitious use of fig leaves. *J Burn Care Res* 33 (2012): e309–12.

Anthony, F.A., Laboda, H.M., Costlow, M.E. Psoralen-fatty acid adducts activate melanocyte protein kinase C: A proposed mechanism for melanogenesis induced by 8-methoxypsoralen and ultraviolet A light. *Photodermatol Photoimmunol Photomed* 13 (1997): 9–16.

Archier, E., Devaux, S., Castela, E. et al. Carcinogenic risks of psoralen UV-A therapy and narrowband UV-B therapy in chronic plaque psoriasis: A systematic literature review. *J Eur Acad Dermatol Venereol* 26 (Suppl 3) (2012): 22–31.

Balato, N., Giordano, C., Montesano, M., Lembo, G. 8-Methoxypsoralen-induced photo-onycholysis. *Photodermatology* 1 (1984): 202–3.

Bordin, F. Photochemical and photobiological properties of furocoumarins and homologues drugs. *International Journal of Photoenergy* 1 (1999): 1–6.

Bylaite, M., Grigaitiene, J., Lapinskaite, G.S. Photodermatoses: Classification, evaluation and management. *Br J Dermatol* 161 (Suppl 3) (2009): 61–68.

Chandran, N.S, Aw, D.C. Drug-induced photo-onycholysis: An often-neglected phenomenon. *Intern Med J* 43 (2013): 1349–50.

Commission Directive 2000/33/EC of 25 April 2000.

Corasaniti, M.T., Maiuolo, J., Maida, S. et al. Cell signaling pathways in the mechanisms of neuroprotection afforded by bergamot essential oil against NMDA-induced cell death in vitro. *Br J Pharmacol* 151 (2007): 518–29.

Cosmetic Ingredient Review Expert Panel. Final report on the safety assessment of *Hypericum perforatum*. *Int J Toxicol* 20 Suppl 2 (2001): 31–9.

Costa, R., Dugo, P., Navarra, M., Raymo, V., Dugo, G., Mondello, L. Study on the chemical composition variability of some processed bergamot (Citrus bergamia) essential oils. *Flavour Fragr J* 25 (2010): 4–12.

Council Directive 67/548/EEC, 2004. https://osha.europa.eu/en/legislation/directives/58.

Crockett, S.L. Essential oil and volatile components of the genus *Hypericum* (Hypericaceae). *Nat Prod Commun* 5 (2010): 1493–506.

Dall'Acqua, F., Vedaldi, D., Bordin, F, Rodighiero, G. New studies on the interaction between 8-methoxypsoralen and DNA in vitro. *J Invest Dermatol* 73 (1979): 191–7.

Dijoux, N., Guingand, Y., Bourgeois, C. et al. Assessment of the phototoxic hazard of some essential oils using modified 3T3 neutral red uptake assay. *Toxicol In Vitro* 20 (2006): 480–89.

Dubakiene, R., Kupriene, M. Scientific problems of photosensitivity. *Medicina (Kaunas)* 42 (2006): 619–24.

Dubertret, L., Serraf-Tircazes, D., Jeanmougin, M., Morlière, P., Averbeck, D., Young, A.R. Phototoxic properties of perfumes containing bergamot oil on human skin: Photoprotective effect of UVA and UVB sunscreens. *J Photochem Photobiol B* 7 (1990): 251–59.

Franceschi, E., Grings, M.B., Frizzo, C.D. et al. Phase behavior of lemon and bergamot peel oils in supercritical CO_2. *Fluid Phase Equilibria* 226 (2004): 1–8.

Gambichler, T., Altmeyer, P., Hoffmann, K. *Role of Clothes in Sun Protection: Cancers of the Skin.* Berlin: Springer (2002), 15–25.

Gasparro, F.P., Dall'Amico, R., Goldminz, D., Simmons, E., Weingold, D. Molecular aspects of extracorporeal photochemotherapy. *Yale J Biol Med* 62 (1989): 579–93.

Hann, S.K., Park, Y.K., Im, S., Byun, S.W. Angelica-induced phytophotodermatitis. *Photodermatol Photoimmunol Photomed* 8 (1991): 84–85.

Hawk, J.L. *Photodermatology*. London: Arnold (1999).

Herbal Medicinal Products Committee of European Medicines Agency. Reflection paper on the risks associated with furocoumarins contained in preparations of Angelica archangelica L. EMEA/HMPC/317913/06 (2007).

Herbal Medicinal Products Committee of European Medicines Agency. Assessment report on *Citrus bergamia* Risso et Poiteau, aetheroleum. EMA/HMPC/56155/2011 (2012).

Kaddu, S., Kerl, H., Wolf, P. Accidental bullous phototoxic reactions to bergamot aromatherapy oil. *J Am Acad Dermatol* 45 (2001): 458–61.

Kejlova, K., Jirova, D., Bendova, H., Gajdoš, P., Kolářová, H. Phototoxicity of essential oils intended for cosmetic use. *Toxicol In Vitro* 24 (2010): 2084–89.

Kutlubay, Z., Sevim, A., Engin, B., Tüzün, Y. Photodermatoses, including phototoxic and photoallergic reactions (internal and external). *Clin Dermatol* 32 (2014) (1): 73–9.

Laskin, J.D., Lee, E., Laskin, D.L., Gallo, M.A. Psoralens potentiate ultraviolet light-induced inhibition of epidermal growth factor binding. *Proc Natl Acad Sci USA* 83 (1986): 8211–15.

Lehmann, P., Schwarz, T. Photodermatoses: Diagnosis and treatment. *Dtsch Arztebl Int* 108 (2011): 135–41.

Linde, K., Berner, M.M., Kriston, L. St John's wort for major depression. *Cochrane Database Syst Rev* (2008): CD000448.

Lugovic, L., Situm, M., Ozanic-Bulic, S., Sjerobabski-Masnec, I. Phototoxic and photoallergic skin reactions. *Coll Antropol* 31 (Suppl 1) (2007): 63–67.

Marzulli, F.N., Maibach, H.I. Perfume phototoxicity. *J Soc Cosmet Chem* 21 (1970): 695–715.

Medeiros, V.L., Lim, H.W. Sunscreens in the management of photodermatoses. *Skin Therapy Lett* 15 (2010): 1–3.

Messer, A., Raquet, N., Lohr, C., Schrenk, D. Major furocoumarins in grapefruit juice II: Phototoxicity, photogenotoxicity, and inhibitory potency vs. cytochrome P450 3A4 activity. *Food Chem Toxicol* 50 (2012): 756–60.

Moreau J.F., English, J.C. 3rd, Gehris, R.P. Phytophotodermatitis. *J Pediatr Adolesc Gynecol* 27 (2014): 93–4.

Naganuma, M., Hirose, S., Nakayama, Y., Nakajima, K., Someya, T. A study of the phototoxicity of lemon oil. *Arch Dermatol Res* 278 (1985): 31–36.

Navarra, M., Mannucci, C., Delbò, M., Calapai, G. Citrus bergamia essential oil: From basic research to clinical application. *Front Pharmacol* 6 (2015): 36.

Nigg, H.N., Nordby, H.E., Beier, R.C., Dillman, A., Macias, C., Hansen, R.C. Phototoxic coumarins in limes. *Food Chem Toxicol* 31 (1993): 331–35.

OECD Guidelines for the Testing of Chemicals, Section 4 (2014). http://www.oecd-ilibrary.org /environment/test-no-442d-in-vitro-skin-sensitisation_9789264229822-en;jsessionid =4n68qmqsjq3f.x-oecd live-02.

Opdyke, D. Monographs on fragrance raw materials. *Food Cosmet Toxicol* 17 (1979): 357–90.

Oppenheim, M. Local sensitization of the skin to Grenz rays by bergamot oil. *J Invest Dermatol* 8 (1947): 255–62.

Ostertag E, Becker T, Ammon J, Bauer-Aymanns H, Schrenk D. Effects of storage conditions on furocoumarin levels in intact, chopped, or homogenized parsnips. *J Agric Food Chem* 24 (2002): 2565–70.

Placzek, M., Fromel, W., Eberlein, B, Gilbertz, K.P., Przybilla, B. Evaluation of phototoxic properties of fragrances. *Acta Derm Venereol* 87 (2007): 312–16.

Raquet, N., Schrenk, D. Application of the equivalency factor concept to the phototoxicity and genotoxicity of furocoumarin mixtures. *Food Chem Toxicol* 68 (2014): 257–66.

Sams, W.M. Photodynamic action of lime oil (*Citrus aurantifolia*). *Arch Dermatol* 44 (1941): 571–87.

Santana, L., Uriarte, E., Roleira, F., Milhazes, N., Borges, F. Furocoumarins in medicinal chemistry. Synthesis, natural occurrence and biological activity. *Curr Med Chem* 11 (2004): 3239–61.

Schiener, R., Brockow, T., Franke, A., Salzer, B., Peter, R.U., Resch, K.L. Bath PUVA and saltwater baths followed by UV-B phototherapy as treatments for psoriasis: A randomized controlled trial. *Arch Dermatol* 143 (2007): 586–96.

Solis, R.R., Dotson, D.A., Trizna, Z. Phytophotodermatitis: A sometimes difficult diagnosis. *Arch Fam Med* 9 (2000): 1195–96.

Spielmann, H., Balls, M., Dupuis, J. et al. The International EU/COLIPA In Vitro Phototoxicity Validation Study: Results of phase II (blind trial). Part 1: The 3T3 NRU phototoxicity test. *Toxicol In Vitro* 12 (1998): 305–27.

Stern, R.S., Beer, J.Z., Mills, D.K. Lack of consensus among experts on the choice of UV therapy for psoriasis. *Arch Dermatol* 135 (1999): 1187–92.

Venugopala, K.N., Rashmi, V., Odhav, B. Review on natural coumarin lead compounds for their pharmacological activity. *Biomed Res Int* 2013 (2013): 963248.

Yanga, Y., Xiong, X., Yang, X. et al. Establishment and use of 3t3 NRU assay for assessment of phototoxic hazard of cosmetic products. *AATEX* 14 (2007): 515–18.

Zala, L., Omar, A., Krebs, A. Photo-onycholysis induced by 8-methoxypsoralen. *Dermatology* 154 (1977): 203–15.

Zaynoun, S.T., Aftimos, B.A., Tenekjian, K.K., Kurban, A.K. Berloque dermatitis—A continuing cosmetic problem. *Contact Dermatitis* 7 (1981): 111 6.

Zammit, M.L. Photosensitivity: Light, sun and pharmacy. *J Malta College Pharmacy Pract* 16 (2010): 12–17.

10 Essential Oils
Fragrances and Antioxidants

Rosalia Crupi and Salvatore Cuzzocrea

CONTENTS

10.1 INTRODUCTION

Plants produce a high diversity of secondary metabolites with a prominent function of protecting plants against predators and microbial pathogens due to their biocidal properties against microbes or repellence to herbivores. Some metabolites are also involved in defense mechanisms against abiotic stress (e.g., UV-B exposure) and are important in the interaction of plants with other organisms (e.g., attraction of pollinators) (Schafer and Wink, 2009). It is believed that most of the 100,000 known secondary metabolites are involved in plant chemical defense systems; they seem to have appeared as a response of plants to the interactions with predators throughout the millions of years of coevolution. There are three major groups of secondary metabolites, including terpenes (Figure 10.1a–d), phenylpropenoids, and N- and S-containing compounds. Among these secondary metabolites, it is estimated that more than 3000 essential oils (EOs) are known, of which about 300 are commercially important and used by the flavor and fragrance industries.

10.2 ESSENTIAL OILS: FEATURES AND APPLICATIONS

Essential oils, or aromatic plant essences, are volatile oils that constitute the aroma and flavor components of organic material (Amorati et al., 2013). They can be both beautifully and powerfully fragrant. They are used in a variety of products, such as incense, aromatherapy oils, perfumes, cosmetics, pharmaceuticals, beverages, and foods. They

Classification	Isoprene units	Carbon atoms
Monoterpenes	2	C_{10}
Sesquiterpenes	3	C_{15}
Diterpenes	4	C_{20}
Sesterterpenes	5	C_{25}
Triterpenes	6	C_{30}

(a)

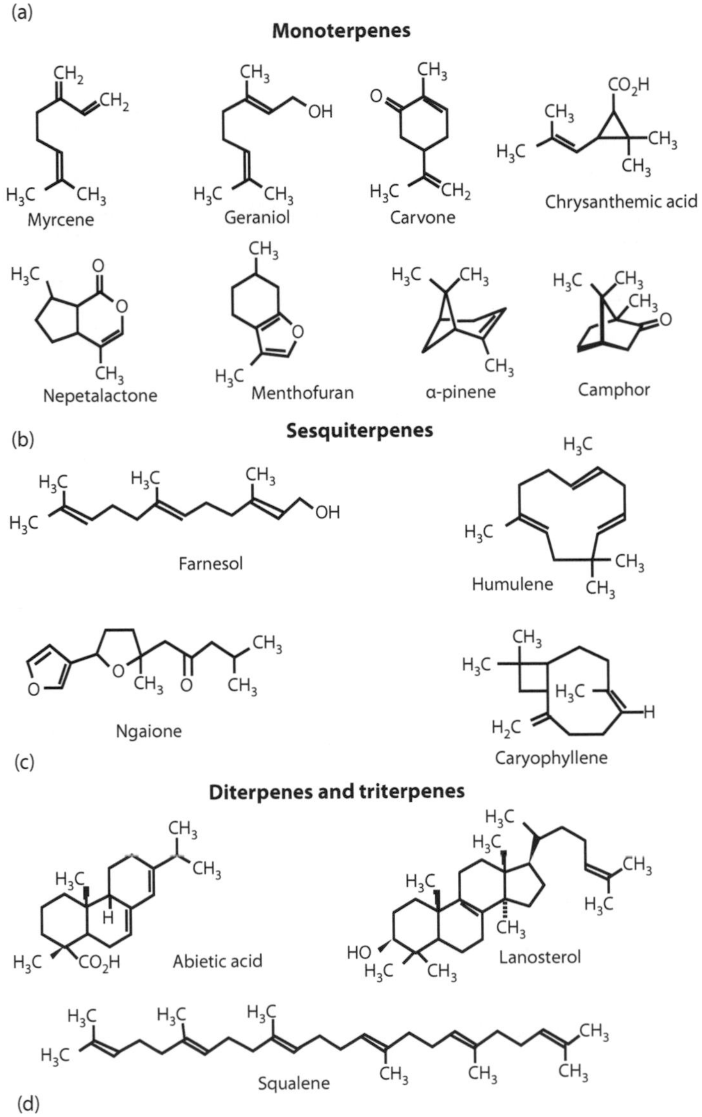

Monoterpenes

Myrcene   Geraniol   Carvone   Chrysanthemic acid

Nepetalactone   Menthofuran   α-pinene   Camphor

(b)

Sesquiterpenes

Farnesol   Humulene

Ngaione   Caryophyllene

(c)

Diterpenes and triterpenes

Abietic acid   Lanosterol

Squalene

(d)

FIGURE 10.1 Classification of the three major groups of secondary metabolites, including terpenes, phenylpropenoids, and N- and S-containing compounds.

can be liquid at room temperature, though a few of them are solid or resinous, and show different colors, ranging from pale yellow to emerald green and from blue to dark brownish red (Amorati et al., 2013). They are synthesized by all plant organs, that is, buds, flowers, leaves, stems, twigs, seeds, fruits, roots, and wood or bark, and are stored in secretory cells, cavities, canals, epidermic cells, or glandular trichomes (Bakkali et al., 2008). The term *essential oil* was used for the first time in the sixteenth century by Paracelsus von Hohenheim, who referred to the effective component of a drug as "Quinta essential" (Rae, 1950). The first reference on the uses of EOs for therapeutic reasons was found in the Ebers papyrus. This document listed in detail more than 800 EO remedies and treatments and showed that myrrh was a favorite ingredient, often mixed with honey and other herbs, because of its ability to inhibit bacterial growth. In addition to their intrinsic benefits to plants and being beautifully fragrant to people, essential oils have been used throughout history in many cultures for their medicinal and therapeutic benefits. Modern scientific study and trends toward more holistic approaches to wellness are driving a revival and new discovery of essential oil health applications. The Egyptians were some of the first people to use aromatic essential oils extensively in medical practice, beauty treatment, food preparation, and religious ceremony. The Romans also used aromatic oils to promote health and personal hygiene. Influenced by the Greeks and Romans, as well as Chinese and Indian Ayurvedic use of aromatic herbs, the Persians began to refine distillation methods for extracting essential oils from aromatic plants. Essential oil extracts were used throughout the dark ages in Europe for their antibacterial and fragrant properties. In modern times, the powerful healing properties of essential oils were rediscovered in 1937 by a French chemist, Rene-Maurice Gattefosse, who healed a badly burned hand with pure lavender oil. The modern use of essential oils has continued to grow rapidly as health scientists and medical practitioners continue to research and validate the numerous health and wellness benefits of therapeutic-grade essential oils. They can be used one oil at a time or in complex blends, depending on user experience and desired benefit. Essential oils are usually administered by one of three methods: diffused aromatically, applied topically, or taken internally as dietary supplements.

10.2.1 AROMATIC USES

Our sense of smell influences many physiological pathways, including the stimulation of hormones and other metabolic processes. Aromatherapy is founded on the body's predictable response to specific olfactory stimuli. Essential oils are widely used in aromatherapy applications. Certain essential oils, when diffused in the air, can be very stimulating, while others can be calming and soothing. Beyond emotional benefits, diffusing essential oils can purify the air of unwanted odors and some airborne pathogens. Low or no-heat essential oil diffusers are recommended, as they do not change the chemical structure of the oil being diffused. Essential oils can also be used as cleansing and purifying additives to laundry and surface cleaners throughout the home.

10.2.2 TOPICAL USES

Due to their natural molecular composition, essential oils are easily absorbed by the skin and can be safely applied topically. Application of essential oils can have immediate, localized benefits to the target area of application. They have restorative and calming properties and can be used effectively with massage and beauty therapy. They are also natural disinfectants. The chemical structure of essential oils also allows them to be absorbed into the bloodstream via the skin for internal benefits throughout the body.

10.2.3 INTERNAL USES

EOs can also be used as dietary supplements supporting a variety of healthy conditions. Some essential oils have powerful antioxidant properties, while others help support healthy inflammatory response in cells. Many essential oils are generally regarded as safe for dietary use, but some oils should not be taken internally.

Essential oils can be extracted using a number of methods, such as steam distillation, hydrodistillation, organic solvent extraction, microwave-assisted distillation, microwave hydrodiffusion and gravity, high-pressure solvent extraction, supercritical CO_2 extraction, ultrasonic extraction, and solvent-free microwave extraction.

10.3 ESSENTIAL OILS: BIOLOGICAL PROPERTIES

EOs from aromatic and medicinal plants have been known to be biologically active, mainly possessing antibacterial, antifungal, and antioxidant properties (Simic et al., 2004). The main components can represent up to 85% of the total, while the remainder is present as traces. The concentration of the specific compound in the total mix of plant oils can be highly variable, depending on factors such as the origin, species and plant organ, climatic conditions and growth, and extraction and storage. The main components of common EOs can be classified in two structural families with respect to the hydrocarbon skeleton: terpenoids, formed by the combination of two (monoterpene), three (sesquiterpene), or four (diterpene) isoprene units, and phenylpropanoids. Both terpenoid and phenylpropanoid families comprise phenolic compounds, sometimes accounted for among principal components of several EOs. The monoterpenes represent 90% of essential oils and have a variety of structures with several activities, such as antimicrobial, anti-inflammatory, and antioxidant. The oil is composed of at least 100 different chemical compounds classified as aldehydes, phenols, oxides, esters, ketones, alcohols, and terpenes. Common terpenes include limonene, which occurs in most citrus oils, and the antiseptic pine, found in pine and terpene oils. Important sesquiterpenes include chamzulene and farnesene, which occur in chamomile oil and have been widely studied for anti-inflammatory and bactericidal properties. The extensive occurrence of ester in essential oil includes linalyl acetate, which is a component of bergamot and lavender, and geranyl acetate, found in sweet marjoram. Other common esters are the bornyl, eugenyl, and lavendulyl acetate. The characteristic fruity aromas of esters are claimed to have sedative and fungicidal properties. Aldehydes are also claimed to have sedative properties, the most common being citralnellal and neral, found in lemon scented oils; citral also has antiseptic properties. Equally pungent to the aldehydes in many instances are the ketones, such as jasmine and funchone, found in jasmine and fennel oil, respectively. Ketones such as camphor, carnone, methone, and pine comphone, found in many proprietary preparations, are effective in upper respiratory tract complaints. However, some ketones are also among the more toxic components of essential oils, such the one found in pennyroyal and buchu. The alcohol within essential oils is generally nontoxic. Commonly occurring terpene alcohols include citronellal found in rose, lemon, and eucalyptus, and geramnial, bornenol, fornenesol, menthol, nerol, and linalool occurring in rose wood and lavender. Alcohol has antiseptic and antiviral properties and in aromatherapy is claimed to have an uplifting quality. A wide range of oxides occur in essential oils, including ascaridol, bisabolol, and bisaleolone oxides and linalool oxide from hyssop. The most important oxide, however, is cineole. Also known as eucalyptus oil, it occurs extensively in other oils, such as bey laurel, rosemary, and cajuput. It is used medicinally for its expectorant properties.

10.4 ANTIOXIDANT ACTIVITY

Free radicals are considered to initiate oxidation that leads to aging and causes diseases in human beings. The human body is equipped with an inherent defense system that can quench free radicals present in almost all cells (Halliwell and Gutteridge, 1990). An imbalance between free radical production and their removal by the body's antioxidant system leads to a phenomenon known as oxidative stress (McCord, 2000). In this situation, an external supply of antioxidants is necessary to regain a balance between free radicals and antioxidants.

EOs, as natural sources of phenolic components, attract investigators to evaluate their activity as antioxidants or free radical scavengers. The essential oils of basil, cinnamon, clove, nutmeg, oregano, and thyme have proved radical scavenging and antioxidant properties in the 2,2-diphenyl-1-picrylhydrazyl (DPPH) radical assay at room temperature (Tuttolomondo et al., 2013). The order of effectiveness was found to be clove >> cinnamon > nutmeg > basil ≥ oregano >> thyme. The essential oil of *Thymus serpyllus* showed a free radical scavenging activity close to that of the synthetic butylated hydroxytoluene (BHT) in a β-carotene/linoleic acid system (Polat et al., 2007). The antioxidant activity was attributed to the high content of the phenolics thymol and carvacrol (20.5% and 58.1%, respectively). *Thymus spathulifolius* essential oil also possessed an antioxidant activity due to the high thymol and carvacrol content (36.5% and 29.8%, respectively) (Tepe et al., 2004). The antioxidant activity of oregano (*Origanum vulgare* L. subsp. *hirtum*) essential oil was comparable to that of α-tocopherol and BHT, but less effective than ascorbic acid (Kulisic et al., 2007). The activity is again attributed to the content of thymol and carvacrol (35.0% and 32.0%, respectively). Although dietary supplementation of oregano oil to rabbits delayed lipid oxidation, this effect was less than that of supplementation with the same concentration of α-tocopheryl acetate (Botsoglou et al., 2004). However, when tested on turkeys, it showed an equivalent performance to the same concentration of α-tocopheryl acetate in delaying iron-induced, lipid oxidation (Papageorgiou et al., 2003). The essential oils of *Salvia cryptantha* and *Salvia multicaulis* have the capacity to scavenge free radicals. The activity of these oils was higher than that of curcumin, ascorbic acid, or BHT (Tepe et al., 2004). The essential oil of *Achillea millefolium* subsp. *millefolium* (Asteraceae) exhibited a hydroxyl radical scavenging effect in the Fe^{3+}–EDTA–H_2O_2 deoxyribose system and inhibited the nonenzymatic lipid peroxidation of rat liver homogenate (Candan et al., 2003). In addition, *Curcuma zedoaria* essential oil was found to be an excellent scavenger for DPPH radical (Lai et al., 2004).

The antioxidant activity of essential oils cannot be attributed only to the presence of phenolic constituents; monoterpene alcohols, ketones, aldehydes, hydrocarbons, and ethers also contribute to the free radical scavenging activity of some essential oils. For instance, the essential oil of *Thymus caespititius*, *Thymus camphoratus*, and *Thymus mastichina* showed antioxidant activity, which in some cases was equal to that of α-tocopherol (Hazzit et al., 2006). Surprisingly, the three species are characterized by high contents of linalool and 1,8-cineole, while thymol and carvacrol are almost absent. The essential oil of lemon balm (*Melissa officinalis* L.) shows an antioxidant and free radical scavenging activity (Mimica-Dukic et al., 2004), with the most powerful scavenging constituents comprising neral/geranial, citronellal, isomenthone, and menthone. Tea tree (*Melaleuca alternifolia*) oil has been suggested as a natural antioxidant alternative for BHT (Kim et al., 2004), with the inherent antioxidant activity attributed mainly to the α-terpinene, γ-terpinene, and α-terpinolene content. EOs isolated from *Mentha aquatica* L., *Mentha longifolia* L., and *Mentha piperita* L. were able to reduce DPPH radicals into the neutral DPPHH form (Mimica-Dukic et al., 2003). The most powerful scavenging constituent was found to be 1,8-cineole for the oil of *M. aquatica*, while menthone and isomenthone were the active principles *of M. longifolia* and *M. piperita*. It is clear that essential oils may be considered potential natural antioxidants and could perhaps be formulated as a part of daily supplements or additives to prevent oxidative stress that contributes to many degenerative diseases.

Moreover, activated oxygen incorporates reactive oxygen species (ROS) that consist of free radicals (1 O_2, $O_2\cdot-$, ·OH, ONOO−) and nonfree radicals (H_2O_2, NO, and R–OOH) (Sultana et al., 2010). ROS are liberated by virtue of stress, and thus an imbalance is developed in the body that damages cells in it and causes health problems (Huang et al., 2005). Moreover, oxidation in processed foods, enriched with fats and oils, during storage leads to spoilage and quality deterioration (Iqbal et al., 2013). The use of synthetic antioxidants such as butylated hydroxyanisole (BHA), butylated hydroxytoluene (BHT), and tertiary butylhydroquinone (TBHQ) has been restricted because of their carcinogenicity and other toxic properties (Siddhuraju and Becker, 2003). Growing evidence has shown an inverse correlation between the intake of dietary antioxidants and the risk of chronic diseases, such as coronary heart disease, cancer, and several other aging-related health concerns (Hussain et al., 2010).

Several EOs have been attributed good antioxidant properties, which can be exploited to protect other materials, such as food, from rancidity (Amorati et al., 2013). Antioxidant properties also play a pivotal role in some EOs' biological activities, which is justified by the involvement of oxidative stress in pathology (Valgimigli et al., 2000). These attributes are due to the inherent ability of some of their components, particularly phenols, to stop or delay the aerobic oxidation of organic matter, although the procedure by which the oil is obtained from the raw material (distillation) limits the content of phenolics in the final matrix because many such compounds are nonvolatile. The antioxidant activity of volatile oils is of great interest because they may preserve foods from the toxic effects of oxidants. Moreover, volatile oils, being also able to scavenge free radicals, may play an important role in some disease prevention, such as brain dysfunction, cancer, heart disease, and immune system decline. Increasing evidence has suggested that these diseases may result from cellular damage caused by free radicals (Miguel, 2010). In industrial processing, mainly synthetic antioxidants are used, in order to prolong the storage stability of food (Gardner et al., 2007). However, the worldwide concern over safety demands for natural antioxidants, which have the advantage of being more widely accepted by consumers, as these are considered nonchemical. In addition, they do not require safety tests before being used, although they are more expensive and less effective than synthetic antioxidants (Daferera et al., 2002). The harmful effect of oxidation on human health has become a serious issue. According to Laguerre et al. (2007), research has confirmed that antioxidants supplied by food products are essential for counteracting this oxidative stress. Antioxidants are able to protect biological systems against oxidative damage, thus helping to prevent cardiovascular, neurologic, and carcinogenic diseases. One solution to this problem is to supplement the diet with antioxidant compounds that are contained in natural plant sources. The source of these compounds is mainly the plant kingdom, and they are mainly phenolic compounds (flavonoids, phenolic acids and alcohols, stilbenes, tocopherols, tocotrienols), ascorbic acid, and carotenoids, which can serve, in some sense, as a type of preventive medicine. In fact, it has been suggested that a high intake of fruits and vegetables could decrease the potential stress caused by reactive oxygen species via a number of mechanisms, including the protection of target molecules (lipids, proteins, and nucleic acids) from oxidative damage (Fernandez-Panchon et al., 2008). Numerous studies have reported the synergistic effects found in antioxidant mixtures (Eberhardt et al., 2000; Augustin et al., 2009). Indeed, combinations of antioxidants may be more effective at reducing reactive oxygen species than pure compounds, especially if the mixture includes both water-soluble and lipid-soluble antioxidants. If this is the case, the mixture will be capable of quenching free radicals in both aqueous and lipid phases (Chen and Tappel, 1996).

10.4.1 Antioxidants: Mechanisms of Action

In literature an antioxidant is a "molecule able to react with radicals" or that provides reducing power so as to counteract the oxidative stress caused by radicals. Based on this definition, antioxidants are compounds capable of slowing or retarding the oxidation of an oxidizable material, even when used in very modest amount (<1%, commonly 1–1000 mg/L) compared to the amount of material they have to protect. Focusing on processes of relevance in biological systems or in food science, the materials to protect are most commonly lipids, proteins, carbohydrates, and to a minor extent, other organic molecules that compose animal or vegetal tissues. Their oxidation occurs by a radical chain reaction mediated by peroxyl radicals (ROO·) that parallels the autoxidation of hydrocarbons (Jones and Saso, 2007). The process, represented in Figure 10.2, is initiated by some radical species that, regardless of its origin or structure, is able to react with the (lipid) substrate RH (most commonly by H atom abstraction) to yield an alkyl radical R·, which will react at a diffusion-controlled rate with oxygen to form a peroxyl radical (ROO·). Cyclically, ROO· attacks another molecule of the substrate to yield a hydroperoxide ROOH (the oxidized substrate) and another radical. The chain reaction proceeds for many cycles before two radical species incidentally quench each other in a so-called termination step. The number of cycles occurring between initiation and termination is named chain length. Compounds capable of impairing this radical chain reaction are called direct antioxidants and are divided into two main groups depending on their mechanism of interference (Jones and Saso, 2007). Preventive antioxidants interfere with the initiation process; that is, they retard the initial formation of radical species (Jones and Saso, 2007). Examples of such are the enzyme catalase and metal chelators such as phytic acid. By blocking redox active metal ions (e.g., Fe^{2+}) in an oxidized form (e.g., Fe^{3+}), metal chelators may prevent the occurrence of Fenton-type chemistry, which is one of the most important radical initiation processes. Several compounds of relevant antioxidant behavior that are not provided, for example, in the protection of lipids in model systems or food products, do nonetheless increase the antioxidant defenses in living systems, for example, by inducing the expression or enhancing the activity of antioxidant enzymes. These compounds are called indirect antioxidants, with relevant examples among natural products (Jones and Saso, 2007). Phenolic compounds, both natural (e.g., α-tocopherol) and synthetic (e.g., BHA), act as antioxidants due to their high reactivity with peroxyl radicals, which are disposed of by formal hydrogen atom transfer. Due to its stability, the product phenoxyl radical will not propagate the radical chain, but rather will wait for a second peroxyl radical and quench it in a very fast radical–radical reaction. Other terpenoid components of essential oils can react rapidly with peroxyl radicals. When EO components are mixed with an oxidizable material such as unsaturated lipids, both the lipids and the EO components will undergo autoxidation and will be subjected to

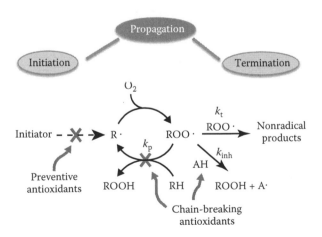

FIGURE 10.2 Oxidation process.

similar degradation. In other words, the substrate to be protected (the lipid) and the potential antioxidant (the EO components) will co-oxidize.

No protection can be expected from the essential oil because products arising from reactions with chain-carrying peroxyl radicals are reactive species able to propagate the oxidative chain.

10.4.2 Antioxidant Activity of Selected EOs

Borneol is a bicyclic monoterpenoid alcohol (Figure 10.3a). Borneol has shown effects such as antibiotic activity (Mai et al., 2003), wound healing activity (Unlu et al., 2002), anti-inflammatory activity by reducing leukocyte migration (Almeida et al., 2013), and antifibrosis activity by decreasing fibroblast growth, inhibiting collagen production, decreasing MMP-2 activity, and inhibiting TIMP-1 production (Dai et al., 2009). It showed no cytotoxicity (Dai et al., 2009), radical scavenging properties (Candan et al., 2003; Kordali et al., 2005), or immunomodulatory effects (Juhas et al., 2008). This monoterpene was able to suppress the proinflammatory cytokine (interleukin [IL]-1β and IL-6) mRNA expression and act as bioactive material in the cellular signal transduction system (Park et al., 2003). It shows antibacterial activity and inhibitory effects on several Gram (−)ve and (+)ve pathogenic microorganisms (Tabanca et al., 2001), antifungal activity (Wenqiang et al., 2006), and antioxidant activity by reducing intracellular ROS generation and attenuating the elevation of nitric oxide (NO), the increase of inducible nitric oxide synthase (iNOS) enzymatic activity, and the upregulation of iNOS expression (Liu et al., 2011). Borneol blocked NF-κB p65 nuclear translocation (Liu et al., 2011) and was shown to be a mast cell membrane stabilizer. Finally, an anti-inflammatory property was shown through

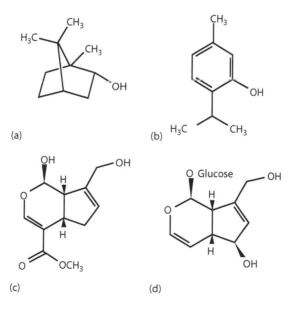

FIGURE 10.3 Example of essential oils: (a) (−)-borneol, (b) thymol, (c) genipin, and (d) aucubin.

fewer ICAM-1 positive vessels, IL-1β positive cells, tumor necrosis factor (TNF)-α positive cells, and a number of neutrophils (Li et al., 2012).

Thymol is a monoterpenoid phenol (Figure 10.3b) that exhibits multiple biological activities. Studies show that thymol modulates prostaglandin synthesis (Anamura et al., 1988); it has an anti-inflammatory effect in incubated human neutrophils (Braga et al., 2006) and beneficial effects on antioxidant status by influence on docosahexaenoic acid (DHA) concentration (Youdim and Deans, 2000). Thymol prevented autoxidation of lipids and the formation of toxic products through the action of reactive nitrogen species.

Genipin is an iridoid compound (Figure 10.3c) and an alternative natural cross-linking agent (Jin et al., 2004). It has shown the ability to form biocompatible and stable cross-linked products as well as low cytotoxicity (Sung et al., 1999).

Moreover, it has been proved that genipin has anti-inflammatory (Nam et al., 2010), wound healing, antioxidative effects and abilities of inhibiting lipid peroxidation and production of nitrogen monoxide (NO) (Wang et al., 2009). Additionally, genipin can increase the mitochondrial membrane potential, increase the ATP levels and close KATP channels, and stimulate insulin secretion. Finally, studies showed that genipin suppresses the α-TN4 lens epithelial cells and subconjunctival fibroblast migration induced by transforming growth factor (TGF)-β (Kitano et al., 2006).

Aucubin is an iridoid glycoside (Figure 10.3d) with a variety of pharmacological effects, such as antimicrobial, anti-inflammatory, and dermal wound healing and *in vitro* antioxidative capacity (Shim et al., 2007). In addition, aucubin showed inhibition of RNA and protein biosynthesis. Further, aucubin inhibits TNF-α-induced secretion and mRNA synthesis, including PAI-1, MCP-1, and IL-6 (Lorente-Cebrian et al., 2013). Furthermore, investigation revealed that aucubin suppressed extracellular signal-regulated kinase (ERK) activation, inhibitory kappa Bα (IκBα) degradation, and subsequent nuclear factor kappa B (NF-κB) activation (Park, 2013). Finally, aucubin was considered a promising chemopreventive agent and was devoid of any cytotoxic activity (Hung et al., 2008).

10.5 CONCLUSIONS

Natural products are in increasing demand from the manufacturers of foods, cosmetics, and pharmaceuticals. Thus, the importance of conducting studies on EOs lies not only in the chemical characterization but also in the possibility of linking the chemical contents with particular bioactive functional properties. The capacity of spices and flavors to minimize disease risk, within the context of culinary use, has not been completely evaluated. There is a strong need to understand the preventive effect of spices and natural flavors for counteracting oxidative damages.

REFERENCES

Almeida, J.R., Souza, G.R., Silva, J.C. et al. Borneol, a bicyclic monoterpene alcohol, reduces nociceptive behavior and inflammatory response in mice. *Sci World J* (2013): 808460.
Amorati, R., Foti, M.C., Valgimigli, L. Antioxidant activity of essential oils. *J Agric Food Chem* 61(46) (2013): 10835–10847.

Anamura, S., Dohi, T., Shirakawa, M., Okamoto, H., Tsujimoto, A. Effects of phenolic dental medicaments on prostaglandin synthesis by microsomes of bovine tooth pulp and rabbit kidney medulla. *Arch Oral Biol* 33(8) (1988): 555–560.

Augustin, K., Frank, J., Augustin, S. et al. Greeen tea extracts lower serum folates in rats at very high dietary concentrations only and do not affect plasma folates in a human pilot study. *J Physiol Pharmacol* 60(3) (2009): 103–108.

Bakkali, F., Averbeck, S., Averbeck, D., Idaomar, M. Biological effects of essential oils: A review. *Food Chem Toxicol* 46(2) (2008): 446–475.

Botsoglou, N.A., Florou-Paneri, P., Christaki, E., Giannenas, I., Spais, A.B. Performance of rabbits and oxidative stability of muscle tissues as affected by dietary supplementation with oregano essential oil. *Arch Anim Nutr* 58(3) (2004): 209–218.

Braga, P.C., Dal Sasso, M., Culici, M., Bianchi, T., Bordoni, L., Marabini, L. Anti-inflammatory activity of thymol: Inhibitory effect on the release of human neutrophil elastase. *Pharmacology* 77(3) (2006): 130–136.

Candan, F., Unlu, M., Tepe, B. Antioxidant and antimicrobial activity of the essential oil and methanol extracts of *Achillea millefolium* subsp. *millefolium* Afan. (Asteraceae). *J Ethnopharmacol* 87(2–3) (2003): 215–220.

Chen, H., Tappel, A. Protection by multiple antioxidants against lipid peroxidation in rat liver homogenate. *Lipids* 31(1) (1996): 47–50.

Daferera, D.J., Tarantilis, P.A., Polissiou, M.G. Characterization of essential oils from Lamiaceae species by Fourier transform Raman spectroscopy. *J Agric Food Chem* 50(20) (2002): 5503–5507.

Dai, J.P., Chen, J., Bei, Y.F., Han, B.X., Wang, S. Influence of borneol on primary mice oral fibroblasts: A penetration enhancer may be used in oral submucous fibrosis. *J Oral Pathol Med* 38(3) (2009): 276–281.

Eberhardt, M.V., Lee, C.Y., Liu, R.H. Antioxidant activity of fresh apples. *Nature* 405(6789) (2000): 903–904.

Fernandez-Panchon, M.S., Villano, D., Troncoso, A.M., Garcia-Parrilla, M.C. Antioxidant activity of phenolic compounds: From in vitro results to in vivo evidence. *Crit Rev Food Sci Nutr* 48(7) (2008): 649–671.

Gardner, C.D., Lawson, L.D., Block, E., Chatterjee, L.M., Kiazand, A., Balise, R.R., Kraemer, H.C. Effect of raw garlic vs commercial garlic supplements on plasma lipid concentrations in adults with moderate hypercholesterolemia: A randomized clinical trial. *Arch Intern Med* 167(4) (2007): 346–353.

Halliwell, B., Gutteridge, J.M. The antioxidants of human extracellular fluids. *Arch Biochem Biophys* 280(1) (1990): 1–8.

Hazzit, M., Baaliouamer, A., Faleiro, M.L., Miguel, M.G. Composition of the essential oils of *Thymus* and *Origanum* species from Algeria and their antioxidant and antimicrobial activities. *J Agric Food Chem* 54(17) (2006): 6314–6321.

Huang, D., Ou, B., Prior, R.L. The chemistry behind antioxidant capacity assays. *J Agric Food Chem* 53(6) (2005): 1841–1856.

Hung, J.Y., Yang, C.J., Tsai, Y.M., Huang, H.W., Huang, M.S. Antiproliferative activity of aucubin is through cell cycle arrest and apoptosis in human non-small cell lung cancer A549 cells. *Clin Exp Pharmacol Physiol* 35(9) (2008): 995–1001.

Hussain, A.I., Anwar, F., Chatha, S.A., Jabbar, A., Mahboob, S., Nigam, P.S. *Rosmarinus officinalis* essential oil: Antiproliferative, antioxidant and antibacterial activities. *Braz J Microbiol* 41(4) (2010): 1070–1078.

Iqbal, T., Hussain, A.I., Chatha, S.A., Naqvi, S.A., Bokhari, T.H. Antioxidant activity and volatile and phenolic profiles of essential oil and different extracts of wild mint (*Mentha longifolia*) from the Pakistani flora. *J Anal Methods Chem* (2013): 536490.

Jin, J., Song, M., Hourston, D.J. Novel chitosan-based films cross-linked by genipin with improved physical properties. *Biomacromolecules* 5(1) (2004): 162–168.

Jones, D.S., Saso, L. Chemistry and biology of antioxidants. *J Pharm Pharmacol* 59(12) (2007): 1671.

Juhas, S., Cikos, S., Czikková, S. et al. Effects of borneol and thymoquinone on TNBS-induced colitis in mice. *Folia Biol* (Praha) 54(1) (2008): 1–7.

Kim, H.J., Chen, F., Wu, C., Wang, X., Chung, H.Y., Jin, Z. Evaluation of antioxidant activity of Australian tea tree (*Melaleuca alternifolia*) oil and its components. *J Agric Food Chem* 52(10) (2004): 2849–2854.

Kitano, A., Saika, S., Yamanaka, O. et al. Genipin suppresses subconjunctival fibroblast migration, proliferation and myofibroblast transdifferentiation. *Ophthalmic Res* 38(6) (2006): 355–360.

Kordali, S., Kotan, R., Mavi, A., Cakir, A., Ala, A., Yildirim, A. Determination of the chemical composition and antioxidant activity of the essential oil of *Artemisia dracunculus* and of the antifungal and antibacterial activities of Turkish *Artemisia absinthium*, *A. dracunculus*, *Artemisia santonicum*, and *Artemisia spicigera* essential oils. *J Agric Food Chem* 53(24) (2005): 9452–9458.

Kulisic, T., Krisko, A., Dragović-Uzelac, V., Milos, M., Pifat, G. The effects of essential oils and aqueous tea infusions of oregano (*Origanum vulgare* L. spp. *hirtum*), thyme (*Thymus vulgaris* L.) and wild thyme (*Thymus serpyllum* L.) on the copper-induced oxidation of human low-density lipoproteins. *Int J Food Sci Nutr* 58(2) (2007): 87–93.

Laguerre, M., Lecomte, J., Villeneuve, P. Evaluation of the ability of antioxidants to counteract lipid oxidation: Existing methods, new trends and challenges. *Prog Lipid Res* 46(5) (2007): 244–282.

Lai, E.Y., Chyau, C.C., Mau, J.L. et al. Antimicrobial activity and cytotoxicity of the essential oil of *Curcuma zedoaria*. *Am J Chin Med* 32(2) (2004): 281–290.

Li, H., Xia, X.H., Liu, M., Zhang, Z.M., Wan, X.L. Metabolomics research on focal cerebral ischemia reperfusion injury in rats' brain treated by musk combined with borneol. *Zhong Yao Cai* 35(8) (2012): 1274–1279.

Liu, R., Zhang, L., Lan, X. et al. Protection by borneol on cortical neurons against oxygen-glucose deprivation/reperfusion: Involvement of anti-oxidation and anti-inflammation through nuclear transcription factor kappaB signaling pathway. *Neuroscience* 176 (2011): 408–419.

Lorente-Cebrian, S., Costa, A.G., Navas-Carretero, S., Zabala, M., Martínez, J.A., Moreno-Aliaga, M.J. Role of omega-3 fatty acids in obesity, metabolic syndrome, and cardiovascular diseases: A review of the evidence. *J Physiol Biochem* 69(3) (2013): 633–651.

Mai, L.M., Lin, C.Y., Chen, C.Y., Tsai, Y.C. Synergistic effect of bismuth subgallate and borneol, the major components of Sulbogin, on the healing of skin wound. *Biomaterials* 24(18) (2003): 3005–3012.

McCord, J.M. The evolution of free radicals and oxidative stress. *Am J Med* 108(8) (2000): 652–659.

Miguel, M.G. Antioxidant and anti-inflammatory activities of essential oils: A short review. *Molecules* 15(12) (2010): 9252–9287.

Mimica-Dukic, N., Bozin, B., Soković, M., Mihajlović, B., Matavulj, M. Antimicrobial and antioxidant activities of three *Mentha* species essential oils. *Planta Med* 69(5) (2003): 413–419.

Mimica-Dukic, N., Bozin, B., Sokovic, M., Simin, N. Antimicrobial and antioxidant activities of *Melissa officinalis* L. (Lamiaceae) essential oil. *J Agric Food Chem* 52(9) (2004): 2485–2489.

Nam, K.N., Choi, Y.S., Jung, H.J. et al. Genipin inhibits the inflammatory response of rat brain microglial cells. *Int Immunopharmacol* 10(4) (2010): 493–499.

Papageorgiou, G., Botsoglou, N., Govaris, A., Giannenas, I., Iliadis, S., Botsoglou, E. Effect of dietary oregano oil and alpha-tocopheryl acetate supplementation on iron-induced lipid oxidation of turkey breast, thigh, liver, and heart tissues. *J Anim Physiol Anim Nutr* (Berl) 87(9–10) (2003): 324–335.

Park, K.S. Aucubin, a naturally occurring iridoid glycoside inhibits TNF-alpha-induced inflammatory responses through suppression of NF-kappa B activation in 3T3-L1 adipocytes. *Cytokine* 62(3) (2013): 407–412.

Park, T.J., Park, Y.S., Lee, T.G., Ha, H., Kim, K.T. Inhibition of acetylcholine-mediated effects by borneol. *Biochem Pharmacol* 65(1) (2003): 83–90.

Polat, Z.A., Tepe, B., Vural, A. In vitro effectiveness of *Thymus sipyleus* subsp. *sipyleus* var. *sipyleus* on *Acanthamoeba castellanii* and its cytotoxic potential on corneal cells. *Parasitol Res* 101(6) (2007): 1551–1555.

Rae, J. Aluminum stearate as a thickener for essential oils. *Manuf Chem Aerosol News* 21(5) (1950): 205.

Schafer, H., Wink, M. Medicinally important secondary metabolites in recombinant microorganisms or plants: Progress in alkaloid biosynthesis. *Biotechnol J* 4(12) (2009): 1684–703.

Shim, K.M., Choi, S.H., Jeong, M.J., Kang, S.S. Effects of aucubin on the healing of oral wounds. *In Vivo* 21(6) (2007): 1037–1041.

Siddhuraju, P., Becker, K. Antioxidant properties of various solvent extracts of total phenolic constituents from three different agroclimatic origins of drumstick tree (*Moringa oleifera* L) leaves. *J Agric Food Chem* 51(8) (2003): 2144–2155.

Simic, A., Soković, M.D., Ristić, M., Grujić-Jovanović, S., Vukojević, J., Marin, P.D. The chemical composition of some Lauraceae essential oils and their antifungal activities. *Phytother Res* 18(9) (2004): 713–717.

Sultana, S., Ripa, F.A., Hamid, K. Comparative antioxidant activity study of some commonly used spices in Bangladesh. *Pak J Biol Sci* 13(7) (2010): 340–343.

Sung, H.W., Huang, R.N., Huang, L.L., Tsai, C.C. In vitro evaluation of cytotoxicity of a naturally occurring cross-linking reagent for biological tissue fixation. *J Biomater Sci Polym Ed* 10(1) (1999): 63–78.

Tabanca, N., Kirimer, N., Demirci, B., Demirci, F., Başer, K.H. Composition and antimicrobial activity of the essential oils of *Micromeria cristata* subsp. *phrygia* and the enantiomeric distribution of borneol. *J Agric Food Chem* 49(9) (2001): 4300–4303.

Tepe, B., Daferera, D., Sökmen, M., Polissiou, M., Sökmen, A. In vitro antimicrobial and antioxidant activities of the essential oils and various extracts of *Thymus eigii* M. Zohary et P.H. Davis. *J Agric Food Chem* 52(5) (2004): 1132–1137.

Tuttolomondo, T., La Bella, S., Licata, M. et al. Biomolecular characterization of wild sicilian oregano: Phytochemical screening of essential oils and extracts, and evaluation of their antioxidant activities. *Chem Biodivers* 10(3) (2013): 411–433.

Unlu, M., Daferera, D., Dönmez, E., Polissiou, M., Tepe, B., Sökmen, A. Compositions and the in vitro antimicrobial activities of the essential oils of *Achillea setacea* and *Achillea teretifolia* (Compositae). *J Ethnopharmacol* 83(1–2) (2002): 117–121.

Valgimigli, L., Valgimigli, M., Gaiani, S., Pedulli, G.F., Bolondi, L. Measurement of oxidative stress in human liver by EPR spin-probe technique. *Free Radic Res* 33(2) (2000): 167–178.

Wang, G.F., Wu, S.Y., Rao, J.J. et al. Genipin inhibits endothelial exocytosis via nitric oxide in cultured human umbilical vein endothelial cells. *Acta Pharmacol Sin* 30(5) (2009): 589–596.

Wenqiang, G., Shufen, L., Ruixiang, Y., Yanfeng, H. Comparison of composition and antifungal activity of *Artemisia argyi* Levl. et Vant inflorescence essential oil extracted by hydrodistillation and supercritical carbon dioxide. *Nat Prod Res* 20(11) (2006): 992–998.

Youdim, K.A., Deans, S.G. Effect of thyme oil and thymol dietary supplementation on the antioxidant status and fatty acid composition of the ageing rat brain. *Br J Nutr* 83(1) (2000): 87–93.

Section III

Rational Basis for Aromatherapy

11 Aromatherapy and Neurotransmission

Behavioral and Neurochemical Studies

Luigi Antonio Morrone, Laura Rombolà,
Diana Amantea, Maria Tiziana Corasaniti,
and Giacinto Bagetta

CONTENTS

11.1   INTRODUCTION

Aromatherapy is the use of concentrated essential oils extracted from herbs, flowers, and other plant parts to treat various diseases (Segen, 1998). This complementary therapy is becoming increasingly popular worldwide, and a number of essential oils are currently in use in the management of chronic pain, depression, anxiety, some cognitive disorders, insomnia, and stress-related disorders (see Perry and Perry, 2006; Setzer, 2009; Umezu, 2012). However, although essential oils are currently in use to treat various mental disorders, their central nervous system (CNS)–acting effects have not been clarified, and the pharmacology of the essential oils and their single chemical constituents remains largely undiscovered. Among the properties of pure fragrance compounds and essential oils, the emotional and behavioral modulations, although there are many anecdotal or empirically speculated efficacious effects, are often difficult to examine and demonstrate in scientifically controlled conditions. Individual constituents reach the blood, cross the blood–brain barrier, and enter the CNS following inhalation, dermal application (Brooker et al., 1997), intraperitoneal or subcutaneous injection, and oral administration (Orafidiya et al., 2004). The inhalation of essential oils can induce effects through the CNS (e.g., lung absorption and bloodstream transport) or stimulation of the olfactory system and secondary activation of brain regions. For example, it is well known that olfaction influences the behavior of mammals, and the olfactory system has a direct or indirect connection to a variety of CNS components, including the hypothalamus, hippocampus, and limbic system (Broughan, 2002; Edge, 2003; Weier and Beal, 2004). Consequently, the inhalation of fragrance produces a variety of physiological effects, including brain (Lorig, 2000; see Kiecolt-Glaser et al., 2008), endocrine (Komori et al., 1995a; see Kiecolt-Glaser et al., 2008), and immune (Haze et al., 2002; see Kiecolt-Glaser et al., 2008) functions. Thus, it can be hypothesized that inhalation of an essential oil can be used as a therapeutic intervention for correcting a reversible malfunction of the body by direct activation of a targeted brain pathway (see Zhao et al., 2005). In consideration of the diffusion of aromatherapy, in the last decades many studies on essential oils and related compounds have been conducted, and some studies have suggested that essential oils affect the modulation of the central neurotransmitter system. This review discusses the most current knowledge on the neurochemical effects of the most popular essential oils in experimental studies.

11.2   ANGELICA

Angelica is an important genus in the family Umbelliferae (or Apiaceae) and is extremely polymorphic in fruit anatomy, leaf morphology, and subterranean structures (Vasil'eva and Pimenov, 1991; see Li et al., 2013). The dried radixes of *Angelica gigas*, *Angelica sinensis*, and *Angelica acutiloba* have been used in folk medicine for the treatment of gynecological diseases such as menoxenia and anemia (see Zhao et al., 2005), whereas *Angelica archangelica* has been used in traditional and folk medicine as a remedy for nervous headaches, anxiety, fever, skin rashes, wounds, rheumatism, and toothaches (see Kumar et al., 2012). The results of some animal studies provided evidence for the involvement of the CNS in the effects of *Angelica* spp. For example, a total methanolic extract of *A. gigas* significantly inhibited acetylcholinesterase (AChE) activity (Kang et al., 2001) and mitigated the amnesia induced by scopolamine administration in mice (Kang et al., 2003). Moreover, INM-176, a standardized ethanolic extract of *A. gigas*, also inhibited AChE activity in the hippocampal tissue *in vitro* and *ex vivo* (Park et al., 2012a). Interestingly, INM-176 attenuated the Aβ(1-42) protein-induced astrocyte activation in the hippocampus, as well as cholinergic neuronal damage in the CA3 region of the hippocampus and the nucleus basalis of Meynert and exhibited antiamnesic effects (Park et al., 2012a). INM-176 also exhibited neuroprotective activities against lipopolysaccharide (LPS)-induced neuronal damage *in vitro* and *in vivo* (Park et al., 2012b). In primary microglial cells, INM-176 significantly inhibited LPS-induced nitric oxide release and expression of tumor necrosis factor-α and interleukin-1β. The expression levels of inducible nitric oxide synthase and cylcooxygenase-2 in microglial cells were markedly upregulated by LPS, but this increased expression was counteracted by INM-176. LPS-mediated neuronal damage in an organotypic hippocampal slice culture was also attenuated by the administration of INM-176. In addition, LPS-induced cognitive dysfunction in mice, as determined by passive avoidance and Y-maze tasks, was significantly attenuated by the administration of INM-176. Finally, the activation of microglia or astrocytes by LPS in the hippocampal regions of mice was suppressed by INM-176. These results suggest that the neuroprotective and cognition ameliorating effects of INM-176 against LPS-induced damage were mediated, in part, by its anti-inflammatory activities. In addition, angelica administration in rats reduced cognitive impairment during chronic cerebral hypoperfusion through the modulation of brain-derived neurotrophic factor (BDNF) and nerve growth factor (NGF) expression in the hippocampus (Zheng et al., 2008). Accordingly, *A. sinensis* root promoted neurogenesis to facilitate recovery from the cognitive impairment induced by chronic cerebral hypoperfusion (Xin et al., 2013) and ligustilide, a main lipophilic component of phytocomplex, alleviated brain damage, and improved cognitive function in rats in a chronic cerebral hypoperfusion model (Feng et al., 2012). Interestingly, decursin, a major coumarin constituent isolated from *A. gigas*, significantly ameliorated scopolamine-induced amnesia as measured in both the passive avoidance test and the Morris water maze test (Kang et al., 2003). Moreover, decursin significantly inhibited AChE activity by 34% in the hippocampus of treated mice (Kang et al., 2003). These results indicate that decursin may exert antiamnestic activity *in vivo* through inhibition of AChE activity in the hippocampus. Decursinol, another coumarin isolated from *A. gigas*, significantly blunted the Aβ(1-42)-induced decrease in alternation behavior (spatial working memory) in the Y-maze test in mice without change in general locomotor activity, suggesting it may have preventive effects against memory impairment related to Aβ in Alzheimer's disease (Yan et al., 2004). Interestingly, decursin conferred protection *in vitro* against the Aβ(25-35)-induced oxidative damage in the rat pheochromocytoma (PC12) cells, presumably through the induction of nuclear transcription factor Nrf2 and related antioxidant enzymes, but also the antiaggregation of Aβ (Li et al., 2011). More recently, the same authors suggested the involvement of mitogen-activated protein kinases (MAPKs) in the effect of decursin (Li et al., 2013). Fractions of *A. acutiloba* improved the scopolamine-induced impairment of rat's spatial cognition (Hatip-Al-Khatib et al., 2004), and more recently, extracts and constituents from *A. archangelica* (i.e., imperatorin) showed AChE inhibitory activity (Sigurdsson and Gudbjarnason, 2007, 2013). In addition to cognitive effects, inhalation of essential oil from *A. sinensis* exhibited anxiolytic-like effects in several murine tests of anxiety (Chen et al., 2004). Particularly in the elevated plus-maze test, compared to the positive control diazepam, angelica essential oil increased the percentage of open-arm time and reduced the percentage of protected head dips. In the light–dark test, it prolonged the time spent in the light area without altering the locomotor activity of the animals, whereas in the stress-induced hyperthermia test, angelica essential oil inhibited stress-induced hyperthermia. In addition, Min and colleagues (2005) reported that in the social interaction test, angelica essential oil decreased aggressive behaviors and significantly increased social interaction time, whereas in the hole-board test, it significantly increased head-dipping counts and duration. Recently, Kumar and colleagues (2012, 2013) reported that the mixture of coumarins isolated from *A. archangelica* and its constituents imperatorin and isoimperatorin have the potential to reduce anxiety in rats, but it is the mixture that has more significant activity, compared to its individual components. In addition, ligustilide and butylidenephthalide, the major components of the essential oil from *A. acutiloba*, have been shown to reverse the isolation stress-induced decrease in pentobarbital sleep in mice through central noradrenergic or γ-aminobutiric acid (GABA)A receptors (Matsumoto et al., 1998). Some authors have also reported that *A. acutiloba* has analgesic and anti-inflammatory effects (Tanaka et al., 1971; Takahashi et al., 1982), and more recently, Choi and colleagues (2003a) reported that *A. gigas* produces antinociception via acting on the CNS, showing antinociceptive profiles in various pain models, especially inflammatory pain. Interestingly, the same authors reported that decursinol showed antinociceptive activity in various pain models, suggesting that this effect may be mediated by noradrenergic, serotonergic, adenosine A2, and histamine H1 and H2 receptors (Choi et al., 2003b). Moreover, Seo and colleagues (2009) suggested that the analgesic effect of decursinol might be involved in supraspinal cyclooxygenase regulation. Interestingly, Zhao and colleagues (2005) reported that *A. gigas* essential oil attenuated the sensitization of extracellular dopamine levels in the nucleus accumbens and behavioral sensitization induced by repeated nicotine treatment, suggesting that its use may be effective in treating nicotine addiction. In this regard, recently, a small comparative study in humans corroborated these results (Cordell and Buckle, 2013).

11.3   BERGAMOT

The essential oil of bergamot (*Citrus bergamia* Risso et Poiteau) (BEO), a citrus fruit that belongs to the Rutacee growing almost exclusively in Calabria, Italy, is obtained by cold pressing of the epicarp and partly of the mesocarp of the fresh fruit. The essential oil of bergamot comprises a volatile fraction (93%–96% of total) containing monoterpene and sesquiterpene hydrocarbons (such as limonene, α- and β-pinene, β-myrcene, γ-terpinene, terpinolene, sabinene, β-caryophyllene, and β-isabolene) and oxygenated derivatives (such as linalool, neral, geranial, linalyl acetate, neryl acetate, and geranyl acetate) and a nonvolatile fraction (4%–7% of total) containing waxes, polymethoxylated flavones, coumarins, and psoralens (such as bergapten [5-methoxypsoralen] and bergamottine [5-geranyloxypsoralen]) (Mondello et al., 1993; Dugo et al., 2000). BEO is used in aromatherapy to minimize symptoms of stress-induced anxiety and mild mood disorders and chronic pain, though the rational basis for such applications awaits discovery. Recently, *in vivo* studies reported that BEO is endowed with quantifiable and reproducible gross behavioral and electroencephalogram (EEG) spectrum power effects (Rombolà et al., 2009). In particular, systemic administration of increasing volumes of BEO produces dose-dependent increases in locomotor and exploratory activity that correlate with a predominant increase in the energy in the faster-frequency bands of the EEG spectrum. These results are possibly a functional reflection of the ability of the phytocomplex to interfere with mechanisms controlling synaptic levels of neurotransmitters (Bagetta et al.,

2010). In this regard, microdialysis studies demonstrated that for systemic administration, BEO increases extracellular aspartate, glycine, and taurine in the hippocampus of freely moving rats via a Ca2+-dependent mechanism; in fact, in experiments carried out with a cerebrospinal fluid devoid of Ca2+, the latter effect is suppressed, suggesting that the phytocomplex interferes with the exocytotic release of amino acid neurotransmitters (Morrone et al., 2007). The central origin of the effects on both EEG spectrum power and synaptic amino acids evoked by systemic administration of BEO is supported by experiments in which focal administration of the phytocomplex, given at a diluted dose through the microdialysis probe, preferentially increases synaptic glutamate and GABA via a Ca2+-dependent mechanism, as seen after systemic administration, whereas given undiluted, BEO increases all of the amino acids measured via a Ca2+-independent mechanism (Morrone et al., 2007). These different sensitivities of BEO to Ca2+ have multiple explanations. Diverse active compounds, present in the phytocomplex, with different pharmacokinetic profiles may be responsible for the neurochemical changes observed in the CNS after systemic versus focal administration of BEO. In addition, different concentrations of the same active components can be obtained in the hippocampus depending on the route of administration or on the dilution of BEO employed. The effects of bergamot essential oil on the release of amino acid neurotransmitters in rat hippocampus have also been studied by in vitro superfusion of isolated nerve terminals. BEO concentration-dependently enhanced the release of [(3)H]D-aspartate from superfused hippocampal synaptosomes. Similar results were obtained by monitoring the BEO-evoked release of endogenous glutamate. At relatively high concentrations, the BEO-induced [(3)H]D-aspartate release was almost entirely prevented by the glutamate transporter blocker DL-threo-β-benzyloxyaspartic acid (DL-TBOA) and was Ca(2+) independent. At relatively low concentrations the release of [(3)H]D-aspartate was only in part DL-TBOA sensitive and Ca(2+) independent; the remaining portion of release was dependent on extracellular Ca(2+). Interestingly, the monoterpene hydrocarbon-free fraction of the essential oil appeared to be inactive, while the bergapten-free fraction superimposed the releasing effect of BEO, supporting the deduction that psoralens may not be implicated. The behavioral and EEG spectrum power effects of BEO correlate well with its exocytotic and carrier-mediated release of discrete amino acids endowed with neurotransmitter function in the mammalian hippocampus, supporting the deduction that BEO is able to interfere with normal and pathological synaptic plasticity. In this regard, recently, Saiyudthong and Marsden (2011) investigated the effect of BEO administered to rats on both anxiety-related behaviors (elevated plus-maze and hole-board tests) and stress-induced levels of plasma corticosterone in comparison with the effects of diazepam and reported that inhalation of BEO and injection of diazepam significantly increased the percentage of open-arm entries on the elevated plus-maze test and the number of head dips in the hole-board test (Saiyudthong and Marsden, 2011). Interestingly, the ability of BEO to modulate synaptic plasticity is supported by the observed neuroprotection in the course of experimental brain ischemia. In fact, intraperitoneal injection of BEO reduced, in a dose-dependent manner, the brain damage caused by focal cerebral ischemia in rats (Amantea et al., 2009). Intriguingly enough, under these experimental conditions, microdialysis experiments show that BEO does not affect basal amino acid levels in the frontoparietal cortex (penumbra region), whereas it significantly reduces excitatory amino acid, namely, glutamate, efflux typically enhanced in this brain region soon after occlusion of the middle cerebral artery (MCA) (Amantea et al., 2009). The observed minimization of MCA-induced increase in excitatory amino acid levels in the ischemic penumbra can be rationalized on the basis of BEO-induced normalization of the transporter function; whether the latter relates to an inversion of the direction or a blockade of excitatory amino acid transport (Morrone et al., 2007) remains to be established, though a reported free radical scavenging activity (Corasaniti et al., 2007) may contribute. More importantly, reduction of excitatory amino acid accumulation in the ischemic penumbra was accompanied at 24 h by enhanced levels of phosphorylation of the prosurvival gene product Akt and of the downstream kinase GSK-3β, a protein implicated in promoting cell death (Amantea et al., 2009).

11.4 CITRUS AURANTIUM

Essential oil from peel of *Citrus aurantium* (Rutaceae) is commonly used in aromatherapy to treat insomnia, anxiety, and epilepsy, suggesting CNS action (see Costa et al., 2013). Carvalho-Freitas and Costa (2002) reported that essential oil of *C. aurantium* increased the sleeping time induced by barbiturates, the time spent in the open arms of an elevated plus maze, and the latency period of tonic seizures in pentylenetetrazole and maximal electroshock experimental models. Specific tests also indicated that the phytocomplex did not promote deficits in general activity or motor coordination. Subsequently, Pultrini Ade and colleagues (2006) evaluated in two other experimental models the anxiolytic effect of *C. aurantium* essential oil. Particularly in the light–dark box (LDB) test, a single treatment with essential oil augmented the time spent by mice in the light chamber and the number of transitions between the two compartments (Pultrini Ade et al., 2006). On the other hand, there were no observed alterations in the parameters evaluated in the light–dark box after repeated treatment. In the marble-burying test (MBT), the essential oil significantly decreased the number of marbles buried after single and repeated treatments (Pultrini Ade et al., 2006). Moreover, in a study carried out by Leite and colleagues (2008), exposure of rats to *C. aurantium* essential oil caused an anxiolytic effect in these animals in the elevated plus maze. More recently, to gain more insights into the mechanisms underlying the anxiolytic and antidepressant effects of *C. aurantium* essential oil, Costa and colleagues (2013) investigated the putative mechanisms of these effects and the neurochemical changes in specific brain structures of mice after acute treatment with the phytocomplex. The anxiolytic-like activity of the essential oil was investigated in a light–dark box (LDB) and the antidepressant activity was investigated in a forced swim test (FST). To exclude false positive results due to motor impairment, the mice were also submitted to the rotarod test. The results of the LDB revealed a significant increase in the amount of time spent in the light chamber and in exploratory parameters after the administration of a single dose of *C. aurantium* essential oil when compared to the control group. The anxiolytic-like effects of the acute treatments were not antagonized by flumazenil, a benzodiazepine antagonist, but these effects were antagonized by the

5-HT1A-specific antagonist WAY100635, suggesting that the anxiolytic-like activity observed in the LDB procedure after acute dosing was mediated by the serotonergic system (5-HT1A receptors). Interestingly, acute treatment with *C. aurantium* essential oil showed no activity in FST, which is sensitive to antidepressants and had no effect on the ability of the mice to remain on the rotating bar. In addition, acute treatment with *C. aurantium* essential oil did not change the levels of dopamine and serotonin or their metabolites 3,4-dihydroxyphenylacetic acid, homovanillic acid, and 5-hydroxyindoleacetic acid in the cortex, the striatum, the pons, or the hypothalamus (Costa et al., 2013). The major compound present in the phytocomplex was limonene, followed by β-myrcene. Both of these compounds are biologically active in the CNS, as mice treated with these compounds have shown decreases in spontaneous activity, rearing, and grooming in an open-field test, and the compounds increased barbiturate sleeping time (do Vale et al., 2002). However, in the study of Costa and colleagues, limonene did not modify the parameters evaluated in the LDB at a dose corresponding to the level present in the effective dose of the essential oil (Costa et al., 2013). On the other hand, these results corroborate previous reports in which limonene was not able to modify the parameters of anxiolytic-like activity evaluated in the elevated plus-maze procedure (do Vale et al., 2002). These findings strengthen the idea that in herbal preparations, the interactions between compounds often result in biological activity that is greater than the activity of isolated compounds (Galindo et al., 2010).

11.5 LAVENDER

Lavender belongs to the family Labiatae (Lamiacae) and has a variety of therapeutic and cosmetic uses. Traditionally, essential oils distilled from members of the genus *Lavandula* have been used for centuries, with the most commonly used species being *L. angustifolia*, *L. latifolia*, *L. stoechas*, and *L. × intermedia*. Lavender was used as a sedative, antidepressant, anticonvulsant, antispasmodic, analgesic, anti-inflammatory, and to treat cerebrovascular disease (Chu and Kemper, 2001; Cavanagh and Wilkinson, 2002; see Koulivand et al., 2013). Lavender is comprised of more than 100 constituents, among which the primary components are linalool (51%) and linalyl acetate (35%), α-pinene, limonene, 1,8-cineole, cis- and trans-ocimene, 3-octanone, camphor, caryophyllene, terpinen-4-olandlavendulyl acetate, cineole, and flavonoids (Cavanagh and Wilkinson, 2002), which are responsible for its pharmacological activity (Lis-Balchin and Hart, 1999). Although the mechanisms underlying the physiological effects of lavender oil remain unclear, research on the neurobiological consequences of lavender oil has largely focused on neurotransmitter systems in the CNS and associated behavioral alterations. For example, *L. angustifolia* inhalation has been used in folk medicine for the treatment of anxiety, and clinical and animal studies have corroborated its anxiolytic effect. Although its mechanism of action has not been determined, it was reported to be similar to that of benzodiazepines, which increase the inhibitory neurotransmitter GABA in the amygdala (Tisserand, 1988). Although lavender was less effective than benzodiazepines in a mouse anxiety model, it still had antianxiety effects in these animals (Shaw et al., 2011). The exposure to lavender odor may also have an anxiolytic profile in gerbils similar to that of the anxiolytic diazepam (Bradley et al., 2007). In this regard, *in vitro* studies suggested that lavender essential oil and some ingredients as α-pinene could potentiate the effect of GABA at GABAA receptors (Aoshima and Hamamoto, 1999), and their anxiolytic effect could be related to this GABAergic action (Tsang and Ho, 2010). Moreover, Huang et al. (2008) showed in a dual-radioligand binding and electrophysiological study that essential oil inhibited [35S] TBPS binding to the rat forebrain GABAA receptor channel, but had no effect on N-methyl-D-aspartate (NMDA), α-amino-3-hydroxy-5-methyl-4-isoxazolepropionic acid (AMPA), or nicotinic acetylcholine receptors. Electrophysiological analyses with rat cortical primary cultures also demonstrated that lavender oil reversibly inhibited GABA-induced currents in a concentration-dependent manner, whereas no inhibition of NMDA- or AMPA-induced currents was noted. Nevertheless, pretreatment with the GABAA receptor antagonist picrotoxin did not modify the behavioral effect of lavender essential oil in the marble-burying test or alter [(3)H]flunitrazepam binding to the benzodiazepine site on the GABAA receptor (Chioca et al., 2013b). However, Silexan, an essential oil produced from *L. angustifolia* flowers with proven clinical efficacy for the treatment of anxiety disorders (Kasper et al., 2010; Woelk and Schlafke, 2010; Kasper, 2013), showed significant and dose-dependent anxiolytic activity in several pharmacological models that was comparable to that of the standard anxiolytic agent lorazepam (Kumar, 2013). In addition, Silexan amplified pentobarbital-induced sleeping time, but in contrast to diazepam, it was found to be devoid of any significant effect on locomotor activity and muscle-grip performance. Recently, a number of studies using pharmacological and behavioral tools suggested an important role for the serotonergic system in the anxiolytic-like effect of lavender essential oil in mice (Chioca et al., 2013b; Takahashi et al., 2014). Neurochemical analysis of the serotonin (5-HT) turnover rate was performed, and essential oil extracted from *L. officinalis* significantly increased the striatal and hippocampal levels of 5-HT and decreased turnover rates in accordance with the anxiolytic behavioral changes (Takahashi et al., 2014). Linalool, one of the major components of lavender oil, has been the compound most linked to the anxiolytic effect of lavender (Umezu et al., 2006; Linck et al., 2010; Tsang and Ho, 2010; Takahashi et al., 2011; Woronuk et al., 2011). Moreover, some authors suggested that linalyl acetate works synergistically with linalool and that the presence of both is essential for the whole oil to work (Takahashi et al., 2011). Interestingly, although the olfactory system activation plays a pivotal role in the effects of essential oils on CNS, recent studies showed that anosmia does not impair the anxiolytic-like effect of lavender essential oil inhalation in mice (Chioca et al., 2013a; Takahashi et al., 2014). An anticonvulsant effect for hydroalcoholic extract of lavender was reported against chemoconvulsant-induced seizures in male mice. Particularly, lavender inhibited the onset, shortened the duration, and reduced the intensity of seizure attacks (Arzi et al., 2011). Anticonvulsant effects of lavender, together with diminution in spontaneous activity, when combined with other narcotics, have also been reported (Atanossova-Shopova and Roussinov, 1970; Lis-Balchin and Hart, 1999). Inhalation of lavender was also noted to inhibit convulsion induced by pentylenetetrazol, nicotine, or electroshock in mice (Yamada et al., 1994). Interestingly, linalool has been shown to inhibit the convulsion induced by pentylenetetrazol and transcorneal electroshock in different animal models (Elisabetsky et al.,

1999; de Sousa et al., 2010), an effect that may induce via a direct interaction with the glutamatergic NMDA subreceptor as well as GABAA receptors (Elisabetsky et al., 1995; Silva Brum et al., 2001). Beyond the anxiolytic and anticonvulsant effects, folk and traditional therapeutic use of the essential oil of *L. angustifolia* for relaxation, sedation, and pain dates back centuries. Lavender oil is thought to have a sedative effect in mice (Guillemain et al., 1989) and rats (Shaw et al., 2007). In contrast, lavender oil was shown to modulate motor movement and locomotion (Cline et al., 2008) and increase arousal levels (Duan et al., 2007). Furthermore, 2-week lavender oil exposure increased exploratory behavior in female gerbils (Bradley et al., 2007). Because the dopaminergic nervous system has been implicated in the regulation of motor behavior, Kim and colleagues (2009) examined the expression of dopamine receptors (DRs) in response to lavender oil exposure in the olfactory bulb and the striatum of mice. Lavender oil exposure upregulated DRD3 expression at the mRNA and protein levels in a dose-dependent manner in the olfactory bulb, suggesting that altered DRD3 homeostasis may contribute to lavender oil–induced behavioral changes. Furthermore, some studies have suggested that linalool enhances the release of dopamine from rat brain striatum slices (Okuyama et al., 2004) and alters plasma dopamine levels in ovariectomized female rats (Yamada et al., 2005). These observations suggest that lavender oil may exert its physiological effects, at least in part, by disturbing dopaminergic neurotransmission. Interestingly, evidence is accumulating that aromatherapy with lavender oil is efficacious at reducing behavioral and psychological symptoms of dementia (BPSD) (Moss et al., 2003; Lee, 2005; Lin et al., 2007; Jimbo et al., 2009; van der Ploeg et al., 2010); however, the mechanisms underlying these effects of the phytocomplex remain unclear. In this regard, in 2011, Kashani and colleagues reported that aqueous extract of *L. angustifolia* improves the spatial performance of a rat model of Alzheimer's disease. Moreover, Hritcu and colleagues (2012) reported that lavender essential oils from *L. angustifolia* Mill. and *L. hybrida* Rev. improve scopolamine-induced spatial memory impairment in rats and significantly reduce anxiety-like behavior, and inhibited depression in elevated plus-maze and forced swimming tests. In 2013 the same authors suggested the antioxidant and antiapoptotic activities of the lavender essential oils are the major mechanisms for their neuroprotective effects against scopolamine-induced oxidative stress in the rat brain (Hancianu et al., 2013). More recently, Videira and colleagues (2014) observed in a screening procedure for inhibitors of BACE-1 activity that the oil of *L. luisieri* was identified as the most potent among several essential oils. BACE-1 is an aspartic protease involved in the conversion of amyloid precursor protein (APP) to amyloid-β (Aβ) *in vivo*, one of the key steps in the development and progression of Alzheimer's disease.

11.6 LEMON

Lemon (*Citrus limon* L. Burms, Rutaceae) is grown in many parts of the world for juice production. *C. limon* has been shown in several studies to have various biological functions (anti-inflammatory, antiallergic, antiviral, antimutagenic, and anticarcinogenic) (see Campêlo et al., 2011). Furthermore, traditional uses in folk medicine suggest that *C. limon* may have an effect on the CNS. In this regard, its essential oil (lemon essential oil) was found to induce various behavioral responses in rodents. Particularly in rats, it has been reported that lemon odor reduced the immobility time and potentiated the imipramine-induced reduction of immobility time in the forced swim test (Komori et al., 1995). The authors have also reported that lemon odor decreased locomotor activity in the open-field task, suggesting its effects to be different from those of psychostimulants but similar to those of antidepressants. The anti-immobility effect may be mediated by facilitating central dopamine neurotransmission, although there may be the possible involvement of other neuronal systems (Komori et al., 1995).

In mice, it has been reported that lemon oil has antidepressant-like effects with the elevated plus-maze test, the forced swim test, and the open-field task via the suppression of dopamine (DA) activity related to enhanced serotonergic neurons (Rainville et al., 1997). Moreover, Komiya and colleagues (2006) examined the anti-stress action of the essential oil of lemon using the same behavioral models and found that the effect of lemon oil was significantly blocked by pretreatment with flumazenil, a benzodiazepine receptor antagonist, or apomorphine, a nonselective DA receptor agonist. In contrast, agonists or antagonists to the 5-HT receptor and the α-2 adrenergic receptor did not affect the antistress effect of lemon oil. Buspirone, (±)-2,5-dimethoxy-4-iodoamphetamine hydrochloride (DOI), and mianserine blocked the antidepressant-like effect of lemon oil in the forced swimming task, but WAY100635 did not, suggesting that the antidepressant-like effect of lemon oil is closely related to the 5-HTnergic pathway, especially via 5-HT1A receptor (Komiya et al., 2006). Moreover, the inhalation of lemon oil vapor for 90–180 min significantly increased the DA content in the hippocampus (Komiya et al., 2006). Furthermore, the contents of 3,4-dihydroxyphenylacetic acid (DOPAC) in the prefrontal cortex and hippocampus significantly increased following inhalation of lemon oil vapor, whereas the DA/DOPAC ratio was not particularly changed in the hippocampus, striatum, and prefrontal cortex. The inhalation of lemon oil vapor also resulted in a significant increase of 5-HT in the prefrontal cortex, and 5-HIAA contents were more apparently affected by treatment with lemon oil vapor in all three brain regions. Moreover, 5-HIAA/5-HT ratios in the hippocampus and striatum were also enhanced by lemon oil inhalation. Then lemon oil possibly reduced distress by modulating GABAergic, serotonergic, and dopaminergic systems in the brain. This effect might be caused by a suppression of DA activity via enhanced 5-HTnergic neurons under the lemon oil inhalation condition (Komiya et al., 2006). Recently, Yun and colleagues (2014) reported that limonene administration significantly inhibited 5-HT-induced head twitch response in mice and decreased hyperlocomotion induced by methamphetamine injection in rats. In addition, limonene reversed the increase in dopamine levels in the nucleus accumbens of rats given methamphetamine, suggesting that limonene may inhibit stimulant-induced behavioral changes via regulating dopamine levels and 5-HT receptor function (Yun 2014). Interestingly, Fukumoto and colleagues (2006) used brain tissue slices to investigate the effect of compounds in lemon essential oil on monoamine release. They investigated R-limonene, γ-terpinene, and citral, major components of lemon essential oil; S-limonene, an isomer of R-limonene; and metabolites of these compounds. The results obtained suggest that the metabolites of these monoterpene compounds contained in essential oils have a stronger effect on monoamine release from brain tissue than the monoterpene compounds themselves (Fukumoto et al., 2006). Lopes Campêlo and colleagues (2011) instead examined the sedative, anxiolytic, and anti-depressant effects of essential oil of leaves from *C. limon*. The effects of essential oil were evaluated by open-field, elevated plus-maze, rotarod, pentobarbital-induced sleeping time, and forced swimming tests in mice. In the open-field test, after oral administration, it significantly decreased the number of crossings, grooming, and rearing. In the elevated plus-maze test, the phytocomplex increased the time of permanence and the number of entrances in the open arms. On the contrary, the time of permanence and the number of entrances in the closed arms were decreased. In the rotarod test, *C. limon* essential oil did not alter motor coordination and thus was devoid of effects, as related to controls. In the pentobarbital-induced sleeping time test, it significantly increased the animals' sleeping time duration, and in the forced swimming test, the phytocomplex induced a decrease in the immobility time, similarly to that of imipramine (Lopes Campêlo et al., 2011). However, the antidepressant effects of *C. limon* essential oil were not altered by the previous administration of paroxetine. In addition, its effects in the forced swimming test were totally blocked by reserpine pretreatment. Altogether, the results evidenced sedative and anxiolytic effects of *C. limon* essential oil that might involve an action on benzodiazepine-type receptors, and also an antidepressant effect where noradrenergic and serotoninergic mechanisms will probably play a role (Lopes Campêlo et al., 2011). The microdialysis technique was used to study the ability of essential oil from *C. limon* to modulate hippocampal acetylcholine (ACh) release in male and female rats (Ceccarelli et al., 2002). Animals were allowed to inhale this odor while experiencing a persistent nociceptive input (formalin, 5%) or under control conditions (sham injection). In males, exposure to the essential oil did not change the time course and magnitude of the ACh increase induced by pain. Conversely, in females, the pain-induced increase of ACh was delayed and increased by exposure to lemon essential oil (Ceccarelli et al., 2002). Subsequently, the same researchers reported in formalin-treated animals that lemon essential oil decreased licking of the injected paw in both sexes, whereas flinching and flexing were decreased in males and increased in females in the interphase of the formalin test (Aloisi et al., 2002). Interestingly, essential oil increased the c-Fos expression in the arcuate nucleus of the hypothalamus, whereas essential oil and formalin increased c-Fos in the paraventricular nucleus of the hypothalamus and in the dentate gyrus of the hippocampus (Aloisi et al., 2002). In the paraventricular nucleus of the thalamus, formalin induced higher c-Fos than the control in both sexes; when formalin treatment was carried out in the presence of essential oil, c-Fos further increased in males, but remained at control levels in females (Aloisi et al., 2002). These results clearly indicate the ability of lemon essential oil to modulate the behavioral and neuronal responses related to nociception and pain. Furthermore, Ceccarelli and colleagues (2004) investigated in male and female rats behavioral, hormonal, and neuronal responses to prolonged exposure to lemon essential oil. Animals were exposed to the lemon essence for 2 weeks while in their cage. Anxiety was then determined with the elevated plus-maze apparatus, while nociception was evaluated with a phasic thermal pain stimulus (plantar test) and with a chemical pain stimulus (formalin test). In both sexes, prolonged exposure to essential oil decreased the time spent in the open arms of the plus-maze apparatus. Essential oil–exposed males and females showed higher thermal nociceptive thresholds than controls when tested with the plantar test apparatus, whereas exposure induced female-specific decreases in formalin-induced pain behaviors during the formalin test (Ceccarelli et al., 2002). Interestingly, β-endorphin concentrations in the hypothalamus and periaqueductal gray matter were affected by lemon oil. Corticosterone was lower in essential oil–exposed animals of both sexes than in their controls. These results suggest that long-term exposure to lemon essential oil can induce significant, at times sex-specific, changes in neuronal circuits involved in anxiety and pain (Ceccarelli et al., 2004).

11.7   LEMONGRASS

Cymbopogon citratus (DC) Stapf (Poaceae), commonly known as lemongrass, is a popular medicinal plant used for treating different diseases in tropical countries (see Shah et al., 2011) and widely used in traditional medicine as an infusion or decoction for treating nervous disturbances (Carlini et al., 1986). The compounds identified in essential oil of *C. citratus* are mainly terpenes, alcohols, ketones, aldehyde, and esters, but the plant also contains reported phytoconstituents such as flavonoids and phenolic compounds (see Shah et al., 2011). In Mexico, lemongrass is used as a sedative (Tortoriello and Romero, 1992), and in Brazil, an infusion or the cold juice of the leaves has been employed as a sedative and analgesic (Hiruma-Lima et al., 2002). Recently, the anxiolytic-like activity of the essential oil of *C. citratus* was investigated in a light–dark box (LDB) and marble-burying test (MBT), and the antidepressant activity was investigated in a forced swimming test (FST) in mice (Costa et al., 2011). Flumazenil, a competitive antagonist of benzodiazepine binding, and the selective 5-HT1A receptor antagonist WAY100635 was used in experimental procedures to determine the action mechanism of essential oil. Particularly, Costa and colleagues reported anxiolytic-like activity of the essential oil in LDB, and that flumazenil, but not WAY100635, was able to reverse the effect of the phytocomplex in the LDB, indicating that its activity occurs via the GABAA receptor–benzodiazepine complex. Only at higher doses did the essential oil potentiate diethyl ether–induced sleeping time in mice. In the FST and MBT, lemongrass showed no effect. Moreover, the increase in time spent in the light chamber, demonstrated by concomitant treatment with ineffective doses of diazepam (DZP) and the essential oil, revealed a synergistic effect of the two compounds. The lack of activity after long-term treatment in the LDB test might be related to tolerance induction, even in the DZP-treated group. Furthermore, there were no significant differences between groups after either acute or repeated treatments with the essential oil in the rotarod test. In addition, neurochemical evaluation showed no amendments in neurotransmitter levels in the cortex, striatum, pons, and hypothalamus (Costa et al., 2011). Tea obtained from leaves of *C. citratus* is also used for its anxiolytic, hypnotic, and anticonvulsant properties in Brazilian folk medicine (see Blanco et al., 2007). Essential oil was evaluated in mice for sedative or hypnotic activity through pentobarbital sleeping time, anxiolytic activity by elevated plus-maze and light–dark box procedures, and anticonvulsant activity through seizures induced by pentylenetetrazole and maximal electroshock

(Blanco et al., 2007). Lemongrass was effective in increasing the sleeping time, the percentage of entries and time spent in the open arms of the elevated plus maze, and the time spent in the light compartment of the light–dark box. In addition, it delayed clonic seizures induced by pentylenetetrazole and blocked tonic extensions induced by maximal electroshock, indicating the elevation of the seizure threshold or blockage of seizures spread. These effects were observed in the absence of motor impairment evaluated on the rotarod and open-field test (Blanco et al., 2007). Recently, Silva and colleagues (2010) studied the effects of *C. citratus* essential oil on three experimental models of convulsions (pentylenetetrazol, pilocarpine, and strychnine) and on the barbiturate-induced sleeping time on mice. The results showed that lemongrass was more active on the pentylenetetrazol-induced convulsion model and was even more efficient in increasing latency to the first convulsion and latency to death (Silva et al., 2010). Both parameters were potentiated in the presence of a lower dose of diazepam when associated to a lower dose of essential oil. Besides, its anticonvulsant effect was blocked by flumazenil. This effect was somewhat lower on the pilocarpine-induced convulsion, and better effects were seen only with higher doses (Silva et al., 2010). A similar result was observed on the strychnine-induced convulsion model. Lemongrass also potentiated the barbiturate-induced sleeping time, suggesting that the mechanism of action of the anticonvulsant effect of *C. citratus* essential oil is, at least in part, dependent on the GABAergic neurotransmission (Silva et al., 2010).

11.8 *MELISSA*

Melissa officinalis (lemon balm) is a medicinal plant from the Lamiaceae family used traditionally in the treatment of cognitive disorders, anxiety, stress, and sleep disturbance (see Dobetsberger and Buchbauer, 2011). Based on its traditional medicinal use in the treatment of cognitive dysfunction, several studies assessed *M. officinalis* neuroprotective properties. Particularly, it has cholinomimetic and potent antioxidant activity. Total extract of *M. officinalis* and different fractions of it have anticholinesterase activity (Dastmalchi et al., 2009; Sepand et al., 2013), and most of the fractions showed inhibitory activity and were more potent than the extract. The contents of the most potent fraction were identified as cis- and trans-rosmarinic acid isomers and a rosmarinic acid derivative (Dastmalchi et al., 2009). In addition, *M. officinalis* extract shows a potent antioxidant activity, and plant extracts could protect cells against oxidative damage induced by different pro-oxidant agents, which eventually leads to lipid peroxidation by different processes (Pereira et al., 2009). Although the mechanism and constituents involved in neuroprotective properties of *Melissa* are not well known, it is claimed that the main effective components of this plant are polyphenols and terpenoid compounds. The polyphenols that were found in *M. officinalis* extract are caffeic acid derivatives, and among them, rosmarinic acid is the major polyphenol component (see Sepand et al., 2013). Interestingly, rosmarinic acid has high anticholinesterase activity and free radical scavenging activity (Petersen and Simmonds, 2003; Alkam et al., 2007). In addition, it is reported that the *Melissa* extract contains compounds with acetylcholine receptor affinities, and that the affinity for the nicotinic receptor is more than that for the muscarinic receptor (Wake et al., 2000). Interestingly, several studies indicated that the nicotinic receptor stimulation can protect neurons against Aβ-induced toxicity (Kihara et al., 1997; Liu and Zhao, 2004). According to these studies, it can be suggested that the protective effect of *M. officinalis* and acidic fraction against β-amyloid-induced toxicity may be exerted through the nicotinic receptors (Sepand et al., 2013). However, the nature of compounds in *Melissa* extract that have nicotinic receptor affinity was unknown. The extract of *M. officinalis* significantly reduced anxiety-like reactivity in the elevated plus maze dose dependently, but no significant effect was observed in the open-field task (Ibarra et al., 2010). Parallel experiments in independent groups of mice showed that the dose at which it exerted anxiolytic-like effects in the elevated plus maze did not alter exploratory or circadian activities. Concerning the anxiolytic properties of *M. officinalis*, it has been reported that the aqueous or methanol extracts of the phytocomplex exhibited a potent inhibition of GABA transaminase (GABA-T) activity and increased GABA levels in the brain (Awad et al., 2007, 2009). A dual-radioligand binding and electrophysiological study, focusing on a range of ligand-gated ion channels, was performed with a chemically validated essential oil derived from *M. officinalis* that has shown clinical benefit in treating agitation. In addition, the phytocomplex inhibited binding of [35S]tertiary-butylbicyclophosphorothionate ([35S] TBPS) to the rat forebrain GABAA receptor channel, but had no effect on NMDA, AMPA, or nicotinic acetylcholine receptors. Electrophysiological analyses with primary cultures of rat cortical neurons also demonstrated that *M. officinalis* essential oil reversibly inhibited GABA-induced currents in a concentration-dependent manner, whereas no inhibition of NMDA- or AMPA-induced currents was noted (Abuhamdah et al., 2008).

11.9   ROSEMARY

Rosemary (*Rosmarinus officinalis* Linn) is a common household plant grown in many parts of the world. Rosemary leaves are used for food flavoring and have been used in folk medicine in curing or managing several disorders (see al-Sereiti et al., 1999), such as inflammatory diseases, physical and mental fatigue, and treatment of nervous agitation and depression, among other applications (Balmé, 1978; Duke, 2000; Heinrich et al., 2006). The chemical constituents include bitter principle, resin, tannic acid, volatile oils, and flavonoids. The main constituents of essential oil are camphor, 1,8-cineole, α-pinene, borneol, camphene, β-pinene, β-phellandrene, myrcene, and bornyl acetate (Begum et al., 2013; Lakusić et al., 2013). Machado and colleagues (2009) demonstrated that the extract of *R. officinalis* produces an antidepressant-like effect in the mouse tail suspension test and in the forced swimming test. It is noteworthy that the effect produced by the extract of this plant was comparable to the one produced by the classical antidepressant fluoxetine (Machado et al., 2009). In this study, the antidepressant-like effect of the extract of rosemary was completely prevented by pretreatment of mice with the neuronal serotonin store depletor, PCPA, as well as the 5-HT1A and 5-HT2A receptor antagonists, NAN-190 and ketanserin, respectively. In addition, the pretreatment of mice with 5-HT3 receptor agonist mCPBG was able to reverse the antidepressant-like effect of the extract, whereas the 5-HT3 receptor antagonist, MDL72222, administered in combination with the extract, produced a synergistic antidepressant-like effect (Machado et al., 2009). These results provide evidence that the antidepressant-like effect of the extract of *R. officinalis* is dependent on an interaction with the serotonergic system. Moreover, the pretreatment of mice with prazosin (an α1-adrenoceptor antagonist) was able to reverse the antidepressant-like effect of the extract of *R. officinalis*, whereas yohimbine (an α2-adrenoceptor antagonist) was ineffective in reversing the immobility period in mice (Machado et al., 2009). In addition, the selective dopamine D1 receptor antagonist, SCH23390, and the dopamine D2 receptor antagonist, sulpiride, were able to reverse the antidepressant-like effect of the extract of rosemary. Altogether, the results obtained by Machado and colleagues (2009) indicate that the antidepressant-like effect of the extract of *R. officinalis* was mediated by an interaction with the monoaminergic system. Subsequently, the same authors investigated the antidepressant-like effect of ursolic acid isolated from this plant and demonstrated that this ingredient was effective in producing an antidepressant-like effect in the tail suspension test and in the forced swimming test. Moreover, a clear involvement of the dopaminergic system in the antidepressant-like effect of ursolic acid was indicated by the reversal of its effect by the pretreatment of mice with dopamine D1 and D2 receptor antagonists and also by the synergistic antidepressant-like effect afforded by the dopamine D1 and D2 receptor agonists, as well as the antidepressant bupropion (Machado et al., 2012). More recently, Machado and colleagues (2013) also showed that carnosol and betulinic acid were able to cause a similar effect, suggesting that they could, at least in part, be responsible for the antidepressant activity of this plant. Recently, Sasaki and colleagues (2013) reported that *R. officinalis* polyphenols produce an antidepressant-like effect through monoaminergic and cholinergic function modulation. Particularly, to evaluate the antidepressant effect of rosemary, these authors used mice and PC12 cells as an *in vitro* neuronal model. Proteomics analysis of PC12 cells treated with *R. officinalis* polyphenols luteolin, carnosic acid, and rosmarinic acid revealed a significant upregulation of tyrosine hydroxylase (TH) and pyruvate carboxylase (PC), two major genes involved in dopaminergic, serotonergic, and GABAergic pathway regulations. These results were concordant with decreasing immobility time in the tail suspension test and regulation of several neurotransmitters (dopamine, norepinephrine, serotonin, and acetylcholine) and gene expression in mice brain, like TH, PC, and MAPK phosphatase (MKP-1) (Sasaki et al., 2013). Previously, the same group of researchers reported that *R. officinalis*, carnosic acid, and rosmarinic acid exhibited neurotrophic effects in PC12 cells through cell differentiation induction and cholinergic activity enhancement (El Omri et al., 2010). Interestingly, caffeic acid, a constituent of *R. officinalis*, produced antidepressive- and anxiolytic-like effects in two different types of stress models through indirect modulation of the α 1A-adrenoceptor system in mice (Takeda et al., 2003). Extensive research suggests that a number of plants possess cognition-enhancing properties, and rosemary is a promising candidate (Kennedy and Scholey, 2006), as suggested by clinical studies (Moss et al., 2003; Pengelly et al., 2012). In this regard, recently, Ozarowski and colleagues (2013) reported that *R. officinalis* leaf extract improves memory impairment and affects acetylcholinesterase (AChE) and butyrylcholinesterase (BuChE) activities in rat brain. Particularly, it improved long-term memory in scopolamine-induced rats, inhibiting the AChE activity and showing a stimulatory effect on BuChE in both parts of the rat brain. Moreover, rosemary extract produced a lower mRNA BuChE expression in the cortex and simultaneously an increase in the hippocampus (Ozarowski et al., 2013). Orhan and colleagues (2008) also reported that extracts of rosemary displayed significant inhibitory effects on both AChE and BuChE enzymes. The authors went on to identify that the major active component of the essential oil was 1,8-cineole, a terpene previously identified as possessing anti-AChE activity (Perry et al., 2000, 2003; Savelev et al., 2003). Interestingly, previously, Kovar and colleagues (1987) reported that both the inhalation and oral administration of rosemary oil stimulated locomotor activity in mice, and that this was related to serum 1,8-cineole concentration. Interestingly, recently, in human studies, Moss and Oliver (2012) observed that plasma 1,8-cineole correlated with cognitive performance following exposure to rosemary essential oil aroma. In addition, administration of rosmarinic acid on an elevated plus-maze task increased the number of entries in the open arms, suggesting an anxiolytic-like activity when used in lower doses, without affecting the short-term memory and long-term memory retention on inhibitory avoidance tasks (Pereira et al., 2005). Interestingly, Meng and colleagues (2013) reported that carnosic acid, a phenolic diterpene compound found in the labiate herbs rosemary and sage, suppresses $A\beta$(1-40) and (1-42) production by activating α-secretase in cultured SH-SY5Y human neuroblastoma cells. Moreover, Yoshida and colleagues (2014) showed that carnosic acid reduces the production of $A\beta$ peptides (1-40, 1-42, and 1-43) in U373MG human astrocytoma cells at least partially, by activating tumor necrosis factor-α-converting enzyme (TACE).

11.10 SAGE

Salvia is an important genus consisting of about 900 species in the family Lamiaceae. Some species of *Salvia* have been cultivated worldwide for use in folk medicine and for culinary purposes (Imanshahidi and Hosseinzadeh, 2006). *Salvia sclarea* L. (clary sage), occurring in the Mediterranean basin (Dweck, 2000), is one of the most important aromatic plants cultivated worldwide as a source of essential oils. The essential oils or extracts of the aerial part of the *S. sclarea* plant have a broad spectrum of effects: analgesic, anti-inflammatory (Moretti et al., 1997), antioxidant, antifungal (Pitarokili et al., 2002), and antibacterial (Peana et al., 1999; Gülçin, 2004). The main components of clary sage essential oil are sclareol, α-terpineol, geraniol, linalyl acetate, linalool, caryophyllene, neryl acetate, and germacrene-d. Clary oil was found to alleviate stress and have antidepressive effects in a mouse model, effects manifested by activation of paths with dopamine characteristics (Seol et al., 2010). Particularly, the antidepressant effect was assessed using a forced swim test in rats by pretreatment with agonists or antagonists to serotonin, dopamine, adrenaline, and GABA receptors. Rats were treated with essential oils by intraperitoneal injection or inhalation. The antistressor effect of clary oil was significantly blocked by pretreatment with buspirone (a 5-HT1A agonist), SCH-23390 (a D1 receptor antagonist), and haloperidol (a D2, D3, and D4 receptor antagonist), suggesting that the antidepressant-like effect of clary oil is closely associated with modulation of the DAergic pathway. Herrera-Ruiz and colleagues (2006) evaluated in mice the antidepressant- and anxiolytic-like effects of hydroalcoholic extract of *Salvia elegans*. The extract, administered orally, was able to increase the percentage of time spent and the percentage of arm entries in the open arms of the elevated plus-maze, as well as to increase the time spent by mice in the illuminated side of the light–dark test, and to decrease the immobility time of mice subjected to the forced swimming test. The same extract was not able to modify the spontaneous locomotor activity measured in the open-field test (Herrera-Ruiz et al., 2006). Ethanolic extracts from dried leaves of *Salvia officinalis* showed inhibition of [35S] TBPS binding to rat brain membranes *in vitro* (Rutherford et al., 1992). This ligand is considered to bind to the chloride channel of the GABA–benzodiazepine receptor complex in brain tissue. Substances having inhibitory activity were purified and their chemical structure identified as the diterpenes carnosic acid and carnosol. The two compounds did not affect binding of the ligands [3H]muscimol and [3H] diazepam to the GABA–benzodiazepine complex *in vitro*. Saturation experiments of [35S]TBPS binding indicated that carnosic acid decreased the binding affinity (Rutherford et al., 1992). Interestingly, some constituents of *S. officinalis* evidenced *in vitro* affinity to human brain benzodiazepine receptor (Kavvadias et al., 2003). Particularly, the flavones apigenin, hispidulin, and cirsimaritin and the diterpenes 7-methoxyrosmanol and galdosol competitively inhibited 3H-flumazenil binding to the benzodiazepine receptor. In addition, miltirone, a tanshinone isolated from the root of *Salvia miltiorrhiza*, has been characterized as a low-affinity ligand for central benzodiazepine receptors (Lee et al., 1991). The ability of *Salvia* spp. to interfere with neurotransmission is highlighted by a neurochemical study of Cheng and colleagues (1999) in a model of ischemia/reperfusion in the gerbil. The result obtained by microdialysis experiments showed that the extract of *S. miltiorrhiza* reduced the extracellular levels of dopamine, norepinephrine, and serotonin in the striatum of the gerbil probably by attenuating the dysfunctions of monoamine neurotransmitters that occurred during ischemia (Cheng et al., 1999). Members of the sage family, such as *S. officinalis* and *S. lavandulaefolia*, have a long history of use as memory-enhancing agents coupled with cholinergic properties. In this regard, extracts of *Salvia* spp. and individual monoterpenoid constituents have been shown to inhibit the enzyme acetylcholinesterase *in vitro* (Perry et al., 2000, 2001; Ferreira et al., 2006) and *in vivo* (Perry et al., 2002). Particularly *in vitro*, the essential oil, α-pinene, 1,8-cineole, and camphor were found to be uncompetitive reversible inhibitors (Perry et al., 2000), whereas *in vivo* activity has been confirmed with the observation that a 5-day oral administration to rats of *Salvia lavandulaefolia* essential oil led to dose-dependent decreases in AChE activity in the striatum and also in the hippocampus (Perry et al., 2002). This activity may potentially be relevant to the amelioration of the cognitive deficits associated with Alzheimer's disease (Akhondzadeh et al., 2003; Tildesley et al., 2003, 2005; Scholey et al., 2008; Moss et al., 2010; da Rocha et al., 2011; Kennedy et al., 2011; Perry and Howes, 2011). Interestingly, Wong and colleagues (2010) reported that cryptotanshinone, an acetylcholinesterase inhibitor from *S. miltiorrhiza*, improved learning in rats with scopolamine-induced cognitive impairment in the Morris water maze task. Moreover, extracts of *S. elegans* displayed displacement at muscarinic acetylcholine receptors (Wake et al., 2000).

11.11 *SPIRANTHERA ODORATISSIMA*

Spiranthera odoratissima A. St. Hillaire (Rutaceae) is a shrub that is found in Brazil, especially in the central region, and popularly known as manacá. In folk medicine, it is used to treat renal and hepatic diseases, stomachache, headaches, and rheumatism (see Nascimento et al., 2012). The aqueous fraction from the ethanolic extract of manacá leaves showed analgesic and anti-inflammatory activities in the acetic acid–induced writhing, croton oil–induced ear edema, and carrageenan-induced peritonitis models (Matos et al., 2003). The antinociceptive and anti-inflammatory activities of *S. odoratissima* were assessed more recently using a formalin test in carrageenan-induced paw edema (Nascimento et al., 2012). In this study, manacá reduced the licking time only in the later phase of the formalin test and showed anti-inflammatory activity by reducing the paw edema, migration cell, myeloperoxidase activity, capillary permeability, and TNF-α levels. Similar results were obtained with the ethanolic extract of manacá roots, which are also characterized by the CNS depressant activity (Matos et al., 2004). The evaluation of the effects of the hexane fraction from the ethanolic extract of *S. odoratissima* leaves on the murine CNS indicates that this fraction has active substances that increase the sleep time in a pentobarbital-induced sleep test (Matos et al., 2004, 2006). Recently, Galdino and colleagues (2012) evaluated the neuropharmacological activity of the essential oil obtained from *S. odoratissima* leaves and its major component, β-caryophyllene, on the murine CNS with special attention to possible anxiolytic-like effects and the underlying mechanisms involved. Upon subcutaneous and intraperitoneal administration of essential oil, decreases in spontaneous ambulations and environmental alienations were observed; at higher doses, palpebral ptosis and analgesia were also observed. These effects on general behavioral tests are suggestive of central depressant drugs (Galdino et al., 2012). The results obtained in the rotarod test showed that *S. odoratissima*, unlike diazepam, had no significant effect on motor coordination, and the results obtained in the open-field task support this lack of alteration in motor coordination. Interestingly, essential oil treatment increased the preference for the central area, enhancing the crossing number and the time spent in the central area of the apparatus. An increase in these parameters could be indicative of anxiolytic-like effects (Prut and Belzung, 2003). In addition, in the study of Galdino and colleagues, *S. odoratissima* essential oil increased the entries into and time spent in the open arms of the elevated plus maze without altering the number of entries into closed arms, and also increased the number of head dips without altering the number of squares crossed in the hole-board test, indicating an anxiolytic-like effect without motor impairment. Moreover, the results obtained in the light–dark box test corroborate the anxiolytic-like effect shown in the hole-board and elevated plus-maze tests. These effects of the phytocomplex were not significantly altered by flumazenil treatment, indicating that essential oil's anxiolytic-like effects do not involve the benzodiazepine site of the GABAA receptor. However, the effects were significantly decreased when mice were pretreated with NAN-190, a 5-HT1A receptor antagonist. Meanwhile, the anxiolytic-like effect of β-caryophyllene was not significantly altered by either flumazenil or NAN-190 pretreatment, suggesting that non-GABAA–benzodiazepine, non-5-HT1A receptors are involved. Interestingly, Gertsch and colleagues (2008) demonstrated that β-caryophyllene binds selectively to cannabinoid receptor 2, acting as a full agonist. In addition, recent results from mice with genetically modified CB2 suggest that CB2 signaling is involved in the regulation of emotional behaviors, including anxiety (Marco et al., 2011); thus, the cannabinoid system may be involved in the anxiolytic-like effects of β-caryophyllene. More recently, Klauke and colleagues (2014) demonstrated that β-caryophyllene also exerts analgesic effects in mouse models of inflammatory and neuropathic pain in a CB2 receptor–dependent manner. The possibility of using the essential oil of *S. odoratissima* that acts on two systems (serotonergic and cannabinoid) may widen the spectrum of cellular targets, thus resulting in a more favorable clinical effect (Galdino et al., 2012).

11.12 THYME

Thyme (*Thymus vulgaris* L., Lamiaceae) is an aromatic and medicinal plant native to the western Mediterranean region of Europe that has been used in folk medicine, phytopharmaceutical preparations, food preservatives, and as an aromatic ingredient (see Fachini-Queiroz et al., 2012). *Thymus vulgaris* essential oil is a mixture of monoterpenes, and major bioactive compounds of the extract are thymol and its phenol isomer carvacrol (Hudaib et al., 2002; Amiri, 2012). Thymol exhibits multiple biological activities, and it is known for its antimicrobial and antioxidant properties (see García et al., 2006). Its main therapeutic application is still in dental preparations to kill odor-producing bacteria; furthermore, some previous studies suggested that thymol may have an effect on the CNS (Credner, 1960; Ashford et al., 1963). Interestingly, more recently, thymol was shown to have a direct agonist effect on heterologously expressed human GABAA receptors resembling that of the anaesthetic propofol (Mohammadi et al., 2001). In this regard, Priestley and colleagues (2003) reported that thymol potentiates the actions of GABA at three recombinant human GABAA receptors of different subunit compositions, and also at a recombinant insect ionotropic GABA receptor. Modulation of the human α1β3γ2s, α6β3γ2s, and α1β1γ2s GABAA receptors and *Drosophila melanogaster* RDL$_{ac}$ homomers was dose dependent over a similar concentration range, suggesting a non-subunit-selective action, although it appears that thymol is less potent on mammalian GABAA receptors than on the insect model ionotropic GABA receptor (Priestley et al., 2003). At all subunit combinations, potentiation was observed at concentrations where thymol elicited either zero or minimal agonist activity, indicating that the enhanced response to GABA is likely to be the result of a positive allosteric action of thymol. Subsequently, Sánchez and colleagues (2004) reported enhanced GABAA receptor–operated chloride channel activity and increased binding affinity of [(3)H]flunitrazepam in the presence of thymol. Moreover, García and colleagues (2006) reported that thymol enhanced GABA-induced chloride influx at concentrations lower than those exhibiting direct activity in the absence of GABA. This direct effect was inhibited by competitive and noncompetitive GABAA receptor antagonists. Thymol also increased [(3)H]flunitrazepam binding and showed a tendency to increase [(3)H] muscimol binding (García et al., 2006). Altogether, these results confirm that thymol is a positive allosteric modulator of the GABAA. The effect of thymol, as positive control, on [(35)S] TBPS binding at the GABAA receptor in primary cultures of cortical neurons corroborates the previous data (García et al., 2008). Huang and colleagues (2005) also investigated the effects of thymol on ion currents in pituitary GH(3) cells showing a stimulatory action of terpene on Ca(2+)-activated K(+) currents. Carvacrol, the major natural constituent in the essential oil fraction of aromatic plants belonging to the family Lamiaceae, such as thyme and oregano, possesses antimicrobial, antifungal, and antioxidant activities (Alma et al., 2003; Horosová et al., 2006; Bozin et al., 2007), as well as antimutagenic and anticarcinogenic effects (Arcila-Lozano et al., 2004). A recent study showed that this phytochemical protects liver against ischemia/reperfusion (I/R) injury in rats (Canbek et al., 2008). Due to its lipophilicity and capacity to readily cross membranes, such as the blood–brain barrier (Savelev et al., 2004), this volatile molecule can accumulate in the brain, interacting with different receptor sites in CNS, showing centrally active properties (Hotta et al., 2010; Trabace et al., 2011). Recent findings showed that carvacrol inhibits the transient receptor potential (TRP) cation channel, subfamily M, member 7 (TRPM7) of the TRP family expressed in both HEK cells and CA3–CA1 hippocampal primary cultured cells (Parnas et al., 2009). Interestingly, it was demonstrated that TRPM7 is an essential mediator of anoxic neuronal death (Parnas et al., 2009). Therefore, inhibition of TRPM7 is expected to reduce cell death following ischemia and brain damage. It has been recently shown that carvacrol may play a role to protect against cerebral I/R injury (Yu et al., 2012). Lamiaceae species are a rich source of various natural AChE inhibitors and antioxidants that could be useful in the prevention and treatment of Alzheimer's and other related diseases (Vladimir-Knežević et al., 2014). In this regard, Jukic and colleagues (2007) examined *in vitro* the inhibitory activity exerted by the main constituents of essential oil obtained from *T. vulgaris* L. on AChE and found that carvacrol exerts a strong AChE inhibitory effect 10 times stronger than that exerted by its isomer thymol, although thymol and carvacrol have very similar structures. However, in a recent study by Kaufmann and colleagues (2011), a monoterpene myrtenal showed the highest efficacy as an inhibitor of AChE. Interestingly, Azizi and colleagues (2012), in two rat models of dementia (by administration of Aβ(25-35) or scopolamine), reported that thymol and carvacrol relieve cognitive impairments caused by increased Aβ levels or cholinergic hypofunction, suggesting that anticholinesterase, antioxidant, and anti-inflammatory activities may be the mechanisms contributing toward their beneficial effects in these models. In addition, recent experimental data indicated that carvacrol induces anxiolytic-like effects and antidepressant-like properties in tasks for anxiety and depression behavior in mice (Melo et al., 2010, 2011). It is likely that the bioactivity of this specific compound, having the ability to modulate mood and cognitive processes, involves several neurotransmitter systems in the brain. In this regard, recently, Zotti and colleagues (2013) investigated the possible alterations induced by low chronic and high acute doses of carvacrol on monoaminergic transmission in the prefrontal cortex (PFC) and hippocampus (HIPP) of male Wistar rats. The results from this study provided evidence for a modulatory activity of carvacrol on dopaminergic and serotonergic transmissions. Particularly, results indicated that rats treated with carvacrol displayed impaired serotonergic transmission in both brain areas considered in the study. Moreover, carvacrol significantly reduced dopamine levels in HIPP, while increased levels of dopamine were observed in PFC (Zotti et al., 2013).

REFERENCES

Abuhamdah, S., Huang, L., Elliott, M.S. et al. 2008. Pharmacological profile of an essential oil derived from *Melissa officinalis* with anti-agitation properties: Focus on ligand-gated channels. *J Pharm Pharmacol*, 60(3): 377–84.

Akhondzadeh, S., Noroozian, M., Mohammadi, M., Ohadinia, S., Jamshidi, A.H., and Khani, M. 2003. *Salvia officinalis* extract in the treatment of patients with mild to moderate Alzheimer's disease: A double blind, randomized and placebo-controlled trial. *J Clin Pharm Ther*, 28(1): 53–59.

Alkam, T., Nitta, A., Mizoguchi, H., Itoh, A., and Nabeshima, T. 2007. A natural scavenger of peroxynitrites, rosmarinic acid, protects against impairment of memory induced by Abeta (25-35). *Behav Brain Res*, 180: 139–45.

Alma, M.H., Mavi, A., Yildirim, A., Digrak, M., and Hirata, T. 2003. Screening chemical composition and *in vitro* antioxidant and antimicrobial activities of the essential oils from *Origanum syriacum* L. growing in Turkey. *Biol Pharm Bull*, 26(12): 1725–29.

Aloisi, A.M., Ceccarelli, I., Masi, F., and Scaramuzzino, A. 2002. Effects of the essential oil from citrus lemon in male and female rats exposed to a persistent painful stimulation. *Behav Brain Res*, 36: 127–35.

al-Sereiti, M.R., Abu-Amer, K.M., and Sen, P. 1999. Pharmacology of rosemary (*Rosmarinus officinalis* Linn.) and its therapeutic potentials. *Indian J Exp Biol*, 37(2): 124–30.

Amantea, D., Fratto, V., Maida, S. et al. 2009. Prevention of glutamate accumulation and upregulation of phospho-Akt may account for neuroprotection afforded by bergamot essential oil against brain injury induced by focal cerebral ischemia in rat. *Int Rev Neurobiol*, 85: 389–405.

Amiri, H. 2012. Essential oils composition and antioxidant properties of three thymus species. *Evid Based Complement Alternat Med*, 2012: 728065.

Aoshima, H., and Hamamoto, K. 1999. Potentiation of GABAA receptors expressed in *Xenopus* oocytes by perfume and phytoncid. *Biosci Biotechnol Biochem*, 63: 743–48.

Arcila-Lozano, C.C., Loarca-Piña, G., Lecona-Uribe, S., González de Mejía, E. 2004. Oregano: Properties, composition and biological activity. *Arch Latinoam Nutr*, 54(1): 100–11.

Arzi, A., Ahamehe, M., and Sarahroodi, S. 2011. Effect of hydroalcoholic extract of *Lavandula officinalis* on nicotine-induced convulsion in mice. *Pakistan J Biol Sci*, 14(11): 634–40.

Ashford, A., Sharpe, C.J., and Stephens, F.F. 1963. Thymol basic ethers and related compounds: Central nervous system depressant action. *Nature*, 197: 969–71.

Atanossova-Shopova, S., and Roussinov, K.S. 1970. On certain central neurolotropic effects of lavender essential oil. *Bull Inst Physiol*, 8: 69–76.

Awad, R., Levac, D., Cybulska, P., Merali, Z., Trudeau, V.L., and Arnason, J.T. 2007. Effects of traditionally used anxiolytic botanicals on enzymes of the gamma-aminobutyric acid (GABA) system. *Can J Physiol Pharmacol*, 85(9): 933–42.

Awad, R., Muhammad, A., Durst, T., Trudeau, V.L., and Arnason, J.T. 2009. Bioassay-guided fractionation of lemon balm (*Melissa officinalis* L.) using an *in vitro* measure of GABA transaminase activity. *Phytother Res*, 23(8): 1075–81.

Azizi, Z., Ebrahimi, S., Saadatfar, E., Kamalinejad, M., and Majlessi, N. 2012. Cognitive-enhancing activity of thymol and carvacrol in two rat models of dementia. *Behav Pharmacol*, 23(3): 241–49.

Bagetta, G. Morrone, L.A., Rombolà, L. et al. 2010. Neuropharmacology of the essential oil of bergamot. *Fitoterapia*, 81(6): 453–61.

Balmé, F. 1978. *Plantas medicinais* (5th ed.). São Paulo: Hemus.

Begum, A., Sandhya, S., Shaffath Ali, S., Vinod, K.R., Reddy, S., and Banji, D. 2013. An in-depth review on the medicinal flora *Rosmarinus officinalis* (Lamiaceae). *Acta Sci Pol Technol Aliment*, 12(1): 61–73.

Berliocchi, L., Russo, R., Levato, A. et al. 2009. (–)-Linalool attenuates allodynia in neuro-pathic pain induced by spinal nerve ligation in c57/bl6 mice. *Int Rev Neurobiol*, 85: 221–35.

Blanco, M.M., Costa, C.A., Freire, A.O., Santos, J.G., and Costa, I.M. 2007. Neurobehavioral effect of essential oil of *Cymbopogon citratus* in mice. *Phytomedicine*, 16: 265–70.

Bozin, B., Mimica-Dukic, N., Samojlik, I., and Jovin, E. 2007. Antimicrobial and antioxidant properties of rosemary and sage (*Rosmarinus officinalis* L. and *Salvia officinalis* L., Lamiaceae) essential oils. *J Agric Food Chem*, 55(19): 7879–85.

Bradley, B.F., Starkey, N.J., Brown, S.L., and Lea, R.W. 2007. Anxiolytic effects of *Lavandula angustifolia* odour on the Mongolian gerbil elevated plus maze. *J Ethnopharmacol*, 111: 517–25.

Brooker, D.J., Snape, M., Johnson, E., Ward, D., and Payne M. 1997. Single case evaluation of the effects of aromatherapy and massage on disturbed behaviour in severe dementia. *Br J Clin Psychol*, 36: 287–96.

Broughan, C. 2002. Odours, emotions, and cognition: How odours may affect cognitive per-formance. *Int J Aromather*, 12: 92–98.

Campêlo, L.M., Gonçalves, F.C., Feitosa, C.M., and de Freitas, R.M. 2011. Antioxidant activ-ity of *Citrus limon* essential oil in mouse hippocampus. *Pharm Biol*, 49(7): 709–15.

Canbek, M., Uyanoglu, M., Bayramoglu, G. et al. 2008. Effects of carvacrol on defects of ischemia-reperfusion in the rat liver. *Phytomedicine*, 15: 447–52.

Carlini, E.A., Contar, J.D.P., Silva-Filho, A.R., Silveira-Filho, N.G., Frochtengarten, M.L., and Bueno, O.F.A. 1986. Pharmacology of lemongrass (*Cymbopogon citratus* STAPF). I. Effects of teas prepared from the leaves on laboratory animals. *J Ethnopharmacol*, 17: 37–64.

Carvalho-Freitas, M.I.R., and Costa, M. 2002. Anxiolytic and sedative effects of extracts and essential oil from *Citrus aurantium* L. *Biol Pharm Bull*, 25: 1629–33.

Cavanagh, H.M., and Wilkinson, J.M. 2002. Biological activities of lavender essential oil. *Phytother Res*, 16(4): 301–8.

Ceccarelli, I., Masi, F., Fiorenzani, P., and Aloisi, A.M. 2002. Sex differences in the cit-rus lemon essential oil-induced increase of hippocampal acetylcholine release in rats exposed to a persistent painful stimulation. *Neurosci Lett*, 330(1): 25–28.

Ceccarelli, I., Lariviere, W.R., Fiorenzani, P., Sacerdote, P., and Aloisi, A.M. 2004. Effects of long-term exposure of lemon essential oil odor on behavioral, hormonal and neuronal parameters in male and female rats. *Brain Res*, 1001(1–2): 78–86.

Chen, S.W., Min, L., Li, W.J., Kong, W.X., Li, J.F., and Zhang, Y.J. 2004. The effects of angelica essential oil in three murine tests of anxiety. *Pharmacol Biochem Behav*, 79(2): 377–82.

Cheng, J., Kuang, P., Wu, W., and Zhang, F. 1999. Effects of transient forebrain ischemia and radix Salviae miltiorrhizae (RSM) on extracellular levels of monoamine neurotrans-mitters and metabolites in the gerbil striatum: An *in vivo* microdialysis study. *J Tradit Chin Med*, 19(2): 135–40.

Chioca, L.R., Antunes, V.D., Ferro, M.M., Losso, E.M., and Andreatini, R. 2013a. Anosmia does not impair the anxiolytic-like effect of lavender essential oil inhalation in mice. *Life Sci*, 92(20–21): 971–75.

Chioca, L.R., Ferro, M.M., Baretta, I.P. et al. 2013b. Anxiolytic-like effect of lavender essential oil inhalation in mice: Participation of serotonergic but not GABAA/benzodiazepine neuro-transmission. *J Ethnopharmacol*, 147(2): 412–18.

Choi, S.S., Han, K.J., Lee, H.K., Han, E.J., and Suh, H.W. 2003a. Antinociceptive profiles of crude extract from roots of *Angelica gigas* NAKAI in various pain models. *Biol Pharm Bull*, 26(9): 1283–88.

Choi, S.S., Han, K.J., Lee, J.K. et al. 2003b. Antinociceptive mechanisms of orally adminis-tered decursinol in the mouse. *Life Sci*, 73(4): 471–85.

Chu, C.J., and Kemper, K.J. 2001. *Lavender (Lavandula spp.).* Boston: Longwood Herbal Task Force.

Cline, M., Taylor, J.E., Flores, J., Bracken, S., McCall, S., and Ceremuga, T.E. 2008. Investigation of the anxiolytic effects of linalool, a lavender extract, in the male Sprague–Dawley rat. *AANA J*, 76: 47–52.

Corasaniti, M.T., Maiuolo, J., Maida, S. et al. 2007. Cell signaling pathways in the mechanisms of neuroprotection afforded by bergamot essential oil against NMDA induced cell death *in vitro. Br J Pharmacol*, 151: 518–29.

Cordell, B., and Buckle, J. 2013. The effects of aromatherapy on nicotine craving on a U.S. campus: A small comparison study. *J Altern Complement Med*, 19(8): 709–13.

Costa, C.A., Kohn, D.O., de Lima, V.M., Gargano, A.C., Flório, J.C., and Costa, M. 2011. The GABAergic system contributes to the anxiolytic-like effect of essential oil from *Cymbopogon citratus* (lemongrass). *J Ethnopharmacol*, 137(1): 828–36.

Costa, C.A., Cury, T.C., Cassettari, B.O., Takahira, R.K., Flório, J.C., and Costa, M. 2013. *Citrus aurantium* L. essential oil exhibits anxiolytic-like activity mediated by 5-HT(1A)-receptors and reduces cholesterol after repeated oral treatment. *BMC Complement Altern Med*, 23: 13–42.

Credner, K. 1960. Studies on the central depressor features of some thymol ethers. *Arzneimittelforschung*, 10: 170–74.

da Rocha, M.D., Viegas, F.P., Campos, H.C. et al. 2011. The role of natural products in the discovery of new drug candidates for the treatment of neurodegenerative disorders II: Alzheimer's disease. *CNS Neurol Disord Drug Targets*, 10(2): 251–70.

Dastmalchi, K., Ollilainen, V., Lackman, P. et al. 2009. Acetylcholinesterase inhibitory guided fractionation of *Melissa officinalis* L. *Bioorg Med Chem*, 17: 867–71.

de Sousa, D.P., Nóbrega, F.F.F., Santos, C.C.M.P., and de Almeida, R.N. 2010. Anticonvulsant activity of the linalool enantiomers and racemate: Investigation of chiral influence. *Nat Prod Commun*, 5(12): 1847–51.

Dobetsberger, C., and Buchbauer, G. 2011. Actions of essential oils on the central nervous system: An updated review. *Flavour Frag J*, 26: 300–16.

do Vale, T.G., Furtado, E.C., Santos, J.G., Jr., and Viana, G.S. 2002. Central effects of citral, myrcene and limonene, constituents of essential oil chemotypes from *Lippia alba* (Mill.) n.e. Brown. *Phytomedicine*, 9(8): 709–14.

Duan, X., Tashiro, M., Wu, D. et al. 2007. Autonomic nervous function and localization of cerebral activity during lavender aromatic immersion. *Technol Health Care*, 15: 69–78.

Dugo, P., Mondello, L., Dugo, L., Stancanelli, R., and Dugo, G. 2000. LC-MS for the identification of oxygen heterocyclic compounds in citrus essential oils. *J Pharm Biomed Anal*, 24: 147–50.

Duke, J.A. 2000. *Handbook of Medicinal Herbs.* Boca Raton, FL: CRC Press.

Dweck, A.C. 2000. The folklore and cosmetics use of various *Salvia* species. In *Sage: The Genus Salvia*, ed. S.E. Kintzios. Amsterdam: Harwood Academic Publishers, pp. 1–25.

Edge, J. 2003. A pilot study addressing the effect of aromatherapy massage on mood, anxiety and relaxation in adult mental health. *Complement Ther Nurs Midwifery*, 9: 90–97.

Elisabetsky, E., Marschner, J., and Souza, D.O. 1995. Effects of linalool on glutamatergic system in the rat cerebral cortex. *Neurochem Res*, 20: 461–65.

Elisabetsky, E., Brum, L.F.S., and Souza, D.O. 1999. Anticonvulsant properties of linalool in glutamate-related seizure models. *Phytomedicine*, 6(2): 107–13.

El Omri, A., Han, J., Yamada, P., Kawada, K., Ben Abdrabbah, M., and Isoda, H. 2010. *Rosmarinus officinalis* polyphenols activate cholinergic activities in PC12 cells through phosphorylation of ERK1/2. *J Ethnopharmacol*, 131(2): 451–58.

Fachini-Queiroz, F.C., Kummer, R., Estevão-Silva, C.F. et al. 2012. Effects of thymol and carvacrol, constituents of *Thymus vulgaris* L. essential oil, on the inflammatory response. *Evid Based Complement Alternat Med*, 2012: 657026.

Feng, Z., Lu, Y., Wu, X. et al. 2012. Ligustilide alleviates brain damage and improves cognitive function in rats of chronic cerebral hypoperfusion. *J Ethnopharmacol*, 144(2): 313–21.

Ferreira, A., Proenca, C., Serralheiro, M., and Araujo, M. 2006. The *in vitro* screening for acetylcholinesterase inhibition and antioxidant activity of medicinal plants from Portugal. *J Ethnopharmacol*, 108: 31–37.

Fukumoto, S., Sawasaki, E., Okuyama, S., Miyake, Y., and Yokogoshi, H. 2006. Flavor components of monoterpenes in citrus essential oils enhance the release of monoamines from rat brain slices. *Nutr Neurosci*, 9(1–2): 73–80.

Galdino, P.M., Nascimento, M.V., Florentino, I.F. et al. 2012. The anxiolytic-like effect of an essential oil derived from *Spiranthera odoratissima* A. St. Hil. leaves and its major component, β-caryophyllene, in male mice. *Prog Neuropsychopharmacol Biol Psychiatry*, 38(2): 276–84.

Galindo, L.A., Pultrini Ade, M., and Costa, M. 2010. Biological effects of *Ocimum gratissimum* L. are due to synergic action among multiple compounds present in essential oil. *J Nat Med*, 64(4): 436–41.

García, D.A., Bujons, J., Vale, C., and Suñol, C. 2006. Allosteric positive interaction of thymol with the GABAA receptor in primary cultures of mouse cortical neurons. *Neuropharmacology*, 50(1): 25–35.

García, D.A., Vendrell, I., Galofré, M., and Suñol, C. 2008. GABA released from cultured cortical neurons influences the modulation of t-[(35)S]butylbicyclophosphorothionate binding at the GABAA receptor: Effects of thymol. *Eur J Pharmacol*, 600(1–3): 26–31.

Gertsch, J., Leonti, M., Raduner, S. et al. 2008. Beta-caryophyllene is a dietary cannabinoid. *Proc Natl Acad Sci USA*, 105(26): 9099–104.

Guillemain, J., Rousseau, A., and Delaveau, P. 1989. Neurodepressive effects of the essential oil of *Lavandula angustifolia* Mill. *Ann Pharm Fr*, 47(6): 337–43.

Gülçin, I. 2004. Evaluation of the antioxidant and antimicrobial activities of clary sage (*Salvia sclarea* L.). *Turk J Agric For*, 28: 25–33.

Hancianu, M., Cioanca, O., Mihasan, M., and Hritcu, L. 2013. Neuroprotective effects of inhaled lavender oil on scopolamine-induced dementia via anti-oxidative activities in rats. *Phytomedicine* 20(5): 446–52.

Hatip-Al-Khatib, I., Egashira, N., Mishima, K. et al. 2004. Determination of the effectiveness of components of the herbal medicine Toki-shakuyaku-san and fractions of *Angelica acutiloba* in improving the scopolamine-induced impairment of rat's spatial cognition in eight-armed radial maze test. *J Pharmacol Sci*, 96(1): 33–41.

Haze, S., Sakai, K., and Gozu, Y. 2002. Effects of fragrance inhalation on sympathetic activity in normal adults. *Jpn J Pharmacol*, 90: 247–53.

Heinrich, M., Kufer, J., Leonti, M., and Pardo-de-Santayana, M. 2006. Ethnobotany and ethnopharmacology: Interdisciplinary links with the historical sciences. *J Ethnopharmacol*, 107: 157–60.

Herrera-Ruiz, M., García-Beltrán, Y., Mora, S. et al. 2006. Antidepressant and anxiolytic effects of hydroalcoholic extract from *Salvia elegans*. *J Ethnopharmacol*, 107(1): 53–58.

Hiruma-Lima, C.A., Guimarães, E.M., Santos, C.M., and Di Stasi, L.C., 2002. Commelinidae medicinais. In *Plantas Medicinais na Amazônia e na Mata Atlântica*, ed. L.C. Di Stasi and C.A. Hiruma-Lima. São Paulo: Editora UNESP, pp. 41–50.

Horosová, K., Bujnáková, D., and Kmet, V. 2006. Effect of oregano essential oil on chicken lactobacilli and *E. coli*. *Folia Microbiol* (Praha), 51(4): 278–80.

Hotta, M., Nakata, R., Katsukawa, M., Hori, K., Takahashi, S., and Inoue, H. 2010. Carvacrol, a component of thyme oil, activates PPAR alpha and gamma and suppresses COX-2 expression. *J Lipid Res*, 51, 132–39.

Hritcu, L., Cioanca, O., and Hancianu, M. 2012. Effects of lavender oil inhalation on improving scopolamine-induced spatial memory impairment in laboratory rats. *Phytomedicine*, 19(6): 529–34.

Huang, M.H., Wu, S.N., and Shen, A.Y. 2005. Stimulatory actions of thymol, a natural product, on Ca(2+)-activated K(+) current in pituitary GH(3) cells. *Planta Med*, 71(12): 1093–98.

Huang, L., Abuhamdah, S., Howes, M.J. et al. 2008. Pharmacological profile of essential oils derived from *Lavandula angustifolia* and *Melissa officinalis* with anti-agitation properties: Focus on ligand-gated channels. *J Pharm Pharmacol*, 60(11): 1515–22.

Hudaib, M., Speroni, E., Di Pietra, A.M., and Cavrini, V. 2002. GC/MS evaluation of thyme (*Thymus vulgaris* L.) oil composition and variations during the vegetative cycle. *J Pharm Biomed Anal*, 29(4): 691–700.

Ibarra, A., Feuillere, N., Roller, M., Lesburgere, E., and Beracochea, D. 2010. Effects of chronic administration of *Melissa officinalis* L. extract on anxiety-like reactivity and on circadian and exploratory activities in mice. *Phytomedicine*, 17(6): 397–403.

Imanshahidi, M., and Hosseinzadeh, H. 2006. The pharmacological effects of *Salvia* species on the central nervous system. *Phytother Res*, 20(6): 427–37.

Jimbo, D., Kimura, Y., Taniguchi, M., Inoue, M., and Urakami, K. 2009. Effect of aromatherapy on patients with Alzheimer's disease. *Psychogeriatrics*, 9(4): 173–79.

Jukic, M., Politeo, O., Maksimovic, M., and Milos, M. 2007. *In vitro* acetylcholinesterase inhibitory properties of thymol, carvacrol and their derivatives thymoquinone and thymohydroquinone. *Phytother Res*, 21: 259–61.

Kang, S.Y., Lee, K.Y., Sung, S.H., Park, M.J., and Kim, Y.C. 2001. Coumarins isolated from *Angelica gigas* inhibit acetylcholinesterase: Structure-activity relationships. *J Nat Prod*, 64(5): 683–85.

Kang, S.Y., Lee, K.Y., Park, M.J. et al. 2003. Decursin from *Angelica gigas* mitigates amnesia induced by scopolamine in mice. *Neurobiol Learn Mem*, 79(1): 11–18.

Kashani, M.S., Tavirani, M.R., Talaei, S.A., and Salami, M. 2011. Aqueous extract of lavender (*Lavandula angustifolia*) improves the spatial performance of a rat model of Alzheimer's disease. *Neurosci Bull*, 27(2): 99–106.

Kasper, S. 2013. An orally administered *Lavandula* oil preparation (Silexan) for anxiety disorder and related conditions: An evidence based review. *Int J Psychiatry Clin Pract*, 17 (Suppl 1): 15–22.

Kasper, S., Gastpar, M., Müller, W.E. et al. 2010. Silexan, an orally administered *Lavandula* oil preparation, is effective in the treatment of 'subsyndromal' anxiety disorder: A randomized, double-blind, placebo controlled trial. *Int Clin Psychopharmacol*, 25(5): 277–87.

Kaufmann, D., Dogra, A.K., and Wink, M. 2011. Myrtenal inhibits acetylcholinesterase, a known Alzheimer target. *J Pharm Pharmacol*, 63(10): 1368–71.

Kavvadias, D., Monschein, V., Sand, P., Riederer, P., and Schreier, P. 2003. Constituents of sage (*Salvia officinalis*) with *in vitro* affinity to human brain benzodiazepine receptor. *Planta Med*, 69(2): 113–17.

Kennedy, D.O., and Scholey, A.B. 2006. The psychopharmacology of European herbs with cognition-enhancing properties. *Curr Pharm Des*, 12(35): 4613–23.

Kennedy, D.O., Dodd, F.L., Robertson, B.C. et al. 2011. Monoterpenoid extract of sage (*Salvia lavandulaefolia*) with cholinesterase inhibiting properties improves cognitive performance and mood in healthy adults. *J Psychopharmacol*, 25(8): 1088–100.

Kiecolt-Glaser, J.K., Graham, J.E., Malarkey, W.B., Porter, K., Lemeshow, S., and Glaser, R. 2008. Olfactory influences on mood and autonomic, endocrine, and immune function. *Psychoneuroendocrinology*, 33(3): 328–39.

Kihara, T., Shimohama, S., Sawada, H. et al. 1997. Nicotinic receptor stimulation protects neurons against beta-amyloid toxicity. *Ann Neurol*, 42: 159–63.

Kim, Y., Kim, M., Kim, H., and Kim, K. 2009. Effect of lavender oil on motor function and dopamine receptor expression in the olfactory bulb of mice. *J Ethnopharmacol*, 125(1): 31–35.

Klauke, A.L., Racz, I., Pradier, B. et al. 2014. The cannabinoid CB2 receptor-selective phyto-cannabinoid beta-caryophyllene exerts analgesic effects in mouse models of inflammatory and neuropathic pain. *Eur Neuropsychopharmacol*, 24(4): 608–20.

Komiya, M., Takeuchi, T., and Harada, E. 2006. Lemon oil vapor causes an anti-stress effect via modulating the 5-HT and DA activities in mice. *Behav Brain Res*, 172: 240–49.

Komori, T., Fujiwara, R., Tanida, M., and Nomura, J. 1995a. Potential antidepressant effects of lemon odor in rats. *Eur Neuropsychopharmacol*, 5: 477–80.

Komori, T., Fujiwara, R., Tanida, M., Nomura, J., and Yokoyama, M.M. 1995b. Effects of citrus fragrance on immune function and depressive states. *Neuroimmunomodulation*, 2: 174–80.

Koulivand, P.H., Ghadiri, M.K., and Gorji, A. 2013. Lavender and the nervous system. *Evid Based Complement Alternat Med*, 2013: 1–11.

Kovar, K.A., Gropper, B., Friess, D., and Ammon, H.T.P. 1987. Blood levels of 1,8-cineole and locomotor activity of mice after inhalation and oral administration of rosemary oil. *Planta Med*, 53: 315–19.

Kumar, V. 2013. Characterization of anxiolytic and neuropharmacological activities of Silexan. *Wien Med Wochenschr*, 163(3–4): 89–94.

Kumar, D., Bhat, Z.A., and Shah, M.Y. 2012. Anti-anxiety activity of successive extracts of *Angelica archangelica* Linn. on the elevated t-maze and forced swimming tests in rats. *J Tradit Chin Med*, 32(3): 423–29.

Kumar, D., Bhat, Z.A., Kumar, V., and Shah, M.Y. 2013. Coumarins from *Angelica archangelica* Linn. and their effects on anxiety-like behavior. *Prog Neuropsychopharmacol Biol Psychiatry*, 40: 180–86.

Lakušić, D., Ristić, M., Slavkovska, V., and Lakušić, B. 2013. Seasonal variations in the composition of the essential oils of rosemary (*Rosmarinus officinalis*, Lamiaceae). *Nat Prod Commun*, 8(1): 131–34.

Lee, S.Y. 2005. The effect of lavender aromatherapy on cognitive function, emotion, and aggressive behavior of elderly with dementia. *Taehan Kanho Hakhoe Chi*, 35(2): 303–12.

Lee, C.M., Wong, H.N., Chui, K.Y., Choang, T.F., Hon, P.M., and Chang, H.M. 1991. Miltirone, a central benzodiazepine receptor partial agonist from a Chinese medicinal herb *Salvia miltiorrhiza*. *Neurosci Lett*, 127(2): 237–41.

Leite, M.P., Fassin, J., Jr., Baziloni, E.M.F., Almeida, R.N., Mattei, R., and Leite, J.R. 2008. Behavioral effects of essential oil of *Citrus aurantium* L. inhalation in rats. *Rev Bras Farmacogn*, 18: 661–66.

Li, L., Li, W., Jung, S.W., Lee, Y.W., and Kim, Y.H. 2011. Protective effects of decursin and decursinol angelate against amyloid β-protein-induced oxidative stress in the PC12 cell line: The role of Nrf2 and antioxidant enzymes. *Biosci Biotechnol Biochem*, 75(3): 434–42.

Li, L., Du, J.K., Zou, L.Y., Wu, T., Lee, Y.W., and Kim, Y.H. 2013. Decursin isolated from *Angelica gigas* Nakai rescues PC12 cells from amyloid β-protein-induced neurotoxicity through Nrf2-mediated upregulation of heme oxygenase-1: Potential roles of MAPK. *Evid Based Complement Alternat Med*, 2013: 467245.

Lin, P.W., Chan, W.C., Ng, B.F., and Lam, L.C. 2007. Efficacy of aromatherapy (*Lavandula angustifolia*) as an intervention for agitated behaviours in Chinese older persons with dementia: A crossover randomized trial. *Int J Geriatr Psychiatry*, 22: 405–10.

Linck, V.M., da Silva, A.L., Figueiró, M., Caramão, E.B., Moreno, P.R., and Elisabetsky, E. 2010. Effects of inhaled linalool in anxiety, social interaction and aggressive behavior in mice. *Phytomedicine*, 17: 679–83.

Lis-Balchin, M., and Hart, S. 1999. Studies on the mode of action of the essential oil of lavender (*Lavandula angustifolia* P. Miller). *Phytother Res*, 6: 540–42.

Liu, Q., and Zhao, B. 2004. Nicotine attenuates beta-amyloid peptide-induced neurotoxicity, free radical and calcium accumulation in hippocampal neuronal cultures. *Br J Pharmacol*, 141: 746–54.

Lopes Campêlo, L.M., Gonçalves e Sá, C., de Almeida, A.A. et al. 2011. Sedative, anxiolytic and antidepressant activities of *Citrus limon* (Burn) essential oil in mice. *Pharmazie*, 66(8): 623–27.

Lorig, T.S. 2000. The application of electroencephalographic techniques to the study of human olfaction: A review and tutorial. *Int J Psychophysiol*, 36(2): 91–104.

Machado, D.G., Bettio, L.E.B., Cunha, M.P. et al. 2009. Antidepressant-like effect of the extract of *Rosmarinus officinalis* in mice: Involvement of the monoaminergic system. *Prog Neuropsychopharmacol Biol Psychiatry*, 33: 642–50.

Machado, D.G., Neis, V.B., Balen, G.O. et al. 2012. Antidepressant-like effect of ursolic acid isolated from *Rosmarinus officinalis* L. in mice: Evidence for the involvement of the dopaminergic system. *Pharmacol Biochem Behav*, 103(2): 204–11.

Machado, D.G., Cunha, M.P., Neis, V.B. et al. 2013. Antidepressant-like effects of fractions, essential oil, carnosol and betulinic acid isolated from *Rosmarinus officinalis* L. *Food Chem*, 136(2): 999–1005.

Marco, E.M., García-Gutiérrez, M.S., Bermúdez-Silva, F.J. et al. 2011. Endocannabinoid system and psychiatry: In search of a neurobiological basis for detrimental and potential therapeutic effects. *Front Behav Neurosci*, 5: 63.

Matos, L.G., Santos, L.D.A.R, Vilela, C.F. et al. 2003. Atividade analgésica e/ou antiinflamatória da fração aquosa do extrato etanólico das folhas da Spiranthera odoratissima A. St. Hillaire (manacá). *Rev Bras Farmacognosia*, 3: 15–16.

Matos, L.G., Pontes, I.S., Tresvenzol, L.M., Paula, J.R., and Costa, E.A. 2004. Analgesic and anti-inflammatory activity of the ethanolic extract from *Spiranthera odoratissima* A. St. Hillaire (manacá) roots. *Phytother Res*, 18(12): 963–66.

Matos, L.G., Galdino, P.M., Maldaner, R.R., Costa, E.A., and Paula, J.R. 2006. Estudo das atividades no sistema nervoso central da fração hexânica do extrato etanólico das folhas da *Spiranthera odoratissima*. Presented at Anais do XIX Simpósio de Plantas Medicinais do Brasil, Salvador, Brazil.

Matsumoto, K., Kohno, S., Ojima, K., Tezuka, Y., Kadota, S., and Watanabe, H. 1998. Effects of methylenechloride-soluble fraction of Japanese angelica root extract, ligustilide and butylidenephthalide, on pentobarbital sleep in group-housed and socially isolated mice. *Life Sci*, 62(23): 2073–82.

Melo, F.H., Venancio, E.T., de Sousa, D.P. et al. 2010. Anxiolytic-like effect of carvacrol (5-isopropyl-2-methylphenol) in mice: Involvement with GABAergic transmission. *Fundam Clin Pharmacol*, 24: 437–43.

Melo, F.H., Moura, B.A., de Sousa, D.P. et al. 2011. Antidepressant-like effect of carvacrol (5-isopropyl-2-methylphenol) in mice: Involvement of dopaminergic system. *Fundam Clin Pharmacol*, 25: 362–67.

Meng, P., Yoshida, H., Matsumiya, T. et al. 2013. Carnosic acid suppresses the production of amyloid-β 1-42 by inducing the metalloprotease gene TACE/ADAM17 in SH-SY5Y human neuroblastoma cells. *Neurosci Res*, 75(2): 94–102.

Min, L., Chen, S.W., Li, W.J. et al. 2005. The effects of angelica essential oil in social interaction and hole-board tests. *Pharmacol Biochem Behav*, 81(4): 838–42.

Mohammadi, B., Haeseler, G., Leuwer, M., Dengler, R., Krampfl, K., and Bufler, J. 2001. Structural requirements of phenol derivatives for direct activation of chloride currents via GABA(A) receptors. *Eur J Pharmacol*, 421(2): 85–91.

Mondello, L., Stagno d'Alcontres, I., Del Duce, R., and Crispo, F. 1993. On the genuineness of citrus essential oils. XL. The composition of the coumarins and psoralens of calabrian bergamot essential oil (*Citrus bergamia* Risso). *Flavour Fragr J*, 8: 17–24.

Moretti, M.D.L., Peana, A.T., and Satta, M.A. 1997. A study of antiinflammatory and peripheral analgesic actions of *Salvia sclarea* oil and its main constituents. *J Essent Oil Res*, 9: 199–204.

Morrone, L.A., Rombolà, L., Corasaniti, M.T. et al. 2007. The essential oil of bergamot enhances the levels of amino acid neurotransmitters in the hippocampus of rat: Implication of monoterpene hydrocarbons. *Pharmacol Res*, 55: 255–62.

Moss, M., and Oliver, L. 2012. Plasma 1,8-cineole correlates with cognitive performance following exposure to rosemary essential oil aroma. *Ther Adv Psychopharmacol*, 2(3): 103–13.

Moss, M., Cook, J., Wesnes, K., and Duckett, P. 2003. Aromas of rosemary and lavender essential oils differentially affect cognition and mood in healthy adults. *Int J Neurosci*, 113(1): 15–38.

Moss, L., Rouse, M., Wesnes, K.A., and Moss, M. 2010. Differential effects of the aromas of *Salvia* species on memory and mood. *Hum Psychopharmacol*, 25(5): 388–96.

Nascimento, M.V., Galdino, P.M., Florentino, I.F. et al. 2012. Anti-inflammatory effect of *Spiranthera odoratissima* A. St.-Hil. leaves involves reduction of TNF-α. *Nat Prod Res*, 26(23): 2274–79.

Okuyama, S., Sawasaki, E., and Yokogoshi, H. 2004. Conductor compounds of phenylpentane in *Mycoleptodonoides aitchisonii* mycelium enhance the release of dopamine from rat brain striatum slices. *Nutr Neurosci*, 7: 107–11.

Orafidiya, L.O., Agbani, E.O., Iwalewa, E.O., Adelusola, K.A., and Oyedapo, O.O. 2004. Studies on the acute and sub-chronic toxicity of the essential oil of *Ocimum gratissimum* L. leaf. *Phytomedicine*, 11: 71–76.

Orhan, I., Aslan, S., Kartal, M., Sener, B., and Baser, K.H.C. 2008. Inhibitory effect of Turkish *Rosmarinus officinalis* L. on acetylcholinesterase and butyrylcholinesterase enzymes. *Food Chem*, 108: 663–68.

Ozarowski, M., Mikolajczak, P.L., Bogacz, A. et al. 2013. *Rosmarinus officinalis* L. leaf extract improves memory impairment and affects acetylcholinesterase and butyrylcholinesterase activities in rat brain. *Fitoterapia*, 91: 261–71.

Park, S.J., Jung, J.M., Lee, H.E. et al. 2012a. The memory ameliorating effects of INM-176, an ethanolic extract of *Angelica gigas*, against scopolamine- or Aβ(1-42)-induced cognitive dysfunction in mice. *J Ethnopharmacol*, 143(2): 611–20.

Park, S.J., Jung, H.J., Son, M.S. et al. 2012b. Neuroprotective effects of INM-176 against lipopolysaccharide-induced neuronal injury. *Pharmacol Biochem Behav*, 101(3): 427–33.

Parnas, M., Peters, M., Dadon, D. et al. 2009. Carvacrol is a novel inhibitor of *Drosophila* TRPL and mammalian TRPM7 channels. *Cell Calcium*, 45: 300–39.

Peana, A.T., Moretti, M.D., and Juliano, C. 1999. Chemical composition and antimicrobial action of the essential oils of *Salvia desoleana* and *S. sclarea*. *Planta Med*, 65: 752–54.

Pengelly, A., Snow, J., Mills, S.Y., Scholey, A., Wesnes, K., and Butler, L.R. 2012. Short-term study on the effects of rosemary on cognitive function in an elderly population. *J Med Food*, 15(1): 10–17.

Pereira, P., Tysca, D., Oliveira, P., da Silva Brum, L.F., Picada, J.N., and Ardenghi, P. 2005. Neurobehavioral and genotoxic aspects of rosmarinic acid. *Pharmacol Res*, 52(3): 199–203.

Pereira, R.P., Fachinetto, R., de Souza Prestes, A. et al. 2009. Antioxidant effects of different extracts from *Melissa officinalis*, *Matricaria recutita* and *Cymbopogon citratus*. *Neurochem Res*, 34: 973–83.

Perry, N.S.L., and Perry, E.K. 2006. Aromatherapy in the management of psychiatric disorders: Clinical and neuropharmacological perspectives. *CNS Drugs*, 20: 257–80.

Perry, E., and Howes, M.J. 2011. Medicinal plants and dementia therapy: Herbal hopes for brain aging? *CNS Neurosci Ther*, 17(6): 683–98.

Perry, N.S.L., Houghton, P., Theobald, A., Jenner, P., and Perry, E.K. 2000. *In vitro* inhibition of human erythrocyte acetylcholinesterase *by Salvia lavandulaefolia* essential oil and constituents terpenes. *J Pharmacol*, 52: 895–902.

Perry, N.S.L., Houghton, P.J., Sampson, J., Theobald, A.E. et al. 2001. *In vitro* activities of *S. lavandulaefolia* (Spanish sage) relevant to treatment of Alzheimer's disease. *J Pharmacy Pharmacol*, 53: 1347–56.

Perry, N.S.L., Houghton, P.J., Jenner, P., Keith, A., and Perry, E.K. 2002. *Salvia lavandulaefolia* essential oil inhibits cholinesterase *in vivo*. *Phytomedicine*, 9: 48–51.

Perry, N.S.L., Bollen, C., Perry, E.K., and Bollard, C. 2003. *Salvia* for dementia therapy, review of pharmacological activity and pilot tolerability clinical trial. *Pharmacol Biochem Behav*, 75: 651–58.

Petersen, M., and Simmonds, M.S. 2003. Rosmarinic acid. *Phytochemistry*, 62: 121–25.

Pitarokili, D., Couladis, M., Petsikos-Panayotarou, N., and Tzakou, O. 2002. Composition and antifungal activity on soil-borne pathogens of the essential oil of *Salvia sclarea* from Greece. *J Agric Food Chem*, 50: 6688–91.

Priestley, C.M., Williamson, E.M., Wafford, K.A., and Sattelle, D.B. 2003. Thymol, a constituent of thyme essential oil, is a positive allosteric modulator of human GABA(A) receptors and a homo-oligomeric GABA receptor from *Drosophila melanogaster*. *Br J Pharmacol*, 140(8): 1363–72.

Prut, L., and Belzung, C. 2003. The open field as a paradigm to measure the effects of drugs on anxiety-like behaviors: A review. *Eur J Pharmacol*, 463: 3–33.

Pultrini Ade, M., Galindo, L.A., and Costa, M., 2006. Effects of the essential oil from *Citrus aurantium* L. in experimental anxiety models in mice. *Life Sci*, 78: 1720–25.

Rainville, P., Duncan, G.H., Price, D.D., Carrier, B., and Bushnell, M.C. 1997. Pain affect encoded in human anterior cingulate but not somatosensory cortex. *Science*, 277: 968–71.

Rombolà, L., Corasaniti, M.T., Rotiroti, D. et al. 2009. Effects of systemic administration of the essential oil of bergamot (BEO) on gross behaviour and EEG power spectra recorded from the rat hippocampus and cerebral cortex. *Funct Neurol*, 24: 107–12.

Rutherford, D.M., Nielsen, M.P., Hansen, S.K., Witt, M.R., Bergendorff, O., and Sterner, O. 1992. Isolation and identification from *Salvia officinalis* of two diterpenes which inhibit t-butylbicyclophosphoro[35S]thionate binding to chloride channel of rat cerebrocortical membranes *in vitro*. *Neurosci Lett*, 135(2): 224–26.

Saiyudthong, S., and Marsden, C.A. 2011. Acute effects of bergamot oil on anxiety-related behaviour and corticosterone level in rats. *Phytother Res*, 25(6): 858–62.

Sánchez, M.E., Turina, A.V., García, D.A., Nolan, M.V., and Perillo, M.A. 2004. Surface activity of thymol: Implications for an eventual pharmacological activity. *Colloids Surf B Biointerfaces*, 34(2): 77–86.

Sasaki, K., El Omri, A., Kondo, S., Han, J., and Isoda, H. 2013. *Rosmarinus officinalis* polyphenols produce anti-depressant like effect through monoaminergic and cholinergic functions modulation. *Behav Brain Res*, 238: 86–94.

Savelev, S., Okello, E., Perry, N.S.L., Wilkins, R.M., and Perry, E.K. 2003. Synergistic and antagonistic interactions of anticholinesterase terpenoids in *Salvia lavandulaefolia* essential oil. *Pharmacol Biochem Behav*, 75: 661–68.

Savelev, S.U., Okello, E.J., and Perry, E.K. 2004. Butyryl- and acetyl-cholinesterase inhibitory activities in essential oils of *Salvia* species and their constituents. *Phytother Res*, 18, 315–24.

Scholey, A.B., Tildesley, N.T., Ballard, C.G. et al. 2008. An extract of *Salvia* (sage) with anticholinesterase properties improves memory and attention in healthy older volunteers. *Psychopharmacology* (Berl), 198(1): 127–39.

Segen, J.C. 1998. *Dictionary of Alternative Medicine*. Stamford, CT: Appleton and Lange.

Seo, Y.J., Kwon, M.S., Park, S.H. et al. 2009. The analgesic effect of decursinol. *Arch Pharm Res*, 32(6): 937–43.

Seol, G.H., Shim, H.S., Kim, P.J. et al. 2010. Antidepressant-like effect of *Salvia sclarea* is explained by modulation of dopamine activities in rats. *J Ethnopharmacol*, 1: 187–90.

Sepand, M.R., Soodi, M., Hajimehdipoor, H., Soleimani, M., and Sahraei, E. 2013. Comparison of neuroprotective effects of *Melissa officinalis* total extract and its acidic and non-acidic fractions against a β-induced toxicity. *Iran J Pharm Res*, 12 (2): 415–23.

Setzer, W.N. 2009. Essential oils and anxiolytic aromatherapy. *Nat Prod Commun*, 4(9): 1305–16.

Shah, G., Shri, R., Panchal, V., Sharma, N., Singh, B., and Mann, A.S. 2011. Scientific basis for the therapeutic use of *Cymbopogon citratus*, Staph (lemon grass). *J Adv Pharm Tech Res*, 2: 3–8.

Shaw, D., Annett, J.M., Doherty, B., and Leslie, J.C. 2007. Anxiolytic effects of lavender oil inhalation on open-field behaviour in rats. *Phytomedicine*, 14: 613–20.

Shaw, D., Norwood, K., and Leslie, J.C. 2011. Chlordiazepoxide and lavender oil alter unconditioned anxiety-induced c-fos expression in the rat brain. *Behav Brain Res*, 1: 1–7.

Sigurdsson, S., and Gudbjarnason, S. 2007. Inhibition of acetylcholinesterase by extracts and constituents from *Angelica archangelica* and *Geranium sylvaticum*. *Z Naturforsch C*, 62(9–10): 689–93.

Sigurdsson, S., and Gudbjarnason, S. 2013. Effect of oral imperatorin on memory in mice. *Biochem Biophys Res Commun*, 441(2): 318–20.

Silva, M.R., Ximenes, R.M., da Costa, J.G., Leal, L.K., de Lopes, A.A., and Viana, G.S. 2010. Comparative anticonvulsant activities of the essential oils (EOs) from *Cymbopogon winterianus* Jowitt and *Cymbopogon citratus* (DC) Stapf. in mice. *Naunyn Schmiedebergs Arch Pharmacol*, 381(5): 415–26.

Silva Brum, L.F., Elisabetsky, E., and Souza, D. 2001. Effects of linalool on [3H] MK801 and [3H] muscimol binding in mouse cortical membranes. *Phytother Res*, 15(5): 422–25.

Takahashi, M., Cyong, J.C., Toita, S., Shindo, M., and Cho, S. 1982. Suppression of adjuvant arthritis by oral administration of oriental herbs II. *Kitasato Arch Exp Med*, 55(1–2): 39–45.

Takahashi, M., Satou, T., Ohashi, M., Hayashi, S., Sadamoto, K., and Koike, K. 2011. Interspecies comparison of chemical composition and anxiolytic-like effects of lavender oils upon inhalation. *Nat Prod Commun*, 6(11): 1769–74.

Takahashi, M., Yamanaka, A., Asanuma, C., Asano, H., Satou, T., and Koike, K. 2014. Anxiolytic-like effect of inhalation of essential oil from *Lavandula officinalis*: Investigation of changes in 5-HT turnover and involvement of olfactory stimulation. *Nat Prod Commun*, 9(7): 1023–26.

Takeda, H., Tsuji, M., Miyamoto, J., Masuya, J., Iimori, M., and Matsumiya, T. 2003. Caffeic acid produces antidepressive- and/or anxiolytic-like effects through indirect modulation of the alpha 1A-adrenoceptor system in mice. *Neuroreport*, 14(7): 1067–70.

Tanaka, S., Kano, Y., Tabata, M., and Konoshima, M. 1971. Effects of "Toki" (*Angelica acutiloba* Kitagawa) extracts on writhing and capillary permeability in mice (analgesic and antiinflammatory effects). *Yakugaku Zasshi*, 91(10): 1098–104.

Tildesley, N.T., Kennedy, D.O., Perry, E.K. et al. 2003. *Salvia lavandulaefolia* (Spanish sage) enhances memory in healthy young volunteers. *Pharmacol Biochem Behav*, 75(3): 669–74.

Tildesley, N.T., Kennedy, D.O., Perry, E.K., Ballard, C.G., Wesnes, K.A., Scholey, A.B. 2005. Positive modulation of mood and cognitive performance following administration of acute doses of Salvia lavandulae folia essential oil to healthy young volunteers. *Physiol Behav*. 83(5): 699–709.

Tisserand, R. 1988. Lavender beats benzodiazepines. *Int J Aromather*, 1: 1–2.

Tortoriello, J., and Romero, O. 1992. Plants used by Mexican traditional medicine with presumable sedative properties: An ethnobotanical approach. *Arch Med Res*, 23: 111–16.

Trabace, L.Z.M., Morgese, M.G., Tucci, P. et al. 2011. Estrous cycle affects the neurochemical and neurobehavioral profile of carvacrol-treated female rats. *Toxicol Appl Pharmacol*, 255: 169–75.

Tsang, H.W., and Ho, T.Y. 2010. A systematic review on the anxiolytic effects of aromatherapy on rodents under experimentally induced anxiety models. *Rev Neurosci*, 21: 141–52.

Umezu, T. 2012. Evaluation of the effects of plant-derived essential oils on central nervous system function using discrete shuttle-type conditioned avoidance response in mice. *Phytother Res*, 26(6): 884–91.

Umezu, T., Nagano, K., Ito, H., Kosakai, K., Sakaniwa, M., and Morita, M. 2006. Anticonflict effects of lavender oil and identification of its active constituents. *Pharmacol Biochem Behav*, 85: 713–21.

van der Ploeg, E.S., Eppingstall, B., and O'Connor, D.W. 2010. The study protocol of a blinded randomised-controlled cross-over trial of lavender oil as a treatment of behavioural symptoms in dementia. *BMC Geriatr*, 10: 49.

Vasil'eva, M.G., and Pimenov, M.G. 1991. Karyo taxonomical analysis in the genus *Angelica* (Umbelliferae). *Plant Syst Evol*, 177: 117–38.

Videira, R., Castanheira, P., Grãos, M. et al. 2014. Dose-dependent inhibition of BACE-1 by the monoterpenoid 2,3,4,4-tetramethyl-5-methylenecyclopent-2-enone in cellular and mouse models of Alzheimer's disease. *J Nat Prod*, 77(6): 1275–79.

Vladimir-Knežević, S., Blažeković, B., Kindl, M., Vladić, J., Lower-Nedza A.D., and Brantner, A.H. 2014. Acetylcholinesterase inhibitory, antioxidant and phytochemical properties of selected medicinal plants of the Lamiaceae family. *Molecules*, 19(1): 767–82.

Wake, G., Court, J., Pickering, A., Lewis, R., Wilkins, R., and Perry, E. 2000. CNS acetylcholine receptor activity in European medicinal plants traditionally used to improve failing memory. *J Ethnopharmacol*, 69: 105–14.

Weier, K.M., and Beal, M.W. 2004. Complementary therapies as adjuncts in the treatment of postpartum depression. *J Midwifery Womens Health*, 49: 96–104.

Woelk, H., and Schlafke, S. 2010. A multi-center, double-blind, randomised study of the lavender oil preparation Silexan in comparison to lorazepam for generalized anxiety disorder. *Phytomedicine*, 17(2): 94–99.

Wong, K.K, Ho, M.T., Lin, H.Q. et al. 2010. Cryptotanshinone, an acetylcholinesterase inhibitor from *Salvia miltiorrhiza*, ameliorates scopolamine-induced amnesia in Morris water maze task. *Planta Med*, 76(3): 228–34.

Woronuk, G., Demissie, Z., Rheault, M., and Mahmoud, S. 2011. Biosynthesis and therapeutic properties of *Lavandula* essential oil constituents. *Planta Med*, 77(1): 7–15.

Xin, J., Zhang, J., Yang, Y., Deng, M., and Xie, X. 2013. Radix *Angelica sinensis* that contains the component Z-ligustilide promotes adult neurogenesis to mediate recovery from cognitive impairment. *Curr Neurovasc Res*, 10(4): 304–15.

Yamada, K., Mimaki, Y., and Sashida, Y. 1994. Anticonvulsive effects of inhaling lavender oil vapour. *Biol Pharm Bull*, 17(2): 359–60.

Yamada, K., Mimaki, Y., and Sashida, Y. 2005. Effects of inhaling the vapor of *Lavandula burnatii* super-derived essential oil and linalool on plasma adrenocorticotropic hormone (ACTH), catecholamine and gonadotropin levels in experimental menopausal female rats. *Biol Pharm Bull*, 28: 378–79.

Yan, J.J., Kim, D.H., Moon, Y.S. et al. 2004. Protection against beta-amyloid peptide-induced memory impairment with long-term administration of extract of *Angelica gigas* or decursinol in mice. *Prog Neuropsychopharmacol Biol Psychiatry*, 28(1): 25–30.

Yoshida, H., Meng, P., Matsumiya, T. et al. 2014. Carnosic acid suppresses the production of amyloid-β 1-42 and 1-43 by inducing an α-secretase TACE/ADAM17 in U373MG human astrocytoma cells. *Neurosci Res*, 79: 83–93.

Yu, H., Zhang, Z.L., Chen, J. et al. 2012. Carvacrol, a food-additive, provides neuroprotection on focal cerebral ischemia/reperfusion injury in mice. *PLoS One*, e33584.

Yun, J. 2014. Limonene inhibits methamphetamine-induced locomotor activity via regulation of 5-HT neuronal function and dopamine release. *Phytomedicine*, 21(6): 883–87.

Zhao, R.J., Koo, B.S., Kim, G.W. et al. 2005. The essential oil from *Angelica gigas* NAKAI suppresses nicotine sensitization. *Biol Pharm Bull*, 28(12): 2323–26.

Zheng, P., Zhang, J., Liu, H., Xu, X., and Zhang, X. 2008. Angelica injection reduces cognitive impairment during chronic cerebral hypoperfusion through brain-derived neurotrophic factor and nerve growth factor. *Curr Neurovasc Res*, 5(1): 13–20.

Zotti, M., Colaianna, M., Morgese, M.G. et al. 2013. Carvacrol: From ancient flavoring to neuromodulatory agent. *Molecules*, 18(6): 6161–72.

12 Rational Basis for Research and Development of Essential Oils in Pain Trials

*Laura Rombolà, Luigi Antonio Morrone,
Chizuko Watanabe, Hirokazu Mizoguchi,
Tsukasa Sakurada, Laura Berliocchi,
Maria Tiziana Corasaniti, Giacinto Bagetta,
and Shinobu Sakurada*

CONTENTS

12.1 INTRODUCTION

Pain is a common and serious health problem worldwide. Pain affects all populations, regardless of age, sex, income, race/ethnicity, or geography (Goldberg and McGee, 2011). Those who experience pain can experience acute, chronic, or intermittent pain, or a combination of the three. Particularly, chronic pain affects approximately 20% of the adult European population and is more frequent in women and older people (Gupta et al., 2012; see Van Hecke et al., 2013). Unfortunately, pain management in the community remains generally unsatisfactory and rarely under the control of currently available analgesics (Cherubino et al., 2012). Chronic pain leads to physical and psychological dysfunctions, including, but not limited to, depression, anxiety, stress, inability to work, disrupted social relationships, and suicidal thoughts (Cecchi et al., 2009; see Goldberg and McGee, 2011; Gorczyca et al., 2013; Fadgyas-Stanculete et al., 2014; Novy and Aigner, 2014; Strobel et al., 2014). Despite advances in pain management, pain continues to be undertreated, and some studies suggest viewing pain using a multidimensional and holistic approach (see Tang and Tse, 2014). Consequently, a variety of pharmacological and nonpharmacological treatments have been investigated (see Boldt et al., 2014; Kizhakkeveettil et al., 2014). Although drugs are the most effective available means to control pain, patients suffering from pain can benefit from complementary medicines (see Boldt et al., 2014; Crawford et al., 2014; Kizhakkeveettil et al., 2014). Among the latter, a number of clinical research works have reported promising findings in reducing pain in adults and infants with aromatherapy, a branch of herbal medicine (Pruthi et al., 2010; Hadi and Hanid, 2011; Çetinkaya and Başbakkal, 2012; Sasannejad et al., 2012; Olapour et al., 2013; Sadeghi Aval Shahr et al., 2014). Interestingly, aromatherapy can be effective in relieving pain, but also in reducing side effects of analgesics (Kim et al., 2006, 2007; Soltani et al., 2013). However, several clinical studies report contradictory findings (Kim et al., 2006; De Jong et al., 2012; Masaoka et al., 2013), with some suggesting that exposure to odors may not lead to pain relief (Martin et al., 2006). Pain is a complex experience consisting of sensory-discriminative, affective-motivational, and cognitive-evaluative dimensions with the activation of multiple neurons across the pain system and the interaction between the thalamus and cortex, as well as limbic system (Price, 2000; Yalcin et al., 2014). For example, the anterior cingulate cortex neurons are activated by painful stimulation and are involved in affective responses to pain (Ikeda et al., 2014). Accordingly, the analgesic effects induced by inhalation of essential oils could be attributed to their cognitive effects at the level of different cerebral areas involved in the descending inhibitory system. The capacity of the essential oils to affect cerebral areas involved in pain and cognitive processes could represent a challenge in pain treatment, for example, in management of pain in dementia (Ballard et al., 2009; Wells et al., 2010). Untreated pain is a major contributor to reduced quality of life and disability, and can lead to increased behavioral and psychological symptoms of dementia (Corbett et al., 2012; Achterberg et al., 2013).

Moreover, massage with essential oils induces analgesic effects enlightening upon the peripheral action of essential oils on primary sensory neurons (Yip and Tam, 2008).

Despite the large use of essential oils in traditional and complementary medicine, as well as primary care settings, evidence for the efficacy and mechanistic understanding of aromatherapy in treating medical conditions remains poor, with a particular lack of studies employing rigorous methodology in clinical trials. Replication, longer follow-up, and larger trials (Germann et al., 2013) are needed to accrue the necessary evidence for therapeutic use of essential oils.

In this review preclinical results on the analgesic effects of some essential oils extracted from different aromatic plants are analyzed, and they are a springboard for the oils' rational use in forthcoming clinical trials.

12.2   ESSENTIAL OILS AND PRECLINICAL RESULTS

12.2.1   *LAVANDULA* SPECIES

Lavandula (lavender) is a flowering plant from the Lamiaceae family, native of the western Mediterranean region. *Lavandula* species and their essential oils have been used in complementary medicine for several centuries as sedatives, antidepressants, anticonvulsants, antispasmodics, antimicrobials, and analgesics and anti-inflammatories (Chu and Kemper, 2001; Cavanagh and Wilkinson, 2002; see Koulivand et al., 2013). Lavender oil has been particularly attributed with mood-enhancing and analgesic properties in healthy subjects and in experimental nociception (see Kim et al., 2006; Stea et al., 2014). In a formalin test, oral administration in mice of *Lavandula angustifolia* Mill. essential oil, 1 hour prior to formalin injection, dose-dependently inhibited the licking response to the formalin injected paw in the first and second phases of the test (Hajhashemi et al., 2003). The first phase is generated in the periphery through the activation of nociceptive neurons by the direct action of formalin, while in the late phase, a combination of an inflammatory reaction in peripheral tissue and functional changes in the dorsal horn of the spinal cord is involved (Tjolsen et al., 1992). The capacity of the phytocomplex to inhibit both phases of the test indicates antinociceptive and anti-inflammatory properties. *L. angustifolia* essential oil also produced a dose-dependent inhibition of the inflammatory pain in mice in acetic acid–induced abdominal writhing (Hajhashemi et al., 2003), a visceral inflammatory pain model (Barber and Gottschlich, 1992). Moreover, the anti-inflammatory activity of lavender oil was confirmed in rat by the reduction of the paw edema following injection of carrageenan (Hajhashemi et al., 2003). Altogether, these results confirm the traditional use of *L. angustifolia* for the treatment of painful and inflammatory conditions. More recently, Huang and colleagues (2012) have reported that lavender inhibits lipopolysaccharide (LPS)-induced inflammatory reaction in human monocyte THP-1 cells. Particularly, the authors observed inhibition of the production of interleukin-1β (IL-1β) and superoxide anion and downregulation of LPS-induced protein levels of both phospho-NF-κB and membrane Toll-like receptor 4. In addition, results showed that the phytocomplex increased heat shock protein 70 (HSP70) expression in LPS-stimulated THP-1 cells, suggesting that the essential oil–inhibited LPS-induced inflammatory effect might be associated with the expression of HSP70 (Huang et al., 2012). Lavender oil also revealed an interesting analgesic activity after inhalation, at doses devoid of sedative side effects (Barocelli et al., 2004). Particularly, *Lavandula hybrida* Reverchon "Grosso" essential oil significantly reduced the acetic acid writhing response in a naloxone-sensitive manner. In addition, in the hot-plate test the analgesic activity observed after oil inhalation was inhibited by naloxone, atropine, and mecamylamine pretreatment, suggesting the involvement of opioidergic as well as cholinergic pathways (Barocelli et al., 2004). Interestingly, Barocelli and colleagues (2004) reported a remarkable gastroprotective effect of oral lavender oil on acute ethanol-induced gastric lesions, while it did not protect against indomethacin-induced gastric ulcers for either oral administration or inhalation; the latter evidence suggests that gastroprotection afforded by lavender oil is not due to interference with the constitutive arachidonic acid metabolic cascade. Major constituents present in the volatile fraction of *Lavandula* species are the terpenes, 1,8-cineol, limonene, linalool, and linalyl acetate (Hajhashemi et al., 2003; Barocelli et al., 2004; Lakusić et al., 2014), which showed antinociceptive and anti-inflammatory activities (see Guimarães et al., 2013).

Several studies indicate that 1,8-cineol induced anti-inflammatory effects through the inhibition of cyclooxygenase (COX), suppression of arachidonic acid metabolism, and cytokine (tumor necrosis factor [TNF]-α and IL-1β) production (Santos and Rao, 2000; Juergens et al., 2004). Zhou and colleagues (2007) showed that 1,8-cineol might suppress the expression of many genes important for inflammation by inhibiting early growth response factor-1 (Egr-1) synthesis and nuclear localization. 1,8-Cineol produced cooling sensations by directly activating the transient receptor potential (TRP) channel TRPM8, which contributes to its analgesic activity (Behrendt et al., 2004; Proudfoot et al., 2006). Limonene also showed a significant antinociceptive effect in different models of pain (Do Amaral et al., 2007; Piccinelli et al., 2014) by the writhing test and the second phase of the formalin test, but not the hot-plate test (Do Amaral et al., 2007). Interestingly, limonene-induced antinociception in the second phase of the formalin test was insensitive to naloxone. The antinociceptive effect of limonene was attributed to the anti-inflammatory activity responsible for a decrease of cytokine release and cell migration, in addition to a potent antioxidant effect (Hirota et al., 2010). Linalool and its metabolic precursor, linalyl acetate, was endowed with analgesic activity in several models of pain (Peana et al., 2003, 2004a,b; Berliocchi et al., 2009; Sakurada et al., 2009, 2011). However, at variance with lavender oil, both linalool and linalyl acetate produced only scarce or no analgesic effect in the two pain models adopted in the study of Barocelli and colleagues (2004). The latter results were in apparent contrast with the data yielded by Peana and colleagues (2003, 2004a), and this may stem from the use of different doses in identical tests. Linalool decreased thermal hyperalgesia induced by carrageenan, L-glutamate, and prostaglandin E_2 (Peana et al., 2004b). Different receptors and K^+ channels contribute to the analgesic effects of linalool (Peana et al., 2003, 2004a; Sakurada et al., 2011) other than a local anesthetic activity and a negative modulation of glutamate transmission (Elisabetsky et al., 1999; Ghelardini et al., 1999; Silva Brum et al., 2001). Moreover, an anti-inflammatory activity of linalool was due to its ability to reduce nitric oxide (NO) production or release, and this was confirmed by the inhibitory effect on nitrite accumulation *in vitro* (Peana et al., 2006), as well as its capacity to prevent lipid peroxidation (Celik and Ozkaya, 2001).

12.2.2 *CITRUS* SPECIES

Citrus species (Rutaceae) are the most widely grown fruit crops (see Donmez et al., 2013). Some species of *Citrus* have a broad spectrum of biological activities, including antibacterial, antifungal, antiviral, antioxidant, analgesic, and anti-inflammatory (see Campêlo et al., 2011). Research-based results with different species of *Citrus* essential oils indicate central and peripheral effects. Aroma interferes with cerebral areas involved in pain and emotional control (Aloisi et al., 2002; Ceccarelli et al., 2002, 2004; Ikeda et al., 2014). Local application of the oils, through lipophilic compounds, such as linalool and linalyl acetate (Berliocchi et al., 2009; Sakurada et al., 2009; Batista et al., 2010), β-caryophyllene (Kuwahata et al., 2012; Katsuyama et al., 2013), or naringenin (Straub et al., 2013; Hu and Zhao, 2014), induces anti-inflammatory and antinocicpeptive effects, amplifying opioid response on sensitive neurons (Bagetta et al., 2010; Sakurada et al., 2011; Kuwahata et al., 2013). In the formalin test, inhalation of *Citrus lemon* essential oil induced sex-specific changes in neuronal circuits involved in anxiety and pain (Aloisi et al., 2002; Ceccarelli et al., 2002, 2004). In female rats, lemon oil decreased the second phase of licking in the injected paw, and this analgesic effect was associated with an altered degree of neuronal activation in limbic structures (Aloisi et al., 2002). This phytocomplex increased c-Fos expression in the arcuate nucleus of the hypothalamus, whereas lemon oil and formalin increase c-Fos in the paraventricular nucleus of the hypothal-amus and in the dentate gyrus of the hippocampus (Aloisi et al., 2002). Interestingly, in the paraventricular nucleus, formalin induced higher c-Fos than control in both sexes; when formalin was injected with the phytocomplex, c-Fos further increased in males, but remained at control levels in females (Aloisi et al., 2002). These same authors observed a decreased content of β-endorphin in the periaqueductal gray mat-ter (PAG) in rats exposed to lemon odor. Altogether, these results suggest that lemon oil affects brain areas involved in the modulation of nociceptive input.

More recently, Ikeda and colleagues (2014) have evaluated the influence of lemon oil on pain sensitivity in mice, suggesting that the analgesic effect of lemon odor is mediated by the descending inhibitory system via the periaqueductal gray-rostral ventromedial medulla pathway. The origin of the latter inhibitory system may be the dopamine-related activation of the anterior cingulate cortical neurons by the lemon odor (Ikeda et al., 2014). Moreover, oral administration of lemon oil produced a dose-dependent inhibition of the inflammatory pain in mice as determined by a sig-nificant reduction in acetic acid–induced abdominal writhing (Campêlo et al., 2011). The latter effect was reversed by pretreatment with naloxone, suggesting the involve-ment of the opioid system.

The essential oil of bergamot (*Citrus bergamia* Risso et Poiteau) has been used by folk medicine as an antiseptic and anthelmintic and to facilitate wound healing. *In vitro* studies demonstrated cytotoxic effects, potential protective activity on tumor cells (Berliocchi et al., 2011; Russo et al., 2013, 2015), and an increase in the oxida-tive metabolism in human polymorphonuclear leukocytes (Cosentino et al., 2014). In normal rats, bergamot oil produces a dose-related sequence of sedative and stimula-tory behavioral effects (Rombolà et al., 2009) and affects synaptic transmission by modulating release of specific amino acid neurotransmitters (Morrone et al., 2007) that could underlie its neuroprotective (Amantea et al., 2009), anxiolytic (Saiyudthong and Marsden, 2011), and analgesic effects (see Bagetta et al., 2010). In formalin and capsaicin tests, intraplantar injection of bergamot essential oil produced a significant antinociceptive effect (Sakurada et al., 2009; Katsuyama et al., 2015). The injection of capsaicin into the hindpaw induced an immediate, short-lasting, nociceptive response (approximately 5 min) (Sakurada et al., 1992). Capsaicin acts on transient receptor potential vanilloid type-1 (TRPV-1) receptors located mainly on C-fiber-type nociceptors (Szallasi, 2006) and releases endogenous tachykinins (Sakurada et al., 1992), substance P or neurokinin A, and glutamate from primary sensory neu-rons in the dorsal spinal cord (Holzer 1991; Sakurada et al., 1998). In the nociceptive tests, bergamot oil acts on sensitization of the afferent nerve fibers; in fact, the administration in the contralateral paw did not induce analgesia (Sakurada et al., 2009; Katsuyama et al., 2015). This local antinociceptive effect is mediated, at least in part, by interaction with the peripheral opioid system; in fact, pretreatment with naloxone or naloxone methyl iodide, an opioid receptor antagonist unable to cross the blood–brain barrier, reverted the effect of the oil (Sakurada et al., 2011; Katsuyama et al., 2015). Intrathecal injection of morphine induces dose-dependent antinociception in the capsaicin test (Sakurada et al., 1994), but it is known that drugs that interfere with opioid receptors cause central adverse effects. Synergistic antinociceptive effects were observed after intraplantar injection of an inactive dose of bergamot essential oil with systemic or intrathecal low doses of morphine (Sakurada et al., 2011). Likely, after systemic or central administration, morphine acts, respectively, at the spinal or supraspinal level, while the phytocomplex acts locally, amplifying the effects mediated by opioid receptors. Interestingly, bergamot essential oil contains linalool and linalyl acetate in high concentrations, and intraplantar injection of *Citrus sinensis* essential oil, known to contain extremely small amounts of linalool and linalyl acetate, did not induce antinociceptive effects (Sakurada et al., 2009). These results confirm the antinociceptive effects observed with the monoterpenes in capsaicin and formalin tests (Sakurada et al., 2011; Katsuyama et al., 2015) and in the inflammatory pain model induced by complete Freund's adjuvant (CFA) (Batista et al., 2010). Moreover, local injection of bergamot essential oil induces analgesic effects in different neuropathic pain models in mice (Bagetta et al., 2010; Kuwahata et al., 2013). Peripheral nerve damage injury produces long-lasting, heterogeneous pain conditions referred to as neuropathic pain, which is manifested by hyperalgesia, as well as allodynia, with the perception of typically innocuous stimuli being painful (Jensen and Finnerup, 2014). Subchronic systemic administration of bergamot essential oil has been shown to attenuate mechanical allodynia (Bagetta et al., 2010) in the spinal nerve ligation (SNL) model of neuropathic pain (Kim and Chung, 1992), and this has been attributed, at least in part, to the anti-inflammatory action of linalool at the spinal level (Berliocchi et al., 2009; Batista et al., 2010). In a partial sciatic nerve injury (PSNI) model (Seltzer et al., 1990), intraplantar injection of the phytocomplex in the injured paw induced a local antiallodynic effect; in fact, the administration of the oil in the controlateral hindpaw did not attenuate nociceptive response (Kuwahata et al., 2013). Similar results were also observed after local injection of linalool, although the effects induced by the monoterpene were longer lasting. Neuropathic pain has often been reported to be resistant to opioids, including morphine; in fact, neither systemic nor intrathecal (i.t.) morphine is effective in experimental models of neuropathic pain. In mice with PSNI, a large dose of morphine is required to achieve an antiallodynic effect similar to that obtained with a much lower dose in the capsaicin test (Sakurada et al., 2011). In neuropathic mice, intraplantar injection of very low doses of morphine induced a dose-dependent analgesic effect when combined with inactive doses of bergamot essential oil or linalool (Kuwahata et al., 2013). This latter effect results from interactions with primary afferent neurons, and this is important since unwanted side effects in the central nervous system (CNS) are avoided. Several studies indicate that astrocytes and microglia in the CNS are activated by noxious stimuli, including nerve injury and inflammation, and play an important role in the maintenance of long-term chronic pain (McMahon and Malcangio, 2009) via the activation of multiple signaling pathways, such as extracellular-signal-regulated kinase (ERK) and mitogen-activated protein kinase (MAPK). Intraplantar injection of bergamot essential oil or linalool reduces ERK activation in the lumbar spinal cord, suggesting that the antiallodynic effect observed with these natural products is also mediated by a modulation of the MAPK signaling pathways (Kuwahata et al., 2013). Recently, it was reported that intraplantar injection of β-caryophyllene, an ingredient of bergamot essential oil and common constituent of the essential oils of several plants, including *Cannabis* (Gertsch et al., 2008), exerted dose-dependent analgesic effects in inflammatory (Katsuyama et al., 2013) and neuropathic (Kuwahata et al., 2012) pain models. The analgesic effect is CB2 receptor dependent since it was minimized by AM630, a selective CB2 antagonist, but not by AM251, a selective CB1 antagonist. In the capsaicin test, the combination of ineffective doses of β-caryophyllene and morphine increased antinociception, and this effect was reversed by pretreatment with naloxone hydrochloride, while pretreatment with β-endorphin antisera did not show significant effects (Katsuyama et al., 2013). These data suggest that the enhanced effect of the combination is mediated through simultaneous activation of both central and peripheral opioid receptors. The possible underlying mechanism could be due to a functional enhancement between the separate sites of action following systemic or spinal injection of morphine acting at the supraspinal or spinal level. Morphine binds mainly μ-opioid receptors, and β-caryophyllene acts at the peripheral level, further increasing the release of the endogenous β-endorphin through CB2 receptor–mediated events (Katsuyama et al., 2013). Considering other *Citrus* species, Sood and colleagues (2009) reported that *Citrus decumana* peel extract shows significant antioxidant activity *in vitro* and produces a significant decrease in paw volume and pain when compared with diclofenac and morphine, respectively. Recently, some studies reported that flavonoids in *Citrus* fruits possess anti-inflammatory and antinociceptive properties. Particularly, intrathecal administration of naringenin dose-dependently attenuated the mechanical allodynia and thermal hyperalgesia induced by SNL and significantly inhibited expression of inflammatory mediators in neuropathic pain (Hu and Zhao, 2014). Interestingly, Straub and colleagues (2013) suggested that flavonoids such as naringenin and hesperetin, which selectively inhibit TRPM3, significantly reduced the sensitivity of mice to noxious heat and pregnenolone sulfate–induced chemical pain.

12.2.3 Ocimum Species

The genus *Ocimum* (Lamiaceae) has a long history of use as culinary and medicinal herbs. Particularly, *Ocimum basilicum* Linn. has been used traditionally for the treatment of anxiety, diabetes, cardiovascular diseases, headaches, and nerve pain and as an anticonvulsant and anti-inflammatory, and it has also been used in a variety of neurodegenerative disorders (see Bora et al., 2011; Nascimento et al., 2015). Antinociceptive and antinflammatory activity of *O. basilicum* was observed in the formalin test, where the phytocomplex reduced paw licking time in the first and second phases. In the hot-plate test, the essential oil significantly increased the latency at the low dose injected, and this effect was reverted by naloxone (Venâncio et al., 2011). Systemic administration of *O. basilicum* oil was also effective in reducing the abdominal contractions in the writing test (Venâncio et al., 2011). The authors suggested that the peripheral and central antinociceptive effects of the phytocomplex are related to the biosynthesis inhibition of pain mediators, such as prostaglandins and prostacyclins, and its ability to interact with opioid receptors (Venâncio et al., 2011). More recently, in a mice fibromyalgia model, Nascimento and colleagues (2015) reported that oral treatment with *O. basilicum* essential oil, isolated or complexed with β-cyclodextrin, at all doses tested, produced a significant reduction of mechanical hyperalgesia and increased Fos protein expression in the central nervous system, suggesting an analgesic effect on chronic noninflammatory pain such as fibromyalgia. In zymosan synovitis associated with hyperalgesia in animal models of knee arthritis (Gegout et al., 1994), the essential oil obtained by hydrodistillation from *Ocimum americanum* L. inhibited leukocyte influx into the synovial space and reduced paw edema and interferon-γ levels (Yamada et al., 2013). The chemical composition of the oils obtained from *O. basilicum* L. and *O. americanum* L. indicated that linalool and 1,8-cineol were among the main compounds present in the volatile fraction (Bassolé et al., 2010; Yamada et al., 2013). Recently, the antinociceptive properties of *Ocimum gratissimum* essential oil and two of its active principles, eugenol and myrcene, were tested in thermal and inflammatory models of pain (Paula-Freire et al., 2013). Mice acutely received oral administration of the oil, eugenol or myrcene, morphine, and corn oil. The highest doses of the drugs significantly increased the latency to lick the paw in the hot-plate test and were effective in minimizing pain in the first and second phases of the formalin test (Paula-Freire et al., 2013). Interestingly, the antinociceptive effect shown by all drugs tested in the hot-plate test was reverted by naloxone. Conversely, in the writhing test, *Ocimum micranthum* essential oil inhibited the contractions induced by acetic acid, and this effect was not reversed by naloxone (Lino et al., 2005). Pretreatment with L-arginine reversed the antinociception, suggesting an involvement of the nitric oxide system (Lino et al., 2005). Moreover, *O. micranthum* oil did not show a significant antiedema effect in the carrageenan and dextran models (Lino et al., 2005). Pinho and colleagues (2012) reported for the phytocomplex antinociceptive and antispasmodic properties but did not observe any activity in the hot-plate test. One of the major components of the volatile fraction of *Ocimum* species is the CB2 receptor selective agonist β-caryophyllene (Gertsch et al., 2008). CB2-selective agonists induced good antinociceptive effects in several animal models of pain and failed to show psychoactive effects (see Maione et al., 2013). Oral administration of β-caryophyllene produced potent anti-inflammatory effects in wild-type mice but not in mice lacking CB2 receptors (Gertsch et al., 2008). Similar effects are reported by Klauke and colleagues (2014), confirming an anti-inflammatory activity of β-caryophyllene in the late phase of the formalin test after oral administration. These same authors indicated that subchronic treatment with β-caryophyllene reduced mechanical allodynia and thermal hyperalgesia in the partial spinal nerve ligation model of neuropathic pain. These effects were not observed in CB2$^{-/-}$ neuropathic mice (Klauke et al., 2014). More recently, Paula-Freire and colleagues (2014) reported that sesquiterpene trans-caryophyllene administration significantly minimized pain in acute and chronic pain models. Interestingly, the antinociceptive effect observed during the hot-plate test was reversed by naloxone and AM630, indicating the participation of both the opioid and endocannabinoid systems. Trans-caryophyllene treatment also decreased the IL-1β levels in the chronic constriction injury (CCI) of the sciatic nerve in mice, a chronic pain model. In this same model of pain, subchronic administration of *Ocimum sanctum* and its saponin-rich fraction significantly attenuated CCI-induced neuropathic pain, as well as decreased the oxidative stress and calcium levels (Kaur et al., 2015).

12.2.4 CROTON SPECIES

Croton is a large genus of Euphorbiaceae, comprising around 1300 species of trees, shrubs, and herbs distributed in tropical and subtropical regions of both hemispheres. Several species have a long-standing role in the traditional use of medicinal plants in Africa, Asia, and South America in the treatment of constipation, digestive problems, ulcers, dysentery, intestinal worms, diabetes, hypercholesterolemia, weight loss, malaria, fever, inflammation, pain, hypertension, and cancer (see Salatino et al., 2007). Crude leaf extracts of *Croton cajucara* Benth exhibited a significant antinociceptive effect in rats (Campos et al., 2002). Particularly, phytocomplexes demonstrated significant inhibition of acetic acid–induced writhing and the second phase response of formalin, but did not manifest a significant effect in the hot-plate test (Campos et al., 2002). Similarly, *Croton sonderianus* essential oil showed antinociceptive activity against chemical nociception induced in mice by intraperitoneal acetic acid, subplantar capsaicin, or formalin, though it lacked efficacy against thermal nociception (Santos et al., 2005). Ethanol extract of *Croton crassifolius* also showed no significant antinociceptive activity in the hot-plate test, although it significantly reduced acetic acid–induced writhing and caused marked dose-related inhibition of formalin-induced pain in the second phase (Zhao et al., 2012). Conversely, for oral administration, the volatile oil of *Croton nepetaefolius* promoted a dose-dependent antinociceptive effect in the hot-plate test (Abdon et al., 2002). The antinociception caused by *C. sonderianus* oil seems to be unrelated to motor impairment or sedation since in rotarod and barbiturate sleeping time tests it showed no significant effects (Santos et al., 2005). The authors suggested that the phytocomplex produced antinociception possibly involving glibenclamide-sensitive K-ATP+ channels (Santos et al., 2005). The analgesic effects of *C. sonderianus* oil were observed at low doses with respect to other *Croton* species, and this could be attributed to the level of β-caryophyllene present in this essential oil. The capacity of *C. nepetaefolius* oil to suppress thermal nociception was attributed to the large amounts of 1,8-cineol present in the volatile fraction (Santos et al., 2005). Furthermore, the results obtained by some studies suggested that *Croton celtidifolius* possesses antinociceptive properties since the phytocomplex fractions and particularly 63SF, a proanthocyanidin-rich fraction, significantly reduced the writhing induced by acetic acid and the nociception in both phases of the formalin test (DalBó et al., 2005; Nardi et al., 2006). Moreover, the same authors suggested that the 63SF exerted antinociceptive effects by enhancing the activity of descending control, possibly by direct stimulation of dopaminergic D_2 receptors (DalBó et al., 2006). *C. cajucara* Benth essential oil dose-dependently inhibited carrageenan-induced edema and chronic inflammation in the cotton pellet granuloma model (Bighetti et al., 1999). Particularly, the anti-inflammatory effect observed was comparable to that obtained with diclofenac. Interestingly, at the same dose, *C. cajucara* oil showed antiulcerogenic activity similar to that seen with an equal dose of cimetidine (Hiruma-Lima et al., 2002). The diterpene trans-dehydrocrotonin, isolated from the bark of *C. cajucara* Benth, produced a significant inhibition of carrageenin-induced paw edema and cotton pellet granuloma in rats. It also inhibited the writhings induced in mice by acetic acid, but did not show a significant effect in the hot-plate test in mice (Carvalho et al., 1996).

An antinociceptive effect of the volatile oil of *Croton zehntneri* was likely associated with its anti-inflammatory activity (Oliveira et al., 2001). Moreover, the aqueous extract of *Croton malambo* bark administered intraperitoneally showed antinociceptive and anti-inflammatory effects comparable to those of acetylsalicylic acid and sodium diclofenac (Suárez et al., 2003).

12.2.5 SALVIA SPECIES

Salvia is a genus consisting of about 900 species in the family Lamiaceae that is used in folk medicine to treat different peripheral and central diseases. Imanshahidi and Hosseinzadeh (2006) reviewed the pharmacological effects of different *Salvia* species on the central nervous system. *Salvia leriifolia* leaf extract showed a significant antinociceptive effect in the hot-plate test reversed by naloxone, but it was ineffective to reduce nociceptive stimulus in the tail flick test, indicating that the spinal mechanism is not involved (Hosseinzadeh et al., 2003). Anti-inflammatory effects were observed in a vascular permeability test induced by acid acetic and in xylene-induced ear edema (Hosseinzadeh et al., 2003). Similar results were reported in the chronic inflammatory model using the cotton pellet test. However, the analgesic effects of *S. leriifolia* were observed following administration of high systemic doses of the extract. Conversely, antinociceptive effects in the hot-plate test are shown with *Salvia limbata*, *Salvia hypoleuca*, and *Salvia macrosiphon* at low doses (Karami et al., 2013). Hydroalcoholic extract from *Salvia officinalis* leaves inhibited, after oral administration, the number of writhings induced by acetic acid, and in the formalin test, it reduced both neurogenic and inflammatory phases. Naloxone reversed the antinociceptive effect, suggesting participation of the opioid system (Rodrigues et al., 2012). In glutamate, capsaicin and cinnamaldehyde (agonist of transient receptor potential A1 [TRPA1]) models, the nociception and paw edema were reduced by *S. officinalis* extract (Rodrigues et al., 2012). Carnosol and ursolic acid or oleanolic acid contained in this plant appear to contribute to the antinociceptive property of the extract, possibly through a modulatory influence on TRPA1 receptors (Rodrigues et al., 2012). Similar results were obtained with aqueous and butanol extracts of *S. officinalis*, although at the highest doses (Qnais et al., 2010). These authors indicated that both extracts exhibited an antinociceptive effect against formalin-induced nociception and the hot-plate test, as well as anti-inflammatory activity against carrageenan-induced paw edema and formation of cotton pellet granuloma (Qnais et al., 2010). In addition, essential oil of *Salvia sclarea* showed analgesic effects on the capsaicin-induced nociceptive response in rats (Sakurada et al., 2009). Jung and colleagues (2009) also reported that the ethanol extract of *Salvia plebeia* exhibited anti-inflammatory activities in vascular permeability and air-pouch models and displayed antinociceptive activities in the writhing response model in mice. Recently, scientific interest was addressed to study the pharmacological properties of salvinorin A, a diterpene present in *Salvia divinorum* and agonist of κ-opioid receptors (KORs) (Cunningham et al., 2011). Anti-inflammatory effects were observed in LPS-stimulated murine macrophages where salvinorin A reduced TNF-α and restored the LPS-increased levels of IL-10, a regulatory cytokine that acts by limiting the inflammatory response (Aviello et al., 2011). Moreover, salvinorin A reduced nitrite levels, and this was reversed by naloxone, nor-binaltorphimine (selective KOR antagonist), and rimonabant (CB1 receptor antagonist), suggesting that the anti-inflammatory effect of salvinorin A could be mediated by opioid and cannabinoid systems (Aviello et al., 2011). An anti-inflammatory effect of the diterpene was also shown in mice in LPS- and carrageenan-induced paw edema (Aviello et al., 2011). Salvinorin A partially reduced the first phase of formalin-induced nociceptive behavior, and it completely abolished the second one (Aviello et al., 2011). Subchronic treatment with the diterpene was also effective in reducing formalin-induced ipsilateral allodynia (Guida et al., 2012). Salvinorin A reduced the formalin-mediated microglia and astrocyte activation and modulated pro- and anti-inflammatory mediators in the spinal cord (Guida et al., 2012). Moreover, salvianolic acid B, the most characteristic constituent of *Salvia miltiorrhiza* Bge, was effective against mechanical hyperalgesia in an animal model of neuropathic pain where a peripheral mononeuropathy was produced by a chronic constriction injury of the sciatic nerve (Isacchi et al., 2011).

REFERENCES

Abdon, A.P., Leal-Cardoso, J.H., Coelho-de-Souza, A.N. et al. 2002. Antinociceptive effects of the essential oil of *Croton nepetaefolius* on mice. *Med Biol Res*, 35(10): 1215–19.

Achterberg, W.P., Pieper, M.J., van Dalen-Kok, A.H. et al. 2013. Pain management in patients with dementia. *Clin Interv Aging*, 8: 1471–82.

Aloisi, A.M., Ceccarelli, I., Masi, F., and Scaramuzzino, A. 2002. Effects of the essential oil from *Citrus lemon* in male and female rats exposed to a persistent painful stimulation. *Behav Brain Res*, 136: 127–35.

Amantea, D., Fratto, V., Maida, S. et al. 2009. Prevention of glutamate accumulation and upregulation of phospho-Akt may account for neuroprotection afforded by bergamot essential oil against brain injury induced by focal cerebral ischemia in rat. *Int Rev Neurobiol*, 85: 389–405.

Aviello, G., Borrelli, F., Guida, F. et al. 2011. Ultrapotent effects of salvinorin A, hallucinogenic compound from *Salvia divinorum*, on LPS-stimulated murine macrophages and its anti-inflammatory action in vivo. *J Mol Med* (Berl), 89(9): 891–902.

Bagetta, G., Morrone, L.A., Rombolà, L. et al. 2010. Neuropharmacology of the essential oil of bergamot [Review]. *Fitoterapia*, 81: 453–61.

Ballard, C.G., Gauthier, S., Cummings, J.L. et al. 2009. Management of agitation and aggression associated with Alzheimer disease [Review]. *Nat Rev Neurol*, 5(5): 245–55.

Barber, A., and Gottschlich, R. 1992. Opioid agonists and antagonists: An evaluation of their peripheral actions in inflammation. *Med Res Rev*, 12(5): 525–62.

Barocelli, E., Calcina, F., Chiavarini, M. et al. 2004. Antinociceptive and gastroprotective effects of inhaled and orally administered *Lavandula hybrida* Reverchon "Grosso" essential oil. *Life Sci*, 76(2): 213–23.

Bassolé, I.H., Lamien-Meda, A., Bayala, B. et al. 2010. Composition and antimicrobial activities of *Lippia multiflora* Moldenke, *Mentha* × *piperita* L., and *Ocimum basilicum* L. essential oils and their major monoterpene alcohols alone and in combination. *Molecules*, 15(11): 7825–39.

Batista, P.A., Werner, M.F.P., Oliveira, E.C. et al. 2010. The antinociceptive effect of (–)-linalool in models of chronic inflammatory and neuropathic hypersensitivity in mice. *J Pain*, 11: 1222–29.

Behrendt, H.J., Germann, T., Gillen, C. et al. 2004. Characterization of the mouse cold-menthol receptor TRPM8 and vanilloid receptor type-1 VR1 using a fluorometric imaging plate reader (FLIPR) assay. *Br J Pharmacol*, 141: 737–45.

Berliocchi, L., Russo, R., Levato, A. et al. 2009. (–)-Linalool attenuates allodynia in neuro-pathic pain induced by spinal nerve ligation in c57/bl6 mice. *Int Rev Neurobiol*, 85: 221–35.

Berliocchi, L., Ciociaro, A., Russo, R. et al. 2011. Toxic profile of bergamot essential oil on survival and proliferation of SH-SY5Y neuroblastoma cells. *Food Chem Toxicol*, 11: 2780–92.

Bighetti, E.J., Hiruma-Lima, C.A., Gracioso, J.S., and Brito, A.R. 1999. Antiinflammatory and antinociceptive effects in rodents of the essential oil of *Croton cajucara* Benth. *J Pharm Pharmacol*, 51(12): 1447–53.

Boldt, I., Eriks-Hoogland, I., Brinkhof, M.W. et al. 2014. Non-pharmacological interven-tions for chronic pain in people with spinal cord injury. *Cochrane Database Syst Rev*, 11: CD009177.

Bora, K.S., Arora, S., and Shri, R. 2011. Role of *Ocimum basilicum* L. in prevention of ische-mia and reperfusion-induced cerebral damage, and motor dysfunctions in mice brain. *J Ethnopharmacol*, 137(3): 1360–65.

Campêlo, L.M., de Almeida, A.A., de Freitas, R.L. et al. 2011. Antioxidant and anti-nociceptive effects of *Citrus limon* essential oil in mice. *J Biomed Biotechnol*. doi: 10.1155/2011/678673.

Campos, A.R., Albuquerque, F.A., Rao, V.S., Maciel, M.A., and Pinto, A.C. 2002. Investigations on the antinociceptive activity of crude extracts from *Croton cajucara* leaves in mice. *Fitoterapia*, 73(2): 116–20.

Carvalho, J.C., Silva, M.F., Maciel, M.A. et al. 1996. Investigation of anti-inflammatory and antinociceptive activities of trans-dehydrocrotonin, a 19-nor-clerodane diterpene from *Croton cajucara*. Part 1. *Planta Med*, 62(5): 402–4.

Cavanagh, H.M., and Wilkinson, J.M. 2002. Biological activities of lavender essential oil. *Phytother Res*, 16(4): 301–8.

Ceccarelli, I., Masi, F., Fiorenzani, P., and Aloisi, A.M. 2002. Sex differences in the cit-rus lemon essential oil-induced increase of hippocampal acetylcholine release in rats exposed to a persistent painful stimulation. *Neurosci Lett*, 330: 25–28.

Ceccarelli, I., Lariviere, W.R., Fiorenzani, P. et al. 2004. Effects of long-term exposure of lemon essential oil odor on behavioral, hormonal and neuronal parameters in male and female rats. *Brain Res*, 1001(1–2): 78–86.

Cecchi, F., Sgalambro, A., Baldi, M. et al. 2009. Microvascular dysfunction, myocardial isch-emia, and progression to heart failure in patients with hypertrophic cardiomyopathy. *J Cardiovasc Transl Res*, 2(4): 452–61. doi: 10.1007/s12265-009-9142-5.

Celik, S., and Ozkaya, A. 2001. Effects of intraperitoneally administered lipoic acid, vitamin E, and linalool on the level of total lipid and fatty acids in guinea pig brain with oxida-tive stress induced by H2O2. *J Biochem Mol Biol*, 35: 547–52.

Çetinkaya, B., and Başbakkal, Z. 2012. The effectiveness of aromatherapy massage using lavender oil as a treatment for infantile colic. *Int J Nurs Pract*, 18(2): 164–69. doi: 10.1111/j.1440-172X.2012.02015.x.

Cherubino, P., Sarzi-Puttini, P., Zuccaro, S.M., and Labianca, R. 2012. The management of chronic pain in important patient subgroups. *Clin Drug Investig*, 32(Suppl 1): 35–44. doi: 10.2165/11630060-000000000-00000.

Chu, C.J., and Kemper, K.J. 2001. *Lavender (Lavandula spp.)*. Boston: Longwood Herbal Task Force.

Corbett, A., Husebo, B., Malcangio, M. et al. 2012. Assessment and treatment of pain in people with dementia. *Nat Rev Neurol*, 8(5): 264–74.

Cosentino, M., Luini, A., Bombelli, R. et al. 2014. The essential oil of bergamot stimulates reactive oxygen species production in human polymorphonuclear leukocytes. *Phytother Res*, 28(8): 1232–39.

Crawford, C., Lee, C., Buckenmaier, C. et al. 2014. Active Self-Care Therapies for Pain (PACT) Working Group. The current state of the science for active self-care complementary and integrative medicine therapies in the management of chronic pain symptoms: Lessons learned, directions for the future. *Pain Med*, Suppl 1: S104–13.

Cunningham, C.W., Rothman, R.B., and Prisinzano, T.E. 2011. Neuropharmacology of the naturally occurring kappa-opioid hallucinogen salvinorin A. *Pharmacol Rev*, 63(2): 316–47.

DalBó, S., Jürgensen, S., Horst, H. et al. 2005. Antinociceptive effect of proanthocyanidins from *Croton celtidifolius* bark. *J Pharm Pharmacol*, 57(6): 765–71.

DalBó, S., Jürgensen, S., Horst, H. et al. 2006. Analysis of the antinociceptive effect of the proanthocyanidin-rich fraction obtained from *Croton celtidifolius* barks: Evidence for a role of the dopaminergic system. *Pharmacol Biochem Behav*, 85(2): 317–23.

De Jong, J.R., Vlaeyen, J.W., van Eijsden, M. et al. 2012. Reduction of pain-related fear and increased function and participation in work-related upper extremity pain (WRUEP): Effects of exposure in vivo. *Pain*, 153(10): 2109–18. doi: 10.1016/j.pain.2012.07.001.

Do Amaral, J.F., Silva, M.I.G., Neto, M.R.A. et al. 2007. Antinociceptive effect of the monoterpene R-(+)-limonene in mice. *Biol Pharm Bull*, 30: 1217–20.

Donmez, D., Simsek, O., Izgu, T. et al. 2013. Genetic transformation in citrus. *Scientific World Journal*. doi: 10.1155/2013/491207.

Elisabetsky, E., Brum, L.F., and Souza, D.O. 1999. Anticonvulsant properties of linalool in glutamate-related seizure models. *Phytomedicine*, 6: 107–13.

Fadgyas-Stanculete, M., Buga, A.M., Popa-Wagner, A., and Dumitrascu, D.L. 2014. The relationship between irritable bowel syndrome and psychiatric disorders: From molecular changes to clinical manifestations. *J Mol Psychiatry*, 2(1): 4. doi: 10.1186/2049-9256-2-4.

Gegout, P., Gillet, P., Chevrier, D. et al. 1994. Characterization of zymosan-induced arthritis in the rat: Effects on joint inflammation and cartilage metabolism. *Life Sci*, 55(17): 321–26.

Germann, P.G., Schuhmacher, A., Harrison, J. et al. 2013. How to create innovation by building the translation bridge from basic research into medicinal drugs: An industrial perspective. *Hum Genomics*, 5: 7–5.

Gertsch, J., Leonti, M., Raduner, S. et al. 2008. Beta-caryophyllene is a dietary cannabinoid. *Proc Natl Acad Sci USA*, 105(26): 9099–104.

Ghelardini, C., Galeotti, N., Salvatore, G., and Mazzanti, G. 1999. Local anaesthetic activity of the essential oil of *Lavandula angustifolia*. *Planta Medica*, 65: 700 3.

Goldberg, D.S., and McGee, S.J. 2011. Pain as a global public health priority. *BMC Public Health*. doi: 10.1186/1471-2458-11-770.

Gorczyca, R., Filip, R., and Walczak, E. 2013. Psychological aspects of pain. *Ann Agric Environ Med*, spec. no. 1: 23–27.

Guida, F., Luongo, L., Aviello, G. et al. 2012. Salvinorin A reduces mechanical allodynia and spinal neuronal hyperexcitability induced by peripheral formalin injection. *Mol Pain*, 8: 60. doi: 10.1186/1744-8069-8-60.

Guimarães, A.G., Quintans, J.S., and Quintans, L.J. 2013. Monoterpenes with analgesic activity: A systematic review. *J Phytother Res*, 27(1): 1–15.

Gupta, S., Gupta, M., Nath, S., and Hess, GM. 2012. Survey of European pain medicine practice. *Pain Physician* 15(6): E983–94.

Hadi, N., and Hanid, A.A. 2011. Lavender essence for post-cesarean pain. *Pak J Bio Sci*, 14: 664–67.

Hajhashemi, V., Ghannadi, A., and Sharif, B.J. 2003. Anti-inflammatory and analgesic properties of the leaf extracts and essential oil of *Lavandula angustifolia* Mill. *Ethnopharmacology*, 89(1): 67–71.

Hirota, R., Roger, N.N., Nakamura, H. et al. 2010. Anti-inflammatory effects of limonene from yuzu (*Citrus junos* Tanaka) essential oil on eosinophils. *J Food Sci*, 75: 87–92.

Hiruma-Lima, C.A., Gracioso, J.S., Bighetti, E.J. et al. 2002. Effect of essential oil obtained from *Croton cajucara* Benth. on gastric ulcer healing and protective factors of the gastric mucosa. *Phytomedicine*, 9(6): 523–29.

Holzer, P. 1991. Capsaicin: Cellular targets, mechanisms of action, and selectivity for thin sensory neurons. *Pharmacol Rev*, 43: 143–201.

Hosseinzadeh, H., Haddadkhodaparast, M.H., and Arash, A.R. 2003. Antinociceptive, anti-inflammatory and acute toxicity effects of *Salvia leriifolia* Benth seed extract in mice and rats. *Phytother Res*, 17(4): 422–25.

Hu, C.Y., and Zhao, Y.T. 2014. Analgesic effects of naringenin in rats with spinal nerve ligation-induced neuropathic pain. *Biomed Rep*, 2(4): 569–73.

Huang, M.Y., Liao, M.H., Wang, Y.K. et al. 2012. Effect of lavender essential oil on LPS-stimulated inflammation. *Am J Chin Med*, 40(4): 845–59.

Ikeda, H., Takasu, S., and Murase, K. 2014. Contribution of anterior cingulated cortex and descending pain inhibitory system to analgesic effect of lemon odor in mice. *Mol Pain*. doi: 10.1186/1744-8069_10-14.

Imanshahidi, M., and Hosseinzadeh, H. 2006. The pharmacological effects of *Salvia* species on the central nervous system. *Phytother Res*, 20(6): 427–37.

Isacchi, B., Fabbri, V., Galeotti, N. et al. 2011. Salvianolic acid B and its liposomal formulations: Anti-hyperalgesic activity in the treatment of neuropathic pain. *Eur J Pharm Sci*, 44(4): 552–58.

Jensen, T.S., and Finnerup, N.B. 2014. Allodynia and hyperalgesia in neuropathic pain: Clinical manifestations and mechanisms (Review). *Lancet Neurol* 13(9): 924–35. doi: 10.1016/S1474-4422(14)70102-4.

Juergens, U.R., Engelen, T., Racke, K. et al. 2004. Inhibitory activity of 1,8-cineol (eucalyptol) on cytokine production in cultured human lymphocytes and monocytes. *Pulm Pharmacol Ther*, 17: 281–87.

Jung, H.J., Song, Y.S., Lim, C.J., and Park, E.H. 2009. Anti-inflammatory, anti-angiogenic and anti-nociceptive activities of an ethanol extract of *Salvia plebeia* R. Brown. *J Ethnopharmacol*, 126(2): 355–60.

Karami, M., Shamerani, M.M., Hossini, E. et al. 2013. Antinociceptive activity and effect of methanol extracts of three *Salvia* spp. on withdrawal syndrome in mice. *Adv Pharm Bull*, 3(2): 457–59.

Katsuyama, S., Mizoguchi, H., Kuwahata, H. et al. 2013. Involvement of peripheral cannabinoid and opioid receptors in β-caryophyllene-induced antinociception. *Eur J Pain*, 17(5): 664–75.

Katsuyama, S., Otowa, A., Kamio, S. et al. 2015. Effect of plantar subcutaneous administration of bergamot essential oil and linalool on formalin-induced nociceptive behavior in mice. *Biomed Res*, 36(1): 47–54.

Kaur, G., Bali, A., Singh, N., and Jaggi, A.S. 2015. Ameliorative potential of *Ocimum sanctum* in chronic constriction injury-induced neuropathic pain in rats. *An Acad Bras Cienc*, 87(1): 417–429.

Kim, S.H., and Chung, J.M. 1992. An experimental model for peripheral neuropathy produced by segmental spinal nerve ligation in the rat. *Pain*, 50(3): 355–63.

Kim, J.T., Wajda, M., Cuff, G. et al. 2006. Evaluation of aromatherapy in treating postoperative pain: Pilot study. *Pain Pract*, 6: 273–77.

Kim, J.T., Ren, C.J., Fielding, G.A. et al. 2007. Treatment with lavender aromatherapy in the post-anesthesia care unit reduces opioid requirements of morbidly obese patients undergoing laparoscopic adjustable gastric banding. *Obes Surg*, 17: 920–25.

Kizhakkeveettil, A., Rose, K., and Kadar, G.E. 2014. Integrative therapies for low back pain that include complementary and alternative medicine care: A systematic review. *Glob Adv Health Med*, 3(5): 49–64.

Klauke, A.L., Racz, I., Pradier, B. et al. 2014. The cannabinoid CB2 receptor-selective phyto-cannabinoid beta-caryophyllene exerts analgesic effects in mouse models of inflammatory and neuropathic pain. *Eur Neuropsychopharmacol*, 24(4): 608–20.

Koulivand, P.H., Khaleghi Ghadiri, M., and Gorji, A. 2013. Lavender and the nervous system. *Evid Based Complement Alternat Med*, 2013: 681304. doi: 10.1155/2013/681304.

Kuwahata H., Katsuyama S., Komatsu T. et al. 2012. Local peripheral effects of β-caryophyllene through CB2 receptors in neuropathic pain in mice. *Pharmacol Pharm*, 3: 397–403.

Kuwahata, H., Komatsu, T., Katsuyama, S. et al. 2013. Peripherally injected linalool and bergamot essential oil attenuate mechanical allodynia via inhibiting spinal ERK phosphorylation. *Pharmacol Biochem Behav*, 103(4): 735–41.

Lakusić, B., Lakusić, D., Ristić, M. et al. 2014. Seasonal variations in the composition of the essential oils of *Lavandula angustifolia* (Lamiacae). *Nat Prod Commun*, 9(6): 859–62.

Lino, C.S., Gomes, P.B., Lucetti, D.L. et al. 2005. Evaluation of antinociceptive and antiinflammatory activities of the essential oil (EO) of *Ocimum micranthum* Willd. from northeastern Brazil. *Phytother Res*, 19(8): 708–12.

Maione, S., Costa, B., and Di Marzo, V. 2013. Endocannabinoids: A unique opportunity to develop multi target analgesics. *Pain*. doi: 10.1016/j.pain.2013.03.023.

Martin, G.J., Heck, G., Djamaris-Zainal, R., and Martin, M.L. 2006. Isotopic criteria in the characterization of aromatic molecules. 2. Influence of chemical elaboration process. *J Agric Food Chem*, 54(26): 10120–28.

Masaoka, Y., Takayama, M., Yajima, H., Kawase, A. et al. 2013. Analgesia is enhanced by providing information regarding good outcomes associated with an odor: Placebo effects in aromatherapy. *Evid Based Complement Alternat Med*. doi: 10.1155/2013/921802.

McMahon, S.B., and Malcangio, M. 2009. Current challenges in glia-pain biology. *Neuron*, 64: 46–54.

Morrone, L.A., Rombolà, L., Corasaniti, M.T. et al. 2007. The essential oil of bergamot enhances the levels of amino acid neurotransmitters in the hippocampus of rat: Implication of monoterpene hydrocarbons. *Pharmacol Res*, 55: 255–62.

Nardi, G.M., Dalbó, S., Monache, F.D., Pizzolatti, M.G., and Ribeiro-do-Valle, R.M. 2006. Antinociceptive effect of *Croton celtidifolius* Baill (Euphorbiaceae). *J Ethnopharmacol*, 107(1): 73–78.

Nascimento, S.S., Araújo, A.A.S., Brito, R.G. et al. 2015. Cyclodextrin-complexed *Ocimum basilicum* leaves essential oil increases Fos protein expression in the central nervous system and produce an antihyperalgesic effect in animal models for fibromyalgia. *Int J Mol Sci*, 16: 547–63.

Novy, D.M., and Aigner, C.J. 2014. The biopsychosocial model in cancer pain. *Curr Opin Support Palliat Care*, 8(2): 117–23. doi: 10.1097/SPC.0000000000000046.

Olapour, A., Behaeen, K., Akhondzadeh, R. et al. 2013. The effect of inhalation of aromatherapy blend containing lavender essential oil on cesarean postoperative pain. *Anesth Pain Med*, 3: 203–7.

Oliveira, A.C., Leal-Cardoso, J.H., Santos, C.F., Morais, S.M., and Coelho-de-Souza, A.N. 2001. Antinociceptive effects of the essential oil of *Croton zehntneri* in mice. *Braz J Med Biol Res*, 34(11): 1471–74.

Paula-Freire, L.I.G., Andersen, M.L., Molska, G.R. et al. 2013. Evaluation of the antinociceptive activity of *Ocimum gratissimum* L. (Lamiaceae) essential oil and its isolated active principles in mice. *Phytother Res*, 27: 1220–24.

Paula-Freire, L.I., Andersen, M.L., Gama, V.S., Molska, G.R., and Carlini, E.L. 2014. The oral administration of trans-caryophyllene attenuates acute and chronic pain in mice. *Phytomedicine*, 21(3): 356–62.

Peana, A.T., D'Aquila, P.S., Chessa, M.L. et al. 2003. (–)-Linalool produces antinociception in two experimental models of pain. *Eur J Pharmacol*, 460: 37–41.

Peana, A.T., De Montis, M.G., Nieddu, E. et al. 2004a. Profile of spinal and supra-spinal antinociception of (–)-linalool. *Eur J Pharmacol*, 485: 165–74.

Peana, A.T., De Montis, M.G., Sechi, S. et al. 2004b. Effects of (–)-linalool in the acute hyper-algesia induced by carrageenan, L-glutamate and prostaglandin E2. *Eur J Pharmacol*, 497: 279–84.

Peana, A.T., Marzocco, S., Popolo, A., and Pinto, A. 2006. (–)-Linalool inhibits in vitro NO formation: Probable involvement in the antinociceptive activity of this monoterpene compound. *Life Sci*, 78: 719–23.

Piccinelli, A.C., Santos, J.A., Konkiewitz, E.C. et al. 2014. Antihyperalgesic and anti-depressive actions of (R)-(+)-limonene, α-phellandrene, and essential oil from *Schinus terebinthifolius* fruits in a neuropathic pain model. *Nutr Neurosci*, Epub 18(5): 217–224.

Pinho, J.P., Silva, A.S., Pinheiro, B.G. et al. 2012. Antinociceptive and antispasmodic effects of the essential oil of *Ocimum micranthum*: Potential anti-inflammatory properties. *Planta Med*, 78: 681–85.

Price, D.D. 2000. Psychological and neural mechanisms of the affective dimension of pain. *Science*, 288: 1769–72.

Proudfoot, C.J., Garry, E.M., Cottrell, D.F. et al. 2006. Analgesia mediated by the TRPM8 cold receptor in chronic neuropathic pain. *Curr Biol*, 16: 1591–605.

Pruthi, S., Wahner-Roedler, D.L., Torkelson, C.J. et al. 2010. Vitamin E and evening primrose oil for management of cyclical mastalgia: A randomized pilot study. *Altern Med Rev*, 15: 59–67.

Qnais, E.Y., Abu-Dieyeh, M., Abdulla, F.A., and Abdalla, S.S. 2010. The antinociceptive and anti-inflammatory effects of *Salvia officinalis* leaf aqueous and butanol extracts. *Pharm Biol*, 48(10): 1149–56.

Rodrigues, M.R., Kanazawa, L.K., das Neves, T.L. et al. 2012. Antinociceptive and anti-inflammatory potential of extract and isolated compounds from the leaves of *Salvia officinalis* in mice. *J Ethnopharmacol*, 139(2): 519–26.

Rombolà, L., Corasaniti, M.T., Rotiroti, D. et al. 2009. Effects of systemic administration of the essential oil of bergamot (BEO) on gross behaviour and EEG power spectra recorded from the rat hippocampus and cerebral cortex. *Funct Neurol*, 24: 107–12.

Russo, R., Ciociaro, A., Berliocchi L. et al. 2013. Implication of limonene and linalyl ace-tate in cytotoxicity induced by bergamot essential oil in human neuroblastoma cells. *Fitoterapia*, 89(1): 48–57.

Russo, R., Corasaniti, M.T., Bagetta, G., Morrone, L.A. 2015. Exploitation of cytotoxicity of some essential oils for translation in cancer therapy. *Evid Based Complement Alternat Med*. doi: 10.1155/2015/397821.

Sadeghi Aval Shahr, H., Saadat, M., Kheirkhah, M., and Saadat, E. 2014. The effect of self-aromatherapy massage of the abdomen on the primary dysmenorrhea. *J Obstet Gynaecol*, 25: 1–4.

Saiyudthong, S., and Marsden, CA. 2011. Acute effects of bergamot oil on anxiety-related behaviour and corticosterone level in rats. *Phytother Res*, 25: 858–62.

Sakurada, T., Katsumata, K., Tan-No, K. et al. 1992. The capsaicin test in mice for evaluating tachykinin antagonists in the spinal cord. *Neuropharmacology*, 31: 1279–85.

Sakurada, T., Yogo, H., Katsumata, K. et al. 1994. Differential antinociceptive effects of sendide, and morphine in the capsaicin test. *Brain Res*, 649: 319–22.

Sakurada, T., Wako, K., Sugiyama, A. et al. 1998. Involvement of spinal NMDA receptors in capsaicin-induced nociception. *Pharmacol Biochem Behav*, 59: 339–45.

Sakurada, T., Kuwahata, H., Katsuyama, H. et al. 2009. Intraplantar injection of bergamot essential oil into the mouse hindpaw: Effects on capsaicin-induced nociceptive behaviors. *Int Rev Neurobiol*, 85: 235–46.

Sakurada, T., Mizoguchi, H., Kuwahata, H. et al. 2011. Intraplantar injection of bergamot essential oil induces peripheral antinociception mediated by opioid mechanism. *Pharmacol Biochem Behav*, 97(3): 436–43.

Salatino, A., Faria Salatino, M.L., and Negri, G. 2007. Traditional uses, chemistry and pharmacology of *Croton* species (Euphorbiaceae). *J Braz Chem Soc*, 18(1).

Santos, F.A., and Rao, V.S.N. 2000. Anti-inflammatory and antinociceptive effects of 1,8-cineole, a terpenoid oxide present in many plant essential oils. *Phytother Res*, 14: 240–44.

Santos, F.A., Jeferson, F.A., Santos, C.C. et al. 2005. Antinociceptive effect of leaf essential oil from *Croton sonderianus* in mice. *Life Sci*, 77(23): 2953–63.

Sasannejad, P., Saeedi, M., Shoeibi, A. et al. 2012. Lavender essential oil in the treatment of migraine headache: A placebo-controlled clinical trial. *Eur Neurol*, 67: 288–91.

Seltzer Z., Dubner R., and Shir Y. 1990. A novel behavioral model of neuropathic pain disorders produced in rats by partial sciatic nerve injury. *Pain*, 43: 205–18.

Silva Brum, L.F., Elisabetsky, E., and Souza, D. 2001. Effects of linalool on [^{3}H] MK801 and [^{3}H] muscimol binding in mouse cortical membranes. *Phytother Res*, 15: 422–25.

Soltani, R., Soheilipour, S., Hajhashemi, V. et al. 2013. Evaluation of the effect of aromatherapy with lavender essential oil on post-tonsillectomy pain in pediatric patients: A randomized controlled trial. *Int J Pediatric Otorhinol*, 77: 1579–81.

Sood, S., Arora, B., Bansal, S. et al. 2009. Antioxidant, anti-inflammatory and analgesic potential of the *Citrus decumana* L. peel extract. *Inflammopharmacology*, 17(5): 267–74.

Stea, S., Beraudi, A., and De Pasquale, D. 2014. Essential oil for complementary treatment of surgical patients: State of the art. *Evid Based Complement Alternat Med*. doi: 10.1155/2014/726341.

Straub, I., Krügel, U., Mohr, F. et al. 2013. Flavanones that selectively inhibit TRPM3 attenuate thermal nociception in vivo. *Mol Pharmacol*, 84(5): 736–50.

Strobel, C., Hunt, S., Sullivan, R. et al. 2014. Emotional regulation of pain: The role of noradrenaline in the amygdala. *Sci China Life Sci*, 57(4): 384–90. doi: 10.1007/s11427-014-4638-x.

Suárez, A.I., Compagnone, R.S., Salazar-Bookaman, M.M. et al. 2003. Antinociceptive and anti-inflammatory effects of *Croton malambo* bark aqueous extract. *J Ethnopharmacol*, 88(1): 11–14.

Szallasi, A. 2006. Small molecule vanilloid TRPV1 receptor antagonists approaching drug status: Can they live up to the expectations? *Naunyn Schmiedebergs Arch Pharmacol*, 373: 273–86.

Tang, S.K., and Tse, M.Y. 2014. Aromatherapy: Does it help to relieve pain, depression, anxiety, and stress in community-dwelling older persons? *Biomed Res Int*. doi: 10.1155/2014/430195.

Tjolsen, A., Berge, O.G., Hunskaar, S. et al. 1992. The formalin test: An evaluation of the method. *Pain*, 51(1): 5–17.

Van Hecke, O., Torrance, N., and Smith, B.H. 2013. Chronic pain epidemiology and its clinical relevance. *Br J Anaesth*. doi: 10.1093/bja/aet123.

Venâncio, A.M., Onofre, A.S., Lira, A.F. et al. 2011. Chemical composition, acute toxicity, and antinociceptive activity of the essential oil of a plant breeding cultivar of basil (*Ocimum basilicum* L.). *Planta Med*, 77(8): 825–29.

Wells, R.E., Phillips, R.S., Schachter, S.C., and McCarthy, E.P. 2010. Complementary and alternative medicine use among US adults with common neurological conditions. *J Neurol*, 257(11): 1822–31.

Yalcin, I., Barthas, F., and Barrot, M. 2014. Emotional consequences of neuropathic pain: Insight from preclinical studies. *Neurosci Biobehav Rev*, 47: 154–64.

Yamada, A.N., Grespan, R., Yamada, Á.T. et al. 2013. Anti-inflammatory activity of *Ocimum americanum* L. essential oil in experimental model of zymosan-induced arthritis. *Am J Chin Med*, 41(4): 913–26.

Yip, Y.B., and Tam, A.C. 2008. An experimental study on the effectiveness of massage with aromatic ginger and orange essential oil for moderate-to-severe knee pain among the elderly in Hong Kong. *Complement Ther Med*, 16: 131–38.

Zhao, J., Fang, F., Yu, L., Wang, G., and Yang L. 2012. Anti-nociceptive and anti-inflammatory effects of *Croton crassifolius* ethanol extract. *J Ethnopharmacol*, 142(2): 367–73.

Zhou, J., Wang, X., Tang, F. et al. 2007. Inhibitory effect of 1,8-cineol (eucalyptol) on Egr-1 expression in lipopolysaccharide stimulated THP-1 cells. *Acta Pharmacol Sin*, 28: 908–12.

13 Pain Relief by Local Peripheral Injection of Beta-Caryophyllene through Cannabinoid 2 Receptor

Soh Katsuyama, Takaaki Komatsu,
Giacinto Bagetta, Shinobu Sakurada,
and Tsukasa Sakurada

CONTENTS

13.1 INTRODUCTION

Aromatherapy usually uses aromatic essential oils, which are highly volatile organic compounds extracted by distillation from plants to achieve physical and psychological health. Plants are used for various purposes, including their cosmetic, nutritive, and biomedical properties. Plant-derived drugs have played an important role in health and wellness benefits. Plant essential oils are typically composed of volatile aromatic terpenes and phenylpropanoids. The natural sesquiterpene beta-caryophyllene (BCP) is a major plant volatile found in large amounts in the essential oils of many different spice and food plants, such as clove, oregano, thyme, black pepper, and cinnamon (Legault and Pichette, 2007), all of which have been used as natural remedies and fragrances. BCP has been shown to produce marked anti-inflammatory activity against carrageenan- and prostaglandin E_1–induced edema in rats as well as antiarthritic activity (Martin et al., 1993; Baricevic et al., 2001; Agarwal and Rangari, 2003). There is evidence that oral administration of BCP is sufficient to display anti-inflammatory effects on dextran sulfate sodium–induced colitis in mice (Beltramo, 2009 for review). Moreover, BCP is known to be a major component in the essential oil of the marijuana plant *Cannabis sativa* L. (Hendriks et al., 1975), while Δ^9-tetrahydrocannabinol, the active constituent of marijuana, binds with high affinity to cannabinoid (CB) receptors, cloned and determined as the CB_1 and CB_2 receptor subtypes (Matsuda et al., 1990; Munro et al., 1993). There is accumulated evidence that the activation of both CB_1 and CB_2 receptors elicits antinociception in mice and rats through not only central, but also peripheral mechanisms involving CB_1 and CB_2 receptors (for review, Hohmann, 2002; Malan et al., 2002; Anand et al., 2009). Further studies show that the activation of CB_2 receptors stimulates the release from keratinocytes of β-endorphin, an endogenous opioid (Ibrahim et al., 2005). In addition, there is evidence that the activation of peripheral μ-opioid receptors in local tissue is effective at attenuating neuropathic pain (Obara et al., 2004; Guan et al., 2008). This review will focus on elucidating the pain relief functions of beta-caryophyllene and peripheral CB_2 receptor.

13.2 CANNABINOID 2 RECEPTOR

Two subtype CB receptors, CB_1 and CB_2, have been identified (Matsuda et al., 1990; Munro et al., 1993). The CB_1 receptor is localized predominantly in the brain (central receptor), whereas the CB_2 receptor is in peripheral cells and tissues derived from the immune system (peripheral receptor) (Ameri, 1999 for review). CB_2 receptors are coupled with Gi/Go-type protein, negatively to adenylyl cyclase and positively to mitogen-activated protein (MAP) kinase cascades (Di Marzo and De Petrocellis, 2006). Inwardly rectifying potassium channels can also serve as a signaling mechanism for the CB_2 receptor (Ho et al., 1999). In pathological pain states, CB_2 messenger RNA is also detected in the lumbar dorsal horn concurrently with the appearance of activated microglia (Zhang et al., 2003). CB_2 receptor–selective agonists produce peripheral antinociception, but do not cause the effects of CNS (Malan et al., 2001), suggesting that selective activation of CB_2 receptors may achieve the goal of peripheral pain relief without CNS effects. CB_2 receptor modulation has been implicated in processes as diverse as analgesia, fibrosis, bone growth, and atherosclerosis (Mackie and Ross, 2008). Effects of CB_2 receptor–selective agonists that suppress peripheral antinociception in different pain models are summarized in Table 13.1.

13.3 BETA-CARYOPHYLLENE

A natural selective agonist for CB_2 receptors is the plant volatile sesquiterpene BCP, which represents a dietary phytocannabinoid (Gertsch et al., 2008, 2010). Orally administered BCP (5 mg/kg) produces strong anti-inflammatory and analgesic

TABLE 13.1

CB₂ Receptor–Selective Agonists Suppress Peripheral Antinociception in Different Pain Models

Drug	Dose	Pain Model	Reference
JWH-133	5–15 µg/50 µl/rat, paw	Carrageenan/inflammatory	Elmes et al., 2004
	5–15 µg/50 µl/rat, paw	Neuropathic pain	Elmes et al., 2004
	30.5–91.6 nmol/30 µl/ mouse, paw	Neuropathic pain	Hervera et al., 2010
	31 or 92 nmol/30 µl/ mouse, paw	Neuropathic pain	Hervera et al., 2012
	15–300 µg/30 µl/mouse, paw	Complete Freund's adjuvant/inflammatory	Negrete et al., 2011
AM1241	0.33–3.3 mg/kg/rat, paw	Plantar/thermal	Malan et al., 2001
	33 µg/kg/rat, paw	Carrageenan/inflammatory	Nackley et al., 2003
	1–4 mg/kg/rat, paw	Carrageenan/inflammatory	Quartilho et al., 2003
	33 or 330 µg/kg/rat, paw	Carrageenan/inflammatory	Nackley et al., 2004
	33 µg/kg/rat, paw	Carrageenan/inflammatory	Gutierrez et al., 2007
	33 µg/kg/rat, paw	Capsaicin/inflammatory	Hohmann et al., 2004
	0.6–6 µmol/kg/rat, paw	Complete Freund's adjuvant/inflammatory	Hsieh et al., 2011

effects in wild-type mice but not in CB₂ receptor knockout mice, which is a clear indication that it may be a functional CB₂ ligand (Gertsch et al., 2008). The BCP is a major plant volatile found in large amounts in the essential oils of many different spice and food plants, such as clove, oregano, thyme, black pepper, and cinnamon (Legault and Pichette, 2007), all of which have been used as natural remedies and fragrances. It is widely used in seasoning mixture, in various food products, and in soups and detergents (Sabulal et al., 2006). BCP is also often used in cosmetics and is a Food and Drug Administration (FDA)–approved food additive and component of *Cannabis sativa* and Sativex, an approved drug in European countries and Canada (Sibbald, 2005). Several studies have demonstrated that BCP- or BCP-containing plants (Russo, 2011) possess biological activities, including antioxidant (Alma et al., 2003; Singh et al., 2006), antibacterial (Michielin et al., 2009), gastroprotective (Tambe et al., 1996), anti-inflammatory (Medeiros et al., 2007; Gertsch et al., 2008; Klauke et al., 2013), anticarcinogenic (Legault and Pichette, 2007; Loizzo et al., 2008), antifibrotic (Calleja et al., 2013), local anesthetic (Ghelardini et al., 2001) and anxiolytic-like (Galdino et al., 2012) activity. Antinociceptive effects of BCP were also observed after local peripheral (Kuwahata et al., 2012; Katsuyama et al., 2013), oral (Paula-Freire et al., 2013; Klauke et al., 2013) administration. BCP also exhibits neuroprotective effects (Chang et al., 2013) and inhibits inflammatory and tissue damage (Bento et al., 2011; Horváth et al., 2012). Biological activities of CB_2 receptor–selective agonist BCP are summarized in Figure 13.1.

13.4 LOCAL PERIPHERAL ANTINOCICEPTIVE EFFECTS OF BETA-CARYOPHYLLENE

Recently, our research group investigated whether local intraplantar injection of BCP would produce antinociception in a capsaicin-induced acute pain model or a partial sciatic nerve ligation (PSNL)–induced mechanical allodynia model in mice. We assessed the involvement of the peripheral CB or opioid mechanism (Kuwahata et al., 2012; Katsuyama et al., 2013).

13.4.1 ANTINOCICEPTIVE EFFECT OF LOCAL INTRAPLANTAR INJECTION OF BCP WAS ASSAYED BY THE CAPSAICIN TESTS IN MICE

The capsaicin test is widely used as a model of pain in animals (Sakurada et al., 1992, 1993; Pelissier et al., 2002) and humans (Hughes et al., 2002). Sakurada et al. (1994) also reported in mice that subcutaneous injection of capsaicin into the hindpaw produced a short-lasting paw-licking/biting response, which was dose-dependently inhibited by intrathecal injection of morphine. Activation of primary afferent nociceptors by capsaicin causes the release of nociceptive neurotransmitters from the dorsal spinal cord *in vivo* and *in vitro* (Gamse et al., 1979; Sorkin and McAdoo, 1993; Ueda et al., 1993). In addition, it has been shown that capsaicin

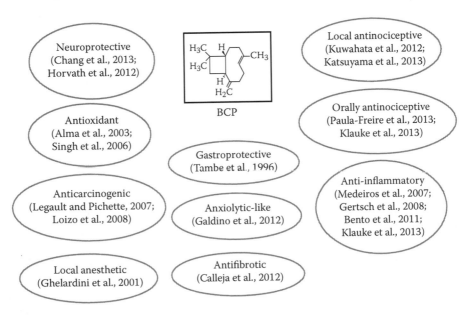

FIGURE 13.1 Biological activities of CB_2 receptor–selective agonist beta-caryophyllene (BCP).

excites the C-fiber population of nociceptive afferents, since capsaicin acts on transient vanilloid type-1 receptors located in C-fiber-type nociceptors (Di Marzo et al., 2002; Szallasi et al., 2007). BCP was injected 10 min prior to local intraplantar injection of capsaicin injection, and the induced paw-licking/biting was observed for 5 min after capsaicin injection. BCP or jojoba wax was injected 10 min before capsaicin at the same site via an intraplantar route to evaluate the antinociceptive effects. Behavioral alterations following local intraplantar injection of jojoba wax as control were not statistically different when compared to the nonpretreated group. BCP (18.0 μg/paw) into the hindpaw ipsilateral to the capsaicin injection significantly reduced nociceptive behavior when compared to the jojoba wax–treated control group. The lower doses of BCP (2.25 and 4.5 μg/paw) did not attenuate the duration of nociceptive behavior relative to the jojoba wax control. To ensure that the effects of local intraplantar injection of BCP were local and not due to systemic diffusion of BCP, BCP (18.0 μg/paw) was injected into the hindpaw contralateral to the capsaicin injection. Capsaicin-induced nociceptive response following injection of BCP in the contralateral hindpaw was not statistically different when compared to the jojoba wax–treated control group. To test whether the antinociceptive effect of BCP was mediated by cannabinoid systems, animals were pretreated subcutaneously (s.c.) with AM251, a selective CB_1 receptor antagonist, or AM630, a selective CB_2 receptor antagonist. The selective CB_2 receptor antagonist AM630 (1.0 mg/kg) reversed the inhibitory effects of BCP on the capsaicin-induced behavioral response. The selective CB_1 receptor antagonist AM251 (3.0 mg/kg) gave no significant effect on BCP-induced antinociception. In another group of mice, AM251 or AM630 was injected directly into the same site on the hindpaw before local intraplantar injection of BCP. Pretreatment with AM630 (2.5 μg/paw) could also significantly antagonize antinociceptive effects of BCP (18.0 μg/paw), whereas AM251 (7.5 μg/paw) was without effect on BCP-induced antinociception. To determine whether the antinociceptive effect of BCP was mediated by opioid systems, animals were pretreated s.c. with naloxone hydrochloride or naloxone methiodide 15 min before injection of BCP (18.0 μg/paw). The opioid receptor antagonist naloxone hydrochloride (8.0 mg/kg, s.c.) dose-dependently reversed the inhibitory effect of BCP on the capsaicin-induced behavioral response. In another group of mice, naloxone hydrochloride was injected directly into the same site on the hindpaw before intraplantar injection of BCP. Pretreatment with naloxone hydrochloride (10.0 μg/paw) could also significantly antagonize the antinociceptive effect of BCP. Pretreatment with naloxone methiodide (8.0 mg/kg, s.c.), a peripherally acting opioid receptor antagonist, resulted in a significant antagonistic effect on BCP-induced antinociception. The selective μ-opioid receptor antagonist, β-funaltrexamine (β-FNA) (20.0 mg/kg, s.c.), preinjected 24 h before BCP injection, significantly prevented the inhibitory effect of BCP on the capsaicin-induced nociceptive response. In another group of mice, β-FNA was injected directly into the same site on the hindpaw before local intraplantar injection of BCP. Local pretreatment with β-FNA (50.0 μg/paw) could also significantly antagonize the antinociceptive effect of BCP. However, pretreatment with the selective δ- and κ-opioid receptor antagonists, NTI and nor-BNI (s.c. and intraplantar), did not prevent the BCP-induced antinociceptive effect. Pretreatment with antisera against β-endorphin resulted in a dilution-related antagonistic effect

TABLE 13.2
Antinociceptive Effect of Local Intraplantar Injection of BCP Was Assayed by the Capsaicin Tests in Mice

Drugs	Licking/Biting Response (sec/5 min)
Vehicle + capsaicin (1.6 µg/20 µl/mouse, paw)	80.6 ± 5.47
Effect of BCP (18 µg/20 µl/mouse, paw)	31.3 ± 3.13[a]
BCP + AM630 (1 mg/kg, s.c.)	76.6 ± 4.51[b]
BCP + AM630 (2.5 µg/20 µl/mouse, paw)	76.3 ± 6.11[b]
BCP + AM251 (3 mg/kg, s.c.)	38.6 ± 3.52
BCP + AM251 (7.5 µg/20 µl/mouse, paw)	33.1 ± 7.44
BCP + naloxone (8 mg/kg, s.c.)	77.2 ± 9.64[b]
BCP + naloxone (10 µg/20 µl/mouse, paw)	74.9 ± 7.92[b]
BCP + naloxone methiodide (8 mg/kg, s.c.)	71.3 ± 8.32[b]
BCP + β-FNA (20 mg/kg, s.c.)	79.2 ± 4.17[b]
BCP + β-FNA (50 µg/20 µl/mouse, paw)	78.0 ± 5.37[b]
BCP + naltrindole (3 mg/kg, s.c.)	29.2 ± 4.28
BCP + naltrindole (7.5 µg/20 µl/mouse, paw)	29.7 ± 4.67
BCP + nor-BNI (10 mg/kg, s.c.)	33.2 ± 4.48
BCP + nor-BNI (25 µg/20 µl/mouse, paw)	32.2 ± 5.37
BCP + antisera against β-endorphin (1:50/20 µl/mouse, paw)	76.2 ± 4.37[b]

[a] $P < 0.01$ when compared with vehicle + capsaicin.
[b] $P < 0.01$ when compared with BCP.

on BCP-induced antinociception (Table 13.2). In summary, the present study has demonstrated for the first time that local intraplantar injection of BCP could reduce the nociceptive behavioral response induced by capsaicin injection into the hindpaw. This mechanism allows for the local activation of CB_2 receptors induced by BCP, which may produce peripheral local release of endogenous β-endorphin from keratinocytes, thereby leading to antinociceptive effects of opioid.

13.4.2 ANTIALLODYNIC EFFECT OF LOCAL INTRAPLANTAR INJECTION OF BCP WAS ASSAYED BY THE PSNL-INDUCED MECHANICAL ALLODYNIA MODEL IN MICE

Injury to the sciatic nerve in mice as well as rats produces a prolonged mechanical allodynia and thermal hyperalgesia (Seltzer et al., 1990; Malmberg and Basbaum, 1998). This experimental model has established a reliable and objective method to access neuropathic pain. We confirmed that PSNL produced a rapid-onset and prolonged mechanical allodynia in mice. The responsiveness to mechanical stimuli was determined on days 1–35 after PSNL. Compared with the sham-operated mice, PSNL resulted in mechanical allodynia demonstrated by a significantly lower threshold to von Frey filaments from day 7 to day 28 post-PSNL. The maximal decrease in withdrawal threshold after PSNL was observed on day 7. On day 7 post-PSNL, local intraplantar injection of BCP (18.0 μg/paw) dose-dependently increased the mechanical response threshold on the nerve-injured side. The effect of BCP reached a maximum at 5 min and lasted for 15 min on the nerve-ligated side. Jojoba wax control, injected into the nerve-ligated side, did not affect the mechanical thresholds. To ensure that the effects of local intraplantar injection of BCP were local and not due to systemic diffusion, BCP (18.0 μg/paw) was injected into the contralateral hindpaw. The mechanical threshold following local intraplantar injection of BCP in the contralateral hindpaw was not statistically different when compared with the jojoba wax control group in PSNL mice. To determine if the antiallodynic effect of BCP was mediated by peripheral CB systems, animals were pretreated systemically with AM251 (3.0 mg/kg, s.c.), a selective CB_1 receptor antagonist, and AM630 (1.0 mg/kg, s.c.), a selective CB_2 receptor antagonist, 30 min before local intraplantar injection of BCP (18.0 μg/paw). The selective CB_2 receptor antagonist, AM630, significantly reversed the inhibitory effects of BCP on the PSNL-induced mechanical allodynia, whereas the selective CB_1 receptor antagonist, AM251, gave no effect. In further experiments, AM251 and AM630 were pretreated directly into the same site on the hindpaw prior to local intraplantar injection of BCP. Local intraplantar injection of pretreatment with AM630 (4.0 μg/paw) could also significantly antagonize antiallodynic effects of BCP, whereas AM251 (12.0 μg/paw) gave no effect (Table 13.3). In conclusion, i.pl. injection of BCP reduced the mechanical allodynia by the PSNL model in mice. The antiallodynic effects of BCP were antagonized by s.c. and i.pl. pretreatment with the selective CB_2 receptor antagonist, AM630, but not by the selective CB_1 receptor antagonist, AM251. The results suggest that a local effect of BCP on cutaneous nociceptors is mediated through CB_2 receptors. BCP is predicted to be effective in treating allodynia without the central side effects of cannabinoid-based drugs retaining activity at the CB_1 receptor.

TABLE 13.3
Antiallodynic Effect of Local Intraplanar Injection of BCP Was Assayed by the PSNL-Induced Mechanical Allodynia Model in Mice

Drugs	Withdrawal Threshold (g/5 sec)
Sham operation	2.68 ± 0.83
Vehicle	0.78 ± 0.13
Effect of BCP (18 μg/20 μl/mouse, paw)	2.40 ± 0.34^a
BCP + AM630 (1 mg/kg, s.c.)	0.71 ± 0.18^b
BCP + AM630 (4 μg/20 μl/mouse, paw)	0.85 ± 0.12^b
BCP + AM251 (3 mg/kg, s.c.)	2.15 ± 0.41
BCP + AM251 (12 μg/20 μl/mouse, paw)	2.26 ± 0.35

[a] $P < 0.01$ when compared with vehicle.
[b] $P < 0.01$ when compared with BCP.

REFERENCES

Agarwal, R.B., and Rangari, V.D. Phytochemical investigation and evaluation of anti-inflammatory and anti-arthritic activities of essential oil of *Strobilanthus ixiocephala* Benth. *Indian J Exp Biol* 41 no. 8 (2003): 890–94.

Alma, M.H., Mavi, A., Yildirim, A., Digrak, M., and Hirata, T. Screening chemical composition and *in vitro* antioxidant and antimicrobial activities of the essential oils from *Origanum syriacum* L. growing in Turkey. *Biol Pharm Bull* 26 no. 12 (2003): 1725–29.

Ameri, A. The effects of cannabinoids on the brain. *Prog Neurobiol* 58 no. 4 (1999): 315–48.

Anand, P., Whiteside, G., Fowler, C.J., and Hohmann, A.G. Targeting CB_2 receptors and the endocannabinoid system for the treatment of pain. *Brain Res Rev* 60 no. 1 (2009): 255–66.

Baricevic, D., Sosa, S., Della Loggia, R. et al. Topical anti-inflammatory activity of *Salvia officinalis* L. leaves: The relevance of ursolic acid. *J Ethnopharmacol* 75 no. 2–3 (2001): 125–32.

Beltramo, M. Cannabinoid type 2 receptor as a target for chronic pain. *Mini Rev Med Chem* 9 no. 8 (2009): 11–25.

Bento, A.F., Marcon, R., Dutra, R.C. et al. β-Caryophyllene inhibits dextran sulfate β-Cβ-caryophyllene inhibits dextran sulfate sodiβ-caryophyllene inhibits dextran sulfate sodium-induced colitis in mice through CB2 receptor activation and PPARγ pathway. *Am J Pathol* 178 no. 3 (2011): 1153–66.

Calleja, M.A., Vieites, J.M., Montero-Meterdez, T. et al. The antioxidant effect of β-caryophyllene protects rat liver from carbon tetrachloride-induced fibrosis by inhibiting hepatic stellate cell activation. *Br J Nutr* 109 no. 3 (2013): 394–401.

Chang, H.J., Kim, J.M., Lee, J.C., Kim, W.K., and Chun, H.S. Protective effect of β-caryophyllene, a natural bicyclic sesquiterpene, against cerebral ischemic injury. *J Med Food* 16 no. 6 (2013): 471–80.

Di Marzo, V., and De Petrocellis, L. Plant, synthetic, and endogenous cannabinoids in medicine. *Annu Rev Med* 57 (2006): 553–74.

Di Marzo, V., Blumberg, P.M., and Szallasi, A. Endovanilloid signaling in pain. *Curr Opin Neurobiol* 12 no. 4 (2002): 372–79.

Elmes, S.J., Jhaveri, M.D., Smart, D., Kendall, D.A., and Chapman, V. Cannabinoid CB2 receptor activation inhibits mechanically evoked responses of wide dynamic range dorsal horn neurons in naïve rats and in rat models of inflammatory and neuropathic pain. *Eur J Neurosci* 20 no. 9 (2004): 2311–20.

Galdino, P.M., Nascimento, M.V., Florentino, I.F. et al. The anxiolytic-like effect of an essential oil derived from *Spiranthera odoratissima* A. St. Hil. leaves and its major component, β-caryophyllene, in male mice. *Prog Neuropsychopharmacol Biol Psychiatry* 38 no. 2 (2012): 276–84.

Gamse, R., Molnar, A., and Lembeck, F. Substance P release from spinal slices by capsaicin. *Life Sci* 25 no. 7 (1979): 629–36.

Gertsch, J., Leonti, M., Raduner S. et al. Beta-caryophyllene is a dietary cannabinoid. *Proc Natl Acad Sci USA* 105 no. 26 (2008): 9099–104.

Gertsch, J., Pertwee, R.G., and Di Marzo, V. Phytocannabinoids beyond the Cannabis plant: Do they exist? *Br J Pharmacol* 160 no. 3 (2010): 523–29.

Ghelardini, C., Galeotti, N., Di Cesare Mannelli, L., Mazzanti, G., and Bartolini, A. Local anaesthetic activity of beta-caryophyllene. *Farmaco* 56 no. 5–7 (2001): 387–89.

Guan, Y., Johanek, L.M., Hartke, T.V. et al. Peripherally acting mu-opioid receptor agonist attenuates neuropathic pain in rats after L5 spinal nerve injury. *Pain* 138 no. 2 (2008): 318–29.

Gutierrez, T., Farthing, J.N., Zvonok, A.M., Makriyannis, A., and Hohmann, A.G. Activation of peripheral cannabinoid CB1 and CB2 receptors suppresses the maintenance of inflammatory nociception: A comparative analysis. *Br J Pharmacol* 150 no. 2 (2007): 153–63.

Hendriks, H., Malingre, T., Battermann, S., and Boss, R. Mono- and sesquiterpene hydrocarbons of essential oil of *Cannabis sativa*. *Phytochemistry* 14 (1975): 814–15.

Hervera, A., Negrete, R., Leánez, S., Martín-Campos, J., and Pol, O. The role of nitric oxide in the local antiallodynic and antihyperalgesic effects and expression of delta-opioid and cannabinoid-2 receptors during neuropathic pain in mice. *J Pharmacol Exp Ther* 334 no. 3 (2010): 887–96.

Hervera, A., Leánez, S., and Pol, O. The inhibition of the nitric oxide-cGMP-PKG-JNK signaling pathway avoids the development of tolerance to the local antiallodynic effects produced by morphine during neuropathic pain. *Eur J Pharmacol* 685 no. 1–3 (2012): 42–51.

Ho, B.Y., Uezono, Y., Takada, S., Takase, I., and Izumi, F. Coupling of the expressed cannabinoid CB1 and CB2 receptors to phospholipase C and G protein-coupled inwardly rectifying K+ channels. *Recept Channels* 6 no. 5 (1999): 363–74.

Hohmann, A.G. Spinal and peripheral mechanisms of cannabinoid antinociception: Behavioral, neurophysiological and neuroanatomical perspectives. *Chem Phys Lipids* 121 no. 1–2, (2002): 173–90.

Hohmann, A.G., Farthing, J.N., Zvonok, A.M., and Makriyannis, A. Selective activation of cannabinoid CB2 receptors suppresses hyperalgesia evoked by intradermal capsaicin. *J Pharmacol Exp Ther* 308 no. 2 (2004): 446–53.

Horváth, B., Mukhopadhyay, P., Kechrid, M. et al. β-Caryophyllene ameliorates cisplatin-induced nephrotoxicity in a cannabinoid 2 receptor-dependent manner. *Free Radic Biol Med* 52 no. 8 (2012): 1325–33.

Hsieh, G.C., Pai, M., Chandran, P. et al. Central and peripheral sites of action for CB_2 receptor mediated analgesic activity in chronic inflammatory and neuropathic pain models in rats. *Br J Pharmacol* 162 no. 2 (2011): 428–40.

Hughes, A., Macleod, A., Growcott, J., and Thomas, I. Assessment of the reproducibility of intradermal administration as a model for inducing human pain. *Pain* 99 no. 1–2 (2002): 323–31.

Ibrahim, M.M., Porreca, F., Lai, J. et al. CB_2 cannabinoid receptor activation produces antinociception by stimulating peripheral release of endogenous opioids. *Proc Natl Acad Sci USA* 102 no. 8 (2005): 3093–98.

Katsuyama, S., Mizoguchi, H., Kuwahata, H. et al. Involvement of peripheral cannabinoid and opioid receptors in β-caryophyllene-induced antinociception. *Eur J Pain* 17 no. 5 (2013): 664–75.

Klauke, A.L., Racz, I., Pradier, B. et al. The cannabinoid CB2 receptor-selective phytocannabinoid beta-caryophyllene exerts analgesic effects in mouse models of inflammatory and neuropathic pain. *Eur Neuropsychopharmacol* 24 no. 4 (2013): 608–20.

Kuwahata, H., Katsuyama, S., Komatsu, T. et al. Local peripheral effects of β-caryophyllene through CB_2 receptors in neuropathic pain in mice. *Pharmacol Pharm* 3 no. 4 (2012): 397–403.

Legault, J., and Pichette, A. Potentiating effect of beta-caryophyllene on anticancer activity of alpha-humulene, isocaryophyllene and paclitaxel. *J Pharm Pharmacol* 59 no. 12 (2007): 1643–47.

Loizzo, M.R., Tundis, R., Menichini, F., Saab, A.M., Statti, G.A., and Menichini, F. Antiproliferative effects of essential oils and their major constituents in human renal adenocarcinoma and amelanotic melanoma cells. *Cell Prolif* 41 no. 6 (2008): 1002–12.

Mackie, K., and Ross, R.A. CB_2 cannabinoid receptors: New vistas. *Br J Pharmacol* 153 no. 2 (2008): 177–78.

Malan, T.P., Ibrahim, M.M., Deng, H. et al. CB_2 cannabinoid receptor-mediated peripheral antinociception. *Pain* 93 no. 3 (2001): 239–45.

Malan, T.P., Ibrahim, M.M., Vanderah, T., Makriyannis, A., and Porreca, F. Inhibition of pain responses by activation of CB_2 cannabinoid receptors. *Chem Phys Lipids* 121 no. 1–2 (2002): 191–200.

Malmberg, A.B., and Basbaum, A.I. Partial sciatic nerve injury in the mouse as a model of neuropathic pain: Behavioral and neuroanatomical correlates. *Pain* 76 no. 1–2 (1998): 215–22.

Martin, S., Padilla, E., Ocete, M.A., Galvez, J., Jimenez, J., and Zarzuelo, A. Anti-inflammatory activity of the essential oil of *Bupleurum fruticescens*. *Planta Med* 59 no. 6 (1993): 533–36.

Matsuda, L.A., Lolait, S.J., Brownstein, M.J., Young, A.C., and Bonner, T.I. Structure of a cannabinoid receptor and functional expression of the cloned cDNA. *Nature* 346 no. 6284 (1990): 561–64.

Medeiros, R., Passos, G.F., Vitor, C.E. et al. Effect of two active compounds obtained from the essential oil of *Cordia verbenacea* on the acute inflammatory responses elicited by LPS in the rat paw. *Br J Pharmacol* 151 no. 5 (2007): 618–27.

Michielin, E.M., Salvador, A.A., Riehl, C.A., Smânia, A., Jr., Smânia, E.F., and Ferreira, S.R. Chemical composition and antibacterial activity of *Cordia verbenacea* extracts obtained by different methods. *Bioresour Technol* 100 no. 24 (2009): 6615–23.

Munro, S., Thomas, K.L., and Abu-Shaar, M. Molecular characterization of a peripheral receptor for cannabinoids. *Nature* 365 no. 6441 (1993): 61–65.

Nackley, A.G., Makriyannis, A., and Hohmann, A.G. Selective activation of cannabinoid CB(2) receptors suppresses spinal Fos protein expression and pain behavior in a rat model of inflammation. *Neuroscience* 119 no. 3 (2003): 747–57.

Nackley, A.G., Zvonok, A.M., Makriyannis, A., and Hohmann, A.G. Activation of cannabinoid CB2 receptors suppresses C-fiber responses and windup in spinal wide dynamic range neurons in the absence and presence of inflammation. *J Neurophysiol* 92 no. 6 (2004): 3562–74.

Negrete, R., Hervera, A., Leánez, S., Martín-Campos, J.M., and Pol, O. The antinociceptive effects of JWH-015 in chronic inflammatory pain are produced by nitric oxide-cGMP-PKG-KATP pathway activation mediated by opioids. *PLoS One* 6 no. 10 (2011): e26688.

Obara, I., Przewlocki, R., and Przewlocka, B. Local peripheral effects of μ-opioid receptor agonists in neuropathic pain in rats. *Neurosci Lett* 360 no. 1–2 (2004): 85–89.

Paula-Freire, L.I., Andersen, M.L., Gama, V.S., Molska, G.R., and Carlini, E.L. The oral administration of trans-caryophyllene attenuates acute and chronic pain in mice. *Phytomedicine* 21 no. 3 (2013): 356–62.

Pelissier, T., Pajot, J., and Dallel, R. The orofacial capsaicin test in rats: Effects of different capsaicin concentrations and morphine. *Pain* 96 no. 1–2 (2002): 81–87.

Quartilho, A., Mata, H.P., Ibrahim, M.M. et al. Inhibition of inflammatory hyperalgesia by activation of peripheral CB2 cannabinoid receptors. *Anesthesiology* 99 no. 4 (2003): 955–60.

Russo, E.B. Taming THC: Potential cannabis synergy and phytocannabinoid-terpenoid entourage effects. *Br J Pharmacol* 163 no. 7 (2011): 1344–64.

Sabulal, B., Dan, M., J, A.J. et al. Caryophyllene-rich rhizome oil of *Zingiber nimmonii* from south India: Chemical characterization and antimicrobial activity. *Phytochemistry* 67 no. 22 (2006): 2469–73.

Sakurada, T., Katsumata, K., Tan-No, K., Sakurada, S., and Kisara, K. The capsaicin test in mice for evaluating tachykinin antagonists in the spinal cord. *Neuropharmacology* 31 no. 12 (1992): 1279–85.

Sakurada, T., Katsumata, K., Manome, Y., Tan-No, K., Sakurada, S., Kisara, K., and Ohba M. Antinociceptive effects in the formalin and capsaicin tests after intrathecal administration of substance P analogues in mice. *Eur J Pharmacol* 242 no. 1 (1993): 47–52.

Sakurada, T., Yogo, H., Katsumata, K. et al. Differential antinociceptive effects of sendide, a NK$_1$-receptor antagonist, and morphine in the capsaicin test. *Brain Res* 649 no. 1–2 (1994): 319–22.

Seltzer, Z., Dubner, R., and Shir, Y. A novel behavioral model of neuropathic pain disorders produced in rats by partial sciatic nerve injury. *Pain* 43 no. 2 (1990): 205–18.

Sibbald, B. Conditional okay for cannabis prescription drug. *CMAJ* 172 no. 13 (2005): 1672.

Singh, G., Marimuthu, P., de Heluani, C.S., and Catalan, C.A. Antioxidant and biocidalactivities of *Carum nigrum* (seed) essential oil, oleoresin, and their selected components. *J Agric Food Chem* 54 no. 1 (2006): 174–81.

Sorkin, L.S., and McAdoo, D.J. Amino acids and serotonin are released into the lumbar spinal cord of the anesthetized cat following intradermal capsaicin injections. *Brain Res* 607 no. 1–2 (1993): 89–98.

Szallasi, A., Cortright, D.N., Blum, C.A., and Eid, S.R. The vanilloid receptor TRPV1: 10 years from channel cloning to antagonist proof-concept. *Nat Rev* 6 no. 5 (2007): 357–72.

Tambe, Y., Tsujiuchi, H., Honda, G., Ikeshiro, Y., and Tanaka, S. Gastric cytoprotection of the non-steroidal anti-inflammatory sesquiterpene, beta-caryophyllene. *Planta Med* 62 no. 5 (1996): 469–70.

Ueda, M., Kuraishi, Y., and Satoh, M. Detection of capsaicin-evoked release of glutamate from spinal dorsal horn slices of rat with on-line monitoring system. *Neurosci Lett* 155 no. 2 (1993): 179–82.

Zhang, J., Hoffert, C., Vu, H.K., Groblewski, T., Ahmad, S., and O'Donnell, D. Induction of CB2 receptor expression in the rat spinal cord of neuropathic but not inflammatory chronic pain models. *Eur J Neurosci* 17 no. 12 (2003): 2750–54.

14 Essential Oils, the Immune System, and Inflammation

Franca Marino, Raffaella Bombelli,
and Marco Cosentino

CONTENTS

14.1 INTRODUCTION

According to the chemical definition, an essential oil (EO) is a concentrated hydrophobic liquid containing volatile aromatic compounds from plants and is characterized by its volatile properties; this last characteristic justifies other terms used to define EO, such as volatile oil, ethereal oil, aetherolea, or simply "oil of" the plant from which it was extracted, for example, eucalyptus oil and rose oil. Among the herbal materials, according to the definition of the World Health Organization (WHO), the essential oils are "the scented liquid taken from certain plants using steam or pressure. Essential oils contain the natural chemicals that give the plant its 'essence' (specific odour and flavour). Essential oils are used in perfumes, food flavourings, medicine, and aromatherapy."

EOs contain the true essence of the plant from which they were derived, and usually, through different kinds of processes, these oils are highly concentrated. The most common characteristics of the different EOs are that they can provide valuable psychological and physical effects. Effects can be achieved by inhalation or application of the oil on the skin. EOs are commonly used for cooking as well as for therapeutics. The EO of *Mentha* (which contains different esters, such as menthone, menthyl acetate, menthofuran, and 1,8-cineol) represents the most ancient oil used, with archaeological evidence placing its use to ten thousand years ago, and much evidence indicates different types of effects that support its use to treat symptoms such as nausea, vomiting, abdominal pain, indigestion, irritable bowels, and swelling; more recently, evidence in animal models has shown that this oil may have protective effects against radiation used in patients during cancer radiotherapy (Baliga and Rao, 2010) or per se can have antiproliferative effects (Faridi et al., 2011).

In recent years, interest in these "natural" products has been increasing, in particular regarding their possible alternative uses as therapeutic agents with respect to conventional drugs, for example, in inflammatory and infectious disease and depression (Guilhon et al., 2011; Conrad and Adams, 2012; Sasannejad et al., 2012; Sienkiewicz et al., 2012). The most common constituents of EOs are terpenoids, monoterpenes, sesquiterpenes, and the oxygenated derivatives, and the chemical characteristics, including low molecular weight, permit them to diffuse across biological membranes and exert their biological effects (Chao et al., 2005).

14.1.1 ESSENTIAL OILS AND IMMUNE SYSTEM

The documented use of EOs in therapy dates back to ancient times: Pliny the Elder (79 CE, an ancient Roman natural philosopher who wrote *Naturalis Historia*) wrote that the Greeks and Romans used EOs for treating some diseases; for example, extracts from peppermint were widely used, and even now, these extracts are used in medicine throughout the world (Moreno et al., 2002). Not only peppermint oil, but also some other plant-derived EOs are extensively used for their clinical properties. At present, more than 300 different products obtained from diverse plants are commercially important, and in particular, interest has been focused on the pharmaceutical, cosmetic, and perfume industries. In addition, EOs are widely used as natural remedies, in massage, in aromatherapy, or as food preservatives and additives (Mitoshi et al., 2012). For some EOs the interest is well established for treatment of several organ diseases, and most of them show the ability to directly or indirectly modulate immune functions (Carrasco et al., 2009). For example, it has been confirmed that EOs obtained from parsley suppress humoral responses and reduce macrophage activity (Yousofi et al., 2012). Frequently EO exerts opposite effects on the two arms of immunity: EO from *Eugenia caryophyllata* (in particular eugenol) is known to have antiseptic and analgesic activity, as well as activity against oral bacteria associated with dental caries, and its application may result in immunostimulant effects by increasing lymphocyte activity (Halder et al., 2011). In addition, this EO reduced cell-mediated immune responses showing an anti-inflammatory action (Markowitz et al., 1992). Another effect that has been found to be common for different EOs is their anticancer activity, for example, the cancer cytotoxicity of *Melaleuca alternifolia* oil (known as tea tree) that shows anticancer activity by modulation of neutrophil and dendritic cell infiltration in cancer tissues

(Ireland et al., 2012). EOs are also known for their immunostimulant properties; for example, the oil extracted from *Zingiber officinale*, *Salvia officinalis*, and *Syzygium aromaticum* restores immune responses in cyclophosphamide-immunosuppressed mice (Carrasco et al., 2009). The most common EOs are able to differently modulate functions of the immune cells. For example, tea tree oil (TTO) obtained from *Melaleuca alternifolia* showed anti-inflammatory properties through effects on specific cell types. TTO reduced peripheral blood mononuclear cell (PBMC) proliferation *in vitro*, nickel-induced antigen cell presentation (Pearce et al., 2005), and reactive oxygen species (ROS) generation, which led to an increase of interleukin (IL)-4 and IL-10 production in human PBMCs without affecting neutrophil chemotaxis (Caldefie-Chézet et al., 2006). Lavender EO exerted anti-inflammatory activity in an animal model of bronchial asthma in which the increased number of immune cells in bronchoalveolar lavage (BAL) is directly associated with the severity of disease. In the animal model of allergic asthma, lavender EO potently reduced IL-5 and IL-13 (two inflammatory cytokines abundant in BAL) and cell number in BAL, and reduced the total cell number and eosinophil number in the peribronchial and perivascular tissue, showing beneficial effects not only in immune response but also in tissue hyperplasia (Ueno-Iio et al., 2014).

The general aim of this chapter is to discuss the ability of EOs to affect the immune response. To this end, EOs will be considered complex multicomponent compounds obtained from plants by usage of different techniques (as above discussed). Studies on individual compounds isolated from EOs and tested for their specific ability to affect immune function have been excluded from the present review.

14.2   INNATE IMMUNE SYSTEM

The innate immune system, usually considered the first line of defense against invading microorganisms, has been recently reconsidered a system involved in several noninfectious inflammatory diseases, including atherosclerosis (Libby et al., 2013) and its complications (Swirski and Nahrendorf, 2013; Courties et al., 2014). Innate immunity is actively involved in some chronic diseases, such as inflammatory bowel disease (Levine and Segal, 2013), metabolic syndrome and diabetes (Coppieters and von Herrath, 2014; Lee, 2014), and liver inflammation and disease (Liaskou et al., 2012; Meli et al., 2014). In addition, more recently, the innate immune system has been recognized to also play a role in several diseases of the central nervous system, like multiple sclerosis and other demyelinating diseases (Mayo et al., 2012; Hernández-Pedro et al., 2013) and neurodegenerative diseases (Boutajangout and Wisniewski, 2013), and in psychiatric disorders (Jones and Thomsen, 2013).

Innate immunity orchestrates the first phases of cancer development, promoting the formation of premalignant lesions and accelerating, for example, pancreatic cancer development (Inman et al., 2014), contributing to tumor recognition (van den Boorn and Hartmann, 2013; Marcus et al., 2014), and represents a barrier to organ transplantation (Farrar et al., 2013). Activation of noxious stimuli of the innate immune system occurs through the pattern recognition receptors (PRRs) that can be activated by both exogenous pathogen-associated molecular patterns (PAMPs) and endogenous danger-associated molecular patterns (DAMPs).

14.2.1 Cells of the Innate Immune Response

Structural organization of innate immunity includes effector molecules such as complement (Noris and Remuzzi, 2013) and antibacterial (Zanetti, 2004) peptides, as well as effector cells that include monocytes and macrophages, granulocytes (neutrophils, eosinophils, and basophils), mast cells, dendritic cells, natural killer (NK) cells, and γδ T lymphocytes. The latter class of cells are unconventional T cells that, like NK cells, functionally and phenotypically belong to both the innate and the adaptive immune system and connect both systems to each other. They represent about 1%–10% of circulating T cells, play a role in infective disease, and seem to be involved in the inhibition of tumor growth and development (Mak and Ferrick, 1998; Carding and Egan, 2002).

14.2.1.1 Monocytes and Macrophages

Granulocytes, monocytes and macrophages, and dendritic cells (DCs) are named myeloid cells. Physiologically, these cells are present in blood and in the lymphatic system; in specific conditions they are rapidly recruited into sites of tissue damage and infection under specific stimuli represented by different chemokines. Their primary role is in the protective immunity. Other functions ascribed to these cells are the control of development, homeostasis, and tissue repair (De Kleer et al., 2014).

Among myeloid cells, monocytes and macrophages show different phenotypes, homeostatic turnover, and functions in different tissues (Geissmann et al., 2010). Monocytes have long been considered a developmental intermediate between bone marrow precursors and tissue macrophages. However, renewed interest in recent years has revealed that, in particular, human monocytes carry out specific effector functions during inflammation (De Kleer et al., 2014) and are usually classified in CD14++CD16 classical monocytes or intermediate CD14++CD16+ cells. Monocytes are endowed with chemokine receptors and PRR that modulate their migration from blood to produce inflammatory mediators such as tumor necrosis factor (TNF)-α, nitric oxide, and ROS (De Kleer et al., 2014). Another important role exerted by macrophages is the antitumor activity. Moreover, they contribute to septic shock and organ destruction in many inflammatory and autoimmune-mediated diseases (Petros et al., 1991).

The monocytes and macrophages are widely used as a target model for *in vitro* or *ex vivo* evaluation of EOs. Both human and animal models were widely employed to test the ability of these compounds to affect immune responses. Here we report studies on animals characterizing the properties of EOs to modulate *in vivo* this innate branch of immune response, while Table 14.1 shows the effects observed in *in vitro* studies. The most common animals employed in these studies are rats and mice.

Considering tumor models, EOs often showed the ability to modulate the innate arm of the immune response. For example, they increased the phagocytic activity without showing myelotoxicity, the most common side effect of many antitumoral drugs (Serafino et al., 2008). In addition, another approach usually employed to test the ability of these compounds to affect immune response is their ability to interfere with cytokine production. In particular, *eucalyptus oil* (known from ancient times for its therapeutic effects or, more precisely, the most abundant

TABLE 14.1

In Vitro **Models of Animal and Human Cells Showing the Ability of EOs to Affect Monocyte and Macrophage Function**

Plant	Functions Investigated	Cell Models	Effect	References
		Animal		
Abies koreana	LPS-induced NO and PGE2 production; TNF-α, IL-1β, and IL-6 production	Murine macrophages	Inhibition/reduction	Yoon et al., 2009a
Achillea millefolium	iNOS and COX-2 activity; TNF-α and IL-6 production	RAW 264.7 murine macrophage cell line	Downregulation	Chou et al., 2013
Anthemis wiedemanniana	LPS-induced NO production	RAW 264.7 murine macrophage cell line	Inhibition	Conforti et al., 2012
Artemisia capillaries	LPS-induced NO and PGE-2 production; iNOS and COX-2 activity; NF-kB and MAPK pathways	RAW 264.7 murine macrophage cell line	Inhibition	Cha et al., 2009
Artemisia fukudo	TNF-α, IL-1β, and IL-6 production	RAW 264.7 murine macrophage cell line	Inhibition/reduction	Yoon et al., 2010b
Cannabis sativa	LPS-induced cytokine production; CB2 receptor-type involvement	Monocytes	Inhibition	Gertsch et al., 2008
Cinnamomum osmophloeum	LPS-induced pro-inflammatory cytokine production	J774A.1 mouse macrophage cell line	Reduction	Chao et al., 2005, 2008
	LPS-induced NO and PGE2 production	RAW 264.7 murine macrophage cell line	Inhibition	Tung et al., 2008, 2010
	LPS-induced IL-1β and IL-6 production	RAW 264.7 murine macrophage cell line	Inhibition	Chao et al., 2005
	LPS-induced NO and PGE2 production	RAW 264.7 murine macrophage cell line	Inhibition	Tung et al., 2010

(Continued)

TABLE 14.1 (CONTINUED)
***In Vitro* Models of Animal and Human Cells Showing the Ability of EOs to Affect Monocyte and Macrophage Function**

Plant	Functions Investigated	Cell Models	Effect	References
		Animal		
Citrus medica	LPS-induced NO production; iNOS and COX-2 activity; PGE2 production; MAPK transduction pathways	RAW 264.7 murine macrophage cell line	Inhibition/ reduction	Kim et al., 2013
Cleistocalyx operculatus	TNF-α and IL-1β production; NF-kB pathways	RAW 264.7 murine macrophage cell line	Inhibition/ reduction	Dung et al., 2009
Crytpomeria japonica	NO production Pathogen-induced pro-inflammatory cytokines	RAW 264.7 murine macrophage cell line	Reduction	Yoon et al., 2009b
Curcuma longa	SOD, GSH, and GSH reductase	Mice blood	Increase	Vijayastelter et al., 2011
	GSH-S-transferase; SOD	Mice liver	Increase	
Cymbopogon citratus	IL-1β and IL-6 production	Mouse macrophages	Inhibition	Sforcin et al., 2009
Lemongrass (linalool)	LPS-induced NO	J774A.1 mouse macrophage cell line	Inhibition	Peana et al., 2006
	LPS-induced COX-2 promoter activity	BAEC bovine endothelial cell line	Suppression	Katsukawa et al., 2010
Distichoselinum tenuifolium	LPS-stimulated NO production	RAW 264.7 murine macrophage cell line	Reduction	Tavares et al., 2010
1,8-Cineole	Cytokine	Monocytes	Inhibition	Sadlon and Lamson, 2010
Farfugium japonicum	LPS-stimulated NO and PGE2 production; iNOS and COX-2 mRNA levels	RAW 264.7 murine macrophage cell line	Reduction	Kim et al., 2008
Illicium anisatum	NO and PGE2 production; mRNA and protein iNOS and COX-2 levels	RAW 264.7 murine macrophage cell line	Inhibition/ suppression	Kim et al., 2009

(Continued)

TABLE 14.1 (CONTINUED)
In Vitro **Models of Animal and Human Cells Showing the Ability of EOs to Affect Monocyte and Macrophage Function**

Plant	Functions Investigated	Cell Models	Effect	References
		Animal		
Lindera umbellata	LPS-induced NO production; IL-6 and iNOS mRNA levels	RAW 264.7 murine macrophage cell line	Inhibition/ reduction	Maeda et al., 2013
Liquidambar formosana	LPS-induced NO production; COX-2 expression; TNF-α, IL-6, and IL-1β release	J774A.1 mouse macrophage cell line	Inhibition	Hua et al., 2014
Magnolia seboldii	LPS-induced NO production	Rat macrophages	Inhibition	Lim et al., 2002
Mentha longifolia	LPS-induced NO and TNF-α production	J774A.1 mouse macrophage cell line	Inhibition	Karimian et al., 2013
	LPS-induced NO production; PGE2	Rat macrophages	Inhibition	Lim et al., 2002
Neolitsea sericea	LPS-induced TNF-α, IL-1β, and IL-6 production	RAW 264.7 murine macrophage cell line	Reduction	Yoon et al., 2010a
	NF-kB and MAPK pathways		Inhibition	
Oenanthe crocata	LPS-induced NO; iNOS activity	RAW 264.7 murine macrophage cell line	Inhibition	Valente et al., 2013
Ocotea quixos	LPS-induced NO production; COX-2 expression; TNF-α, IL-6, and IL-1β production	J774A.1 murine macrophage cell line	Inhibition/ reduction	Ballabeni et al., 2010
Origanum vulgare	Oxidized LDL-induced cytokine production (TNF-α, IL-1β, and IL-6)	THP-1 derived macrophages	Inhibition	Ocana-Fuentes et al., 2010
	IL-10 production		Increase	

(*Continued*)

TABLE 14.1 (CONTINUED)
In Vitro Models of Animal and Human Cells Showing the Ability of EOs to Affect Monocyte and Macrophage Function

Plant	Functions Investigated	Cell Models	Effect	References
		Animal		
Petroselinum crispum	NO production	Unstimulated and stimulated murine macrophages	Inhibition	Karimi et al., 2012; Yousofi et al., 2012
Salvia officinalis	LPS-induced NO production	Murine macrophages	Inhibition	Abu-Darwish et al., 2013
Syzigium aromaticum	IL-1β and IL-6 production	Murine macrophages	Inhibition	Rodrigues et al., 2009; Bachiega et al., 2012
	TNF-α, IL-12, and IL-6 production		Increase	Dibazar et al., 2014
	LPS-induced TNF-α, IL-12, and IL-6 production		Reduction	Dibazar et al., 2014
Tanagetes minuta	ROS production; NADH oxidase and iNOS activity; TNF-α mRNA expression	Murine macrophages	Inhibition	Karimian et al., 2014
Thymus vulgaris	LPS-induced NO production; iNOS synthesis	J774A.1 murine macrophage cell line	Reduction	Vigo et al., 2004
Zataria multiflora	H_2O_2 production; LPS-induced NO production	Murine macrophages	Inhibition	Kavoosi et al., 2012
Zingiber officinalis	LPS-induced IL-1β production; superoxide, hydroxyl radical, and lipid peroxidation	Murine inflammation model—peritoneal macrophages	Inhibition/reduction	Zhou et al., 2006
	IL-1α production	Murine macrophages; tumor animal model	Reduction	Zhou et al., 2006
Zingiber cassumunar	NO production	RAW 264.7 murine macrophage cell line	Inhibition	Kaewchoothong et al., 2012

(Continued)

TABLE 14.1 (CONTINUED)

In Vitro **Models of Animal and Human Cells Showing the Ability of EOs to Affect Monocyte and Macrophage Function**

Plant	Functions Investigated	Cell Models	Effect	References
		Human		
Eucalyptus globulus	Phagocytic activity	Human macrophages	Stimulation	Serafino et al., 2008
Melaleuca alternifolia	Superoxide production	Human monocytes	Decrease	Brand et al., 2001
	TNF α, IL-10, IL-1β, and PGE2 production	LPS-stimulated human monocytes	Suppression	Hart et al., 2000
	Cytokines production; NF-kB and MAPK pathways	Human monocytes	Suppression	Nogueira et al., 2014; Carson et al., 2006
	Phagocytic ability; CD11b expression	Human myelocitic cell line HL-60	Increase	Budhiraja et al., 1999
	ROS production (H₂O₂ level)	Human blood leukocytes	Increase in unstimulated cells and decrease in PMA-stimulated cells	Caldefie-Chézet et al., 2006
Ocotea quixos	Forskolin-stimulated cAMP	SK-N-MC human neural lymph node cell line	Increase	Ballabeni et al., 2010

compound present in this oil, i.e., eucalyptol [1,8-cineole]) reduced the myelotoxicity observed during 5-fluorouracil treatment in a model of immunosuppressed rat (Serafino et al., 2008).

As above described, cytokine production is strongly affected by different natural compounds, and often these immunomodulatory effects are investigated in an animal model of inflammation in order to test the possible therapeutic application of these compounds as anti-inflammatory drugs. *Z. officinale* has been shown to be able to reduce IL-1α production in the hypersensitivity response to 2,4-dinitro-1-fluorobenzene in sensitized mice (Zhou et al., 2006).

Lemongrass (*Cymbopogon citratus*) is known to exert some therapeutic effects, and most of these effects are ascribed to the abundant content in monoterpenes such as linalool oxide, neral oil, epoxy-linalool oxide, α-pinene, camphene, myricene, geranial, and citronella. All these compounds are known to contribute to the typical effects of lemongrass, such as insecticidal, antimicrobial, and other documented effects (Sforcin et al., 2009). Beside these effects, other effects on immune function were specifically ascribed to linalool and epoxy-linalool oxide; in particular, these compounds were able to inhibit in mouse macrophages, both *in vivo* and *in vitro*, IL-1β and IL-6 production, resulting in anti-inflammatory activities (Sforcin et al., 2009). It has been showed that linalool *in vivo* reduced the development of carrageenan-induced edema and hyperalgesia, probably through the same mechanisms exerted *in vitro* (inhibition of NO production) (Peana et al., 2006).

The ability of TTO to exert some therapeutic effects is well documented. *Melaleuca alternifolia*, the plant from which TTO is obtained, contains different components such as α-terpineol, and this component seems to be involved in the reduction of the mechanical carrageenan-induced hypernociception and the TNF-α and prostaglandin E-2 (PGE-2) production. In addition, in a pleurisy mice model, TTO reduces the lipopolysaccharide (LPS)-induced macrophage NO production (de Oliveira et al., 2012), and in mice immunized with complete Freund's adjuvant, it increases spleen macrophage production (Nam et al., 2008).

The isolated fraction of neem oil from *Azadirachta indica*, named NIM-76, has been proved to have immunomodulating properties, and after intraperitoneal (i.p.) administration in rat, it decreased the peritoneal leukocyte count while *ex vivo* led to the increase of macrophage activity measured as the phagocytosis index (SaiRam et al., 1997).

Curcuma longa L. is one of the main spices belonging to the family of Zingiberaceae, known in most regions of southern Asia and traditionally used in Ayurveda and Chinese medicine. The EO present in this plant (for the most part extract from the rhizome of the plant by steam distillation) showed different activities both *in vivo* and *in vitro*. One month administration of turmeric EO *in vivo*, in mice, significantly increased superoxide dismutase, glutathione, and glutathione reductase enzyme levels in blood and glutathione-S-transferase and superoxide dismutase enzymes in liver; in addition, it dramatically decreased paw thickness in carrageenan and dextran-induced acute inflammation, as well as formalin-induced chronic inflammation, and showed a significant antinociceptive activity (Vijayastelter et al., 2011).

Similar anti-inflammatory properties were found by *in vivo* administration of EO from *Z. officinale*: in the mice model of carrageenan and dextran-induced paw edema, the EO was able to increase the antioxidant enzyme levels (catalase, superoxide dismutase, and glutathione reductase) in blood and serum. In a model of formalin-induced paw edema, it was able to suppress the inflammatory response, and finally, in a model of acetic acid–induced writhing, it led to reduction of the writhing movements (Jeena et al., 2013).

Similarly, the EO from *Protium strumosum*, *Grandifolium*, *Lewellyni*, and *Hebetatum* and the resin EO of *Protium heptaphyllum* increased the lymphocyte count in an *in vivo* model of pleurisy while reducing extravasation of protein and the infiltration of granulocytes and eosinophils (Siani et al., 1999).

In recent years, a possible therapeutic role for EOs has been proposed. Namely, there is a possibility to include this compound in order to reduce the inflammatory cascade in an *in vitro* model of atherosclerosis. In an *in vitro* model (THP-1 derived macrophages), EO of *Origanum vulgare* was able to revert TNF-α, IL-1β, and IL-6 production induced by oxidized low density lipoprotein (LDL) and increase the production of the anti-inflammatory cytokine IL-10 (Ocana-Fuentes et al., 2010).

14.2.1.2 Granulocytes

The granulocyte name derives from the presence in the cytoplasm of these cells of specific granules; granulocytes are the most abundant (40%–75%) type of white blood cells in mammals, and on the basis of their staining characteristics, they are divided into different subtypes: neutrophils (the most abundant, representing 40%–80% of total leukocytes in normal conditions), eosinophils, and basophils. All three cell subtypes form part of the polymorphonuclear cell family. Neutrophils are the major cell arm of the innate immune system and represent the phagocytic cells recruited into the site of infection to kill pathogens; more recently, increasing evidence suggests that neutrophils play a key role in the progression of noninfectious disease, as well as in conditions characterized by chronic inflammation (Mócsai, 2013; Mayadas et al., 2014). The key role of neutrophils in the defense against bacterial infections is clearly exemplified by the increased susceptibility to infections after chemotherapy, resulting in severe neutropenia (Brown et al., 2006). The major role ascribed to basophils is protection against infections with parasites (Karasuyama and Yamanishi, 2014), while eosinophils are considered end-stage cells involved in host protection against parasites and control mechanisms associated with allergy and asthma (Rothenberg and Hogan, 2006). Numerous lines of evidence have shown that these cells can be considered pleiotropic multifunctional leukocytes involved in the initiation and propagation of various inflammatory disease, and also key modulators of innate and adaptive immunity (Rothenberg and Hogan, 2006). Therefore, the investigation of possible modulator effects by EO on functions of these cells can represent new possible therapeutic targets.

There is extensive evidence showing the ability of EOs to modulate some properties of granulocytes, in particular the neutrophil subsets, and the most common activities tested are the inflammatory responses elicited by these cells in response to activating stimuli. To this end, both *in vivo* and *in vitro* models were used. As *in vivo* models, carrageenan-induced paw edema and examination of the number of cells in exudates are widely employed (Passos et al., 2007). Table 14.2 reports *in vitro* studies that have shown the ability of EOs to interfere with granulocyte activities in isolated cells from both animals and humans. The ability of these compounds to modulate *in vivo* granulocyte functions in both animal models of disease and humans will be discussed further in this section.

14.2.1.2.1 In Vivo *Studies on Animal Models of Disease*

Frequently EOs were tested in animal models *in vivo*: i.p. administration of the isolated fraction of neem oil from *Azadirachta indica*, named NIM-76, significantly increased the percentage of neutrophils in the blood without affecting their phagocytic activity and the total number of leukocytes (SaiRam et al., 1997).

The carrageenan model is frequently used also to test analgesic properties of substances when pain is the result of an inflammatory condition. For example, α-terpineol, one of the most common monoterpenes present in EOs, includes some analgesics and anti-inflammatory properties. In animal models of nociception induced by carrageenan, α-terpineol reduced neutrophil count in the inflamed region (de Oliveira et al., 2012); in a mouse model of inflammation, geranium,

TABLE 14.2
***In Vitro* Models on Animal and Human Cells Showing the Ability of EOs to Affect Granulocyte Functions**

Plant	Functions Investigated	Cell Models	Effect	Reference
		Animal		
Cordia verbenacea	Neutrophil influx; NF-kB	Neutrophils from rat model of inflammation	Inhibition	Medeiros et al., 2007
Myrciaria tenella	LPS-stimulated migration	Rat leukocytes	Reduction	Apel et al., 2010
Calycorectes sellowianus	LPS-stimulated migration	Rat leukocytes	Reduction	Apel et al., 2010
Matricharia camomilla *Vanillosmopsis erythropappa*	Mieloperoxidase release	PMA-stimulated neutrophils from rat model of inflammation	Decrease	Rocha et al., 2011
		Human		
Cymbopogon citrattus, Thymus vulgaris, Pogostemon cablin, Mentha spicata, Malaleuca alternifolia, Lavandula angustifolia, Pelargonium asperum, Juniperus communis, Matricaria camomilla	TNF-α and LPS-induced neutrophils adhesion	Human neutrophils	Suppression	Abe et al., 2003
Minthostachys verticillata	β-Hexosaminidase release	Basophils from allergic patients	Decrease	Cariddi et al., 2011
Citrus lemon, Ravensara aromatica, Aloe barbadiensis, Niaouly	Eosinophils and neutrophils in rhinocytogram	Eosinophils and neutrophils from patients with allergic rhinopathy	Decrease	Ferrara et al., 2012
Citrus junus	ROS and MCP-1 production; NF-kB and MAPK activity; chemotaxis	Human eosinophilic leukemia HL-60	Inhibition	Hirota et al., 2010
Citrus aurantium bergamia	ROS production	Human neutrophils	Increase	Cosentino et al., 2014
Mentha piperita	ROS production	Human neutrophils	No effects	Cosentino et al., 2009

lemongrass, spearmint oil, and TTO were able to revert recruitment of granulo-cytes in the tissue (Abe et al., 2004). Another typical model of inflammatory dis-ease is the mouse model of colitis, in which the animals are i.p. treated with several kinds of agents in order to induce inflammation of the colon. In this model, the EOs of *Lavandula intermedia* (in particular the 1,8-cineole and borneol-enriched EOs) were able to reduce infiltration of macrophages and neutrophils in the inflamed tissue as well as levels of iNOS (oxidative damage mediator), pro-inflammatory cytokines interferon (IFN)-γ and IL-22, and mRNA expression of macrophage inflammatory protein (MIP)-2α, a chemokine that promotes recruitment of neutro-phils (Baker et al., 2012).

Some other EOs, such as citral, geraniol, citronelol, carvone, and linalool, obtained from different plants (*Cymbopogon citratus* [lemongrass], *Thymus vulgaris* [thyme red], *Pogostemon cablin* [patchouli], *Mentha spicata* [spearmint], *Eucalyptus globu-lus* [eucalyptus], *Melaleuca alternifolia* [TTO], *Lavandula angustifolia* [true laven-der], *Pelargonium asperum* [geranium bourbon], *Juniperus communis* [juniper], and *Matricaria chamomilla* [German chamomilla]), are able to modulate granulocyte functions in different modes (Abe et al., 2003).

14.2.1.2.2 In Vivo *Studies on Humans*

The most frequent studies conducted in humans regard the ability of EOs to show antitumor or antimicrobial activities, and therefore they are not included in this sec-tion. Besides these, the use of EOs in humans is for the most part devoted to the treatment of allergic diseases, in particular allergic diseases of the respiratory tract (González Pereyra et al., 2005; Cariddi et al., 2011).

The extract of *Citrus lemon*, rich in different EOs, was used as topical application (nasal spray) in patients suffering from allergic rhinopathy. In these subjects, it was shown that daily administration of nasal spray rich in lemongrass and *Ravensara* oil, together with other compounds, dramatically decreased the presence of eosino-phils and neutrophils in rhinocytogram and similarly decreased all other symptoms related to rhinopathy (nasal obstruction, rhinorrhea, sneezing, and turbinate hyper-trophy) (Ferrara et al., 2012).

14.2.1.3 Mast Cells

Mast cells (MCs), first described by Paul Erlich in 1878, are long-lived, multifunc-tional immune cells characterized by large granules and usually resident in most tissues of the body, with a particularly high density in the airways; the presence in the airways permits these cells to respond to external triggers and kick-start an inflammatory response (Erjefält, 2014). The most common function of MCs is their activation in allergies and the cross-linkage of surface-bound immunoglobulin (Ig) E, which induces rapid degranulation and release of mediators such as histamine and manifestation of an acute phase of allergic reaction. In addition, the MCs are involved in the extravasation of plasma, showing a severe immunological response and production of cytokines that facilitate the subsequent leukocyte recruitment and development of local inflammation (Persson et al., 1998).

The principal effects exerted by EOs on MC functions have been characterized on local inflammation, for example, their ability to induce edema. EOs obtained from *Pilocarpus spicatus* can induce a local edematous reaction through a mechanism that seems to involve the activation of the phospholipase A2 cascade (Silva and Rao, 1992). Other typical uses of plant-derived oils are reported in asthma, a typical disease of the airway with hyperresponsiveness that affects millions of people in the world, in which it is known that MCs play a key role (Erjefält, 2014). In this context, EOs of *Pistacia integerrima* have shown a potent ability to suppress the degranulation of MCs and reduce ROS generation (Shirole et al., 2014). Allergic rhinitis, another typical inflammatory disease of the respiratory tract, is characterized by intense MC degranulation and an increased number of MCs (and, as above described, other cells of innate immunity, like eosinophils and neutrophils) in the rhinocytogram. Lemon pulp extract, known to be rich in flavonoids (flavanone glycosides, hesperidin and eriocitrin) (Caristi et al., 2003), added together with EOs of *Ravensara* and *Niaouly*, reduced the mast cell number in the rhinocytogram of patients suffering from allergic rhinopathy and impaired dramatically the MC degranulation (Ferrara et al., 2012); the same inhibitory effect has been observed with EOs from chamomile, lemongrass, and sandalwood (Mitoshi et al., 2012). Inhibitory effects not only on MC degranulation, but also on the ability of these cells to infiltrate in the derma, were shown in a mouse model of atopic dermatitis; in this case, the EOs obtained from a tropical tree, *Chamaecypris obtuse*, rich in several types of terpenes (sabinene, limonene, bornul acetate, borneol + α-terpineol, and elemol), reduced IgE serum levels and the number of infiltrating MCs in the inflamed skin (Joo et al., 2010).

14.2.1.4 Dendritic Cells and Natural Killer Cells

Dendritic cells (DCs) specialize in the processing and presenting of antigen, and their major role is the initiation and regulation of adaptive immune responses. They are involved in the development of immunological memory and tolerance (De Kleer et al., 2014). The DC possess high phagocytic activity as immature cells and high cytokine-producing capacity as mature cells, and they are able to migrate into the lymphoid organs and regulate T cell responses in both the steady state and during infection (Mellman and Steinman, 2001).

The natural killer (NK) cells are the first line of defense against invading pathogens and cancer and are included in the group of innate lymphoid cells (Ivanova et al., 2014). Usually they are grouped on the basis of their functional relevance in three categories. The NK cells are always present in all mucosal tissues and play a pivotal role in the defense against bacterial, fungal, viral, and parasitic infections (Hall et al., 2013).

Data about possible effects of EO on functions of DC and NK are very few and limited to studies on healthy subjects or on patients with cancer or inflammatory diseases of the skin or on an animal models of tumor or local inflammation. EOs (in particular phytocides) from *Chamaecyparis obtusa* (Japanese cypress, hinoki cypress, or hinoki) increase the NK activity in healthy subjects (Li et al., 2009). A similar result is obtained in healthy subjects exposed to Ayurvedic treatment with sesame oil, which increases the NK number and in general possesses immunostimulant effects (Uebaba et al., 2008). EOs present in the same plant can have different effects on the immune response. For example, as above discussed, one of the compounds present in the EO from *Zanthoxylum rhoifolium*, the terpene β-caryophyllene, seemed to increase animal survival in the Ehrlich ascites tumor model, in particular by increasing the total number of NK, while on the contrary, α-humulene, α-pinene, and β-pinene were ineffective (da Silva et al., 2007). TTO (*Melaleuca alternifolia*) increased the activity of different immune cells, inducing, for example, the accumulation of DC and other immune cells in the site of inflammation, and in addition expressed antitumor activity *in vivo* (Ireland et al., 2012). All these properties suggest possible therapeutic applications of this plant extract in immune-mediated diseases in which these cells play a key role.

14.3 ADAPTIVE IMMUNITY

Adaptive immunity is the branch of the immune system with specific immune competence and is sometimes called acquired immunity. It is organized by highly specialized cells that eliminate or prevent pathogen growth. The main aim of this branch of the immune response is the creation of immunological memory after an initial response to a specific pathogen, leading to an enhanced response to subsequent encounters with that same pathogen. This crucial step represents the basis of vaccination. Like the innate system, the adaptive system includes both humoral and cellular immunity as well (Martinez and Lynch, 2013).

The immunological memory occurs during the lifetime due to exposure to pathogen organisms, and the acquired response is said to be adaptive because it prepares the body's immune system for future confrontations with invading organisms. Adaptive immunity is characterized by some key features: recognition of specific non-self antigens, thanks to the presence of specific receptors able to distinguish non-self antigens from self antigens during the process of antigen presentation. The generated response is personalized and organized for the maximal elimination of specific pathogens or pathogen-infected cells. Cells of adaptive immunity are characterized by a wide number of receptors (T cell receptor [TCR] and B cell receptor [BCR]), able to recognize any non-self antigen and responsible for the development of immunological memory (Gonzalez et al., 2011).

14.3.1 CELLS OF THE ADAPTIVE IMMUNITY

Classically, the cells of adaptive immunity are considered to be organized into two major classes: T and B lymphocytes, which have been shown to have an extremely diverse repertoire of antigen-specific recognition receptors that facilitate the identification and elimination of pathogens and develop the immunological memory against pathogen reinfection (Dunkelberger and Song, 2010).

Lymphocytes represent one of the subpopulations of white blood cells in the immune system of vertebrates, which includes NK cells (which function in cell-mediated, cytotoxic innate immunity, as discussed above), T cells (cell-mediated, cytotoxic adaptive immunity), and B cells (humoral, antibody-driven adaptive immunity). Specifically, the name *lymphocyte* includes T and B cells (the major cellular components of the adaptive immune response). The main source of T and B lymphocytes is the primary lymphoid tissues (thymus and bone marrow, respectively) (Abbas and Lichtman, 2003).

The physiological role of T cells is to recognize antigens presented by specialized antigen-presenting cells (APCs), through cooperation of TCR and CD3 molecules expressed on their surface, with major histocompatibility complex II (MHC-II) molecules expressed on the surface of APCs. Recognition of antigen by TCRs will start the downstream cascade, resulting in cell activation and response (Smith-Garvin et al., 2009).

The B lymphocytes are distinguished from T cells and NK cells by the presence of a protein on the outer surface named B cell receptor (BCR). The role of this protein is to allow a B cell to bind to a specific antigen. The principal functions of B cells are to secrete antibodies against antigens to perform the role of antigen-presenting cells and release cytokines. B cells can develop into memory B cells after activation by antigen (Mauri and Bosma, 2012). Recently, a suppressive role of this cell was described (Mizoguchi et al., 2002) through the production of IL-10, which suppresses inflammatory responses in experimental autoimmune encephalomyelitis, collagen-induced arthritis, and colitis (Fillatreau et al., 2002; Mauri et al., 2003).

14.3.2 ESSENTIAL OILS AND ADAPTIVE IMMUNITY

The capacity of EOs to interfere with cell functions has been explored for many compounds of both natural and synthetic origin, investigating their possible application as potential new drugs or adjuvant drugs. Various EOs have different effects on adaptive immune response. A large amount of important effects described for EOs on lymphocyte functions come from studies of autoimmune diseases and the ability of these compounds to show immunostimulant or immunosuppressive effects (Khiewkhern et al., 2013).

As above discussed, TTO shows different immunomodulating effects on both innate and adaptive immunity. *In vitro*, it has been shown that TTO inhibited PBMC proliferation of cells obtained from venous blood of nickel-sensitive subjects and *in vivo* (topical application) reduced the flare area and erythema index (the area of local inflammation after nickel exposure) (Pearce et al., 2005). In addition, TTO reduced ROS generation and increased Th2 cytokine production in human PBMCs (Caldefie-Chézet et al., 2006), suggesting an anti-inflammatory profile. Some EOs showed different and frequently opposite effects on the key immune responses. Camphor and borneol, two monoterpenes presents in EOs of different plants, increased rat thymocyte viability and at the same time reduced ROS production (Cherneva et al., 2012).

EO improves health and lessen symptoms in atopic asthma; in particular, the EO from lavender is known to have antibacterial activity and sedative effects (Cavanagh and Wilkinson, 2002). In addition, it has been shown that this EO reduces the total cell infiltrate in BAL and the cytokine production in asthmatic subjects (Ueno-lio et al., 2014).

Parsley (*Petroselinum crispum*) is traditionally used to treat different kinds of disease, such as allergy, autoimmune, and chronic diseases. Recently, anti-inflammatory properties of its EOs were observed *in vitro*; specifically in mouse splenocytes, the phytohaemagglutinin (PHA)-induced proliferation was concentration-dependently inhibited by parsley, suggesting the ability of this oil to affect immune function (Yousofi et al., 2012).

EOs also show ability to bind to specific receptors and exert, through this binding, specific immune properties. The sesquiterpene (E)-β-caryophyllene, abundant in different plants such as oregano, cinnamon, and black pepper and recently found in *Cannabis sativa*, binds the cannabinoid receptor (CB) 2 and, through this binding, can exert some immunomodulatory effects, such as LPS-induced inhibition of TNF-α and IL-1β production in human whole blood (the observed effects were reverted by the CB2 antagonist AM630) (Gertsch et al., 2008).

14.3.2.1   T and B Lymphocytes

The effects of EO were widely investigated on different T lymphocyte functions. Only few data of literature describe studies on the function of B cells. T lymphocytes produce key cytokines involved in the immune response; conventionally, the T-helper (Th) 1 subset is considered the cells that primarily produce pro-inflammatory cytokines, such as IFN-γ and IL-2, while the Th2 cell subset is the T lymphocytes that mainly produce anti-inflammatory cytokines like IL-4 and IL-10 (Romagnini, 1995). EOs, obtained from various plants, are able to modulate the Th1–Th2 balance. In addition, some compounds exerted different effects on the various lymphocyte subsets; for example, immunostimulatory effects were observed by the i.p. administration of EO from *Melaleuca viridiflora*. Further, in mice immunized with Freund's adjuvant, this EO increased the surface expression of CD25, lymphocyte proliferation, and IFN-γ secretion without affecting the B lymphocyte response (Nam et al., 2008).

Interestingly, the EOs obtained from the same plants were able to differently modulate the immune response depending on the varieties of plants: for example, the EOs from two different qualities of *Mentha piperita* (RAC541 and Laimburg) were investigated for their immune effects on both the innate immunity (neutrophils) and the acquired immunity (PBMCs). It has been shown that in human PBMCs, the RAC541 qualities increased PHA-induced proliferation, while Laimburg oils reduced the IL-4 production, suggesting that the composition of the EOs can be influenced by the region or period of cultivation (Cosentino et al., 2009).

EOs can be administered in different forms. A recent paper described positive effects of massage of cancer patients with EOs. In patients with colorectal cancer, an improvement of immune response and subsequent reduction of symptoms related to chemotherapy and disease have been shown; in particular, patients that have received a Thai massage with coconut and ginger oil have shown a renewed total lymphocyte count, increased CD4/CD8 T lymphocyte ratio, and reduced symptoms related to disease and chemotherapy (Khiewkhern et al., 2013). EOs from ginger oil alone exerted different effects on immune functions: a positive effect of ginger was shown in an animal model of tumor, in which *Z. officinale* improved the immune response both *in vivo* and *in vitro*. In particular, EOs from *Z. officinale* increased the percentage of suppressor T cells and reduced the T cell proliferation, affecting both cell-mediated immune response and nonspecific cell proliferation. Positive effects of the compound were also found in the animal model, in which the EO reduced the organ index of the thymus and spleen during tumor growth (Zhou et al., 2006). On the contrary, the same products have been shown to increase the organ index in mice with tumor in different tumor models (Liu and Zhou, 2002), reduce lymphocyte mitogen and alloantigen-induced cell proliferation in mice (Wilasrusmee et al., 2002a), and affect lymphocyte function in humans, by decreasing lymphocyte proliferation and inhibiting IL-2 and IL-10 production (Wilasrusmee et al., 2002b).

EOs are also widely used for their anti-inflammatory activity in different diseases in which a T cell response is considered crucial, for example, through the production of specific mediators. EO from parsley exerts immunosuppressive effects; recently, it was hypothesized that the immunosuppressive ability is due to the inhibition of PHA-induced T cell proliferation and the reduction of LPS-induced B cell stimulation in mice (Karimi et al., 2012). Immunomodulating effects were also observed by the volatile oil extracted from *Nigella sativa*, known to have a wide spectrum of activity, including antimicrobial, antiviral, and anti-inflammatory (Asp, 2001). In a rat model, treatment with this EO led to an increase in the number of lymphocytes and monocytes (Islam et al., 2004); on the contrary, in an animal model of lung inflammation the lymphocyte number was reduced. In this latter model, the observed effect seems to be associated with a reduction of plasma levels of IL-4 and IFN-γ and regulation of the Th1–Th2 balance (Boskabady et al., 2011). Similar inhibitory effects on lymphocyte proliferation and increased cell apoptosis were observed in the use of EOs present in oregano (*Origanum vulgare*) that contain carvacol and eugenol (Bimczok et al., 2008). In JURKAT and THP-1 cell lines this EO increased Ca++ mobilization, an intracellular signalling cascade related to increased cell activity, and initiated cell proliferation and cytokine production (Singer and Koretzky, 2002; Chan et al., 2005). Antiproliferative and pro-apoptotic effects on isolated lymphocytes from the blood of mouse and rats were observed by the EOs obtained from fruits of *Pterodon polygalaeflorus* (Leguminosae or Fabacea), a native tree from the central region of Brazil, popularly named sucupira branca, suggesting an anti-inflammatory effect (Velozo et al., 2013).

The effects of EOs on different diseases can be better explained when isolated compounds are analyzed for their activity. Only as an example we report here some cases for the confirmation of the evidence, although in this chapter we have excluded the studies reporting the effects of single compounds.

I.p. administration of the sesquiterpene β-elemene (isolated from herb *Rhizoma zedoariae*) showed positive effects both *in vitro* and *in vivo* in a mouse model of multiple sclerosis, autoimmune encephalomyelitis (EAE). In this model, β-elemene reduced the presence of the immune cells in the central nervous system (CNS), improved axonal loss in the spinal cord, and inhibited *in vitro* lymphocyte proliferation and the release of IL-17 and IL-6, suggesting a neuroprotective effect. Hence, in this way its possible use has been confirmed not only in cancer (Yang et al., 1999; Tan et al., 2000), where it seems to facilitate the restoration of immune response (Wu et al., 1999), but also in demyelinating diseases (Zhang et al., 2011).

Immunostimulant effects were observed by the EO present in frankincense oil (*Boswellia carteri*), in which the main constituents are α-pinene, octyl acetate, and α-thujene (depending on the origin of the plants). These compounds increased human lymphocyte proliferation, and this effect was comparable to that induced by the well-known immunostimulants, such as the *Echinacea purpurea* extract and levamisole (Mikhaeil et al., 2003). In healthy subjects, EO from *Minthostachys verticillata* (a traditional herbal medicine from South America) increased lymphocyte proliferation measured as cluster formation (González Pereyra et al., 2005).

Effects in the regulation of the cell functions were also observed in the case of inhalation of EO: exposition to vapor of volatile aromatic phytoncides (obtained from hinoki cypress) affected the lymphocyte number in healthy subjects (Li et al., 2009).

Another plant with immunomodulating properties is *Azadirachta indica*: the isolated fraction of neem oil, named NIM-76, when administered i.p. in rat, increased lymphocyte proliferation without affecting primary or secondary antibody levels (SaiRam et al., 1997).

The lymphocyte can also be activated in inflammatory response elicited by allergens, and EOs are able to also affect these reactions. For example, in healthy subjects and allergic patients, the EO obtained from *Minthostachys verticillata* stimulated lymphocyte proliferation, in particular limonene alone or in combination with monoterpene (present in EO), which was able to decrease the IL-13 production (Cariddi et al., 2011).

14.4 CLINICAL PERSPECTIVES

As extensively discussed above, the use of EO in therapy dates back to ancient times, and Greeks and Romans have documented the use of EO in the treatment of many diseases. In fact, from the ancient age, EOs have been widely used for their activity as antiseptic, antifungal, antimicrobial, and antiparasitical substances (Alma et al., 2003; Amer and Mehlhorn, 2006; Bozin et al., 2006) and for their anti-inflammatory activity, but the mechanisms through which these effects were exerted remained obscure for a long time, and in some cases still are. At present, we know that a large amount of EO exerts the ability to interfere with the immune response and show immunomodulating properties. Frequently, EOs induce opposite effects, showing activity that can be immunostimulant or immunosuppressive, or they exert their function on the two arms of an immune response separately or together (Markowitz et al., 1992; Carrasco et al., 2009; Halder et al., 2011).

The most ancient use of EO documented was in fighting infective diseases, in particular bacterial infections. In addition, EOs are known to have antiseptic and analgesic activity as well as activity against infection from oral bacteria associated with dental caries (Halder et al., 2011).

In recent years, different EOs obtained from diverse plants have been employed or proposed for their anticancer activity, for example, TTO, for which anticancer activity (in particular in tumors in which immune cells play a key role) has been shown through its ability to modulate tumor infiltration by neutrophils and DCs and expressing more limited side effects than conventionally used anticancer drugs (Ireland et al., 2012).

Another typical application of EO is in respiratory diseases, in particular those connected with allergies. EOs obtained from lavender exerted anti-inflammatory activity in an animal model of bronchial asthma (Ueno-Iio et al., 2014). More recently, EOs like sesquiterpene β-elemene (isolated from *Rhizoma zedoariae*, a Chinese medicinal herb) were considered for potential applications in neurodegenerative diseases. Namely, in an animal model of multiple sclerosis, the EAE, this EO showed positive effects in both *in vitro* and *in vivo* studies, suggesting a neuroprotective effect (Zhang et al., 2011).

In conclusion, the evidence present in literature and at least partially reported in this chapter suggests that EOs represent valid therapeutic tools and, at the same time, low-cost therapeutics in treating different kinds of diseases (Bakkali et al., 2008; Ireland et al., 2012). In addition, in order to better clarify effects exerted by EOs in different diseases, it should be remembered that most of the studies were done with isolated compounds and not with the whole oil because the individual compounds, depending on the mode of application or administration, exhibit better tolerability and fewer problems. It would be more than useful to propose specific clinical trials aimed at better comprehension of the mechanisms by which activity of EO is exerted in different diseases and to promote the use of these ancient remedies in modern medicine.

REFERENCES

Abbas AK, Lichtman AH. *Cellular and Molecular Immunology* (5th ed.). Saunders, Philadelphia, 2003.

Abe S, Maruyama N, Hayama K, Ishibashi H, Inoue S, Oshima H, Yamaguchi H. Suppression of tumor necrosis factor-alpha-induced neutrophil adherence responses by essential oils. *Mediators Inflamm* 2003;12:323–28.

Abe S, Maruyama N, Hayama K, Inouye S, Oshima H, Yamaguchi H. Suppression of neutrophil recruitment in mice by geranium essential oil. *Mediators Inflamm* 2004;13:21–24.

Abu-Darwish MS, Cabral G, Ferreira IV, Goncalves MJ, Cavaleiro C, Cruz MT, Al-bdour TH, Salgueiro L. Essential oil of common sage (*Salvia officinalis* L.) from Jordan: Assessment of safety in mammalian cells and its antifungal and anti-inflammatory potential. *BioMed Res Int* 2013;ID538940.

Alma MH, Mavi A, Yildirim A, Digrak M, Hirata T. Screening chemical composition and in vitro antioxidant and antimicrobial activities of the essential oils from *Origanum syriacum* L. growing in Turkey. *Biol Pharm Bull* 2003;26:1725–29.

Amer A, Mehlhorn H. Larvicidal effects of various essential oils against Aedes, Anopheles, and Culex larvae (Diptera, Culicidae). *Parasitol Res* 2006;99:466–72.

Apel MA, Lima ME, Sobral M, Young MC, Cordeiro I, Schapoval EE, Henriques AT, Moreno PR. Anti-inflammatory activity of essential oil from leaves of *Myrciaria tenella* and *Calycorectes sellowianus*. *Pharm Biol* 2010;48:433–38.

Asp NG. Beyond basic nutrition: Substantiation and communication of health benefits in the context of balanced diet. *Ann Nutr Metab* 2001;45(Suppl 1):99.

Bachiega TF, Barreto de Sousa JP, Bastos JK, Sforcin JMJ. Clove and eugenol in noncytotoxic concentrations exert immunomodulatory/anti-inflammatory action on cytokine production by murine macrophages. *Pharm Pharmacol* 2012;64:610–16.

Baker J, Brown K, Rajendiran E, Yip A, DeCoffee D, Dai C, Molcan E, Chittick A, Ghosh S, Mahmoud S, Gibson DL. Medicinal lavender modulates the enteric microbiota to protect against *Citrobacter rodentium*-induced colitis. *Am J Physiol Gastrointest Liver Physiol* 2012;303:G825–36.

Bakkali F, Averbeck S, Averbeck D, Idaomar M. Biological effects of essential oils: A review. *Food Chem Toxicol* 2008;46:446–75.

Baliga MS, Rao S. Radioprotective potential of mint: A brief review. *J Canc Res Ther* 2010;6:255–62.

Ballabeni V, Tognolini M, Giorgio C, Bertoni S, Bruni R, Barocelli E. *Ocotea quixos* Lam. essential oil: In vitro and in vivo investigation on its anti-inflammatory properties. *Fitoterapia* 2010;81:289–95.

Bimczok D, Rau H, Sewekow E, Janczyk P, Souffrant WB, Rothkotter HJ. Influence of carvacol on proliferation and survival of porcine lymphcoytes and intestinal epithelial cells in vitro. *Toxicol In Vitro* 2008;22:652–58.

Boskabady MH, Vahedi N, Amery S, Khakzad MR. The effect of *Nigella sativa* alone, and in combination with dexamethasone, on tracheal muscle responsiveness and lung inflammation in sulfur mustard exposed guinea pigs. *J Ethnopharmacol* 2011;137:1028–34.

Boutajangout A, Wisniewski T. The innate immune system in Alzheimer's disease. *Int J Cell Biol* 2013;2013:576383.

Bozin B, Mimica-Dukic N, Simin N, Anackov G. Characterization of the volatile composition of essential oils of some Lamiaceae spices and the antimicrobial and antioxidant activities of the entire oils. *J Agric Food Chem* 2006;54:1822–28.

Brand C, Ferrante A, Prager RH, Riley TV, Carson CF, Finlay-Jones JJ, Hart PH. The water soluble components of the essential oil of *Melaleuca alternifolia* (tea tree oil) suppress the production of superoxide by human monocytes but not neutrophils activated in vitro. *Inflamm Res* 2001;50:213–19.

Brown KA, Brain SD, Pearson JD, Edgeworth JD, Lewis SM, Treacher DF. Neutrophils in development of multiple organ failure in sepsis. *Lancet* 2006;368:157–69.

Budhiraja SS, Cullum ME, Sioutis SS, Evangelista L, Habanova ST. Bological activity of *Melaleuca alternifolia* (tea tree) oil component, terpinen-4-ol, in human myelocytic cell line HL-60. *J Manipulative Physiol Ther* 1999;22:447–53.

Caldefie-Chézet F, Fusillier C, Jarde T, Laroye H, Damez M, Vasson MP, Guillot J. Potential anti-inflammatory effects of *Melaleuca alternifolia* essential oil on human peripheral blood leukocytes. *Phytother Res* 2006;20:364–70.

Carding SR, Egan PJ. Gammadelta T cells: Functional plasticity and heterogeneity. *Nat Rev Immunol* 2002;2:336–45.

Cariddi L, Escobar F, Moser M, Panero A, Alaniz F, Zygadlo J, Sabini L, Maldonado A. Monoterpenes isolated from *Minthostachys verticillata* (Griseb.) Epling essential oil modulates immediate-type hypersensitivity responses in vitro and in vivo. *Planta Med* 2011;77:1687–94.

Caristi C, Bellocco E, Panzera V, Toscano G, Vadalà R, Leuzzi U. Flavonoids detection by HPLC-DAD-MS-MS in lemon juices from *Sicilian cultivars*. *J Agric Food Chem* 2003;51:3528–34.

Carrasco FR, Schmidt G, Romero AL, Sartoretto JL, Caparroz-Assef SM, Bersani-Amado CA, Cuman RK. Immunomodulatory activity of *Zingiber officinale* Roscoe, *Salvia officinalis* L. and *Syzygium aromaticum* L. essential oils: Evidence for humor- and cell-mediated responses. *J Pharm Pharmacol* 2009;61:961–67.

Carson CF, Hammer KA, Riley TV. *Melaleuca alternifolia* (tea tree) oil: A review of antimicrobial and other medicinal properties. *Clin Microbiol Rev* 2006;19:50–62.

Cavanagh HM, Wilkinson JM. Biological activities of lavender essential oil. *Phytother Res* 2002;16:301–8.

Cha JD, Moon SE, Kim HY, Lee JC, Lee KY. The essential oil isolated from *Artemisia* capillaries prevents LPS-induced production of NO and PGE2 by inhibiting MAP-mediated pathways in RAW 264.7 macrophages. *Immunol Investig* 2009;38:483–97.

Chan AS, Pang H, Yip EC, Tam YK, Wong YH. Carvacrol and eugenol differentially stimulate intracellular Ca2+ mobilization and mitogen-activated protein kinases in Jurkat T-cells and monocytic THP-1 cells. *Planta Med* 2005;71:634–39.

Chao LK, Hua KF, Hsu HY, Cheng SS, Liu JY, Chang ST. Study on the antiinflammatory activity of essential oil from leaves of *Cinnamomum osmophloeum*. *J Agric Food Chem* 2005;53:7274–78.

Chao LK, Hua KF, Hsu HY, Cheng SS, Lin IF, Chen CJ, Chen ST, Chang ST. Cinnamaldheyde inhibits pro-inflammatory cytokines secretion from monocytes/macrophages through suppression of intracellular signaling. *Food Chem Toxicol* 2008;46:220–31.

Cherneva E, Pavlovic V, Smelcerovic A, Yancheva D. The effect of camphor and borneol on rat thymocyte viability and oxidative stress. *Molecules* 2012;17:10258–66.

Chou ST, Chang WL, Chang CT, Hsu SL, Lin YC, Shih Y. *Cinnamomum cassia* essential oil inhibits α-MSH-induced melanin production and oxidative stress in murine B16 melanoma cells. *Int J Mo. Sci* 2013;14:12978–93.

Conforti F, Menichini F, Formisano C, Rigano D, Senatore F, Bruno M, Rosselli S, Celik S. *Anthemis wiedemanniana* essential oil prevents LPS-induced production of NO in RAW 274.7 macrophages and exerts antiproliferative and antibacterial activities in vitro. *Nat Prod Res* 2012;26:1594–601.

Conrad P, Adams C. The effects of clinical aromatherapy for anxiety and depression in the high risk postpartum woman: A pilot study. *Complement Ther Clin Pract* 2012;18:164–68.

Coppieters KT, von Herrath MG. Metabolic syndrome: Removing roadblocks to therapy: Antigenic immunotherapies. *Mol Metab* 2014;3:275–83.

Cosentino M, Bombelli R, Conti A, Colombo ML, Azzetti A, Bergamaschi A, Marino F, Lecchini S. Antioxidant properties and in vitro immunomodulatory effects of peppermint (*Mentha × piperita* L.) essential oils in human leukocytes. *J Pharm Sci Res* 2009;1:33–43.

Cosentino M, Luini A, Bombelli R, Corasaniti MT, Bagetta G, Marino F. The essential oil of bergamot stimulates reactive oxygen species production in human polymorphonuclear leukocytes. *Phytother Res* 2014;28:1232–39.

Courties G, Moskowitz MA, Nahrendorf M. The innate immune system after ischemic injury: Lessons to be learned from the heart and brain. *JAMA Neurol* 2014;71:233–36.

da Silva SL, Figueiredo PM, Yano T. Chemotherapeutic potential of the volatile oils from *Zanthoxylum rhoifolium* Lam leaves. *Eur J Pharmacol* 2007;576:180–88.

De Kleer I, Willems F, Lambrecht B, Goriely S. Ontogeny of myeloid cells. *Front Immunol* 2014;5:423.

de Oliveira MGB, Marques RB, de Santana MF, Santos ABD, Brito FA, Barreto EO, De Sousa DP, Almeida FR, Badaue-Passos D, Antonioli AR, Quintans-Junior LJ. Alpha-terpineol reduces mechanical hypernociception and inflammatory response. *Basic Clin Pharmacol Toxicol* 2012;111:120–25.

Dibazar SP, Fateh S, Daneshmandi S. Immunomodulatory effects of clove (*Syzygium aromaticum*) constituents on macrophages: In vitro evaluations of aequous and ethanolic components [Online]. *J Immunotoxicol* 2015;12:124–31.

Dung NT, Bajpai VK, Yoon JI, Kang SC. Anti-inflammatory effects of essential oil isolated from the buds of *Cleistocalyx operculatus* (Roxb) Merr and Perry. *Food Chem Toxicol* 2009;47:449–53.

Dunkelberger JR, Song WC. Complement and its role in innate and adaptive immune responses. *Cell Res* 2010;20:34–50.

Erjefält JS. Mast cells in human airways: The culprit? *Eur Respir Rev* 2014;23:299–307.

Faridi U, Sisodia BS, Shukla AK, Shukla RK, Darokar MP, Dwivedi UN, Shasany AK. Proteomics indicates modulation of tubulin polymerization by L-menthol inhibiting human epithelial colorectal adenocarcinoma cell proliferation. *Proteomics* 2011;11:2115–19.

Farrar CA, Kupiec-Weglinski JW, Sacks SH. The innate immune system and transplantation. *Cold Spring Harb Perspect Med* 2013;3:a015479.

Ferrara L, Naviglio D, Armone Caruso A. Cytological aspects on the effects of a nasal spray consisting of standardized extract of citrus lemon and essential oils in allergic rhinopathy. *ISRN Pharm* 2012;2012:404606.

Fillatreau S, Sweenie CH, McGeachy MJ, Gray D, Anderton SM. B cells regulate autoimmunity by provision of IL-10. *Nat Immunol* 2002;3:944–50.

Geissmann F, Manz MG, Jung S, Sieweke MH, Merad M, Ley K. Development of monocytes, macrophages, and dendritic cells. *Science* 2010;327:656–61.

Gertsch J, Leonti M, Raduner S, Racz I, Chen JZ, Xie XQ, Altmann KH, Karsak M, Zimmer A. Beta-caryophyllene is a dietary cannabinoid. *Proc Natl Acad Sci USA* 2008;105:9099–104.

Gonzalez S, González-Rodríguez AP, Suárez-Álvarez B, López-Soto A, Huergo-Zapico L, Lopez-Larrea C. Conceptual aspects of self and nonself discrimination. *Self Nonself* 2011;2:19–25.

González Pereyra ML, Cariddi LN, Ybarra F, Isola MC, Demo MS, Sabini L, Maldonado AM. Immunomodulating properties of *Minthostachys verticillata* on human lymphocytes and basophils. *Rev Alerg Mex* 2005;52:105–12.

Guilhon CC, Raymundo LJ, Alviano DS, Blank AF, Arrigoni-Blank MF, Matheus ME, Cavalcanti SC, Alviano CS, Fernandes PD. Characterization of the anti-inflammatory and antinociceptive activities and the mechanism of the action of *Lippia gracilis* essential oil. *J Ethnopharmacol* 2011;135:406–13.

Halder S, Mehta AK, Mediratta PK, Sharma KK. Essential oil of clove (*Eugenia caryophyllata*) augments the humoral immune response but decreases cell mediated immunity. *Phytother Res* 2011;25:1254–56.

Hall LJ, Murphy CT, Hurley G, Quinlan A, Shanahan F, Nally K, Melgar S. Natural killer cells protect against mucosal and systemic infection with the enteric pathogen *Citrobacter rodentium*. *Infect Immun*, 2013;81:460–69.

Hart PH, Brand C, Carson CF, Riley TV, Prager RH, Finlay-Jones JJ. Terpinen-4-ol, the main component of the essential oil of *Melaleuca alternifolia* (tea tree oil), suppresses inflammatory mediator production by activated human monocytes. *Inflamm Res* 2000;49:619–26.

Hernández-Pedro NY, Espinosa-Ramirez G, de la Cruz VP, Pineda B, Sotelo J. Initial immunopathogenesis of multiple sclerosis: Innate immune response. *Clin Dev Immunol* 2013;2013:413–65.

Hirota R, Roger NN, Nakamura H, Song HS, Sawamura M, Suganuma N. Anti-inflammatory effects of limonene from yuzu (*Citrus junos* Tanaka) essential oil on eosinophils. *J Food Sci* 2010;75:H87–92.

Hua KF, Yang TJ, Chiu HW, Ho CH. Essential oil from leaves of *Liquidambar formosana* ameliorates inflammatory response and lypopolysaccharide-activated mouse macrophages. *Nat Prod Commun* 2014;9:869–72.

Inman KS, Francis AA, Murray NR. Complex role for the immune system in initiation and progression of pancreatic cancer. *World J Gastroenterol* 2014;20:11160–81.

Ireland DJ, Greay SJ, Hooper CM, Kissick HT, Filion P, Riley TV, Beilharz MW. Topically applied *Melaleuca alternifolia* (tea tree) oil causes direct anti-cancer cytotoxicity in subcutaneous tumour bearing mice. *J Dermatol Sci* 2012;67:120–29.

Islam SKN, Begum P, Ahsam T, Huque S, Ahsan M. Immunosuppressive and cytotoxic properties of *Nigella sativa*. *Phytother Res* 2004;18:395–98.

Ivanova D, Krempels R, Ryfe J, Weitzman K, Stephenson D, Gigley JP. NK cells in mucosal defense against infection. *Biomed Res Int* 2014;2014:413982.

Jeena K, Liju V, Kuttan R. Antioxidant, anti-inflammatory and antinociceptive activities of essential oil from ginger. *Indian J Physiol Pharmacol* 2013;57:51–62.

Jones KA, Thomsen C. The role of the innate immune system in psychiatric disorders. *Mol Cell Neurosci* 2013;53:52–62.

Joo SS, Yoo YM, Ko SH, Choi W, Park MJ, Kang HY, Choi KC, Choi IG, Jeung EB. Effects of essential oil from *Chamaecypris obtusa* on the development of atopic dermatitis-like skin lesions and the suppression of Th cytokines. *J Dermatol Sci* 2010;60:122–25.

Kaewchoothong A, Tewtrakul S, Panichayupakaranant P. Inhibitory effect of phenylbutanoid-rich *Zingiber cassumunar* extracts on nitric oxide production by murine macrophages-like RAW 264.7 cells. *Phytother Res* 2012;26:1789–92.

Karasuyama H, Yamanishi Y. Basophils have emerged as a key player in immunity. *Curr Opin Immunol* 2014;31:1–7.

Karimi MH, Ebadi P, Amirghofran Z. Parsley and immunomodulation. *Expert Rev Clin Immunol* 2012;8:295–97.

Karimian P, Kavoosi G, Amirghofran Z. Anti-inflammatory effect of *Mentha longifolia* in lipopolysaccharide-stimulated macrophages: Reduction of nitric oxide production through inhibition of inducible nitric oxide synthase. *J immunotoxicol* 2013;10:393–400.

Karimian P, Kavoosi G, Amirghofran Z. Anti-oxidative and anti-inflammatory effects of *Tagetes minuta* essential oil in activated macrophages. *Asian Pac J Trop Biomed* 2014;4:219–27.

Katsukawa M, Nakata R, Takizawa Y, Hori K, Takahashi S, Inoue H. Citral, a component of lemongrass oil, activates PPARalpha and gamma and suppresses COX-2 expression. *Biochem Biophys Acta* 2010;1801:1214–20.

Kavoosi G, Teixeira da Silva JA, Saharkhiz MJJ. Inhibitory effects of *Zataria multiflora* essential oil and its main components on nitric oxide and hydrogen peroxide production in lipopolysaccharide-stimulated macrophages. *Pharm Pharmacol* 2012;64:1491–500.

Khiewkhern S, Promthet S, Sukprasert A, Eunhpinitpong W, Bradshaw P. Effectiveness of aromatherapy with light Thai massage for cellular immunity improvement in colorectal cancer patients receiving chemotherapy. *Asian Pac J Cancer Prev* 2013;14:3903–7.

Kim JY, Oh TH, Kim BJ, Kim SS, Lee NH, Hyun CG. Chemical composition and anti-inflammatory effects of essential oil from *Farfugium japonicum*. *Flower J Oleo Sci* 2008;11:623–28.

Kim JY, Kim SS, Oh TH, Baik JS, Song G, Lee NH, Hyun CG. Chemical composition, anti-oxidant, anti-elastase and anti-inflammatory activities of *Illicium anisatum* essential oil. *Acta Pharm* 2009;59:289–300.

Kim KN, Ko YJ, Yang HM, Ham YM, Roh SW, Jeon YJ, Ahn G, Kang MC, Yoon WJ, Kim D, Oda T. Anti-inflammatory effect of essential oil and its constituents from fingered citron (*Citrus medica* L. var. *sarcodactylis*) through blocking JNK, ERK and NF-kB signaling pathways in LPS-activated RAW 264.7 cells. *Food Chem Toxicol* 2013;57:126–31.

Lee MS. Role of innate immunity in the pathogenesis of type 1 and type 2 diabetes. *J Korean Med Sci* 2014;29:1038–41.

Levine AP, Segal AW. What is wrong with granulocytes in inflammatory bowel diseases? *Dig Dis* 2013;31:321–27.

Li Q, Kobayashi M, Wakayama Y, Inagaki H, Katsumata M, Hirata Y, Hirata K, Shimizu T, Kawada T, Park BJ, Ohira T, Kagawa T, Miyazaki Y. Effect of phytoncide from trees on human natural killer cell function. *Int J Immunopathol Pharmacol* 2009;22:951–59.

Liaskou E, Wilson DV, Oo YH. Innate immune cells in liver inflammation. *Mediators Inflamm* 2012;2012:949157.

Libby P, Lichtman AH, Hansson GK. Immune effector mechanisms implicated in atherosclerosis: From mice to humans. *Immunity* 2013;38:1092–104.

Lim SS, Shin KH, Ban HS, Kim YP, Jung SH, Kim YJ, Ohuchi K. Effect of the essential oil from the flowers of *Magnolia sieboldii* on the lipopolysaccharide-induced production of nitric oxide and prostaglandin E2 by rat peritoneal macrophages. *Planta Med* 2002;68:459–62.

Liu H, Zhou Y. Effect of alcohol extract of *Zingiber officinale* rose on immunological function of mice with tumor. *Wei Sheng Yan Jiu* 2002;31:208–9.

Maeda H, Yamazaki M, Katagata Y. Kuromoji (*Lindera umbellata*) essential oil inhibits LPS-induced inflammation in RAW 264.7 cells. *Biosci Biotechnol Biochem* 2013;77:482–68.

Mak TW, Ferrick DA. The gammadelta T-cell bridge: Linking innate and acquired immunity. *Nat Med* 1998;4:764–65.

Marcus A, Gowen BG, Thompson TW, Iannello A, Ardolino M, Deng W, Wang L, Shifrin N, Raulet DH. Recognition of tumors by the innate immune system and natural killer cells. *Adv Immunol* 2014;122:91–128.

Markowitz K, Moynihan M, Liu M, Kim S. Biologic properties of eugenol and zinc oxide-eugenol: A clinically oriented review. *Oral Surg Oral Med Oral Pathol* 1992;73:729–37.

Martinez NM, Lynch KW. Control of alternative splicing in immune responses: Many regulators, many predictions, much still to learn. *Immunol Rev* 2013;253:216–36.

Mauri C, Gray D, Mushtaq N, Londei M. Prevention of arthritis by interleukin 10-producing B cells. *J Exp Med* 2003;197:489–501.

Mauri C, Bosma A. immune regulatory function of B cells *Annu Rev Immunol* 2012;30:221–41.

Mayadas TN, Cullere X, Lowell CA. The multifaceted functions of neutrophils. *Annu Rev Pathol* 2014;9:181–218.

Mayo L, Quintana FJ, Weiner HL. The innate immune system in demyelinating disease. *Immunol Rev* 2012;248:170–87.

Medeiros R, Passos GF, Vitor CE, Koepp J, Mazzuco TL, Pianowski LF, Campos MM, Calixto JB. Effect of two active compounds obtained from the essential oil of *Cordia verbenacea* on the acute inflammatory responses elicited by LPS in the rat paw. *Br J Pharmacol* 2007;151:618–27.

Meli R, Mattace Raso G, Calignano A. Role of innate immune response in non-alcoholic fatty liver disease: Metabolic complications and therapeutic tools. *Front Immunol* 2014;5:177. doi: 10.3389/fimmu.2014.00177.

Mellman I, Steinman RM. Dendritic cells: Specialized and regulated antigen processing machines. *Cell* 2001;106:255–58.

Mikhaeil BR, Maatooq GT, Badria FA, Amer MMA. Chemistry and immunomodulatory activity of frankincense oil. *Z Naturforsch* 2003;58c:230–38.

Mitoshi M, Kuriyama I, Nakayama H, Miyazato H, Sugimoto K, Kobayashi Y, Jippo T, Kanazawa K, Yoshida H, Mizushina Y. Effects of essential oils from herbal plants and citrus fruits on DNA polymerase inhibitory, cancer cell growth inhibitory, antiallergic, and antioxidant activities. *J Agric Food Chem* 2012;60:11343–50.

Mizoguchi A, Mizoguchi E, Takedatsu H, Blumberg RS, Bhan AK. Chronic intestinal inflammatory condition generates IL-10-producing regulatory B cell subset characterized by CD1d upregulation. *Immunity* 2002;16:219–30.

Mócsai A. Diverse novel functions of neutrophils in immunity, inflammation, and beyond. *J Exp Med* 2013;210:1283–99.

Moreno L, Bello R, Primo-Yúfera E, Esplugues J. Pharmacological properties of the methanol extract from *Mentha suaveolens* Ehrh. *Phytother Res* 2002;16(Suppl 1):S10–13.

Nam SY, Chang MH, Do JS, Seo HJ, Oh HK. Essential oil of Niaouli preferentially potentiates antigen-specific cellular immunity and cytokine production by macrophages. *Immunopharmacol Immunotoxicol* 2008;30:459–74.

Nogueira MNM, Aquino SG, Rossa C Junior, Spolidorio DMP. Terpinen-4-ol and alpha-terpineol (tea tree oil components) inhibit the production of IL-1beta, IL-6 and IL-10 on human macrophages. *Inflamm Res* 2014;63:769–78.

Noris M, Remuzzi G. Overview of complement activation and regulation. *Semin Nephrol* 2013;33:479–92.

Ocana-Fuentes A, Arranz-Gutierrez E, Senorans FJ, and Reglero G. Supercritical fluid extraction of oregano (*Origanum vulgare*) essentials oils: Anti-inflammatory properties based on cytokine response on THP-1 macrophages. *Food Chem Toxicol* 2010;48:1568–75.

Passos GF, Fernandes ES, da Cunha FM, Ferreira J, Pianowski LF, Campos MM, Calixto JB. Anti-inflammatory and anti-allergic properties of the essential oil and active compounds from *Cordia verbenacea*. *Ethnopharmacology* 2007;110:323–33.

Peana AT, Marzocco S, Popolo A, Pinto A. (–)Linalool inhibits in vitro NO formation: Probable involvement in the antinociceptive activity of this monoterpene compound. *Life Sci* 2006;78:719–23.

Pearce AL, Finlay-Jones JJ, Hart PH. Reduction of nickel-induced contact hypersensitivity reactions by topical tea tree oil in humans. *Inflamm Res* 2005;54:22–30.

Persson CG, Erjefalt JS, Greiff L et al. Plasma-derived proteins in airway defence, disease and repair of epithelial injury. *Eur Respir J* 1998;11:958–70.

Petros A, Bennett D, Vallance P. Effect of nitric oxide synthase inhibitors on hypotension in patients with septic shock. *Lancet* 1991;338:1557–58.

Rocha NFM, de Oliveira GV, de Araujo YR, Vasconcelos Rios ER, Rodrigues Carvalho AM, Vasconcelos LF, Macedo Silveira D, Gomes Soares PM, Pergentino De Sousa D, Florenco de Sousa FC. (–)-Alpha-bisabolol-induced gastroprotection is associated with reduction in lipid peroxidation, superoxide dismutase activity and neutrophil migration. *Eur J Pharm Sci* 2011;44:455–61.

Rodrigues TG, Fernandes A Jr, Sousa JP, Bastos JK, Sforcin JM. In vitro and in vivo effects of clove on pro-inflammatory cytokines production by macrophages. *Nat Prod Res* 2009;23:319–26.

Romagnini S. Biology of human Th1 and Th2 cells. *J Clin Immunol* 1995;136:2348–54.

Rothenberg ME, Hogan SP. The eosinophil. *Annu Rev Immunol* 2006;24:147–74.

Sadlon AE, Lamson DW. Immune-modifying and antimicrobial effects of Eucalyptus oil and simple inhalation devices. *Altern Med Rev* 2010;15:33–47.

SaiRam M, Sharma SK, Ilavazhagan G, Kumar D, Selvamurthy W. Immunomodulatory effects of NIM-76, a volatile fraction from neem oil. *J Ethnopharmacol* 1997;55:133–39.

Sasannejad P, Saeedi M, Shoeibi A, Gorji A, Abbasi M, Foroughipour M. Lavender essential oil in the treatment of migraine headache: A placebo-controlled clinical trial. *Eur Neurol* 2012;67:288–91.

Serafino A, Sinibaldi Vallebona P, Andreola F, Zonfrillo M, Mercuri L, Federici M, Rasi G, Garaci E, Pierimarchi P. Stimulatory effect of eucalyptus essential oil on innate cell-mediated immune response. *BMC Immunol* 2008;9:17. doi: 10.1186/1471-2172-9-17.

Sforcin JM, Amaral JT, Fernandes A, Sousa JPB, Bastos JK. Lemongrass effects on IL-1β and IL-6 production by macrophages. *Nat Prod Res* 2009;23:1151–59.

Shirole RL, Shirole NL, Kshatriya AA, Kulkarni R, Saraf MN. Investigation into the mechanism of action of essential oil of *Pistacia integerrima* for its antiasthmatic activity. *J Ethnopharmacol* 2014;153:541–51.

Siani AC, Ramos MFS, Menezes-de-Lima O, Ribeiro-dos-Santos R, Fernandez-Ferreira E, Soares ROA, Rosas EC, Susunaga GS, Guimaraes AC, Zoghbi MGB, Henriques MGMO. Evaluation of anti-inflammatory-related activity of essential oils from the leaves and resin of species of *Protium*. *J Ethnopharmacol* 1999;66:57–69.

Sienkiewicz M, Łysakowska M, Denys P, Kowalczyk E. The antimicrobial activity of thyme essential oil against multidrug resistant clinical bacterial strains. *Microb Drug Resist* 2012;18:137–48.

Silva JC, Rao VS. Involvement of serotonin and eicosanoids in the rat paw oedema response to the essential oil of *Pilocarpus spicatus*. *Mediators Inflamm* 1992;1:167–69.

Singer AL, Koretzky GA. Control of T cell function by positive and negative regulators. *Science* 2002;296:1639–40.

Smith-Garvin JE, Koretzky GA, Jordan MS. T cell activation. *Annu Rev Immunol* 2009;27:591–619.

Swirski FK, Nahrendorf M. Leukocyte behavior in atherosclerosis, myocardial infarction, and heart failure. *Science* 2013;339:161–66.

Tan P, Zhong W, Cai W. Clinical study on treatment of 40 cases of malignant brain tumor by elemene emulsion injection. *Zhongguo Zhong Xi Yi Jie He Za Zhi* 2000;20:645–48.

Tavares AC, Goncalves MJ, Cruz MT, Cavaleiro C, Lopes MC, Canhoto J, Salgueiro Ribeiro L. Essential oils from *Distichoselinum tenuifolium*: Chemical composition, cytotoxicity, antifungal and anti-inflammatory properties. *J Ethnopharmacol* 2010;130:593–98.

Tung YT, Chua MT, Wang SY, Chang ST. Anti-inflammation activities of essential oil and its constituents from indigenous cinnamon (*Cinnamomum osmophloeum*) twigs. *Bioresour Technol* 2008;99:3908–13.

Tung YT, Yen PL, Lin CY, Chang ST. Anti-inflammatory activities of essential oils and their constituents from different provenances of indigenous cinnamon (*Cinnamomum osmophloeum*) leaves. *Pharm Biol* 2010;48:1130–36.

Uebaba K, Xu FH, Ogawa H, Tatsuse T, Wang BH, Hisajima T, Venkatraman S. Psychoneuroimmunologic effects of Ayurvedic oil-dripping treatment. *J Altern Complement Med* 2008;14:1189–98.

Ueno-lio T, Shibakura M, Yokota K, Aoe M, Hyoda T, Shinohata R, Kanehiro A, Tanimoto M, Kataoka M. Lavender essential oil inhalation suppress allergic air way inflammation and mucous cell hyperplasia in a murine model of asthma. *Life Sci* 2014;108:109–15.

Valente J, Zuzarte M, Goncalves MJ, Lopes MC, Cavaleiro C, Salgueiro L, Cruz MT. Antifungal, antioxidant and anti-inflammatory activities of *Oenanthe crocata* L. essential oil. *Food Chem Toxicol* 2013;62:349–54.

van den Boorn JG, Hartmann G. Turning tumors into vaccines: Co-opting the innate immune system. *Immunity* 2013;39:27–37.

Velozo LS, Martino T, Vigliano MV, Pinto FA, Silva GP, Justo Mda G, Sabino KC, Coelho MG. *Pterodon polygalaeflorus* essential oil modulates acute inflammation and B and T lymphocyte activation. *Am J Chin Med* 2013;41:545–63.

Vigo E, Cepeda A, Gualillo O, Perz-Fernandez R. In-vitro anti-inflammatory effects of *Eucalyptus glubus* and *Thymus vulgaris*: Nitric oxide inhibition in J774A.1 murine macrophages. *J Pharm Pharmacol* 2004;56:257–63.

Vijayastelter BL, Kottarapat J, Ramadasan K. An evaluation of antioxidant, anti-inflammatory, and antinociceptive activities of essential oil from *Curcuma longa*. L. *J Pharmacol* 2011;43:526–31.

Wilasrusmee C, Kittur S, Siddiqui J, Bruch D, Wilasrusmee S, Kittur DS. In vitro immunomodulatory effects of ten commonly used herbs on murine lymphocytes. *J Alternat Complement Med* 2002a;8:467–75.

Wilasrusmee C, Siddiqui J, Bruch D, Wilasrusmee S, Kittur S, Kittur DS. In vitro immunomodulatory effects of herbal products. *Am Surg* 2002b;68:860–64.

Wu W, Liu K, Tang X. Preliminary study on the antitumor immunoprotective mechanisms of β-elemene. *Zhong-hua Zhong Liu Za Zhi* 1999;21:405–8.

Yang H, Wang X, Yu L, Zheng S. Study on the anticancer mechanisms of elemene. *Chin Clin Cancer* 1999;26:4–7.

Yoon WJ, Kim SS, Oh TH, Lee NH, Hyun CG. *Abies koreana* essential oil inhibits drug-resistant skin pathogen growth and LPS-induced inflammatory effects of murine macrophage. *Lipids* 2009a;44:471–76.

Yoon WJ, Kim SS, Oh TH, Lee NH, Hyun CG. *Cryptomeria japonica* essential oil inhibits the growth of drug-resistant skin pathogens and LPS-induced nitric oxide and proinflammatory cytokine production. *J Microbiol* 2009b;58:61–68.

Yoon WJ, Moon JY, Kang JY, Kim GO, Lee NH, Hyun CG. *Neolitsea sericea* essential oil attenuates LPS-induced inflammation in RAW 264.7 macrophages by suppressing NF-κB and MAPK activation. *Nat Prod Commun* 2010a;5:1311–16.

Yoon WJ, Moon JY, Song G, Lee YK, Han MS, Lee JS, Ihm BA, Lee WJ, Hyun CG. *Artemisia fukudo* essential oil attenuates LPS-induced inflammation by suppressing NF-kB and MAPK activation in RAW 264.7 macrophages. *Food Chem Toxicol* 2010b;48:1222–29.

Yousofi A, Daneshmandi S, Soleimani N, Bagheri K, Karimi MH. Immunomodulatory effect of parsley (*Petroselinum crispum*) essential oil on immune cells: Mitogen-activated splenocytes and peritoneal macrophages. *Immunopharmacol Immunotoxicol* 2012;34:303–8.

Zanetti M. Cathelicidins, multifunctional peptides of the innate immunity. *J Leukoc Biol* 2004;75:39–48.

Zhang R, Tian A, Zhang H, Zhou Z, Yu H, Chen L. Amelioration of experimental autoimmune encephalomyelitis by β-elemene treatment is associated with Th17 and Treg cell balance. *J Mol Neurosci* 2011;44:31–40.

Zhou H, Deng Y, Xie Q. The modulatory effects of the volatile oil of ginger on the cellular immune response in vitro and in vivo in mice. *J Ethnopharmacol* 2006;105:301–5.

15 Antimicrobial Effects of Bergamot Essential Oil
From Ancient Medicine to Modern Research

Alfredo Focà and Maria Carla Liberto

CONTENTS

15.1 INTRODUCTION: RECENT RESEARCH ON CITRUS ESSENTIAL OILS

By happy coincidence, the action of phytopharmaceuticals began to come under the focus of international research attention upon the advent of the technology that permitted the isolation of their active ingredients. Citrus essential oils were found to have the following three constituent groups in common:

1. Oxygenated monoterpene, sesquiterpene, and aliphatic compounds (aldehydes, ketones, esters, and alcohols)
2. Monoterpene and sesquiterpene hydrocarbons
3. Nonvolatile residues

Thus, the characteristic fragrance of essential oils was revealed to be due to their oxygenated components.

The various components of bergamot essence—a long-ignored *panacea*—were found to be a large volatile fraction (93%–96%) and a much smaller nonvolatile part (4%–7%). The former is rich in the hydrocarbons terpene and 4,6-terpene and their unoxidized homolog, as well as alcohols (linalool), esters (linalyl acetate), aldehydes, and ketones, with linalool and linalyl acetate being the primary constituents (60%–70%). The nonvolatile fraction is composed of coumarin residues (citroptene, bergaptene, bergaptol, and bergamottin), as well as waxes, steroids, triterpenoids, fatty acids, and flavones.

Studies into the effects of the nonvolatile residues of bergamot oil appear to show that it exerts a depressive effect on the central nervous system (CNS) [1]. Averbeck et al. jointly conducted a safety assessment [2], revealing that neither bergaptene nor the oil itself was phototoxic, photomutagenic, or photocancerogenous at the concentrations used in commercial formulations, thereby reassuring both the users and researchers and, most importantly, paving the way to its industrial and pharmaceutical development.

Among others, Fitzpatrick opened a particularly ingenious line of research, performing in-depth studies on the application of psoralens—photoactive linear isomers of furocoumarin that can be found in the peel of many citrus fruits, in particular bergamot. Furocoumarins are produced by plants mainly to defend themselves against predators, and many are toxic and photomutagenic, absorbing photons and forming photoadducts with pyrimidine [3]. Aqueous solutions of psoralens are extremely sensitive to ultraviolet light (UVA, wavelength 320–420 nm), and in the lab this high-energy state induces the cycloaddition (2 + 2) of other molecules containing double-acceptor bonds. This leads to the formation of cyclobutane rings and a synthetic compound dubbed S-59. In blood components, S-59 has been found to block the replication of a wide variety of pathogens under UVA, without compromising platelet or plasma protein viability. This alone makes psoralens promising candidates for photochemical treatment applications, but they also have two further beneficial features. Indeed, the fact that they lack sequence specificity makes them nonselective for a particular genomic material or organism, that is, potentially versatile. Furthermore, cross-linking of psoralen with nucleic acids—and the consequent inhibition of replication—occurs only in the presence of UVA, making their effects, theoretically at least, easy to control [3].

The literature also contains several investigations into the antiviral action of other psoralens, in particular bergaptene (5-psoralen [5-MOP]) and methoxsalen (8-methoxypsoralen [8-MOP]), both obtained from the nonvolatile residue of bergamot oil. 5-MOP also proves effective in association with high-dose UVA (20–40 J/cm^2), disabling HIV *in vitro* and in cultures of infected leukocytes. 8-MOP, which also requires high doses of UVA (30–60 J/cm^2), seems to have a far wider-ranging antiviral action, deactivating human immunodeficiency virus (HIV), hepatitis B virus (HBV), hepatitis C virus (HCV) murine cytomegalovirus, and feline leukemia virus. These substances are therefore the keystone of continuing research efforts to develop new extracorporeal photopheresis techniques for the treatment of AIDS, not to mention UV decontamination of blood for use in transfusions [4,5].

We, on the other hand, have managed to show the antibacterial and anti-mycotic activities of bergamot essential oil against a wide range of Gram-negative (*Esherichia coli, Pseudomonas aeruginosa, Proteus mirabilis, Providencia stuartii, Klebsiella pneumoniae, Salmonella* spp., *Enterobacter* spp.) and Gram-positive bacteria (*Staphylococcus aureus, Enterococcus* spp., *Streptococcus pneumoniae, Gardnerella vaginalis*) and various *Candida* strains. We found that the essential oil was particularly active against *S. pneumoniae* and, as other authors have shown on strain ATCC 10231 using the agar dilution method, *Candida albicans* [6–8].

Several researchers have widened the scope of investigation to include different formulations of essence of bergamot. Pizzimenti et al., for example, studied the anti-microbial properties of crude bergamot oil and its solid and liquid cold extraction residues on a total of 13 Gram-positive and Gram-negative bacteria and three strains of *C. albicans*, finding that the distillate possessed the greatest inhibitory capacity [9]. Furthermore, the activity of various dilutions of bergamot essential oil has been tested *in vitro* against several microorganisms of the genus *Mycoplasma* (*M. pneumoniae, M. hominis, M. fermentans,* and *M. pirum*) [10], revealing its antimicrobial effect on all strains at 64- to 128-fold dilutions of the initial concentration (0.025 ml).

The antimicrobial effect of the essential oil has also been tested using microwell liquid-phase chromatography [11], which we used as inspiration for another study to test the antibacterial and antimycotic activities of two bergamot essence derivatives (distillate and deterpenate), as well as the oil itself, on various Gram-negative (*E. coli* and *P. aeruginosa*) and Gram-positive (*S. pyogenes pyogenes, Streptococcus aga-lactiae, Staphylococcus epidermidis,* and *S. aureus*) bacterial strains and *Candida* (*Candida albicans* and *Candida* spp.), clinically isolated from skin and mucosal infection sites (mainly oropharyngeal and vaginal). In a preliminary study, we have also evaluated the antiviral activity of the essential oil against herpes simplex type 1, clearly showing its inhibitory capacity on viral proliferation of single-cycle growth curves [8].

15.2 MATERIALS AND METHODS

To evaluate the trend in the growth curves of 79 clinically isolated Gram-positive (26 *S. pyogenes*, 14 *S. agalactiae*, 18 *S. aureus*, and 21 *S. epidermidis*) and 22 Gram-negative (9 *E. coli* and 13 *P. aeruginosa*) bacterial samples, as well as 51 strains of *Candida* (32 *C. albicans*, 6 *C. glabrata*, 4 *C. krusei*, 3 *C. tropicalis*, 2 *C. lusitaniae*, 1 *C. intermedia*, 1 *C. pulcherrima*, 1 *C. guillermondi*, and 1 *C. parapsilosis*), in the presence of different concentrations of bergamot essential oil, kindly donated by the Reggio Calabria Consorzio per le Essenze, we used two automated systems. The first, Bioscreen C (Labsystem, Helsinki, Finland), measures absorbance, and the second, Bactometer (BioMérieux, Marcy-l'Etoile, France), provides impedometric measurements. Identification was performed using ATB Expression (BioMérieux).

The encouraging results of these experiments prompted us to analyze the morphological modifications induced by the test substances in *Candida* yeasts—stained with an acridine orange-based dye—under fluorescence microscopy. We tested the effect of three formulations of the essential oil: crude, deterpenate, and distillate. The crude essence was obtained via cold-pressing the whole fruit or peel, followed by removal of the other constituents (pith, juice, etc.) via high-speed centrifugation, which was performed twice to improve the yield. The distillate was acquired by steam distillation of the essence in a stainless steel vacuum distiller at a temperature not exceeding 45°C–50°C. This process yields a distillate made up of essential oil and water, which are then separated by means of gravity. Deterpenation, on the other hand, is achieved via removal of monoterpene hydrocarbons. This increases the solubility of the essence in alcohol and raises its aromatic content.

These essential oil formulations were emulsified prior to their addition to the liquid media. This was achieved using Tween 20, an inert, nonionic tensioactive agent with no inherent bactericidal activity, at a dilution of 10% [8]. The emulsions were then filtered through 0.22 mm filters, able to remove any bacterial contaminants. Sensitivity tests were also performed on both filtered and unfiltered emulsions, yielding comparable results (data not reported).

15.2.1 Gas Chromatography Analysis of Bergamot Derivatives

The chemical composition of the volatile fraction of the three test substances was assessed via high resolution gas chromatography (HRGC) using a Fison Mega series 5160 gas chromatograph, equipped with a Shimadzu C-R3A data processor and a fused-silica capillary column of 30 m × 0.32 mm inner diameter (ID), covered with 0.40–0.45 mm thick SE-52 film (Mega, Legnano, Italy), courtesy of the University of Catania Institute of Agrarian Industry. The temperature of the column was maintained at 45°C for 6 minutes, and then raised to 180°C in 3°C/minute increments. This was performed at the following settings: index and system, split; detector, flame ionization detector (FID); temperature of the injector and detector, 280°C; carrier He, 95 kPa; volume of test substance injected into the detector, 1 ml [12].

15.2.2 Microwell Dilution of Bergamot Derivatives

Aliquots of 1 ml of the each test substance were placed in sterile glass test tubes and weighed. Thus, 821 mg/ml of essential oil, 780 mg/ml of deterpenate, and 805 mg/ml of distillate were emulsified with Tween 20, giving the respective concentrations of 739, 702, and 724.5 mg/ml. These were then vortexed, and half aliquots of the emulsion were filtered into sterile glass test tubes. The first dilution of the emulsion was performed in an apposite liquid medium (Sabouraud Nutrient Broth, BioMérieux), placing 100 ml of the emulsion in 2 ml of liquid medium (dilution 1:20) and thereby obtaining concentrations of the test substances of 37, 35.1, and 36.2 mg/ml, respectively. Aliquots (100 μl) of the first dilutions (3.7 mg/100 μl, 3.5 mg/100 μl, and 3.6 mg/100 μl, respectively) were dispensed into the first well of the sterile microtitration plate with 50 μl of the liquid medium. Hence, the first wells contained respective concentrations of 1.85 µg/50 µl, 1.75 µg/50 ml, and 1.81 µg/50 µl, corresponding to the first dilution (2.50% of the initial weight). Twofold serial dilutions of the initial sample were then performed up to the 11th well, while the 12th well contained the medium alone as control.

15.2.3 Microbicidal Activity of Bergamot Derivatives

The microorganisms under investigation were prepared in test tubes containing sterile physiological solution, diluting colonies grown on solid medium to obtain a bacterial suspension of turbidity of 0.5 McFarland (roughly 100 million colony-forming units [CFU]/ml). Each microbial suspension was then diluted 1:100 in liquid medium (100 µl bacterial suspension: 9.9 ml broth), and 50 ml aliquots were placed in all microwells of the relevant plate at a final concentration of 5×10^4 CFU/well. Each plate was incubated for 24 hours at 37°C (bacterial strains) or 48 hours at 32°C (*Candida* strains) prior to absorbance measurement using a wavelength of 630 nm.

To determine the minimum bactericidal concentration (MBC) or minimum fungicidal concentration (MFC) of the three test substances, a sterile gauged inoculation loop was used to withdraw 1 ml aliquots from wells subsequent to those in which an increase in turbidity was not visible to the naked eye. These were inoculated in dishes containing sheep blood, McConkey and Sabouraud agars, and incubated for 24 hours at 37°C (bacteria) or 48 hours at 32°C (*Candida*), prior to colony counting.

15.2.4 Absorbance Measurement of Bacterial Inhibition

Bioscreen C, an entirely automated system, was used to monitor bacterial growth in the presence or absence of the three test substances at various concentrations. The system records the variation in absorbance (outer diameter [OD] 600 nm) of a test culture broth every 10 minutes, expressing this as an increase in biomass. It automatically dilutes microbial suspensions and antimicrobial solutions (concentrations ranging from 2.50% to 0.15%) in apposite microwells, maintains the broth at a constant temperature (37°C for bacteria and 32°C for yeasts), and agitates the mixture every 10 minutes. Using this equipment, our inoculates were brought to a turbidity of 0.5 McFarland, as reported for the microwell dilution, and 0.5 ml aliquots of each bergamot oil were diluted in 9.5 ml of broth (1:20 dilution). This mixture (500 µl) was then added to each well of the apposite sterile strip (2.5×10^6 CFU/well). Bioscreen C then dosed the wells with 10 µl of the inoculate (final concentration 5×10^4 CFU/well). Following incubation, 10 µl of each culture broth was seeded onto the solid medium to enable evaluation of its growth curve and therefore any inhibitory effect.

15.2.5 Impedometric Measurement of Bacterial Inhibition

The automated impedometric system Bactometer was also used to provide growth curves based on its evaluation of the percentage in metabolic variation due to the presence of metabolically active microorganisms. It thereby enables us to study the effect of the essence of bergamot and its derivatives on the metabolic activity of the microorganisms. The device features wells containing electrodes used to measure the variations in ions produced during microbial growth. These variations in electric properties of the culture medium arise from the formation of electrically charged molecules (e.g., acids) by the microorganisms actively metabolizing the macromolecules present in the medium. Results are expressed as a percentage metabolic variation, ascribable to the consumption of the medium by the microorganisms.

As per the two previously described experiments, the bacterial and *C. albicans* inoculates were brought to a turbidity of 0.5 McFarland. Volumes (100 μl) of these inoculates were added to 9.9 ml of broth, and 100 μl aliquots of this mixture were used to dose the Bactometer wells, each containing 1 ml of one of the test substances (final concentration 1×10^5 CFU/well), previously subjected to twofold serial dilutions from a concentration of 2.50% to 0.15% in apposite liquid media. At this point the modules containing the bacteria and yeasts were incubated for 24 hours at 37°C or 48 hours at 32°C, respectively. Following incubation, 10 μl of the culture broth was seeded on solid medium, and growth curves were plotted to reveal any change over time due to the presence of the test substances.

15.2.6 Morphological Alterations in *Candida* Colonies

In order to evaluate the effect of the three substances on the morphology of *C. albicans* cells, 10 μl aliquots of the culture in liquid medium (in the presence or absence of one of the test substances) were taken from the Bactometer wells and mixed on a glass slide with 5 μl of acridine orange solution, at a final concentration of 1.44 mg/ml. Samples were protected by coverslips and then observed at 200× and 400× magnifications under fluorescence microscope (Zeiss, Oberkochen, Germany) equipped with an internal camera.

15.2.7 Effect of Bergamot Essence on Herpes Simplex

The antiviral activity of bergamot essence (*Citrus bergamia risso*) against type 1 and type 2 herpes simplex was assessed *in vitro*. Viral DNA extracted from infected cells (continuous-line WISH amniotic cells), treated or not with various doses of the essence, was investigated both quantitatively and qualitatively. Quantitative analysis was performed by real-time polymerase chain reaction (PCR) with the aid of a LightCycler PCR system, which amplifies and monitors the development of the target nuclear acid (denaturing, coupling, and extension) after each cycle by means of fluorescence. The newly amplified product is continuously monitored in the pairing phase via fluorescence resonance energy transfer (FRET) detected by two hybridization probes, one of which is a fluorophore donor. Fluorescein, upon excitation by an external luminous source, emits light, which is detected by the fluorophore acceptor, LC-Red 640, at position 5′ of the amplified nucleic acid.

The presence of the viral DNA or its fractions was analyzed by gas chromatography in WISH cells (maintained at 37°C in Dulbecco's medium in an atmosphere enriched with 5% CO_2) exposed to the action of bergamot essence. Cell cultures (WISH) were infected with the strains of HSV by the single-cycle growth curve approach, in which the virus remains in contact with the cells for a duration sufficient to consent to adsorption (1–2 hours).

Two different concentrations of bergamot essence, 8 µg/ml and 80 µg/ml, were administered before infection, upon infection, and 1 hour after infection. After 24 hours, viral DNA was extracted from treated and untreated cells (automated MagNa Pure system) prior to quantitative and qualitative analysis.

The primers used for real-time PCR were HSV pol F 5′ GCTCGAGTGCG AAAAAACGTTC 3′ and HSV pol A 5′ TGCGGTTGATAAACGCGCAGT 3′ (amplifying a 140 base-pair segment of the viral gene that codes for the protein DNA polymerase). Probes used to detect the FRET product were HSV-2 FLU 5′ GCGCACCAGATCCACGCCCTTGATGAGC-FLUOR and HSV-2 LCR 5′ LC-Red 640-CTTGCCCCCGCAGATGACGCC-phos.

The LC-PCR master mix contained 1× FastStart Taq DNA polymerase reaction buffer (Roche, Basel, Switzerland), which contains a mixture of dNTP (with dUTP in place of dTTP), 3 mM $MgCL_2$, 0.5 µM of each primer, 0.2 µM of probe HSV-2 FLU, and 0.4 µM of probe HSV-2 LCR.

15.3   RESULTS

15.3.1   GAS CHROMATOGRAPHY ANALYSIS OF BERGAMOT DERIVATIVES

Gas chromatography showed that the three analytes contained the following major constituents: the hydrocarbons sabinene, limonene, b-phellandrene, and g-terpinene; the alcohol linalool; the ester linalyl acetate; and aldehydes and ketones, including neral; as well as an epoxide concentration of <0.1%. Linalool is the predominant alcohol, and its antimicrobial activity has consequently been studied before. In fact, a study on the antimicrobial activity of some constituents of essential oils on 18 bacteria demonstrated that linalool is very effective as an antibacterial since it inhibited 17 bacteria [13–15].

15.3.2   MICROBICIDAL ACTIVITY OF BERGAMOT DERIVATIVES

In order to evaluate the antimicrobial activity of the bergamot derivatives on the various bacterial and *Candida* strains, these were incubated according to the methods outlined above; incremental twofold dilutions of the test substances were obtained manually in microwell plates (from 2.50% to 0.15%), as shown in Table 15.1.

The microbicidal effect of each substance on the Gram-positive bacteria was as follows. All test substances, that is, crude essence, deterpenate, and distillate, showed an MBC for the 26 strains of *S. pyogenes*, ranging from 2.50% and 0.62%, and an MBC_{50} of 1.25%. On the 14 strains of *S. agalactiae*, the crude oil displayed an

TABLE 15.1

Fungicidal Effect of Bergamot Derivatives on Clinically Isolated Strains of *Candida*

Microorganism (No. of Strains)	Crude Essence		Deterpenate		Distillate	
	MFC_{50}	MFC Range	MFC_{50}	MFC Range	MFC_{50}	MFC Range
Candida spp. (13)	>2.50	>2.50–0.50	1.25	2.5–0.62	1.25	2.5–1.25

Note: The test substance concentrations used are expressed as a percentage dilution in the medium with which they were supplemented.

MBC range and MBC_{50} of $\geq 2.50\%$, while the deterpenate and distillate both showed an MBC ranging from 2.50% to 1.25%, with an MBC_{50} of 2.50%. In *S. epidermidis* (21 strains), both the essence and the distillate showed an MBC range and MBC_{50} of >2.50%, while the deterpenate had an MBC range of $\geq 2.50\%$ and an MBC_{50} equal to that of the other two substances. Both the MBC range and MBC_{50} in the 18 strains of *S. aureus* were >2.50% for all three substances.

In Gram-negative bacteria, the essential oil had an MBC range and MBC_{50} of >2.50% in *E. coli* (9 strains), while the deterpenate and distillate had an MBC range of between 2.50% and 1.25% and an MBC_{50} of 2.50%. The other Gram-negative bacteria tested, *P. aeruginosa* (13 strains), showed the same behavior as that observed for *S. epidermidis*.

As regards the *Candida* samples (51 strains), the essence showed an MFC range of between >2.50% and 2.50% and an MFC_{50} of >2.50%, the deterpenate had an MFC range of between 2.50% and 0.62% and an MFC_{50} of 1.25%, and finally, the distillate had an MFC range of between 2.50% and 1.25% and an MFC_{50} of 1.25%.

15.3.3 ABSORBANCE MEASUREMENT OF BACTERIAL INHIBITION

Bioscreen C yielded the following results: *S. pneumoniae* was found to be sensitive to the action of the deterpenate and distillate, even at the lowest concentration tested (0.15%), while the essence was only active at higher concentrations (2.50%). *S. epidermidis*, in accordance with the data obtained from the microwell dilution method, was found to be resistant to the action of the three tested substances at various concentrations. *E. coli* was poorly sensitive to all three substances even at concentrations of 2.50%, which nevertheless caused a substantial decrease in the stationary phase with respect to control. Of the three substances tested on *C. albicans*, deterpenate and distillate (Figures 15.1 and 15.2) concentrations as low as 1.25% prolonged the latent phase, delayed the start of the logarithmic growth phase, and lowered the plateau with respect to control, while the crude essence only delayed the

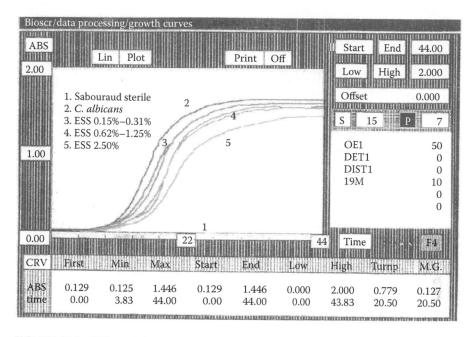

FIGURE 15.1 Effect of different concentrations (0.15%–2.50%) of bergamot essence (ESS) on the growth curve of *C. albicans*, evaluated by means of the Bioscreen system.

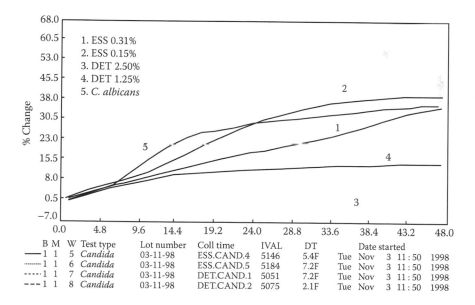

FIGURE 15.2 Effect of different concentrations (0.15%–2.50%) of bergamot essence deterpenate (DET) on the growth curve of *C. albicans*, evaluated by means of the Bactometer system.

start of the logarithmic growth phase and lowered the plateau with respect to control at concentrations of 2.50%.

15.3.4 IMPEDOMETRIC MEASUREMENT OF BACTERIAL GROWTH

The Bactometer system [16,17] used to test the crude essence, deterpenate, and distillate at the different concentrations (2.50%–0.15%) revealed that, with respect to control, all three substances caused a reduction in the percentage metabolic activity of *S. pyogenes* at concentrations as low as 0.15%. In *S. agalactiae*, on the other hand, all three test substances reduced percentage metabolic activity at concentrations as low as 0.31%. In *S. pneumoniae*, the essence and deterpenate caused a reduction in percentage metabolic activity at concentrations as low as 0.15%, while the distillate caused the same effect at concentrations from 0.31%. The essence and distillate reduced the percentage metabolic activity of *S. epidermidis* at concentrations higher than 0.62%, while the deterpenate exerted its effects at concentrations as low as 0.31%. The essence produced a reduction in the percentage metabolic activity of *S. aureus* at concentrations of 0.31% and above, while the deterpenate had the same effect at concentrations above 1.25%, and the distillate as low as 0.62%.

Among the Gram-negative bacteria tested, the percentage metabolic activity of *E. coli* was decreased by concentrations as low as 0.62% when tested with the essence and deterpenate, while the distillate provoked the same effect at concentrations as low as 0.31%. In this case, we repeated the experiment with different inoculates (1×10^5 and 1×10^7 CFU/well) of the microorganisms in question with no measurable effect on the trend of the growth curves.

On *C. albicans*, after 48 hours of incubation, the essence and distillate reduced the percentage metabolic activity at concentrations of 0.62% and above, while the deterpenate caused the same effect even at 0.31%. *C. albicans* was also tested using two different inoculates (1×10^5 and 1×10^7 CFU/well) with no significant effect on the trend of the growth curves (Table 15.1).

15.3.5 MORPHOLOGICAL ALTERATIONS IN CANDIDA COLONIES

Due to the particularly promising results showing the microbicidal effect of the bergamot extracts on the *Candida* yeasts, the morphological changes they provoked in strains of *Candida albicans* were observed under a fluorescence microscope (Figure 15.3). Clinically isolated samples of *Candida* cultured in Sabouraud agar containing incremental concentrations of the three bergamot extracts tested were stained with acridine orange, which revealed an apparent increase in the dimensions of the yeasts exposed to the essential oil. This was accompanied by conspicuous morphological variability and an absence of pseudohyphae and budding cells. Seeding aliquots of the same samples in petri dishes of Sabouraud agar highlighted a direct correlation between concentration of the crude essence and the fungicidal effect.

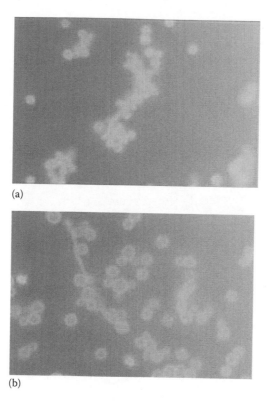

(a)

(b)

FIGURE 15.3 (a) Effect of a concentration of 0.15% bergamot essence on *C. albicans* cell morphology after acridine orange staining. (b) Acridine orange staining of *C. albicans* in a Sabourad culture broth.

In contrast, the deterpenate appeared to exert an absolute fungicidal effect; no morphological alterations were evident, and greater numbers were seen at weaker dilutions (0.15%), but the cells were found to be entirely absent at greater concentrations (2.50%–0.31%). These observations were supported by the colony counts performed after seeding aliquots of the same samples in Sabouraud agar, in which growth was only observed at the highest dilution (0.15%).

The distillate produced effects very similar to those observed of the deterpenate, but at higher concentrations (2.50%–1.25%).

15.3.6 Effect of Bergamot Derivatives on Herpes Simplex

A brief assessment of the antiviral activity of bergamot essential oil on the herpes simplex virus was performed to assess growth inhibition after pretreatment. This inhibition was found to be neither dose nor time dependent. The oil appeared to produce no measurable effect when applied after infection (Figure 15.4).

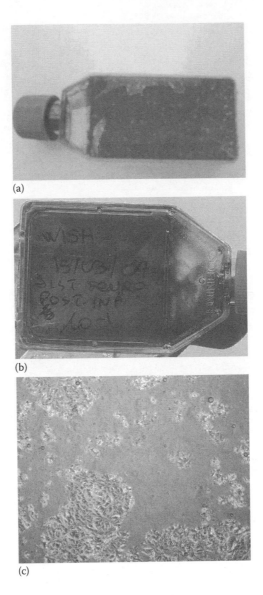

(a)

(b)

(c)

FIGURE 15.4 Titration of the herpes simplex virus. HSV 1 single-cycle growth curve on cell cultures: (a) without bergamot essence treatment, (b) post infection bergamot essence treatment, and (c) cytopathic effects of herpes simplex virus 1 on cell cultures.

15.4 DISCUSSION

The above experiments enabled us to evaluate the respective effects of various concentrations of crude bergamot essential oil and its deterpenate and distillate on both the structure and function of the target microorganisms. Dose–response curves were plotted for a wide variety of Gram-positive and Gram-negative bacteria and yeast strains, particularly those infecting the skin and the oropharangeal and vaginal mucosae, and used to calculate the MBC and MBC_{50} values, that is, the inhibitory effect, of each test substance. The growth–response curves obtained by these means, and all the other experiments performed, demonstrated the significant antibacterial antimicrobial action of all three substances. In particular, the Bioscreen C system provided us with clear evidence of alterations in the growth curves of the bacterial populations caused by the test substances. By correlating these results with those obtained by the traditional method described above, we were able to accurately evaluate the degree of inhibition of each concentration of each of the three test substances. Likewise, the Bactometer provided us with a picture of the interference exerted by the three bergamot derivatives on the metabolism of the bacterial populations, thereby preparing the ground for future experiments to determine the precise mechanism of action of the substances in question. Last but not least, we showed that all three substances provoked profound structural and numerical alterations in several *Candida* colonies stained with acridine orange, another powerful indicator of their antimicrobial effect.

Our results are in line with the data reported in the literature that show correlations between the chemical structure of such compounds and microbicidal activity. The presence of polysaccharides and other hydrophilic substances at the surface of the capsule of the microorganisms examined seems to confer a certain resistance to the microbicidal action of the three substances. This was the case in both Gram-positive staphylococci and Gram-negative bacteria like *Pseudomonadaceae*.

These findings lend weight to previous reports that Gram-positive bacteria are more sensitive to the inhibitory effect of the essential oil than Gram-negative species, a difference ascribed to differences in the structure of the cell wall [8], which is more complex in the latter. That said, many Gram-positive strains of *Staphylococcus* bear highly hydrophilic polysaccharide structures on their surfaces, which, like the cell wall of the Gram-negative bacteria, seem to block the passage of lipophilic substances, that is, the majority of essential oil components, including those in bergamot essence. As regards the yeast strains, the abundance of lipids, in particular sterols, on their exterior envelope may explain their chemical and physical affinity for various components of bergamot oil and its derivatives.

We are certain that bergamot essential oil contains other important active compounds that deserve further chemical and microbiological testing in a wider range of bacterial, viral, and fungal species. It would be especially interesting to determine their respective effects on bacteria that have become resistant to antibiotics using biochips and other microbiological techniques. In the short term, however, it appears that bergamot essence is ripe for applications and commercial exploitation as a disinfectant and in phytocosmeceutical detergents.

15.5   CONCLUSIONS

In conclusion, the data available to date, alongside the notable absence of harmful side effects (e.g., photosensitivity), highlight the potential usefulness of bergamot derivatives in topical antimicrobial applications. In particular, the distillate and deterpenate of the crude essence seem to be especially active against infective agents of the skin and mucosa. Furthermore, the intrinsic characteristics of bergamot essential oil, not least its pleasant, stimulating fragrance and regenerative, soothing action, could considerably broaden its potential field of application. Indeed, evidence that bergamot essence—like other essential oils—and its constituent compounds may have clinically useful psychoactive effects is beginning to emerge [18,19].

To paraphrase our Calabrian colleague Francesco Calabrò, who, admittedly, may have been a little precocious in his predictions, "and it will not be long before our hospital corridors, clinics, surgeries and operating theatres ... rather than being plagued by the acrid odour of disinfectants, will be redolent of the fragrance of bergamot, which is stimulating for patients and visitors alike."

REFERENCES

1. Occhiuto F., F. Limardi, C. Circosta. Effects of nonvolatile residue from the essential oil of Citrus bergamia on the central nervous system. *Int. J. Pharmacognosy*, 33 (1995).
2. Averbeck D., L. Dubutret, P. Morliere, A.L. Young. Genotoxicity of bergapten and bergamot oil in Saccharomyces cerevisiae. *J. Photochem. Photobiol. B*, 7 (1990) 209–229.
3. Fitzpatrick T.B. Gli psoraleni nella clinica medica, Prospettiva della ricerca e dello sviluppo. In *Atti del Congresso Internazionale "Bergamotto98" Stato dell'arte e prospettive*, Reggio Calabria, 1998, pp. 65–84.
4. Lin L., G.P. Wiesehahn, P.A. Morel, L. Corash. Use of 8-methoxypsoralen and long wavelength ultraviolet radiation for decontamination of platelet concentrates. *Blood*, 74 (1989) 517–52.
5. Barre-Senoussi F. et al. Inactivation du virus VIH-1 par l'action du 5-methoxypsoralene associé aux UVA. Unpublished report, Laboratorie des retrovirus, Institut Pasteur Paris, 1991.
6. Frugoni S., M. Ciliberto. Attività antibatterica degli oli essenziali. *Microbiol. Med.*, 11 (1996) 244–45.
7. Hammer K.A., C.F. Carson, T.V. Riley. *In vitro* activity of essential oils, in particular *Melaleuca alternifolia* (tea tree) oil and tea tree oil product, against *Candida* spp. *J. Antimicrob. Chemother.*, 423 (1998) 9221–595.
8. Focà A., M.C. Liberto, G. Matera, G.S. Barreca, A. Pollio, L. Rametti, A. Caliò. Valutazione dell'attività antimicrobica dell'essenza di bergamotto. In *Bergamotto 98; Stato dell'arte*, Reggio Calabria, 1998, pp. 185–207.
9. Pizzimenti F., G. Tulino, A. Marino, A. Cotroneo, A. Verzera, A. Trozzi. Attività antimicrobica e antifungina dell'essenza di bergamotto. In *Atti del Congresso Internazionale "Bergamotto98" Stato dell'arte e prospettive*, Reggio Calabria, 1998, p. 181.
10. Bisignano G., A. Marino, H. Reale, M.P. Furneri, P. Dugo. Attività antimicoplasmatica "*in vitro*" dell'essenza del bergamotto. In *Atti del Congresso Internazionale "Bergamotto98" Stato dell'arte e prospettive*, Reggio Calabria, 1998, pp. 183–84.
11. Camporese A. Aromatogramma in fase liquida su micropiastra: Analisi sperimentale di un nuovo metodo preciso, ripetibile e facilmente automatizzabile. In *Atti del Congresso Nazionale della Società Italiana di Fitoterapia*, Castiglioncello, May 26–28, 1995.
12. Mazza G. Étude sur la composition aromatique de l'huile essentiele de bergamote (*Citrus aurantium* subsp. *bergamia* risso et poiteau engler) par chromatographie gazeuse et spectrométrie de masse. *J. Chromatogr.*, 362 (1986) 87–99.
13. Pattnaik S., V.R. Subramanyam, M. Bapaji, C.R. Kole. Antibacterial and antifungal activity of aromatic constituents of essential oils. *Microbios*, 89 (1997) 39–46.

14. King A.D. Jr., H.G. Bayne, L. Jurd, C. Case. Antimicrobial properties of natural phenols and related compounds: Obtusastyrene and dihydro-obtusastyrene. *Antimicrob. Agents Chemother.*, 1 (1972) 263–67.

15. Russell A.D. et al. In *"S. Block": Disinfection, Sterilization, and Preservation*, p. 717. Lea and Febiger, Philadelphia, PA, 1983.

16. Lewis C.L., Craig C.C., Senecal A.G. Mass and density measurements of live and dead Gram-negative and Gram-positive bacterial populations. *Appl. Environ. Microbiol.*, 80 (2014) 3622–31.

17. Fernández-Escudero I., I. Caro, J. Mateo, J. Tejero, E.J. Quinto. Low variability of growth parameters among six O157:H7 and non-O157:H7 *Escherichia coli* strains. *J. Food Prot.*, 77 (2014) 1988–91.

18. Lv X.N., Z.J. Liu, H.J. Zhang, C.M. Tzeng. Aromatherapy and the central nerve system (CNS): Therapeutic mechanism and its associated genes. *Curr. Drug Targets*, 14 (2013) 872–79.

19. Russo R., M.G. Cassiano, A. Ciociaro, A. Adornetto, G.P. Varano, C. Chiappini, L. Berliocchi, C. Tassorelli, G. Bagetta, M.T. Corasaniti. Role of D-limonene in autograpy induced by bergamot essential oil in SH-SY5Y neuroblastoma cells. *PloS One*, 9 (2014) 113682.

Section IV

Evidence-Based Clinical Use of Aromatherapy

16 Aromatherapy for the Treatment of Neuropsychiatric Symptoms of Dementia

Luca Cravello and Carlo Caltagirone

CONTENTS

16.1 DEMENTIA AND NEUROPSYCHIATRIC SYMPTOMS

The term *dementia* refers to a clinical syndrome characterized by impairment of cognitive functions that is severe enough to interfere with the daily social and working activities. In addition to cognitive decline, noncognitive symptoms affecting the sphere of personality, emotions, perception, and behavior are often present in patients with dementia (Raudino, 2013). These symptoms are a heterogeneous group of psychological reactions and psychiatric behaviors that can be variously associated with each other. They are often fluctuating (i.e., they are not present at each assessment) and may precede the onset of dementia and worsen with the evolution of the disease, contributing to significantly increased disability, morbidity, hospitalization, and economic cost for patient management. Moreover, they are a cause of stress for caregivers (Finkel, 2003).

Over the past 20 years great attention has been paid to noncognitive symptoms of dementia. In 1996, during a consensus conference organized by the International Psychogeriatric Association, the term *behavioral and psychological symptoms of dementia* (BPSD) was officially coined in order to identify the most common behavioral and psychological symptoms related to dementia. These were defined as "symptoms of disturbed perception, thought content, mood, or behavior that frequently occur in patients with dementia" (Small et al., 1997). To date, the expression *neuropsychiatric symptoms* (NPS) is considered more suitable, as it better describes the mixture of purely neurological and psychiatric features (Ballard et al., 2008).

The main neuropsychiatric symptoms are summarized in Table 16.1.

TABLE 16.1

Classification of Neuropsychiatric Symptoms

Symptom Cluster	Type of Symptom
Affective symptoms	Depression/dysphoria, anxiety, exaltation/euphoria, apathy, loss of inhibitions
Psychotic symptoms	Delusions, hallucinations
Behavioral symptoms	Agitation/aggressiveness, inappropriate motor behavior, irritability/lability
Modification in instinctive actions	Sleep disorders, appetite disorders

Source: Dorey, J. M. et al., *CNS Spectr* 13(9): 796–803, 2008.

The study of NPS is of greater importance not only in patients with dementia, but also in subjects in the preclinical phase of dementia, that is, mild cognitive impairment (MCI). Indeed, some of them could represent important risk factors of conversion from MCI to dementia (Monastero et al., 2009).

In Alzheimer's disease (AD), the most common type of dementia, NPS can arise at different times and dominate the evolutionary picture of the disease. Therefore, they need to be carefully researched and evaluated for their treatment. Depression, apathy, and anxiety are the most frequent and important NPS in the early stages of AD, while irritability and delusions prevail in the moderate and severe stages (Geda et al., 2013).

Although they may occur early, only a few neuropsychiatric symptoms are currently considered in the diagnostic guidelines of some forms of dementia: visual hallucinations are often present in dementia with Lewy bodies, and the lack of disease awareness and apathy are considered for the diagnosis of frontotemporal dementia, particularly in the frontal variant.

In various literature studies, the prevalence of NPS varies greatly according to the different forms of dementia: in Alzheimer's disease it ranges from 50% to 80%, in dementia with Lewy bodies it ranges from 40% to 75%, in frontotemporal dementia it is greater than 80%, and in subjects with MCI it varies from 35% to 75%. This large variability is due to specific factors such as the characteristics of the patients (ethnicity, gender, age, and education), the setting of the evaluation (hospital, outpatient clinic, and residential facilities), and finally, the different criteria considered for the NPS diagnosis.

The usual pharmacological management of NPS associated with dementia is based on antipsychotics (typical and atypical). However, this class of drugs has a high risk of important side effects, such as extrapyramidal symptoms, abnormal gait, sedation, increased risk of falls and fractures, increased incidence of delirium, cerebrovascular adverse events, and death (Musicco et al., 2011). Due to the important side effects of pharmacological therapy, nonpharmacological strategies have been proposed for the treatment of NPS in demented patients: among them, aromatherapy might be a potentially effective treatment. Indeed, aromatherapy is one of the most common complementary therapies practiced by healthcare professionals in hospital, hospice, and community settings (Buckle, 2007).

16.2   AROMATHERAPY AND NEUROPSYCHIATRIC SYMPTOMS

In people without dementia, the inhalation of essences used for aromatherapy could have potential beneficial effects, such as promotion of relaxation and sleep, relief of pain, and reduction of depressive symptoms (Forrester et al., 2014). Many patients with dementia have a reduced sense of smell, so it is likely that aromatherapy does not act through the pleasant sensation provided by the fragrant essences used (Jimbo et al., 2009). Thus, it has been postulated that essential oils of aromatherapy, absorbed into the body through digestion, the lining of orifices, olfaction, and the external skin, determine a physical reaction by interacting with hormones and enzymes (Fung et al., 2012). This action may have some effects on specific brain structures, such as the hypothalamus, thalamus and amygdala, that modulate the neuroendocrine system and emotional response. Another possible effect of aromatherapy is related to the ability of essential oils to improve neurotransmission in cholinergic neurons, by inhibiting acetylcholinesterase and increasing acetylcholine, that are implicated in the cognitive decline characteristic of dementia (Arruda et al., 2012). The effect of aromatherapy on brain pathways implicated in both emotional response and cognitive performance might also have a secondary effect on NPS of dementia.

Among the several essential oils that can be used for aromatherapy, only a few have been studied on patients with NPS related to dementia. Lavender (*Lavandula angustifolia*) is the most studied essential oil in demented patients, and some positive results can be drawn from the literature. The first placebo controlled trial on this topic was conducted by Holmes and collaborators (2002) on 15 patients with severe dementia and agitated behavior: after the administration of lavender oil in an aromatherapy stream, 60% of patients showed an improvement, although modest, in agitated behavior (Holmes et al., 2002). In another study, aromatherapy with lavender was found to be well tolerated and resulted in a significant improvement in NPS associated with dementia (Lin et al., 2007). Agitated and aggressive behavior, irritability, and nighttime disturbances were the NPS with the greatest improvement (Lin et al., 2007). Most recently, no positive effects of lavender oil aromatherapy on agitated behavior in dementia were found (O'Connor et al., 2013).

Melissa officinalis is another essence frequently used for aromatherapy in demented people. In a double-blind, placebo-controlled study on patients with severe dementia and associated NPS, aromatherapy with *Melissa* essential oil determined 35% improvement in agitation compared with 11% improvement after placebo treatment, with a highly significant difference. Moreover, quality of life also improved significantly in people receiving aromatherapy with *Melissa* essential oil (Ballard et al., 2002). On the contrary, other authors found no evidence that *Melissa* aromatherapy is superior to placebo or donepezil in the treatment of agitation in people with Alzheimer's disease (Burns et al., 2011).

Other essences (i.e., rosemary, chamomile, marjoram, mandarin, geranium, sweet almond, and thyme) have been used alone or in association for aromatherapy in demented people, with some positive results, such as improvement in cognitive functions (Jimbo et al., 2009), increased independence in daily living activities (Fung et al., 2012), and better relationship with caregivers (Kilstoff and Chenoweth, 1998).

In conclusion, despite the still scarce evidence, aromatherapy could represent a safe and valid alternative for the treatment of NPS related to dementia. Future studies with larger sample size should clarify what are the more efficacious essential oils on these symptoms and the characteristics of patients who can benefit from aromatherapy.

REFERENCES

Arruda, M., Viana, H., Rainha, N. et al. Anti-acetylcholinesterase and antioxidant activity of essential oils from *Hedychium gardnerianum* Sheppard ex Ker-Gawl. *Molecules* 17 (3) (2012): 3082–3092.

Ballard, C. G., O'Brien, J. T., Reichelt, K., Perry, E. K. Aromatherapy as a safe and effective treatment for the management of agitation in severe dementia: The results of a double-blind, placebo-controlled trial with *Melissa*. *J Clin Psychiatry* 63 (7) (2002): 553–558.

Ballard, C., Day, S., Sharp, S. et al. Neuropsychiatric symptoms in dementia: Importance and treatment considerations. *Int Rev Psychiatry* 20 (4) (2008): 396–404.

Buckle, J. Literature review: Should nursing take aromatherapy more seriously? *Br J Nurs* 16 (2) (2007): 116–120.

Burns, A., Perry, E., Holmes, C. et al. A double-blind placebo-controlled randomized trial of *Melissa officinalis* oil and donepezil for the treatment of agitation in Alzheimer's disease. *Dement Geriatr Cogn Disord* 31 (2) (2011): 158–164.

Dorey, J. M., Beauchet, O., Thomas Anterion, C. et al. Behavioral and psychological symptoms of dementia and bipolar spectrum disorders: Review of the evidence of a relationship and treatment implications. *CNS Spectr* 13 (9) (2008): 796–803.

Finkel, S. I. Behavioral and psychologic symptoms of dementia. *Clin Geriatr Med* 19 (4) (2003): 799–824.

Forrester, L. T., Maayan, N., Orrell, M., Spector, A. E., Buchan, L. D., Soares-Weiser, K. Aromatherapy for dementia. *Cochrane Database Syst Rev* 2 (2014): CD003150.

Fung, J. K., Tsang, H. W., Chung, R. C. A systematic review of the use of aromatherapy in treatment of behavioral problems in dementia. *Geriatr Gerontol Int* 12 (3) (2012): 372–382.

Geda, Y. E., Schneider, L. S., Gitlin, L. N. et al. Neuropsychiatric symptoms in Alzheimer's disease: Past progress and anticipation of the future. *Alzheimers Dement* 9 (5) (2013): 602–608.

Holmes, C., Hopkins, V., Hensford, C., MacLaughlin, V., Wilkinson, D., Rosenvinge, H. Lavender oil as a treatment for agitated behaviour in severe dementia: A placebo controlled study. *Int J Geriatr Psychiatry* 17 (4) (2002): 305–308.

Jimbo, D., Kimura, Y., Taniguchi, M., Inoue, M., Urakami, K. Effect of aromatherapy on patients with Alzheimer's disease. *Psychogeriatrics* 9 (4) (2009): 173–179.

Kilstoff, K., Chenoweth, L. New approaches to health and well-being for dementia day-care clients, family carers and day-care staff. *Int J Nurs Pract* 4 (2) (1998): 70–83.

Lin, P. W., Chan, W. C., Ng, B. F., Lam, L. C. Efficacy of aromatherapy (*Lavandula angustifolia*) as an intervention for agitated behaviours in Chinese older persons with dementia: A cross-over randomized trial. *Int J Geriatr Psychiatry* 22 (5) (2007): 405–410.

Monastero, R., Mangialasche, F., Camarda, C., Ercolani, S., Camarda, R. A systematic review of neuropsychiatric symptoms in mild cognitive impairment. *J Alzheimers Dis* 18 (1) (2009): 11–30.

Musicco, M., Palmer, K., Russo, A. et al. Association between prescription of conventional or atypical antipsychotic drugs and mortality in older persons with Alzheimer's disease. *Dement Geriatr Cogn Disord* 31 (3) (2011): 218–224.

O'Connor, D. W., Eppingstall, B., Taffe, J., van der Ploeg, E. S. A randomized, controlled cross-over trial of dermally-applied lavender (*Lavandula angustifolia*) oil as a treatment of agitated behaviour in dementia. *BMC Complement Altern Med* 13 (2013): 315.

Raudino, F. Non-cognitive symptoms and related conditions in the Alzheimer's disease: A literature review. *Neurol Sci* 34 (8) (2013): 1275–1282.

Small, G. W., Rabins, P. V., Barry, P. P. et al. Diagnosis and treatment of Alzheimer disease and related disorders. Consensus statement of the American Association for Geriatric Psychiatry, the Alzheimer's Association, and the American Geriatrics Society. *JAMA* 278 (16) (1997): 1363–1371.

17 Aromatherapy in Dementia and Dementia-Related Neuropsychiatric Disorders

Sergio Fusco, Francesco Corica,
and Andrea Corsonello

CONTENTS

17.1 INTRODUCTION

Disorders of cognition, primarily dementia and delirium, are highly prevalent among older people: the age-standardized prevalence for those >60 years varied in a narrow band, 5%–7% in most world regions, with a higher prevalence in Latin America (8.5%) and a distinctively lower prevalence in the four sub-Saharan African regions (2%–4%). It was estimated that 35.6 million people lived with dementia worldwide in 2010, with numbers expected to almost double every 20 years, to 65.7 million in 2030 and 115.4 million in 2050. In 2010, 58% of all people with dementia lived in countries with low or middle incomes, with this proportion anticipated to rise to 63% in 2030 and 71% in 2050 (Prince et al., 2013).

Dementia itself is a syndrome including symptoms affecting thinking and social abilities severely enough to interfere with daily functioning (Hugo and Ganguli, 2014) caused by diseases and disorders that affect the brain, including Alzheimer's disease (AD) (Holmes et al., 1999; Thies and Bleiler, 2013; Dubois et al., 2014), Parkinson's disease (PD) (Emre et al., 2007), diffuse Lewy body disease (DLBD) (Holmes et al., 1999; Vann Jones and O'Brien, 2014), stroke, and others.

Dementia symptoms vary depending on the cause, but common signs and symptoms include memory loss, difficulty communicating, difficulty with complex tasks, difficulty with planning and organizing, difficulty with coordination and motor functions, problems with disorientation, such as getting lost, personality changes, inability to reason, inappropriate behavior, paranoia, agitation, and hallucinations. The reported prevalence of depression or depressive symptoms in persons with dementia ranges from 0% to 96% (Amore et al., 2007). The Medical Outcomes Study found that depression was more debilitating than other chronic medical disorders, such as diabetes, arthritis, hypertension, and cardiovascular disease (Wells et al., 1989). The treatment of dementia varies through the course of its illness because symptoms evolve over time. Various drugs have been utilized for delaying cognitive decline (Schwarz et al., 2012). Acetylcholinesterase inhibitors have been recommended for use in mild to moderate cases of dementia, while memantine is the only drug recommended for severe cases of dementia. Looking into the morbidity, appropriate utilization of antidementia therapy is highly essential for these patients because these drugs are limited by side effects, short duration of action, and the need for frequent monitoring of blood levels or other laboratory values to prevent toxicity (Patel et al., 2014).

During the natural course of dementia a heterogeneous group of clinical phenomena is subjectively experienced by the patient or observable by an examiner (e.g., caregiver or physician) consisting of several different behavioral disturbances and psychiatric symptoms.

These neuropsychiatric symptoms or behavioral and psychological symptoms of dementia (BPSD) (Finkel et al., 1996) are very common, regardless of the type of dementia, and are present in virtually all patients during the course of their disease (Katona et al., 2007). BPSD often overwhelm families, and lack of treatment increases patient morbidity and almost always leads to institutionalization with an increased cost of care (Ballard and Howard, 2006; Ballard et al., 2009). Even in the early stages of cognitive impairment, neuropsychiatric symptoms are frequent, with estimated rates of 35%–85% in subjects with mild cognitive impairment (MCI) (Monastero et al., 2009). The reported frequency of BPSD largely depends on the type of sample and setting considered. In community dwelling subjects with dementia, neuropsychiatric symptoms are generally less frequent (56%–98%) and severe than in patients recruited in hospital or long-term care facilities (91%–96%) (Cerejeira et al., 2012).

BPSD also increase the risk of caregiver burnout and depression (Kilstoff and Chenoweth, 1998; Feil et al., 2007).

BPSD are difficult to treat with medications, and it is increasingly recognized that pharmacological treatments for dementia should be used as a second-line approach and that nonpharmacological options should, in best practice, be pursued first (Howard et al., 2001; Holmes et al., 2002). Several complementary and alternative medicine (CAM) modalities have received attention as being potentially useful in the management of disruptive behaviors in people with dementia (Fossey et al., 2006; Chenoweth et al., 2009; Jimbo et al., 2009) (Table 17.1). Among these approaches, aromatherapy offers an alternative approach to the risk of pharmacological intervention such as antipsychotics.

TABLE 17.1

Nonpharmacological Therapies for Dementia and Dementia-Related Neuropsychiatric Disorders

Therapies	Methods
Standard therapies	Behavioral therapy
	Reality orientation
	Validation therapy
	Reminiscence therapy
Alternative therapies	Art therapy
	Music therapy
	Activity therapy
	Complementary therapy
	Aromatherapy
	Bright-light therapy
	Multisensory approaches
Brief psychotherapies	Cognitive–behavioral therapy
	Interpersonal therapy

17.2 PHARMACOLOGICAL TREATMENT FOR DEMENTIA

Cholinesterase inhibitors (ChEIs) are the mainstay of treatment of AD (Schwarz et al., 2012). Randomized controlled trials (RCTs) have reported statistically significant, and clinically modest, effects of ChEIs (Birks and Harvey, 2003; Gabelli, 2003; Raskind, 2003). Trials have been short, conducted over 6 months, although effects have been reported, in open-label extensions, to last up to 5 years. There are currently three ChEIs regularly used that are licensed for the treatment of mild to moderate AD: donepezil, galantamine, and rivastigmine. ChEIs have broadly similar side effects. These drugs can increase the risk of falls, extrapyramidal symptoms, cerebrovascular adverse events, and metabolic syndrome (Schneider et al., 2006). Memantine is a partial glutamate receptor antagonist used for the treatment of moderate to severe AD (Schwarz et al., 2012). Despite only being licensed for use in moderate to severe dementia in AD, memantine has been shown to have beneficial effects in slowing deterioration in cognition in patients with mild to moderate AD and vascular dementia too (Versijpt, 2014) (Table 17.2).

Treatment of agitation, when indicated, is usually with sedative or antipsychotic drugs (Sadowsky and Galvin, 2012; Gabryelewicz, 2014). Of all atypical antipsychotics, risperidone has the largest database of double-blind controlled trials to support its efficacy and safety in the treatment of agitation, aggression, and psychosis associated with dementia. Its superiority over placebo for agitation appears to be independent of dementia type, dementia severity, presence of psychosis, or drug-induced somnolence (De Deyn et al., 2005). As atypical antipsychotics have a more favorable side effect profile than typical antipsychotics, there is no compelling reason to recommend the use of more traditional antipsychotics. In fact, it has been reported that risperidone and olanzapine are not associated

TABLE 17.2

Medications for Dementia and Dementia-Related Neuropsychiatric Disorders

Medications	Side Effects
Acetylcholinesterase Inhibitors	
Donepezil Galantamine Rivastigmine	Side effects can include nausea, vomiting, and diarrhea. However, this should settle down within the first two weeks of taking the medication.
Memantine	A common side effect of memantine is dizziness.
Antipsychotics	
Typical antipsychotics Atypical antipsychotics	Increase the risk of a person experiencing cardiovascular diseases, such as stroke or heart attack. Make other symptoms of dementia worse and cause drowsiness. Also, in people who have dementia with Lewy bodies, there is evidence that antipsychotics can cause a range of serious side effects, including rigidity, immobility, and inability to communicate.
Antidepressant	
Tricyclic antidepressants Monamine oxidase inhibitor (MAOI) Selective serotonine reuptake inhibitors (SSRIs)	Cholinergic side effects such as headache, insomnia, and nausea.

with a statistically significant risk of stroke compared with typical antipsychotics (Herrmann et al., 2004). The side effects of these drugs have been well documented and include accelerated cognitive decline, higher cerebrovascular side effects, and increased mortality—risks shared by both first- and second-generation antipsychotics (Jeste et al., 2008). ChEIs are traditionally used to improve cognitive function and appear to confer modest benefits in the overall treatment of neuropsychiatric symptoms (Loy and Schneider, 2006). A meta-analysis demonstrated a small but significant overall advantage of ChEIs compared with placebo over 24–26 weeks with regard to the overall treatment of neuropsychiatric symptoms in Alzheimer's disease (Trinh et al., 2003). Additional support for the benefits of ChEIs on neuropsychiatric symptoms comes from a randomized withdrawal study in which cessation of donepezil in Alzheimer's disease patients was associated with a significant worsening of the total Neuropsychiatric Inventory score within 6 weeks (Holmes et al., 2004). However, there was no short-term benefit for treatment of clinically significant agitation with donepezil over 12 weeks in a large RCT, suggesting that ChEIs do not appear to be useful in the management of acute agitation (Holmes et al., 2007). Regarding memantine, meta- and pooled analyses indicate that memantine confers benefit in the treatment of irritability and lability, agitation and aggression, and to a lesser degree, psychosis over 3–6 months in patients with Alzheimer's disease (Mcshane et al., 2006; Gauthier et al., 2008), and a Cochrane meta-analysis suggested that memantine also conferred a modest but significant benefit in the treatment of neuropsychiatric symptoms in patients with vascular dementia (Mcshane et al., 2006). While this evidence is very encouraging with respect to memantine, there are no RCTs specifically involving patients with clinically significant agitation or aggression.

Symptoms of depression are especially common in the course of dementia. Most clinical trials of antidepressants for depression in dementia have been inconclusive. Pharmacological treatments should probably be reserved for patients with severe depression symptoms (Pollock et al., 2007). To date, mainstream treatment of depression mainly relies on medication with the use of tricyclic antidepressants, monamine oxidase inhibitors (MAOIs), and selective serotonin reuptake inhibitors (SSRIs) (Ohayon and Lader, 2002; Ellen et al., 2007). Unfortunately, nearly one-third of the patients abruptly terminated medication treatment due to the unpleasant cholinergic side effects, such as headache, insomnia, and nausea, which increased cognitive and functional impairments in people with dementia (Smallwood et al., 2001; Nemeroff, 2003).

17.3 MOLECULAR PATHWAYS OF AROMATHERAPY RELEVANT FOR DEMENTIA

Aromatherapy has been used in people with dementia to improve motivation (Macmahon and Kermode, 1998), to promote sleep (Snow et al., 2004), and to reduce disturbed behavior (Brooker et al., 1997; Lin et al., 2007). Aromatherapy has predominantly focused on essential oils believed to have a calming and sedative effect. It is true that many plants have therapeutic properties. For example, the use of acetyl salicylic acid, the active ingredient in aspirin, came from the discovery that chewing willow bark alleviated pain, inflammation, and fever.

However, aromatherapy is based not on the ingestion of various plant-based products, but rather on inhaling their aromas, which are claimed to have a range of therapeutic and psychological properties (Table 17.3).

Several investigations were performed to clarify the mechanism of action of lavender in neuronal tissues. The proposed mechanism of action of the respiratory administration of aromatherapy begins with the absorption of volatile odor molecules through the nasal mucosa.

Odor molecules are then transformed into chemical signals, which travel to the olfactory bulb and then other parts of the limbic system of the brain and the cerebral cortex and the olfactory sensory center at the base of the brain, interacting with the neuropsychological framework to produce characteristic physiological and psychological effects on target tissues (Lis-Balchin and Hart, 1999).

Lavender inhibited lipopolysaccharide-induced inflammatory reaction in human monocyte THP-1 cells (Huang et al., 2012). Antioxidant and relatively weak cholinergic inhibition was reported for lavender (Wang et al., 2012) and linalool (Perry et al., 2000). These findings indicate that several targets relevant to treatment of Alzheimer's disease—anticholinergic, neuroprotective, and antioxidant activities—could be found

TABLE 17.3
Summary of Clinical Trials of Aromatherapy in Patients with Dementia

Essential Oil	Study Design	Outcome
Lemon balm (Melissa) and lavender aroma (Mitchell S. Aromatherapy's effectiveness in disorders associated with dementia. *Int J Aromather* 1993; 4: 20–3).	Placebo-controlled; six patients received treatment oils and six control oil; intervention period: 1 week.	Treatment oils increased functional abilities and communication, and decreased difficult behaviors (no statistical analysis).
Lavender aroma and massage (Smallwood, Brown et al. 2001).	Randomized, controlled; 21 patients; aromatherapy and massage compared with aroma or massage alone; intervention period: 2 weeks.	Aromatherapy with massage significantly reduced frequency of excessive motor behavior.
Lavender aroma (Holmes, Hopkins et al. 2002).	Placebo-controlled; 15 patients; treatment with oil and placebo (water) on alternative days; intervention period: 10 days.	Aromatherapy significantly reduced agitated behavior, as assessed using the Pittsburgh Agitation Scale.
Melissa lotion applied to face and arms (Ballard, O'Brien et al. 2002).	Randomized, controlled; 36 patients received *Melissa* and 36 sunflower oil; intervention period: 4 weeks.	Aromatherapy associated with highly significant reductions in measures on the Cohen Mansfield Agitation Inventory and social withdrawal, together with an increase in constructive activities (dementia care mapping).
Lavender, geranium, and mandarin essential oils in almond oil applied to skin (Kilstoff and Chenoweth 1998).	Open label: 39 patients; treatment over unspecified period; patient, staff and carer interviews/rating.	Aromatherapy increased alertness, contentment, and sleeping at night, and reduced levels of agitation, withdrawal, and wandering.
Direct intake of 60 drops of *Melissa officinalis* (Akhondzadeh, Noroozian et al. 2003).	Randomized, placebo-controlled; 42 patients; AD concomitant disease and other drugs treating dementia were stopped; intervention period: 4 months.	Number of subjects with agitation was significantly less in the treatment group.
2 drops of undiluted oil was placed every 3 h on an absorbent fabric sachet pinned near the collarbone of each subject's shirt (Snow, Hovanec et al. 2004).	Placebo-controlled, within subject design; 7 patients; intervention period: 10 weeks.	No evidence of reduction of agitation in treatment groups. No evidence showed a nonspecific effect for pleasant-smelling substances. No indication of a global placebo effect.

(Continued)

TABLE 17.3 (CONTINUED)
Summary of Clinical Trials of Aromatherapy in Patients with Dementia

Essential Oil	Study Design	Outcome
Inhalation of lavender EO in cosmetic cotton diffused by aroma diffuser (Lin, Chan et al. 2007).	Placebo-controlled crossover randomized study; 70 patients; intervention period: 10 weeks.	Significant reduction of agitation, dysphoria, irritability, aberrant motor behavior, and night-time behavior.
Use of rosemary and lemon essential oils in the morning, and lavender and orange in the evening (Jimbo, Kimura et al. 2009).	Placebo-controlled, within subject design; intervention period: 16 weeks.	Significant improvement in cognitive function and ideational praxis function was observed after aromatherapy.
Melissa oil in base lotion massage into the hands and upper arms 1–2 min twice daily (Burns, Perry et al. 2011).	Double-blind parallel-group placebo-controlled randomized trial; 114 patients; intervention period: 3 months.	No significant difference between or within groups for agitation and functioning in ADL.

in lavender. The neuroprotective effect of lavender oil against cerebral ischemia/reperfusion injury is suggested to be attributed to its antioxidant effects (Wang et al., 2012). Evaluation of the effects of lavender oil on motor activity and its relationship to dopaminergic neurotransmission revealed that intraperitoneal application of lavender significantly increased rotarod activity and enhanced dopamine receptor subtype D3 in the olfactory bulbs of mice (Kim et al., 2009). Lavender oil is also suggested to modulate GABAergic neurotransmission, especially on $GABA_A$ receptors, and enhance the inhibitory tone of the nervous system (Brum et al., 2001). The cholinergic system is suggested to play a role in lavender analgesic, antianxiety, and antidepression effects.

Komiya et al. (2006) studied the antianxiety effect of essential oil from rose, lavender, and lemon. They also researched the linkage of essential oil from lemon with benzodiazepine, 5-hydroxy tryptamine, dopamine, and adrenergic receptor and found essential oil from lemon increasing the nerve energy of 5-hydroxy tryptamine from the suppression the activity of dopamine.

Umezu et al. (2006) studied that dopamine might be involved in the mouse ambulation promoted by peppermint oil and its constituents. Wu et al. (2012) have done a thorough metabolomic study on rat brain tissue and urinary responses to aromatherapy. These metabolic changes include the increased carbohydrates and lowered levels of neurotransmitters (tryptophan, serine, glycine, aspartate, histamine, tyrosine, cysteine, phenylalanine, hypotaurine, histidine, and asparagine), amino acids, and fatty acids in brain.

Lavender extracts display acetylcholinesterase (AChE) activities (Adsersen et al., 2006). The study of Kashani et al. (2011) aimed to evaluate the effects of aqueous extract of lavender (*Lavandula angustifolia*) on the spatial performance of Alzheimer's disease (AD) rats, based on the cholinergic hypothesis that AD patients may have defects in their cholinergic system, which is associated with memory and learning. Indeed, increasing the level of acetylcholine (ACh) in the brain may be an effective therapy for

AD treatment. Male Wistar rats were first divided into control and AD groups. A rat model of AD was established by intracerebroventricular injection of 10 µg of Aβ1-42 20 days prior to administration of the lavender extract. Rats in both groups were then introduced to two stages of task learning (with an interval of 20 days). After the first stage of spatial learning, control and AD animals received different doses (50, 100, and 200 mg/kg) of the lavender extract. In the retrieval test, the lavender-treated animals in both the control and AD groups demonstrated a tendency of better function in memory consolidation. However, the improvement was significant only at the highest dose.

17.4   AROMATHERAPY FOR ANXIETY AND AGITATION

Several animal experiments suggest anxiolytic, sedative, and neuroprotective properties for lavender. It was shown that lavender possesses an anticonflict effect in mice (Umezu, 2000). An experimental study on mice of Chioca et al. (2013) has shown an important role for the serotonergic system in the anxiolytic-like effect of lavender essential oil through the interaction of the GABA/BDZ complex that is the main molecular target of benzodiazepin (BDZ), one of most frequently prescribed anxiolytic drugs, as demonstrated in previous experimental studies (Perry and Perry, 2006; Umezu et al., 2006). Continuous exposure to lavender essential oils for 7 days significantly inhibited anxiety- and depression-like behaviors tested by elevated plus-maze and forced swimming tests in rats (Hritcu et al., 2012). Lavender oil produced significant antianxiety effects in the Geller conflict and the Vogel conflict tests, standards for fast screening of the potential anxiolytic properties of drugs, in mice (Umezu et al., 2006).

Another study has demonstrated the direct action of lavender oil on tryptophan, and helps the relaxation response (Zeilmann et al., 2003). There have been some positive results from controlled trials that have shown statistically significant reductions in agitation, with excellent compliance and tolerability (Ballard et al., 2002). A systematic review by Thorgrimsen et al. cites a study that found that lavender oil placed in a sachet on each side of the pillow for at least 1 hour during sleep seemed to reduce problem behaviors (Thorgrimsen et al., 2003). Several evidence-based guidelines have concluded that aromatherapy may be helpful, and two of the five practice guidelines reviewed by Azermai et al. (2012) recommend it. In line with these studies, the efficacy of a 6-week intake of oral lavender oil preparation, compared to lorazepam, was investigated in adults with generalized anxiety disorder. This study indicates that lavender effectively ameliorates generalized anxiety comparable to 0.5 mg/daily lorazepam (Woelk and Schlafke, 2010). Alleviation of anxiety and mood improvement were reported in 36 patients admitted to an intensive care unit who received lavender oil (diluted to 1% concentration) aromatherapy (Dunn et al., 1995).

17.5   AROMATHERAPY FOR DEPRESSION

In an animal study (De Almeida et al., 2004), lemon essential oil was found to significantly accelerate the metabolic turnover of 5-HT in the prefrontal cortex and striatum. This is similar to the effect of SSRIs, which are commonly used as antidepressants to ameliorate depressive symptoms by increasing serotonin (5-HT) function (Castro et al., 2003). In a pilot, controlled, randomized trial, the effect of citrus fragrance was compared with that of no fragrance in men with depression. The dose of antidepressant drugs was significantly reduced in the active treatment group (Roberts and Williams, 1992).

Perry and Perry (2006) suggested that essential oils such as bergamot, jasmine, lavender, rose, and geranium had antidepressant effects. A clinical investigation points to an antidepressive effect of lavender (Akhondzadeh et al., 2003a). The combined therapy with a tricyclic antidepressant (imipramine) and lavender led to a better and earlier improvement in patients suffering from mild to moderate depression. Anticholinergic side effects of imipramine, such as dry mouth and urinary retention, were observed less often when lavender was administered with imipramine. These results suggest that lavender is an effective adjuvant therapy in combination with imipramine, resulting in a superior and quicker improvement in depressive symptoms.

17.6 LIMITATIONS, SAFETY ISSUES, AND ADVERSE EFFECTS

Essential oils contain potent chemicals and most require dilution before use. Safety issues are related to inappropriate use, excessive use, accidental ingestion, and skin reactions in the allergy-prone. Purity and chemical constituents may vary according to climate, soils, processing, and storage of the essential oils, and certain oils such as pennyroyal and sage should be avoided due to potential toxic effects (Posadzki et al., 2012).

Nevertheless, available evidence in the literature is not sufficient to make a conclusive claim (Burns et al., 2011). In fact, the number of studies in this research field is small. Another problem is related to the presence of confounders on various aspects of the intervention protocol. The administration methods of aromatherapy varied significantly in the studies (Table 17.3). The essential oil used also varied from study to study. Problems of confounding effects might arise from the concurrent use of medications. The last problem was the training of the people that implemented the treatment. The level of training varied remarkably among the studies, from untrained carers or caregiving staff to trained aromatherapists.

17.7 CONCLUSIONS

Substantial evidence exists to recommend aromatherapy for short-term treatment of some neurological disorders. However, long-term trials and observational studies are needed to establish the safety of long-term use as well as overall efficacy in the context of treatment and management of complex patients with dementia and dementia-related neuropsychiatric disorders.

REFERENCES

Adsersen, A., Gauguin, B., Gudiksen, L., Jäger, A. K. Screening of plants used in Danish folk medicine to treat memory dysfunction for acetylcholinesterase inhibitory activity. *J Ethnopharmacol* 104, 3 (2006): 418–22.

Akhondzadeh, S., Kashani, L., Fotouhi, A. et al. Comparison of *Lavandula angustifolia* Mill. Tincture and imipramine in the treatment of mild to moderate depression: A double-blind, randomized trial. *Prog Neuropsychopharmacol Biol Psychiatry* 27, 1 (2003a): 123–27.

Akhondzadeh, S., Noroozian, M., Mohammadi, M., Ohadinia, S., Jamshidi, A. H., Khani, M. *Melissa officinalis* extract in the treatment of patients with mild to moderate Alzheimer's disease: A double blind, randomised, placebo controlled trial. *J Neurol Neurosurg Psychiatry* 74, 7 (2003b): 863–66.

Amore, M., Tagariello, P., Laterza, C., Savoia, E. M. Subtypes of depression in dementia. *Arch Gerontol Geriatr* 44, Suppl 1 (2007): 23–33.

Azermai, M., Petrovic, M., Elseviers, M. M., Bourgeois, J., Van Bortel, L. M., Vander Stichele, R. H. Systematic appraisal of dementia guidelines for the management of behavioural and psychological symptoms. *Ageing Res Rev*, 11, 1 (2012): 78–86.

Ballard, C., Howard, R. Neuroleptic drugs in dementia: Benefits and harm. *Nat Rev Neurosci* 7, 6 (2006): 492–500.

Ballard, C. G., O'Brien, J. T., Reichelt, K., Perry, E. K. Aromatherapy as a safe and effective treatment for the management of agitation in severe dementia: The results of a double-blind, placebo-controlled trial with *Melissa*. *J Clin Psychiatry* 63, 7 (2002): 553–58.

Ballard, C. G., Gauthier, S., Cummings, J. L. et al. Management of agitation and aggression associated with Alzheimer disease. *Nat Rev Neurol* 5, 5 (2009): 245–55.

Birks, J. S., Harvey, R. Donepezil for dementia due to Alzheimer's disease. *Cochrane Database Syst Rev* 3 (2003): CD001190.

Brooker, D. J., Snape, M., Johnson, E., Ward, D., Payne, M. Single case evaluation of the effects of aromatherapy and massage on disturbed behaviour in severe dementia. *Br J Clin Psychol* 36, Pt 2 (1997): 287–96.

Brum, L. F., Elisabetsky, E., Souza, D. Effects of linalool on [(3)H]MK801 and [(3)H] muscimol binding in mouse cortical membranes. *Phytother Res* 15, 5 (2001): 422–25.

Burns, A., Perry, E., Holmes, C. et al. A double-blind placebo-controlled randomized trial of *Melissa officinalis* oil and donepezil for the treatment of agitation in Alzheimer's disease. *Dement Geriatr Cogn Disord* 31, 2 (2011): 158–64.

Castro, E., Tordera, R. M., Hughes, Z. A., Pei, Q., Sharp, T. Use of Arc expression as a molecular marker of increased postsynaptic 5-HT function after SSRI/5-HT1A receptor antagonist co-administration. *J Neurochem* 85, 6 (2003): 1480–87.

Cerejeira, J., Lagarto, L., Mukaetova-Ladinska, E. B. Behavioral and psychological symptoms of dementia. *Front Neurol* 3 (2012): 73.

Chenoweth, L., King, M. T., Jeon, Y. H. et al. Caring for Aged Dementia Care Resident Study (CADRES) of person-centred care, dementia-care mapping, and usual care in dementia: A cluster-randomised trial. *Lancet Neurol* 8, 4 (2009): 317–25.

Chioca, L. R., Ferro, M. M., Baretta, I. P. et al. Anxiolytic-like effect of lavender essential oil inhalation in mice: Participation of serotonergic but not GABAA/benzodiazepine neurotransmission. *J Ethnopharmacol* 147, 2 (2013): 412–18.

De Almeida, R. N., Motta, S. C., de Brito Faturi, C., Catallani, B., Leite, J. R. Anxiolytic-like effects of rose oil inhalation on the elevated plus-maze test in rats. *Pharmacol Biochem Behav* 77, 2 (2004): 361–64.

De Deyn, P. P., Katz, I. R., Brodaty, H., Lyons, B., Greenspan, A., Burns, A. Management of agitation, aggression, and psychosis associated with dementia: A pooled analysis including three randomized, placebo-controlled double-blind trials in nursing home residents treated with risperidone. *Clin Neurol Neurosurg* 107, 6 (2005): 497–508.

Dubois, B., Feldman, H. H., Jacova, C. et al. Advancing research diagnostic criteria for Alzheimer's disease: The IWG-2 criteria. *Lancet Neurol* 13, 6 (2014): 614–29.

Dunn, C., Sleep, J., Collett, D. Sensing an improvement: An experimental study to evaluate the use of aromatherapy, massage and periods of rest in an intensive care unit. *J Adv Nurs* 21, 1 (1995): 34–40.

Ellen, S., Selzer, R., Norman, T., Blashki, G. Depression and anxiety: Pharmacological treatment in general practice. *Aust Fam Physician* 36, 4 (2007): 222–28.

Emre, M., Aarsland, D., Brown, R. et al. Clinical diagnostic criteria for dementia associated with Parkinson's disease. *Mov Disord* 22, 12 (2007): 1689–707; quiz 1837.

Feil, D. G., Maclean, C., Sultzer, D. Quality indicators for the care of dementia in vulnerable elders. *J Am Geriatr Soc* 55, Suppl 2 (2007): S293–301.

Finkel, S. I., Costa E Silva, J., Cohen, G., Miller, S., Sartorius, N. Behavioral and psychological signs and symptoms of dementia: A consensus statement on current knowledge and implications for research and treatment. *Int Psychogeriatr* 8, Suppl 3 (1996): 497–500.

Fossey, J., Ballard, C., Juszczak, E. et al. Effect of enhanced psychosocial care on antipsychotic use in nursing home residents with severe dementia: Cluster randomised trial. *BMJ* 332, 7544 (2006): 756–61.

Gabelli, C. Rivastigmine: An update on therapeutic efficacy in Alzheimer's disease and other conditions. *Curr Med Res Opin* 19, 2 (2003): 69–82.

Gabryelewicz, T. [Pharmacological treatment of behavioral symptoms in dementia patients]. *Przegl Lek*, 71, 4 (2014): 215–20.

Gauthier, S., Loft, H., Cummings, J. Improvement in behavioural symptoms in patients with moderate to severe Alzheimer's disease by memantine: A pooled data analysis. *Int J Geriatr Psychiatry* 23, 5 (2008): 537–45.

Herrmann, N., Mamdani, M., Lanctôt, K. L. Atypical antipsychotics and risk of cerebrovascular accidents. *Am J Psychiatry* 161, 6 (2004): 1113–15.

Holmes, C., Cairns, N., Lantos, P., Mann, A. Validity of current clinical criteria for Alzheimer's disease, vascular dementia and dementia with Lewy bodies. *Br J Psychiatry* 174 (1999): 45–50.

Holmes, C., Hopkins, V., Hensford, C., MacLaughlin, V., Wilkinson, D., Rosenvinge, H. Lavender oil as a treatment for agitated behaviour in severe dementia: A placebo controlled study. *Int J Geriatr Psychiatry* 17, 4 (2002): 305–8.

Holmes, C., Wilkinson, D., Dean, C. The efficacy of donepezil in the treatment of neuropsychiatric symptoms in Alzheimer disease. *Neurology* 63, 2 (2004): 214–19.

Holmes, C., Wilkinson, D., Dean, C. et al. Risperidone and rivastigmine and agitated behaviour in severe Alzheimer's disease: A randomised double blind placebo controlled study. *Int J Geriatr Psychiatry* 22, 4 (2007): 380–81.

Howard, R., Ballard, C., O'Brien, J., Burns, A; UK and Ireland Group for Optimization of Management in Dementia. Guidelines for the management of agitation in dementia. *Int J Geriatr Psychiatry* 16, 7 (2001): 714–17.

Hritcu, L., Cioanca, O., Hancianu, M. Effects of lavender oil inhalation on improving scopolamine-induced spatial memory impairment in laboratory rats. *Phytomedicine* 19, 6 (2012): 529–34.

Huang, M. Y., Liao, M. H., Wang, Y. K., Huang, Y. S., Wen, H. C. Effect of lavender essential oil on LPS-stimulated inflammation. *Am J Chin Med* 40, 4 (2012): 845–59.

Hugo, J., Ganguli, M. Dementia and cognitive impairment: Epidemiology, diagnosis, and treatment. *Clin Geriatr Med* 30, 3 (2014): 421–42.

Jeste, D. V., Blazer, D., Casey, D. et al. ACNP white paper: Update on use of antipsychotic drugs in elderly persons with dementia. *Neuropsychopharmacology* 33, 5 (2008): 957–70.

Jimbo, D., Kimura, Y., Taniguchi, M., Inoue, M., Urakami, K. Effect of aromatherapy on patients with Alzheimer's disease. *Psychogeriatrics* 9, 4 (2009): 173–79.

Kashani, M. S., Tavirani, M. R., Talaei, S. A., Salami, M. Aqueous extract of lavender (*Lavandula angustifolia*) improves the spatial performance of a rat model of Alzheimer's disease. *Neurosci Bull* 27, 2 (2011): 99–106.

Katona, C., Livingston, G., Cooper, C., Ames, D., Brodaty, H., Chiu, E. International Psychogeriatric Association consensus statement on defining and measuring treatment benefits in dementia. *Int Psychogeriatr* 19, 3 (2007): 345–54.

Kilstoff, K., and Chenoweth, L. New approaches to health and well-being for dementia daycare clients, family carers and day-care staff. *Int J Nurs Pract* 4, 2 (1998): 70–83.

Kim, Y., Kim, M., Kim, H., Kim, K. Effect of lavender oil on motor function and dopamine receptor expression in the olfactory bulb of mice. *J Ethnopharmacol* 125, 1 (2009): 31–35.

Komiya, M., Takeuchi, T., Harada, E. Lemon oil vapor causes an anti-stress effect via modulating the 5-HT and DA activities in mice. *Behav Brain Res* 172, 2 (2006): 240–49.

Lin, P. W., Chan, W. C., Ng, B. F., Lam, L. C. Efficacy of aromatherapy (*Lavandula angustifolia*) as an intervention for agitated behaviours in Chinese older persons with dementia: A cross-over randomized trial. *Int J Geriatr Psychiatry* 22, 5 (2007): 405–10.

Lis-Balchin, M., and Hart, S. Studies on the mode of action of the essential oil of lavender (*Lavandula angustifolia* P. Miller). *Phytother Res* 13, 6 (1999): 540–42.

Loy, C., and Schneider, L. Galantamine for Alzheimer's disease and mild cognitive impairment. *Cochrane Database Syst Rev* 1 (2006): CD001747.

Macmahon, S., and Kermode, S. A clinical trial of the effect of aromatherapy on motivational behaviour in a dementia care setting using a single subject design. *Aust J Holist Nurs* 5, 2 (1998): 47–49.

Mcshane, R., Areosa Sastre, A., Minakaran, N. Memantine for dementia. *Cochrane Database Syst Rev* 2 (2006): CD003154.

Monastero, R., Mangialasche, F., Camarda, C., Ercolani, S., Camarda, R. A systematic review of neuropsychiatric symptoms in mild cognitive impairment. *J Alzheimers Dis* 18, 1 (2009): 11–30.

Nemeroff, C. B. Improving antidepressant adherence. *J Clin Psychiatry* 64, Suppl 18 (2003): 25–30.

Ohayon, M. M., and Lader, M. H. Use of psychotropic medication in the general population of France, Germany, Italy, and the United Kingdom. *J Clin Psychiatry* 63, 9 (2002): 817–25.

Patel, M., Joshi, A., Suthar, J., Desai, S. Drug utilization pattern in patients with different types of dementia in western India. *Int J Alzheimers Dis* 2014 (2014): 435202.

Perry, N., and Perry, E. Aromatherapy in the management of psychiatric disorders: Clinical and neuropharmacological perspectives. *CNS Drugs* 20, 4 (2006): 257–80.

Perry, N. S., Houghton, P. J., Theobald, A., Jenner, P., Perry, E. K. In-vitro inhibition of human erythrocyte acetylcholinesterase by *Salvia lavandulaefolia* essential oil and constituent terpenes. *J Pharm Pharmacol*, 52, 7 (2000): 895–902.

Pollock, B. G., Mulsant, B. H., Rosen, J. et al. A double-blind comparison of citalopram and risperidone for the treatment of behavioral and psychotic symptoms associated with dementia. *Am J Geriatr Psychiatry* 15, 11 (2007): 942–52.

Posadzki, P., Alotaibi, A., Ernst, E. Adverse effects of aromatherapy: A systematic review of case reports and case series. *Int J Risk Saf Med* 24, 3 (2012): 147–61.

Prince, M., Bryce, R., Albanese, E., Wimo, A., Ribeiro, W., Ferri, C. P. The global prevalence of dementia: A systematic review and metaanalysis. *Alzheimers Dement* 9, 1 (2013): 63–75.

Raskind, M. A. Update on Alzheimer drugs (galantamine). *Neurologist* 9, 5 (2003): 235–40.

Roberts, A., and Williams, J. M. The effect of olfactory stimulation on fluency, vividness of imagery and associated mood: A preliminary study. *Br J Med Psychol* 65, Pt 2 (1992): 197–99.

Sadowsky, C. H., and Galvin, J. E. Guidelines for the management of cognitive and behavioral problems in dementia. *J Am Board Fam Med* 25, 3 (2012): 350–66.

Schneider, L. S., Dagerman, K., Insel, P. S. Efficacy and adverse effects of atypical antipsychotics for dementia: Meta-analysis of randomized, placebo-controlled trials. *Am J Geriatr Psychiatry* 14, 3 (2006): 191–210.

Schwarz, S., Froelich, L., Burns, A. Pharmacological treatment of dementia. *Curr Opin Psychiatry* 25, 6 (2012): 542–50.

Smallwood, J., Brown, R., Coulter, F., Irvine, E., Copland, C. Aromatherapy and behaviour disturbances in dementia: A randomized controlled trial. *Int J Geriatr Psychiatry* 16, 10 (2001): 1010–13.

Snow, L. A., Hovanec, L., Brandt, J. A controlled trial of aromatherapy for agitation in nursing home patients with dementia. *J Altern Complement Med* 10, 3 (2004): 431–37.

Thies, W., and Bleiler, L. Alzheimer's disease facts and figures. *Alzheimers Dement* 9, 2 (2013): 208–45.

Thorgrimsen, L., Spector, A., Wiles, A., Orrell, M. Aroma therapy for dementia. *Cochrane Database Syst Rev* 3 (2003): CD003150.

Trinh, N. H., Hoblyn, J., Mohanty, S., Yaffe, K. Efficacy of cholinesterase inhibitors in the treatment of neuropsychiatric symptoms and functional impairment in Alzheimer disease: A meta-analysis. *JAMA* 289, 2 (2003): 210–16.

Umezu, T. Behavioral effects of plant-derived essential oils in the geller type conflict test in mice. *Jpn J Pharmacol* 83, 2 (2000): 150–53.

Umezu, T., Nagano, K., Ito, H., Kosakai, K., Sakaniwa, M., Morita, M. Anticonflict effects of lavender oil and identification of its active constituents. *Pharmacol Biochem Behav* 85, 4 (2006): 713–21.

Vann Jones, S. A., and O'Brien, J. T. The prevalence and incidence of dementia with Lewy bodies: A systematic review of population and clinical studies. *Psychol Med* 44, 4 (2014): 673–83.

Versijpt, J. Effectiveness and cost-effectiveness of the pharmacological treatment of Alzheimer's disease and vascular dementia. *J Alzheimers Dis* 42, 0 (2014): S19–25.

Wang, D., Yuan, X., Liu, T. et al. Neuroprotective activity of lavender oil on transient focal cerebral ischemia in mice. *Molecules* 17, 8 (2012): 9803–17.

Wells, K. B., Stewart, A., Hays, R. D. et al. The functioning and well-being of depressed patients: Results from the Medical Outcomes Study. *JAMA*, 262, 7 (1989): 914–99.

Woelk, H., and Schlafke, S. A multi-center, double-blind, randomised study of the lavender oil preparation Silexan in comparison to lorazepam for generalized anxiety disorder. *Phytomedicine* 17, 2 (2010): 94–99.

Wu, Y., Zhang, Y., Xie, G. et al. The metabolic responses to aerial diffusion of essential oils. *PLoS One* 7, 9 (2012): e44830.

Zeilmann, C. A., Dole, E. J., Skipper, B. J., McCabe, M., Low Dog, T., Rhyne, R. L. Use of herbal medicine by elderly Hispanic and non-Hispanic white patients. *Pharmacotherapy* 23, 4 (2003): 526–32.

18 Therapeutic Applications of Aromatherapy in Pediatrics

Samaneh Khanpour Ardestani,
Cecilia Bukutu, and Sunita Vohra

CONTENTS

18.1 INTRODUCTION

Defined as "the controlled use of plant essences for therapeutic purposes," aromatherapy is becoming increasingly popular (Buckle 2003; Ernst et al. 2006). Aromatic plant essences known as essential oils (EOs) are usually mixed with a vegetable "carrier oil" or diluted in alcohol before application (Natural Standard Research Collaboration 2014). EOs may be administered in a variety of ways, including diffusion devices, steaming water or spray bottles, addition to bath water, or topical application by massage or compresses (Fitzgerald and Halcon 2010; Perez 2003). EOs may have effect through olfaction as well as absorption through skin (Buckle 2003; Patricia 2004). While some have suggested internal use (e.g., oral, rectal, and vaginal), others caution against internal administration due to enhanced potential for toxicity (Buckle 2003; Fitzgerald and Halcon 2010). As such, the focus of this chapter is the use and safety of aromatherapy as administered through inhalation, topical application, or as an addition to bath water.

This chapter describes the prevalence of aromatherapy use in pediatric populations as well as issues related to regulation and licensure. It focuses on current evidence in the English literature with regards to safety as well as clinical application and effectiveness of aromatherapy in children. The best available pediatric evidence is described; if no pediatric evidence is available, adult data are discussed. More high-quality pediatric research is needed to inform use.

18.2   EPIDEMIOLOGY OF AROMATHERAPY USE

Aromatherapy is reported to be one of the most popular complementary therapies used by children and adolescents in many parts of the developed world. In a systematic review of surveys focusing on prevalence of complementary therapy use in UK pediatric patients, aromatherapy (19.1%) was rated as the third common modality, after homeopathy (24.9%) and herbal medicine (21.3%) (Posadzki et al. 2013). According to an American survey, adolescents aged 12–18 years reported a lifetime prevalence of aromatherapy use at 18.5% (n = 401) (Braun et al. 2005). A Canadian study showed 16.1% of current aromatherapy use among pediatric specialty outpatients (n = 192) (Adams et al. 2013). In an Australian survey conducted in a tertiary children's hospital in Melbourne (n = 503), aromatherapy was reported by 7% of respondents in the past year (Lim et al. 2005).

Complementary therapies are especially common in children with recurrent, chronic, or serious medical conditions (Adams et al. 2013); the same is true of aromatherapy. The prevalence of complementary therapy use among hospitalized and outpatient children is reported to range between 1.8% and 84% (Meyer et al. 2013). In a Canadian survey of children with neurologic conditions (n = 206), 16% reported they had ever used aromatherapy, while 10.8% reported current aromatherapy use (Galicia-Connolly et al. 2014). Likewise, in another Canadian survey (n = 145), aromatherapy use was reported to be 15% among pediatric cardiology patients (Adams et al. 2014). The prevalence of aromatherapy use may be higher when it is used in combination with massage. A UK study of 49 children with cancer found that 18.8% reported using aromatherapy alone, while 50% reported using aromatherapy coupled with massage (Molassiotis and Cubbin 2004).

18.3   SAFETY

Some assume aromatherapy is safe, as EOs are derived from natural substances (Lis-Balchin 2005). A 2012 systematic review assessed the safety of aromatherapy use by evaluating case reports or case series of adverse effects (AEs) of aromatherapy (Posadzki et al. 2012); clinical trials and reports of unintentional ingestion were excluded. The review included 42 reports describing aromatherapy-related AEs in 71 people. The EOs commonly associated with adverse effects included bergamot, laurel, lavender, peppermint, tea tree oil, and ylang-ylang. The most common reported AE associated with these aromatherapies was contact dermatitis (skin irritation). Although most of the reported AEs associated with the use of aromatherapy were mild to moderate in severity, there were six hospitalizations, two cases of skin grafts, and one death reported. In 40 cases, the causality between the AEs and aromatherapy was considered to be certain or almost certain. Of the 42 included studies, 7 were reports related to AEs of aromatherapy use in children aged 1 month to 18 years. Eucalyptus, bergamot, lavender, and tea tree were the EOs most associated with AEs in children, most often administered topically or through inhalation. Pediatric AEs reported included respiratory distress, acute pulmonary edema, coma, seizures, ataxia, slurred speech, hypotonia, lethargy, nausea, vomiting, metabolic acidosis, prepubertal gynecomastia, and blisters.

The evidence surrounding interaction between EOs and drugs, foods, and other herbal and nonherbal supplements is scant (Natural Standard Research Collaboration 2014). For this reason, it is suggested that EOs be introduced one at a time to children, especially those who are on medications, in order to monitor their reactions (McDowell 2005). Epilepsy is considered a contraindication for use in most aromatherapy literature (Patricia 2004).

TABLE 18.1

General Guidelines to Promote Safe Application of Aromatherapy in Children

1. Identify practitioners with formal aromatherapy training at your center.
2. Discuss potential risks as well as benefits when obtaining consent from parents or guardians.
3. Select EOs that have had few known adverse effects.
4. Ensure product quality.
5. Store EOs in a dark and cool place.
6. Do not use undiluted EOs in any type of administration. (For topical applications doses between 0.1% and 2.5% concentration have been suggested depending on the age and weight of the child.)
7. Check allergy status before applying EOs, particularly in children with a history of allergic dermatitis, skin diseases, asthma, perfume allergy, and respiratory diseases.
8. Consider clinical evidence of effectiveness and child's preference for specific scents before planning treatment sessions.
9. Closely monitor and record child's reactions and responses to therapy.

Source: Adapted from Campbell, L. et al., *Australian Journal of Holistic Nursing* 8 (1): 14–22, 2001; Lee, C. O., *Clinical Journal of Oncology Nursing* 7 (5): 597–98, 2003; McDowell, B. M., *Journal for Specialists in Pediatric Nursing: JSPN* 10 (1): 29–32, 2005; Tisserand, R., and R. Young, *Essential Oil Safety: A Guide for Health Care Professionals*, 2nd ed., Churchill Livingstone: Elsevier Health Sciences, Edinburgh, 2013.

Safety precautions should be taken when storing EOs in the home. Poisoning is a major concern, especially in young children. Over the past 70 years, there have been numerous reports of deaths due to unintended oral intake of EOs in children (Tisserand and Young 2013). Parents and caregivers should be made aware of the risks and cautioned to keep EOs out of the reach of children. Risk of ingestion may be reduced through use of child-resistant packaging and integral drop dispensers. All the EOs included in the product and the diluent carrier oil should be clearly listed on bottle labels (Fitzgerald and Halcon 2010; Tisserand and Young 2013).

General safety guidelines in children have been developed to facilitate a safe application of aromatherapy for health practitioners (Table 18.1).

18.4   REGULATION/LICENSURE

Aromatherapy training, regulation, and licensure are heterogeneous (Ernst et al. 2006). While there is interest from some health professionals to incorporate aromatherapy into their practice (e.g., nurses), lack of standardized training and regulatory oversight regarding clinical practice are viewed as barriers (Hunt et al. 2004). Product quality and variable regulatory oversight are other potential barriers (Lee 2003). The Association Francaise de Normalisation (http://www .afnor.org/en) and the International Organization for Standardization (http:// www.iso.org/iso/home) set standards for product quality and may provide guidelines for use.

Some countries have taken steps to certify or register individuals trained in aromatherapy. For example, in the United States, the National Association for Holistic Aromatherapy is a nonprofit organization with certification programs in aromatherapy (Lee 2003). Trained individuals have the possibility to be registered aromatherapists after passing a registration exam offered by the Aromatherapy Registration Council (http://www.aromatherapycouncil.org). Similarly, the Canadian Federation of Aromatherapists (http://cfacanada.com/) offers certification programs. In the UK, registration is possible through the Aromatherapy Organizations Council (AOC), a core organization for registering aromatherapists (Cooke and Ernst 2000). The International Federation of Aromatherapists (http://www.ifaroma.org), a self-governing body located in the UK, provides training programs worldwide.

18.5   CLINICAL EVIDENCE OF EFFECTIVENESS

While there is a growing body of literature on the therapeutic applications of aromatherapy, rigorous research in children remains scarce. Lee et al. (2012) conducted a review of 10 systematic reviews encompassing 285 primary studies to assess the effectiveness of aromatherapy for any medical condition. The primary studies often had small sample sizes and methodological concerns, such as the absence of appropriate control groups. The authors concluded that there was no compelling evidence regarding effectiveness of aromatherapy in any medical condition due to extensive methodological limitations. In this chapter, we present available evidence and encourage further research to help inform future use.

When evaluating the feasibility of aromatherapy, whether for clinical or research purposes, individual preferences for specific scents must also be considered. Fitzgerald et al. (2007) carried out a pilot study in school-aged children to assess their preferences for selected EOs according to their gender and ethnicity. Thirty-nine Latinos and 48 non-Latino Caucasians (NLCs) were included. Their results showed that lavender (*Lavandula angustifolia*) and ginger (*Zingiber officinalis*) were the least preferred EOs by children. Female participants reported feeling happier when they were smelling sweet orange (*Citrus sinensis*) ($p = .04$). Female Latinos found the smell more calming than NLC girls (56.2% vs. 18.5%). Latino boys described peppermint (*Mentha piperita*) as more energetic than NLC males (65.2% vs. 30%). Almost all children were attracted to aromatherapy as a therapeutic option. The authors concluded that children's preferences were associated with their gender, cultural exposure, and familiarity with scents. In the following sections of this chapter, we provide a critical review of the existing evidence of therapeutic effects of aromatherapy in common medical conditions among children.

18.5.1 INFANTS

18.5.1.1 Apnea

Olfaction is an important sense for newborns to recognize their mothers and discover the world (McDowell 2005). As a consequence, olfactory stimuli have been applied by some investigators to soothe infants in distressing conditions. Vanillin, which is not an essential oil but activates the olfactory system without major impact on the trigeminal system (Bartocci et al. 2000), has been employed in most of these studies. Considered to be a mild and harmless pleasant odor by infants, vanillin is purported to stimulate positive physiological and behavioral reactions (Goubet et al. 2003; Marlier et al. 2005).

Apnea of prematurity, a common condition in preterm neonates, is defined as cessation of breathing movements for more than 20 seconds (or less, if accompanied by reduced oxygen saturation [<88%] or bradycardia [heartrate ≤ 90]). Pharmacological treatments are available, but some infants may experience adverse effects (Marlier et al. 2005). Research evaluating the effect of scent on enhancing respiratory efforts in infants has been pursued.

Marlier et al. (2005) examined the effectiveness of vanillin in preventing apnea. Fourteen premature newborns were diagnosed to have recurrent central apnea resistant to caffeine and doxapram therapy. They underwent a 3-day trial in which each infant was considered to be his or her own control. Measurements were conducted on the first day of the trial as baseline, the second day as the intervention period, and the third day as the posttreatment control. The intervention involved application of 15 drops of saturated solution of vanillin at the margin of infants' pillows every 12 hours. Caffeine and doxapram therapy continued during the study period. Infants were monitored continuously during the trial, and their heart rate, respiratory rate, and oxygen saturation were recorded. In the case of unresolved apnea, usual care was applied by caregivers. Outcome measures were frequency and severity of apnea episodes occurring during the olfactory stimulus intervention period compared to the baseline and posttreatment day. Apnea was defined as any complete cessation of breathing movements for >20 seconds, or less if associated with hypoxia or brady-cardia. Considering all types of apneas, the frequency of episodes decreased to 36% (mean number of events: day before odor application, 34.7; day of odor application, 22.2) and returned to the baseline value (33.2) in the posttreatment day ($p < .001$). A significant reduction of 44% was observed for apnea without bradycardia. Apneas with severe bradycardia were also diminished by 45%. The frequency of apnea epi-sodes with moderate bradycardia did not change significantly. No adverse events occurred during the study period. The authors concluded that premature newborns with central apnea can benefit from vanillin in their incubator. Taking into consider-ation that this study was a 3-day trial with a small sample size, the conclusion should be interpreted cautiously.

The effect of vanillin to prevent apnea in premature neonates was also explored in a randomized clinical trial (RCT) study (Edraki et al. 2013) carried out in Iran. Thirty-six premature infants, who were 2 days old and weighed less than 2500 g, were allocated to receive either olfactory stimulation or no intervention during the 5-day trial. None of the infants had any congenital anomalies, acute infections, or intracranial hemorrhage. The intervention involved pouring of 2 ml of 2% saturated solution of vanillin on a piece of cotton and placing it 20 cm from the infant's head inside the incubator. This procedure was repeated every 12 hours. The control group received usual care; both groups were monitored continuously during the study period. If apnea occurred, routine treatment was provided. The outcome measures were the frequency of apnea episodes, oxygen saturation, and heart rate. The pres-ence of apnea was significantly lower in the intervention group than in the control group on the first, second, and fourth days of the study ($p < .05$). The mean number of apnea episodes during the whole period of the study was 0.4 (SD = 1.4) in the intervention group versus 3.5 (SD = 3.1) in the control group, which was significantly different considering gestational age as a covariate ($p = .001$). The authors observed a 3.1-fold reduction in apnea episodes caused by vanillin with an effect size of 0.72. Adverse events were not discussed. Study limitations include a small sample size and potential lack of generalizability due to numerous exclusion criteria.

18.5.1.2   Resting Energy Expenditure

A study in Israel (Marom et al. 2012) examined the effect of vanillin on the rest-ing energy expenditure (REE) in preterm infants. Their hypothesis was that olfac-tory stimulation increases REE by stimulating "general arousal responses." A pilot crossover RCT was carried out in 20 preterm but otherwise healthy infants of 32–35 weeks gestational age. All infants were in stable clinical condition and were feed-ing breast milk or formula. The study was performed in two consecutive days for each infant, where exposure to vanillin was compared to no scent exposure. On the intervention day, a cloth diaper impregnated with 15 drops of saturated vanillin solu-tion was placed on the opposite side of the infant's incubator. REE was measured by indirect calorimetry. All measurements lasted for 20 minutes and were done at the same time of the day, 1 hour after the last feeding, while infants were asleep. The environmental conditions were the same on both days of the study. REE did not sig-nificantly change by exposure to vanillin (74.5 ± 10.1 kcal/kg/24 hour) in compari-son to no exposure (79.0 ± 11.3 kcal/kg/24 hour) (paired t-test, $p = .16$; Wilcoxon test,

$p = .207$). Although insignificant, REE decreased 6.6% through vanillin exposure in contrast to the investigators' hypothesis. The authors stated that in order to confirm that such a small decline in REE was a true effect, 170 infants were needed to reach statistical significance. Moreover, the clinical significance of such a small observed effect is questionable. Study authors cited limitations of the study, including its small sample size and short time period; adverse events were not discussed, nor it is known if the vanillin dose used was appropriate.

18.5.1.3 Infantile Colic

Infantile colic is defined by spontaneous excessive crying (>3 hours a day, >3 days a week, and >3 weeks) in otherwise healthy, well-nourished infants. It usually starts in the second week after birth and resolves by the fourth month of age (Roberts et al. 2004). While many complementary therapies have been used for infantile colic (Rosen et al. 2007), we only were able to find one study (Cetinkaya and Basbakkal 2012) that looked at the effectiveness of aromatherapy in combination with massage on infantile colic.

In this study, conducted in Turkey (Cetinkaya and Basbakkal 2012), 40 infants (2–6 weeks of age) diagnosed with infantile colic were randomly allocated into intervention and control groups. Mothers were trained to apply the intervention, which included a 5- to 15-minute abdominal massage starting within 1–2 minutes of the colic attack beginning, using 1 ml of lavender oil mixed in 20 ml of almond oil. The control group did not receive any intervention. Five observations were carried out weekly. Each week, mothers were asked to record their infants' crying when it lasted more than 15 minutes. Weekly crying time decreased significantly from the first observation (13.28 ± 2.84 hours/week) to the final observation (6.27 ± 2.16 hours/ week) in the aromatherapy massage group, while it did not change in the control group. The authors concluded that aromatherapy massage with *Lavandula angustifolia* oil may have therapeutic effects on infantile colic. Adverse events were not discussed in this study.

18.5.1.4 Sleep

An RCT (Field et al. 2008) measured the effect of lavender bath oil on reducing stress and crying and enhancing sleep in infants (aged 1 week to 4½ months). Thirty infants were randomly assigned to one of three groups: (1) lavender bath oil, (2) nonaroma bath oil, and (3) lavender bath oil in conjunction with advertising about the beneficial effects of aroma bath on babies in order to enhance the role of maternal expectation. How maternal and infant behavior was measured varied by infant age. Bath behaviors (including if mothers were relaxed, smiling, or touching their babies, as well as if infants were looking at their mother) were recorded by videotaping for older infants ($N = 15$, 2- to 4½-month-old infants). Sleep behaviors, including crying and deep sleep, were recorded for younger children ($N = 15$, 1-week to 2-month-old infants). Additionally, cortisol levels of both mothers and infants were measured in saliva before and 20 minutes after bath. Mothers of group 1 were more relaxed, smiled more, and touched their babies more during bath time. Infants in this group looked more at their mothers as well. Group 1 infants also cried for a shorter duration of time and spent more time in deep sleep in comparison to other groups ($p < .05$). Supporting the behavioral results, cortisol levels of both infants and mothers decreased in group 1. Results of group 3 infants and mothers were between those of the other two groups. Adverse events were not discussed.

18.5.2 PAIN MANAGEMENT IN INFANTS AND CHILDREN

Some EOs comprising lavender (*Lavandula angustifolia*), peppermint (*Mentha piperita*), rosemary (*Rosmarinus officinalis*), lemongrass (*Cymbopogon citratus*) and Roman chamomile (*Chamaemelum nobile*) are purported to have pain-relieving effects (Fitzgerald and Halcon 2010).

An RCT (Goubet et al. 2003) was conducted to assess the effect of a familiar scent in relieving pain in preterm infants. Fifty-one preterm neonates were included and randomly assigned to venipuncture or heel-stick (capillary puncture) groups. Each of these groups was subdivided to three groups afterward. One group ($n = 17$) was familiarized with vanillin scent (0.64 g of vanillin diluted in 100 ml of 85% glycerol, 10 drops were applied on a scarf) the night before the test (average duration 17.37 hour) and exposed to it again during blood sampling. The second group ($n = 17$) was not familiarized but was exposed to vanillin scent during the procedure, and the third group ($n = 17$) had no familiarity or exposure (control group). Crying, grimacing, and head movements were videotaped. In general, infants in the heel-stick group cried for a longer duration of time than the other group ($p < .056$). They cried more during the blood collection procedure compared to the baseline, irrespective of their assignment to vanillin scent groups ($p < .01$). However, the ones familiar with the scent were less agitated after blood sampling ($p < .01$). When considering venipuncture, crying of the vanillin-familiar infants did not significantly increase during the procedure in comparison to the baseline ($p > .1$), unlike the other two groups. Therefore, the authors stated that a familiar scent could influence crying as long as the pain was moderate. Results of grimacing (another index for pain) were almost the same as those for crying in all groups and conditions.

The pain-relieving effect of familiar scents was also examined among full-term newborns in the following three studies. In a study conducted in France (Rattaz et al. 2005), 44 healthy breast-fed newborns (mean gestational age 39.4 weeks) were randomly allocated into four groups: maternal milk ($n = 11$), familiar vanillin ($n = 11$), unfamiliar vanillin ($n = 11$), and control group ($n = 11$). All infants underwent heel stick for phenylketonuria on the third day of life. For the familiar vanillin group, 20 drops of vanillin solution (diluted in glycerol at 0.64%) were applied on a scarf and placed on the infants' crib the day before heel stick (average duration of exposure 22.9 hours), and they were also presented with the same amount during the procedure. The unfamiliar group was only exposed to the same amount of vanillin during the heel-stick procedure. The maternal milk group and control group were presented with maternal milk and distilled water, respectively, in the same manner. Outcome measures (crying, grimacing, and head movements) were assessed by videotaping of infants at baseline (30 seconds), during the procedure (first 60 seconds), and postprocedure (30 seconds). It was indicated that infants in the familiar vanillin and maternal group (considered naturally familiar) cried and grimaced significantly less during the postprocedure period than the infants of the unfamiliar and control groups. However, the difference in crying between these groups was not significant during the heel-stick period. Additionally, infants in the maternal milk group were significantly less agitated (fewer head movements) than the infants in other the groups during the heel-stick procedure.

Goubet and her colleagues (2007) conducted another study to investigate the potential beneficial effect of a familiar odor on healthy full-term breast-fed neonates ($n = 44$). The protocol was similar to that of the previous study (Goubet et al. 2003), but blood was drawn by the heel-stick procedure. Additionally, familiarization with vanillin scent was performed via two methods (the mother or the crib) and the duration was shorter (average of 11 hours). They showed infants in the familiar group had significantly less distress (crying and grimacing) during heel stick than the infants in the other two groups. However, there was no difference in effect regarding route of exposure to familiar scent (i.e., the mother or the crib).

Results of the previous studies (Goubet et al. 2003, 2007) were confirmed in a larger study with the same protocol carried out in Iran (Sadathosseini et al. 2013). One hundred and thirty-five full-term neonates (1–7 days old) were included. The blood collection method was arterial puncture. The average duration of familiarization with vanillin scent was 8.65 hours. The duration of crying, heart rate, and oxygen saturation levels were measured by an observer who was not blinded, but who also was not aware of the purpose of the study. Infants in the familiar scent group cried for a shorter duration than infants in the unfamiliar and control groups ($p < .001$). This difference was not significant between the two other groups ($p = .55$). Moreover, oxygen saturation levels 1 minute after needle removal were higher in the familiar scent group than in the other groups ($p = .04$). The authors concluded that oxygen consumption and crying were decreased by a familiar odor during a painful procedure in neonates.

None of these three studies discussed adverse events. One favorable feature of these studies is that they used the same form of vanillin, which allows the results to be compared (Thiel et al. 2011). The investigators attempted to apply blinding but were unsuccessful due to the intervention characteristics (i.e., recognizable odor of vanillin).

A recent RCT (de Jong et al. 2012) conducted in the Netherlands investigated the effect of aromatherapy massage on reducing distress among infants after craniofacial surgery. Sixty children (mean age 10.8 months, standard deviation [SD] 6.8) were randomly allocated to three groups. The first group received massage (using the M-technique) with carrier oil (almond oil). The second group received M-technique massage with mandarin oil (1% citrus reticulata in carrier oil), and a third group received standard care after surgery. The primary outcomes selected were change in the children's behavior, which was measured by the COMFORT Behavioral (COMFORT-B) Scale, and pain and distress, as measured by numerical rating scales. The children's behaviors were videotaped and assigned scores by a blinded observer. The heart rate and mean arterial pressure (MAP) were also measured as secondary outcomes. Although COMFORT-B scores were increased in all three groups after intervention, the differences observed were not significant.

Heart rate and MAP changed significantly during the three assessment periods, but appeared unrelated to the intervention. The investigators of the study concluded that their results did not support using the M-technique massage with or without aromatherapy to relieve postoperative distress in infants. They explained that they would require 51 more participants to achieve 50% reduction in distress according to the power analysis. The investigators reported there were no adverse events due to the intervention during the 3–6 hours postanesthesia. A strength of this study was videotaping the children's behaviors, which facilitated a blinded outcome assessment.

The analgesic effect of olfactory stimulus with EOs was evaluated in older children as well. Soltani et al. (2013) conducted an RCT to assess the effect of inhalation of lavender oil on children's pain after tonsillectomy surgery. Children aged 6–12 years were randomly assigned to two groups: one group ($n = 24$) received inhaled lavender essential oil plus acetaminophen (10–15 mg/kg/dose, orally) every 6 hours to decrease their pain after surgery; in comparison, the control group ($n = 24$) received only acetaminophen. Outcomes measured for 3 days posttonsillectomy were requirement for daily acetaminophen, awakening at night due to pain, and pain intensity measured by the Visual Analog Scale (VAS). Children in the intervention group had significantly lower frequency of daily use of acetaminophen on all 3 days ($p < .05$), but the frequency of nocturnal awakening and pain intensity were not different between the two groups. Adverse events were not discussed.

18.5.3 ANXIETY/EMOTIONAL DISTRESS

Many claims are made about the healing properties of EOs related to their potential effects on mood, anxiety, sleep, and depression. Some EOs, including lavender, rose, orange, bergamot, lemon, sandalwood, clary sage, Roman chamomile, rose-scented geranium, and jasmine, are frequently used by aromatherapists to reduce stress and anxiety of their clients in different clinical situations (Butje et al. 2008; Setzer 2009).

The effectiveness of clinical aromatherapy on crisis management in adolescents was assessed in a quality improvement study (Fowler 2006). Participants represented a convenience sample of 43 adolescents in a residential treatment center aged between 12 and 19 years with mental health disorders. When the children felt agitated, they were offered 3% solution of a "calming blend" of essential oils (including *Cananga ordorata* [ylang ylang], *Origanum marjorana* [sweet marjoram], and *Citrus bergamia* [bergomot] diluted with jojoba carrier oil) to be used topically (M-technique, bilateral hand massage) or by direct inhalation. They had the choice to use aromatherapy alone or in combination with prescribed "as required" (p.r.n.) medications. At the end of the 3-month study, they were surveyed about their acceptance of aromatherapy. Information regarding prescribed p.r.n. medication and rates of seclusions and restraints were also obtained for a period of 6 months (3 months before and 3 months while in the study). Investigators found that 33 (76.7% of) adolescents used aromatherapy while they were at the center ($p \leq .05$). From the 28 patients that responded to the survey questions, 21 (48.8%) found aromatherapy helpful for calming and relaxation. During 3 months of the study, aromatherapy did not have a significant effect on the rates of prescribed p.r.n. medications or seclusion and restraints. Adverse events were not discussed. As this was a quality improvement study, there was no randomization or blinding.

A randomized single-blinded clinical trial performed in a large midwestern city in the United States (Nord and Belew 2009) evaluated the effectiveness of essential oils on children's postoperative distress. Ninety-four children (with and without developmental disorders) with surgical appointments were included in the study consecutively and randomized to the intervention ($n = 48$) or placebo ($n = 46$) groups. For the intervention group, lavender (thought to have calming and pain-relieving effects) and ginger (thought to reduce nausea and vomiting) were chosen in accordance with consultation with a clinical aromatherapist and a 4-month feasibility study. Jojoba oil was selected as a placebo as it is not known to have any beneficial effects in aromatherapy. Lavender and ginger were administered by inhalation and topically before surgery started and reapplied if surgery was longer than 3 hours; the same dose was used for all subjects. The faces, legs, activity, cry, consolability (FLACC) tool was used as a measurement instrument for pain and distress before application of essential oils and again after surgery was finished. The satisfaction of caregivers and parents was also assessed. Although the mean distress level was lower in the intervention group, there was no statistically significant difference in terms of FLACC score changes between the two groups ($p = .055$). Likewise, caregivers' responses to satisfaction questions were not significantly different between the two groups. Nonetheless, 78% of parents in both groups were willing to use aromatherapy in the future. Due to infrequent nausea and vomiting after surgery, statistical analysis was not performed for these events. The authors stated that no adverse events were reported by the nurses regarding aromatherapy.

A crossover RCT (Jafarzadeh et al. 2013) was conducted in 30 children undergoing dental treatment to investigate the effect of inhalation orange aroma (*Citrus sinensis*) on their anxiety levels. Ten boys and 20 girls aged 6–9 years were included by convenience sampling. Two similar dental appointments (prophylaxis and fissure sealant therapy), 1 week apart, were scheduled for every included subject. An electrical aroma diffuser was used to disperse aroma in the procedure room. For the control group, water was diffused. Pulse rate and salivary cortisol levels were measured as indicators of anxiety before and upon completion of dental treatments. The mean differences of salivary cortisol and pulse rate were 1.047 ± 2.198 nmol/l and 6.73 ± 12.3 minutes, respectively, which were significantly different in the situation using aroma compared to the situation without application of orange aromatherapy ($p < .01$ for both outcomes). Adverse events were not discussed. The investigators suggested that further trials with larger sample sizes were needed.

18.5.4 SLEEP

Twelve autistic children from a residential school in the UK were enrolled in a pilot study (Williams 2006) to investigate the effectiveness of aromatherapy massage for improving their sleep. A within-subject repeated-measure design was developed in which every child underwent three aromatherapy massage sessions, 1 week apart, during the 3 weeks of the study. Massages were offered by an aromatherapist in the last 2 hours before going to bed. Children's legs and feet were massaged by 2% lavender oil diluted in grape seed oil. All included children were observed every half hour during all nights of the study to assess their sleep onset and duration and number of awakenings from sleep. There were no significant differences in any of the measures between the nights with and without application of aromatherapy massage. Although children had significant interindividual differences in terms of falling sleep and the length of time they slept, each child seemed to have a stable sleep pattern during the study period. No more than 22 sleep interruptions were reported, and the average time of sleep duration per child ranged between 6.85 and 8.88 hours. Therefore, the authors concluded that aromatherapy massage had no beneficial effect in autistic children; adverse events were not discussed. They also suggested conducting future studies with larger sample sizes, with a longer time for repeated interventions in a population with more frequent sleep problems.

18.5.5 CANCER

Aromatherapy is used as supportive care for cancer patients in order to relieve their anxiety and emotional distress; alleviate their nausea and vomiting, fatigue, and pain associated with their disease or treatments; and in general increase their quality of life. With respect to effectiveness of aromatherapy, these claims are largely based on observational studies or anecdotal- or case-based reports. Little evidence is available from clinical trials (National Cancer Institute 2015).

A descriptive systematic review was conducted by Boehm et al. (2012) to provide evidence regarding the effectiveness and safety of aromatherapy in patients with cancer. Although the search strategy was not limited to specific ages in this review, no studies conducted in children were retrieved; thus, the entire population was adults. The systematic review included 18 clinical and 12 preclinical studies. Of the 18 clinical studies, 9 were randomized, 2 controlled, 3 uncontrolled, and 4 were case series. The authors concluded that there was a short-term (up to 8 weeks) soothing effect of aromatherapy on anxiety and depression and general well-being of patients with cancer. Some of the trials found improved sleep and better pain control. The quality of the included studies was reported to be medium to low. The main limitations of the included studies were lack of double blinding and use of different types of essential oils. The authors reported that aromatherapy generally carried a low risk. No pediatric data were included, so it is difficult to extrapolate findings to children.

We were able to find only one clinical trial study addressing aromatherapy in pediatric oncology. This placebo-controlled double-blind RCT (Ndao et al. 2012) examined the effect of inhalation aromatherapy on anxiety, nausea, and pain of children undergoing stem cell infusion. Thirty-seven children and adolescents (age 5–21 years old) with malignant and nonmalignant disorders were randomized to receive either bergamot essential oil (*Citrus × bergamia*) ($n = 17$) or placebo (a pleasing scented shampoo) ($n = 20$). Randomization was stratified based on age and transplant type. Four drops per hour of bergamot or placebo were applied using an aromatherapy diffuser during the transplantation session. Children and their parents were assessed at four time points: at recruitment (T1), before infusion (T2), leading to completion of infusion (T3) and 1 hour postinfusion (T4). The primary outcomes were parents and child's state and trait anxiety as measured by the State-Trait Anxiety Inventory (STAI) for parents and the State-Trait Anxiety Inventory for Children (STAIC), children's copying style as measured by the Children's Behavioral Style Scale (CBSS), nausea and pain as assessed by the Visual Analog Scale (VAS); and children's emotional state as measured by the Emotionality Activity Sociability and Impulsivity (EASI) Temperament Survey. Children in the bergamot group had higher state anxiety scores than those in the placebo group upon infusion completion ($p = .01$) and 1 hour postinfusion ($p = .05$). This difference remained significant after controlling for baseline state anxiety ($p < .001$) and baseline pain ($p = .003$). Although parents' anxiety was reduced during and after infusion, the difference between the two groups was not statistically significant. Pain and nausea were decreased in both groups, but the intervention group had significantly higher scores for nausea ($p = .03$). CBSS monitoring scores were significant predictors of state anxiety in children. Adverse events reported by the authors associated with the infusion procedure were greater in the bergamot group (nausea [$n = 4$], vomiting [$n = 2$], and hypertension [$n = 5$]) than in the placebo group (nausea [$n = 1$], vomiting [$n = 1$], hypertension [$n = 1$], headache [$n = 1$], and chest pain [$n = 1$]). The authors concluded that bergamot inhalation aromatherapy did not have a beneficial effect in reducing anxiety and nausea among children and adolescents undergoing stem cell transplantation. To explain their results, the authors cited the study of Fitzgerald et al. (2007), which revealed female children felt happier and more relaxed than males by smelling sweet orange. Taking into account that 73% of the current study population was male, they postulated that this preference may have contributed to the negative results of the study. Moreover, the dose applied in this study may be considered a high dose, which according to Bagetta et al. (2010) might have had a stimulatory rather than calming effect on children. A small sample size, the potential confounding effect of prior aromatherapy use, and different baseline pain scores were among other limitations of this study.

In a case report study, Nancy Frank (2008), a holistic nurse, described her successful experiences regarding aromatherapy use in a pediatric oncology ward. The first case was a school-age girl who had severe anxiety and subsequent vomiting while accessing her portacath by needle. Frank reported that spearmint oil helped the patient to be calm during the procedure and enabled her to tolerate her medications afterward. The other case was a school-age boy who also had anxiety and vomiting before his spinal taps. Spearmint was used and was reported as effective in reducing his anxiety and nausea before the procedure.

18.5.6 DERMATOLOGIC CONDITIONS

18.5.6.1 Eczema

The effectiveness of massage aromatherapy compared to massage alone, in conjunction with standard treatment in childhood atopic eczema, was evaluated in a single pilot study conducted in the UK (Anderson et al. 2000). Sixteen children between 3 and 7 years of age with atopic eczema were randomly allocated to the intervention ($n = 8$) and control ($n = 8$) groups. For the aromatherapy massage group, a blend of three essential oils in an equal proportion was used and was diluted in almond oil to be applied for massage in a 2% solution. A selection of 36 essential oils was presented to mothers. Their selected eight oils were as follows: *Litsea cubeba*, sweet marjoram, spike lavender, frankincense, myrrh, red thyme, benzoin, and German chamomile. Afterward, each mother selected three oils to be used in a blend for her child; thus, each child had a unique blend. Both groups received consultation and massage on a weekly basis by a therapist for 30 minutes. In addition, mothers were taught to bathe and massage their children for 10 minutes every day. Six drops of the same blend for massage were added to the water of the aromatherapy massage group as well. Daytime irritation and night-time disturbance were measured by a numerical scale. Mothers scored the measure every day, 8 weeks before starting the study and for the duration of the study period (8 weeks). A general improvement score was also rated by general practitioners, therapists, and mothers 2 weeks after the end of the study. Daytime irritation and nighttime disturbance were significantly decreased in both groups when comparing the before and after treat-ment scores ($p < .002$). However, these differences, as well as the general improvement scores, did not reach statistical significance when comparing the aromatherapy massage and massage-only group scores. Therefore, no beneficial effect was seen from adding essential oil to massage for childhood atopic eczema. Additionally, improvements in both groups appeared very quickly after the first week of the study and became gradual after that. Thus, a placebo effect due to tactile contact between the mother and child might have played a role in the short-term improvements. It is also noteworthy that employ-ing EOs in a blend makes it difficult to distinguish each EO's individual properties and effects. In a follow-up study, the aromatherapy massage group showed increased night-time disturbances, which could be related to allergic contact dermatitis aggravated by essential oils.

18.5.6.2 Head Lice

Head lice, also known as pediculosis capitis, is the most common pediatric parasitic infection and a potential source of distress (Nutanson et al. 2008). Several reports of resistance to the current pediculicides have propelled researchers to examine the effect of EOs on human lice. Lice-repellent properties of some EOs have been revealed in *in vitro* studies where most promising effects were seen with lavender, eucalyptus, and tea tree oil (Tebruegge et al. 2011). The effectiveness of these EOs in humans is not yet known.

We found one study in children evaluating the effect of a slow-release citronella formulation on head lice. In this placebo-controlled double-blind RCT carried out in Israel (Mumcuoglu et al. 2004), 660 children aged 6–14 years were primarily examined for pediculosis. Healthy children with no dermatologic conditions who had not been treated with pediculicides in the week prior to the beginning of the study were included in the trial: 103 children were randomly allocated to the test solution and 95 to the placebo group. Once the study started, 146 of the included children had nits-only infestation, whereas the remaining 52 were not infested by lice, eggs, or nits. This information was not provided separately for the intervention and placebo groups. Test formulation contained microencapsulated citronella (3.7%) solution. The same formulation without active ingredients in similar packaging was used as the placebo. Parents sprayed one to three puffs (0.3–0.9 ml) of the solution, depending of the length of the child's hair, every morning, 6 days a week. Children were reexamined 2 and 4 months after starting the treatment for louse infestation and potential side effects. A significant decrease in lice infestation was observed after 2 months (12% infestation in the intervention group vs. 50.5% in the placebo group, $p < .0001$). This difference stayed significant in the third examination after 4 months as well (12.4% in the intervention group vs. 33.7% in the placebo group, $p < .0001$). Reinfestation also occurred less frequently in the citronella group than in the placebo one (15.4% vs. 55.1% respectively, $p < .0001$). The authors concluded that the test repellent was three to four times stronger than placebo to protect against infestation. In terms of adverse effects, 4.4% of children and parents did not like the odor of the test solution and 1% had a mild itching and burning sensation.

18.5.7 RESPIRATORY

There is extensive over-the-counter usage of eucalyptus products in children and adults based on the claims regarding their decongestant–expectorant properties in upper respiratory tract infections. Yet, high-quality evidence is lacking (Natural Standard Research Collaboration 2014). We did not find any clinical trial studies in English literature looking at aromatherapy in children with respiratory conditions. Nevertheless, we found two interesting case reports that we describe here.

Hedayat (2008a) presented a case of a 3 year-old female suffering from central core myopathy, restrictive lung disease, and scoliosis, who was admitted to pediatric intensive care and diagnosed with respiratory syncytial virus (RSV) pneumonia and subsequent acute respiratory distress. In intensive care, she received 8 days of N-acetylcysteine (NAC) and dornase alfa therapy, but did not improve. After 8 days, NAC and dornase alfa were discontinued and a blend of essential oils, including *Lavandula latifolia* (spike lavender), *Thymus mastichina* (Spanish marjoram), *Balsam abies* (balsam fir), and *Mentha × piperita* (peppermint), was introduced. Three drops of the blend were nebulized through a fan diffuser every 6 hours into the room, which was passively inhaled by the patient. The oxygen requirement was decreased after 12 hours of introduction of the essential oils to 1.5 liters per minute (LPM), and after 2 days, she was discharged with a pulse oximetry oxygen saturation of 97%.

In another case report (Hedayat 2008b), aromatherapy was beneficial in decreasing the sedative requirement in an 18-month-old previously healthy female who suffered respiratory failure and endotracheal intubation due to adenovirus pneumonia. She failed extubation on day 8 due to subglottic edema. Reintubation was associated with persistent agitation requiring continuous sedative and narcotic infusions. After 45 hours, the mother was permitted to massage her baby during mechanical ventilation with a 7.5% blend of Roman chamomile (*Anthemis nobilis*), sandalwood (*Santalum album*), and galbanum (*Ferrula gummosa*) with jojoba oil (*Simondia chinensis*) as carrier. The patient experienced 50% reduction of sedative requirements after the first topical application. She was discharged 18 days after admission when she had been extubated for 6 days.

18.5.8 NAUSEA AND VOMITING

A Cochrane systematic review (Hines et al. 2012) was conducted to evaluate the effectiveness of aromatherapy on severity and duration of postoperative nausea and vomiting (PONV). Nine studies (six randomized and three controlled clinical trials, total participants = 402) were included. Aromatherapy was compared to saline placebo or standard antiemetic treatments in all studies. Among those, only one study conducted in children (Wang et al. 1999) was identified. The results of six studies evaluating the effect of inhalation of isopropyl alcohol compared to placebo demonstrated reduction in the required rescue antiemetics (relative risk [RR], 0.30; 95% confidence interval [CI], 0.09–1.00; $p = .05$). However, this effect was not further significant when compared to standard antiemetic treatments (RR, 0.66; 95% CI, 0.39–1.13; $p = .13$). Peppermint oil revealed no beneficial effects for reducing PONV. None of the included studies reported any adverse events from aromatherapy. Included studies suffered from medium to high risk of bias, especially incomplete data reporting. The review authors concluded that inhalation of isopropyl alcohol may be effective and harmless to alleviate PONV in adults when standard treatment is not available or contraindicated. For pediatrics, due to limited existing evidence, well-designed large clinical trials have been suggested.

We describe here the single pediatric study included in the systematic review, which was conducted by Wang et al. (1999). Ninety-one children aged 6–16 years who underwent elective outpatient surgery with general anesthesia were included in the study. Thirty-nine of them developed PONV and were randomized to receive either inhaled isopropyl alcohol ($n = 20$) or saline ($n = 19$). If PONV persisted despite three inhalations offered in a 15-minute period, intravenous ondansetron was prescribed. A self-reported VAS was used to measure the severity of nausea. After three times, PONV was relieved significantly in 65% of the children in the experiment group compared to 26% in the placebo group ($p = .03$). However, this improvement was temporary since PONV recurred during the following hour in 54% of the children in the isopropyl alcohol group and 80% of them in the saline group. No adverse events were discussed.

18.6 CONCLUSIONS

Emerging evidence suggests aromatherapy has promising effects to alleviate apnea of prematurity, colic, and pain and improve sleep in infants. Pain relief, anxiolytic and calming effects, lice repellency, and mitigating PONV were also shown in some studies of older children. However, the paucity of pediatric data and the methodological concerns of current evidence suggest more high-quality adequately powered pediatric trials are needed. Safety should not be assumed; it is vital that the presence or absence of adverse events be monitored and reported.

REFERENCES

Adams, D., S. Dagenais, T. Clifford et al. 2013. Complementary and Alternative Medicine Use by Pediatric Specialty Outpatients. *Pediatrics* 131 (2): 225–32. doi: 10.1542/peds.2012-1220; 10.1542/peds.2012-1220.
Adams, D., A. Whidden, M. Honkanen et al. 2014. Complementary and Alternative Medicine: A Survey of Its Use in Pediatric Cardiology. *CMAJ Open* 2 (4): E217–24. doi: 10.9778/cmajo.20130075; 10.9778/cmajo.20130075.

Anderson, C., M. Lis-Balchin, and M. Kirk-Smith. 2000. Evaluation of Massage with Essential Oils on Childhood Atopic Eczema. *Phytotherapy Research: PTR* 14 (6): 452–56. http://ovidsp.ovid.com/ovidweb.cgi?T=JS&PAGE=reference&D=med4&NEWS=N&AN=10960901.

Bagetta, G., L. A. Morrone, L. Rombola et al. 2010. Neuropharmacology of the Essential Oil of Bergamot. *Fitoterapia* 81 (6): 453–61. doi: 10.1016/j.fitote.2010.01.013; 10.1016/j.fitote.2010.01.013.

Bartocci, M., J. Winberg, C. Ruggiero, L. L. Bergqvist, G. Serra, and H. Lagercrantz. 2000. Activation of Olfactory Cortex in Newborn Infants after Odor Stimulation: A Functional Near-Infrared Spectroscopy Study. *Pediatric Research* 48 (1): 18–23. doi: 10.1203/00006450-200007000-00006.

Boehm, K., A. Bussing, and T. Ostermann. 2012. Aromatherapy as an Adjuvant Treatment in Cancer Care: A Descriptive Systematic Review. *African Journal of Traditional, Complementary, and Alternative Medicines: AJTCAM/African Networks on Ethnomedicines* 9 (4): 503–18.

Braun, C. A., L. H. Bearinger, L. L. Halcon, and S. L. Pettingell. 2005. Adolescent Use of Complementary Therapies. *Journal of Adolescent Health: Official Publication of the Society for Adolescent Medicine* 37 (1): 76. doi: 10.1016/j.jadohealth.2004.07.010.

Buckle, J. 2003. *Clinical Aromatherapy: Essential Oils in Practice*. 2nd ed. Philadelphia: Churchill Livingstone: Elsevier Health Sciences.

Butje, A., E. Repede, and M. M. Shattell. 2008. Healing Scents: An Overview of Clinical Aromatherapy for Emotional Distress. *Journal of Psychosocial Nursing and Mental Health Services* 46 (10): 46–52.

Campbell, L., A. Pollard, and C. Roeton. 2001. The Development of Clinical Practice Guidelines for the Use of Aromatherapy in a Cancer Setting. *Australian Journal of Holistic Nursing* 8 (1): 14–22.

Cetinkaya, B., and Z. Basbakkal. 2012. The Effectiveness of Aromatherapy Massage Using Lavender Oil as a Treatment for Infantile Colic. *International Journal of Nursing Practice* 18 (2): 164–169. doi: 10.1111/j.1440-172X.2012.02015.x; 10.1111/j.1440-172X.2012.02015.x.

Cooke, B., and E. Ernst. 2000. Aromatherapy: A Systematic Review. *British Journal of General Practice: Journal of the Royal College of General Practitioners* 50 (455): 493–96.

de Jong, M., C. Lucas, H. Bredero, L. van Adrichem, D. Tibboel, and M. van Dijk. 2012. Does Postoperative 'M' Technique Massage with or without Mandarin Oil Reduce Infants' Distress after Major Craniofacial Surgery? *Journal of Advanced Nursing* 68 (8): 1748–57. doi: 10.1111/j.1365-2648.2011.05861.x; 10.1111/j.1365-2648.2011.05861.x.

Edraki, M., H. Pourpulad, M. Kargar, N. Pishva, N. Zare, and H. Montaseri. 2013. Olfactory Stimulation by Vanillin Prevents Apnea in Premature Newborn Infants. *Iranian Journal of Pediatrics* 23 (3): 261–68.

Ernst, E., M. H. Pittler, B. Wider, and K. Boddy. 2006. *The Desktop Guide to Complementary and Alternative Medicine: An Evidence-Based Approach*. 2nd ed. Edinburgh: Elsevier Mosby.

Field, T., T. Field, C. Cullen et al. 2008. Lavender Bath Oil Reduces Stress and Crying and Enhances Sleep in Very Young Infants. *Early Human Development* 84 (6): 399–401. doi: 10.1016/j.earlhumdev.2007.10.008.

Fitzgerald, M., and L. L. Halcon. 2010. A Pediatric Perspective on Aromatherapy. In *Integrative Pediatrics*, ed. K. Olness and T. Culbert, 123–145. Weil Integrative Medicine Library. Oxford: Oxford University Press.

Fitzgerald, M., T. Culbert, M. Finkelstein, M. Green, A. Johnson, and S. Chen. 2007. The Effect of Gender and Ethnicity on Children's Attitudes and Preferences for Essential Oils: A Pilot Study. *Explore* (New York) 3 (4): 378–85. doi: 10.1016/j.explore.2007.04.009.

Fowler, N. A. 2006. Aromatherapy, used as an Integrative Tool for Crisis Management by Adolescents in a Residential Treatment Center. *Journal of Child and Adolescent Psychiatric Nursing* 19 (2): 69–76. doi: 10.1111/j.1744-6171.2006.00048.x.

Frank, N. L. 2008. Aromatherapy and Pediatric Oncology. *Beginnings* (American Holistic Nurses' Association) 28 (3): 18–19.

Galicia-Connolly, E., D. Adams, J. Bateman et al. 2014. CAM Use in Pediatric Neurology: An Exploration of Concurrent Use with Conventional Medicine. *PloS One* 9 (4): e94078. doi: 10.1371/journal.pone.0094078; 10.1371/journal.pone.0094078.

Goubet, N., C. Rattaz, V. Pierrat, A. Bullinger, and P. Lequien. 2003. Olfactory Experience Mediates Response to Pain in Preterm Newborns. *Developmental Psychobiology* 42 (2): 171–80. doi: 10.1002/dev.10085.

Goubet, N., K. Strasbaugh, and J. Chesney. 2007. Familiarity Breeds Content? Soothing Effect of a Familiar Odor on Full-Term Newborns. *Journal of Developmental and Behavioral Pediatrics: JDBP* 28 (3): 189–94. doi: 10.1097/dbp.0b013e31802d0b8d.

Hedayat, K. M. 2008a. Essential Oil Diffusion for the Treatment of Persistent Oxygen Dependence in a Three-Year-Old Child with Restrictive Lung Disease with Respiratory Syncytial Virus Pneumonia. *Explore* (New York) 4 (4): 264–66. doi: 10.1016/j.explore.2008.04.005; 10.1016/j.explore.2008.04.005.

Hedayat, K. M. 2008b. Reduction of Benzodiazepine Requirements during Mechanical Ventilation in a Child by Topical Application of Essential Oils. *Explore* (New York) 4 (2): 136–38. doi: 10.1016/j.explore.2007.12.005; 10.1016/j.explore.2007.12.005.

Hines, S., E. Steels, A. Chang, and K. Gibbons. 2012. Aromatherapy for Treatment of Postoperative Nausea and Vomiting. *Cochrane Database of Systematic Reviews* 4: CD007598. doi: 10.1002/14651858.CD007598.pub2; 10.1002/14651858.CD007598.pub2.

Hunt, V., J. Randle, and D. Freshwater. 2004. Paediatric Nurses' Attitudes to Massage and Aromatherapy Massage. *Complementary Therapies in Nursing and Midwifery* 10 (3): 194–201. http://ovidsp.ovid.com/ovidweb.cgi?T=JS&PAGE=reference&D=med5&NEWS=N&AN=15279861.

Jafarzadeh, M., S. Arman, and F. F. Pour. 2013. Effect of Aromatherapy with Orange Essential Oil on Salivary Cortisol and Pulse Rate in Children during Dental Treatment: A Randomized Controlled Clinical Trial. *Advanced Biomedical Research* 2: 10–9175.107968. Print 2013. doi: 10.4103/2277-9175.107968; 10.4103/2277-9175.107968.

Lee, C. O. 2003. Clinical Aromatherapy. Part II: Safe Guidelines for Integration into Clinical Practice. *Clinical Journal of Oncology Nursing* 7 (5): 597–98. doi: 10.1188/03.CJON.597-598.

Lee, M. S., J. Choi, P. Posadzki, and E. Ernst. 2012. Aromatherapy for Health Care: An Overview of Systematic Reviews. *Maturitas* 71 (3): 257–60. doi: 10.1016/j.maturitas.2011.12.018; 10.1016/j.maturitas.2011.12.018.

Lim, A., N. Cranswick, S. Skull, and M. South. 2005. Survey of Complementary and Alternative Medicine Use at a Tertiary Children's Hospital. *Journal of Paediatrics and Child Health* 41 (8): 424–27. doi: 10.1111/j.1440-1754.2005.00659.x.

Lis-Balchin, M. 2005. The Safety Issue in Aromatherapy. In *Aromatherapy Science: A Guide for Healthcare Professionals*. London; Chicago: Pharmaceutical Press.

Marlier, L., C. Gaugler, and J. Messer. 2005. Olfactory Stimulation Prevents Apnea in Premature Newborns. *Pediatrics* 115 (1): 83–88. doi: 10.1542/peds.2004-0865.

Marom, R., T. Shedlisker-Kening, F. B. Mimouni et al. 2012. The Effect of Olfactory Stimulation on Energy Expenditure in Growing Preterm Infants. *Acta Paediatrica* (Oslo, Norway: 1992) 101 (1): e11–14. doi: 10.1111/j.1651-2227.2011.02399.x; 10.1111/j.1651-2227.2011.02399.x.

McDowell, B. M. 2005. Nontraditional Therapies for the PICU: Part 1. *Journal for Specialists in Pediatric Nursing: JSPN* 10 (1): 29–32. doi: 10.1111/j.1539-0136.2005.00005.x.

Meyer, S., L. Gortner, A. Larsen et al. 2013. Complementary and Alternative Medicine in Paediatrics: A Systematic Overview/Synthesis of Cochrane Collaboration Reviews. *Swiss Medical Weekly* 143: w13794. doi: 10.4414/smw.2013.13794; 10.4414/smw .2013.13794.

Molassiotis, A., and D. Cubbin. 2004. "Thinking Outside the Box": Complementary and Alternative Therapies Use in Paediatric Oncology Patients. *European Journal of Oncology Nursing: Official Journal of European Oncology Nursing Society* 8 (1): 50–60. doi: 10.1016/S1462-3889(03)00054-1.

Mumcuoglu, K. Y., S. Magdassi, J. Miller et al. 2004. Repellency of Citronella for Head Lice: Double-Blind Randomized Trial of Efficacy and Safety. *Israel Medical Association Journal: IMAJ* 6 (12): 756–59.

National Cancer Institute. Aromatherapy and Essential Oils (PDQ®), Health Professional Version. PDQ Cancer Information Summaries. http://www.cancer.gov/cancertopics /pdq/cam/aromatherapy/healthprofessional (accessed January 30, 2015).

Natural Standard Research Collaboration. Aromatherapy: Natural Standard Professional Monograph. https://naturalmedicines.therapeuticresearch.com/databases/food,-herbs -supplements/professional.aspx?productid=1174 (accessed September 2014).

Ndao, D. H., E. J. Ladas, B. Cheng et al. 2012. Inhalation Aromatherapy in Children and Adolescents Undergoing Stem Cell Infusion: Results of a Placebo-Controlled Double-Blind Trial. *Psycho-Oncology* 21 (3): 247–54. doi: 10.1002/pon.1898; 10.1002 /pon.1898.

Nord, D., and J. Belew. 2009. Effectiveness of the Essential Oils Lavender and Ginger in Promoting Children's Comfort in a Perianesthesia Setting. *Journal of Perianesthesia Nursing: Official Journal of the American Society of Perianesthesia Nurses* 24 (5): 307–12. doi: 10.1016/j.jopan.2009.07.001; 10.1016/j.jopan.2009.07.001.

Nutanson, I., C. J. Steen, R. A. Schwartz, and C. K. Janniger. 2008. Pediculus Humanus Capitis: An Update. *Acta Dermatovenerologica Alpina, Pannonica, Et Adriatica* 17 (4): 147–54, 156–57, 159.

Patricia, M. 2004. Complementary Therapies for Children: Aromatherapy. *Paediatric Nursing* 16 (7): 28–30. doi: 10.7748/paed2004.09.16.7.28.c938.

Perez, C. 2003. Clinical Aromatherapy. Part I: An Introduction into Nursing Practice. *Clinical Journal of Oncology Nursing* 7 (5): 595–96. doi: 10.1188/03.CJON.595-596.

Posadzki, P., A. Alotaibi, and E. Ernst. 2012. Adverse Effects of Aromatherapy: A Systematic Review of Case Reports and Case Series. *International Journal of Risk and Safety in Medicine* 24 (3): 147–61. doi: 10.3233/JRS-2012-0568; 10.3233/JRS-2012-0568.

Posadzki, P., L. Watson, A. Alotaibi, and E. Ernst. 2013. Prevalence of Complementary and Alternative Medicine (CAM) Use in UK Paediatric Patients: A Systematic Review of Surveys. *Complementary Therapies in Medicine* 21 (3): 224–31. doi: 10.1016/j.ctim .2012.11.006; 10.1016/j.ctim.2012.11.006.

Rattaz, C., N. Goubet, and A. Bullinger. 2005. The Calming Effect of a Familiar Odor on Full-Term Newborns. *Journal of Developmental and Behavioral Pediatrics: JDBP* 26 (2): 86–92.

Roberts, D. M., M. Ostapchuk, and J. G. O'Brien. 2004. Infantile Colic. *American Family Physician* 70 (4): 735–40.

Rosen, L. D., C. Bukutu, C. Le, L. Shamseer, and S. Vohra. 2007. Complementary, Holistic, and Integrative Medicine: Colic. *Pediatrics in Review/American Academy of Pediatrics* 28 (10): 381–85. doi: 10.1542/pir.28-10-381.

Sadathosseini, A. S., R. Negarandeh, and Z. Movahedi. 2013. The Effect of a Familiar Scent on the Behavioral and Physiological Pain Responses in Neonates. *Pain Management Nursing: Official Journal of the American Society of Pain Management Nurses* 14 (4): e196–203. doi: 10.1016/j.pmn.2011.10.003; 10.1016/j.pmn.2011.10.003.

Setzer, W. N. 2009. Essential Oils and Anxiolytic Aromatherapy. *Natural Product Communications* 4 (9): 1305–16.

Soltani, R., S. Soheilipour, V. Hajhashemi, G. Asghari, M. Bagheri, and M. Molavi. 2013. Evaluation of the Effect of Aromatherapy with Lavender Essential Oil on Post-Tonsillectomy Pain in Pediatric Patients: A Randomized Controlled Trial. *International Journal of Pediatric Otorhinolaryngology* 77 (9): 1579–81. doi: 10.1016/j.ijporl.2013.07.014; 10.1016/j.ijporl.2013.07.014.

Tebruegge, M., A. Pantazidou, and N. Curtis. 2011. What's Bugging You? An Update on the Treatment of Head Lice Infestation. *Archives of Disease in Childhood: Education and Practice Edition* 96 (1): 2–8. doi: 10.1136/adc.2009.178038; 10.1136/adc.2009.178038.

Thiel, M. T., A. Langler, and T. Ostermann. 2011. Systematic Review on Phytotherapy in Neonatology. *Forschende Komplementarmedizin* (2006) 18 (6): 335–44. doi: 10.1159 /000334712; 10.1159/000334712.

Tisserand, R., and R. Young. 2013. *Essential Oil Safety: A Guide for Health Care Professionals*. 2nd ed. Edinburgh: Churchill Livingstone: Elsevier Health Sciences.

Wang, S. M., M. B. Hofstadter, and Z. N. Kain. 1999. An Alternative Method to Alleviate Postoperative Nausea and Vomiting in Children. *Journal of Clinical Anesthesia* 11 (3): 231–34.

Williams, T. I. 2006. Evaluating Effects of Aromatherapy Massage on Sleep in Children with Autism: A Pilot Study. *Evidence-Based Complementary and Alternative Medicine: eCAM* 3 (3): 373–77. doi: 10.1093/ecam/nel017.

19 Aromatic Plants and Essential Oils in the Treatment and Prevention of Infectious Diseases

*Neda Mimica-Dukić, Natasa Simin,
Ivana Beara, Dejan Orčić, Marija Lesjak,
Marina Francišković, and Emilija Svirčev*

CONTENTS

19.1 INTRODUCTION

The number of new pharmaceutical and dietary products based on natural raw materials has been constantly growing on the global market. More than 60% of the new chemical drugs were inspired by natural products. Scientific research has confirmed a wide range of biological and pharmacological activities for a variety of natural products, regardless of whether they are isolated compounds or complex extracts. In certain therapeutic areas, the productivity is higher: 78% of antibacterials and 74% of anticancer compounds are natural products or have been derived from, or inspired by, a natural product (Newman et al., 2003). Over the past 70 years, a wide range of antimicrobial agents have been discovered and synthesized to combat microbial pathogens, including bacteria, fungi, viruses, and parasites. However, it has clearly been evidenced that many pathogens display antimicrobial resistance, leading to drug resistance. The incidences of antimicrobial resistance have steadily increased globally. Besides increasing morbidity and mortality rates, resistance to antimicrobial agents has resulted in treatment failures and increased health care costs (Howard et al., 2003). The increased resistance to conventional antibiotics is one of the main factors justifying the search for and development of new antimicrobial agents, especially those of natural origin. Among them, essential oils deserve special attention.

Essential oils are complex mixtures of volatile compounds of terpenoid or non-terpenoid origin that can be extracted from different parts of aromatic plants (flower, buds, seed, leaves, and fruits). The composition of an essential oil will vary according to the plant's environment and growing conditions, methods of harvesting, extraction, and storage. Some essential oils contain one or two major constituents, and therapeutic and toxicological properties of the oil can largely be attributed to those compounds. However, other constituents present in low concentrations can be important. The major constituents of an essential oil can also vary in different chemotypes of the same plant species. Aromatic plants and essential oils are widely used in aromatherapy not only for the treatment and prevention of diseases, but also for their effects on mood, emotion, and well-being (Heinrich et al., 2012). The use of aromatic plants and spices in phytotherapy is mostly related to different activities of their essential oils, such as antimicrobial, spasmolytic, carminative, hepatoprotective, antiviral, and anticarcinogenic activities (Blumenthal, 1999; Bruneton, 1999; Wang et al., 2005). In particular, the antimicrobial activity of aromatic plants is the basis of many applications, including raw and processed food preservation (Mišan et al., 2011), pharmaceuticals, alternative medicine, and natural (aromatherapy) therapies (Božin et al., 2006; Mimica-Dukić and Božin, 2007). The antimicrobial activities of essential oils are the results of their various biological activities, such as cytotoxicity, mutagenicity, and phototoxicity. Because of the great number of constituents, essential oils seem to have no specific cellular targets. As typical lipophiles, they pass through the cell wall and cytoplasmic membrane, disrupt the structure of their different layers of polysaccharides, fatty acids, and phospholipids, and permeabilize them. Cytotoxicity appears to include such membrane damage. In bacteria, the permeabilization of the membranes is associated with loss of ions and reduction of membrane potential, collapse of the proton pump, and depletion of the ATP pool (Bakkali et al., 2008; Aleksić et al., 2014). Hence, it is practically impossible for the microorganism to develop resistance to essential oils (Knobloch et al., 1989; Bakkali et al., 2008; Saad et al., 2013). Although essential oils occur in more than 60 plant families, those belonging to the Lamiaceae, Myrtaceae, Apiaceae, Laureaacae, and Asteaceae families are of special significance. Most *in vitro* antimicrobial tests suggest that a considerable number of these plants can be used in the healing of various infectious diseases that are provoked by certain microorganisms (Piccaglia et al., 1993; Inouyea et al., 2001; Bergonzelli et al., 2003; Couladis et al., 2004; Deriu et al., 2007; Mimica-Dukić and Božin, 2008; Rota et al., 2008; Mimica-Dukić et al., 2010; Zanetti et al., 2010; Samojlik et al., 2012; Liao et al., 2013; Zonyane et al., 2013). However, there is still very little information on the results of clinical studies that could confirm their application in clinical therapy. This chapter summarizes numerous *in vitro* and *in vivo* studies of aromatic plants and essential oils, concerning their use in the treatment of various infective diseases.

19.2   RESPIRATORY INFECTIONS

Respiratory tract infections (RTIs) are any infection of the sinuses, throat, airways, or lungs. Specifically, there are two groups of RTIs: upper RTIs, which affect the nose, sinuses, and throat, and lower RTIs, which affect the airways and lungs. Common upper RTIs include the common cold, tonsillitis, sinusitis, laryngitis, and flu. The most common symptom of an upper RTI is a cough. Other symptoms include headaches, a stuffy or runny nose, a sore throat, sneezing, and muscle aches. Common lower RTIs include flu, bronchitis, pneumonia, and tuberculosis. The main symptom of a lower RTI is a cough followed by phlegm and mucus. Other symptoms developed in more serious upper RTIs are a tight feeling in the chest, increased rate of breathing, breathlessness, and wheezing. Generally, RTIs are believed to be one of the main reasons why people visit a general practitioner, while the most widespread respiratory tract infection is the common cold. Mostly RTIs are caused by viruses, such as rhinoviruses, coronaviruses, and influenza viruses, but they can also be caused by a bacterium, such as *Streptococcus pneumonia* or *Mycoplasma pneumoniae*, while tuberculosis is caused by the bacterium *Mycobacterium tuberculosis*. Consequently, most viral RTIs are treated without the need for specific drug treatment other than taking painkillers (paracetamol or ibuprofen) with good hydration and resting. A bacterial RTI is most often treated with antibiotic therapy, and it is the reason for 60% of all antibiotic prescribing in general practice. However, it is generally believed that antibiotics have limited efficacy in treating a large proportion of RTIs. Currently, the greatest concern about antibiotic usage in primary care is the increase in resistance to antibiotics, and this has led to the examination of possible strategies to reduce antibiotic prescribing (Dasaraju and Liu, 1996; NICE Clinical Guideline 69, 2008; Arroll, 2005). In the light of this, there is a growing necessity for replacement of conventional antibiotic therapy in the treatment of RTIs. Good candidates for that purpose are essential oils, which are well known for their antimicrobial properties, both antibacterial and antiviral. Besides antimicrobial activity, essential oils are believed to act as secretolytic and secretomotor drugs. Thus, by increasing serous mucous secretion and mucous discharge, essential oils could consequently reduce symptoms of RTIs (Zhao et al., 2014).

Accordingly, numerous essential oils were tested *in vitro* against bacteria and viruses causing RTIs, and several papers presenting the results of these studies are shown in Table 19.1. Some of the oils are known as traditional RTI remedies, usually applied by steam inhalation. However, clinical and epidemiological studies that confirm the effectiveness of essential oils in treating RTIs *in vivo* in humans are still limited. Namely, there is a case report evidencing successful use of *Eucalyptus globules* Labill. essential oil by inhalation in treatment of tuberculosis (Sherry and Warnke, 2004). Other case reports described successful application of a mixture of *Lavandula latifolia* Medik., *Thymus mastichina* L., *Abies balsamea* (L.) Mill., and *Mentha × piperita* L. essential oils by inhalation in treatment of virus pneumonia (Hedayat, 2008). Apart from these, to the best of our knowledge, no other essential

TABLE 19.1
Selected Essential Oils with *In Vitro* Activity against Microorganisms Causing RTIs

Microorganism	Essential Oil	References
Influenza virus A	*Melaleuca alternifolia* (Maiden & Betche) Cheel	Zai-Chang et al., 2005
	Curcuma longa L.	Garozzo et al., 2011
	Cynanchum stauntonii (Decne.) Schltr. ex H.Lév	Evgeny et al., 2013
	Eucalyptus polybractea (R. Baker)	Liao et al., 2013
S. pneumoniae	*Rosmarinus officinalis* L.	Inouyea et al., 2001
	Melaleuca alternifolia (Maiden & Betche) Cheel	
	Thymus vulgaris L.	
	Cinnamomum verum J. Presl	
	Mentha × *piperita* L.	
	Coriandrum sativum L.	
	Lavandula angustifolia Mill.	
	Eucalyptus polybractea (R. Baker)	
M. pneumoniae	*Melaleuca alternifolia* (Maiden & Betche) Cheel	Harkenthal et al., 2000
M. tuberculosis	*Salvia aratocensis* (J.R.I.Wood & Harley)	Bueno et al., 2011
	Turnera diffusa Willd. ex Schult.	Zanetti et al., 2010
	Lippia Americana L.	
	Myrtus communis L.	

oil was proven to be effective against RTIs in patients. Nevertheless, essential oil of *Mosla dianthera* (Thunb.), an aromatic and medicinal plant from East Asia, was shown to express anti-influenza *in vivo* activity in mice affected with pneumonia (Wu et al., 2012).

Having in mind that some of the oils examined from Table 19.1 showed great *in vitro* activity against microorganisms causing RTIs, further evaluation of their *in vivo* effectiveness and mechanisms of action in treatment of RTIs is absolutely supported.

19.3   URINARY INFECTIONS

Urinary tract infection (UTI) is a very common bacterial infection, particularly in women, babies, and the elderly. More than 150 million UTIs are diagnosed annually, and it is estimated that 1 in 2 women and 1 in 20 men will contract a UTI in their lifetime (Zenati et al., 2014; Medina-Polo et al., 2015).

A UTI is classified according to location, clinical symptoms, and microbiological findings: infection of the upper tract (pyelonephritis) comprises infection of the renal parenchyma and may be associated with systemic sepsis, and infection of the lower tract (cystitis) is located in the bladder alone. Urethritis and male accessory gland infections (prostatitis) are usually observed separately, because their clinical presentations are quite different. A pyelonephritis is always more severe than a cystitis, and may occur as a mild or moderate infection, which usually can be treated by oral antimicrobials in an outpatient. Urosepsis, always more severe than the two former conditions, could eventually lead to uroseptic shock and usually needs initial parenteral therapy and hospitalization (Johansen et al., 2014).

Generally, the most common cause of UTIs is a bacteria, *Escherichia coli*, although in childhood *Klebsiella pneumoniae, Enterobacter* spp., *Enterococcus* spp., and *Pseudomonas* are more frequent than in later life, and there is a higher risk of urosepsis than in adulthood (Stein et al., 2015). Furthermore, *Proteus mirabilis* is a common pathogen responsible for complicated UTIs (Chen et al., 2012), while *Pseudomonas aeruginosa* is also reported to be present in UTIs (Zenati et al., 2014; Medina-Polo et al., 2015). Besides the obvious problem of UTI abundance, the treatment of it becomes a truly difficult task. Namely, the common treatment of UTIs involves antimicrobial agents—antibiotics, but they have been prescribed so extensively that numerous bacteria become resistant, and most failures in healing UTIs are related to multidrug resistance (Gales et al., 2000). Thus, a constant need for new antimicrobial agents points to plant preparations, which have long been safely and effectively used in treatments of all kinds of human infectious diseases, including UTIs (Zenati et al., 2014). According to the literature, more than 1800 species, including medicinal and common food and spice plants, have been tested *in vitro* for their antibacterial activity against various strains of *E. coli*, the pathogen most responsible for UTI development (Mahady et al., 2008). Besides the well-known, traditional, and widespread use of cranberry (*Vaccinium macrocarpon*) tea or juice, bearberry (umbabazane, *Arctostaphylos uva-ursi*) leaf extract, or Saint-John's-wort (*Hypericum perforatum*) extract for prevention and treatment of UTIs, certain attention is directed to essential oils, as renowned antimicrobial agents (Stothers, 2009). Accordingly, numerous essential oils were tested *in vitro* against *E. coli*, and several papers presenting the results of these studies are shown in Table 19.2. Some of the oils are known as traditional UTI remedies, usually used as a bath or massage oil for the lower back or abdominal region, while others have either excellent antibacterial or diuretic properties.

Regarding clinical and epidemiological studies on maintaining a healthy urinary tract by using natural products, the data are very scarce. Namely, some controlled clinical trials were conducted to demonstrate the use of cranberry juice or *uva ursi* extract in reducing the presence of bacteria in urine (Amalaradjou and Venkitanarayanan, 2011), but to the best of our knowledge, no one essential oil was tested in patients. Having in mind that some of the essential oils examined, such as oregano, coriander, or basil, showed great *in vitro* activity against *E. coli*, further evaluation of their *in vivo* effectiveness and mechanisms of action and clinical trials are absolutely supported.

19.4   GENITAL INFECTIONS

Of the genital infections, bacterial vaginosis (BV) is considered the most prevalent vaginal infection in women of reproductive age (Palmeira-de-Oliveira et al., 2013). BV results from an imbalance of the normal vaginal flora, with an overgrowth of anaerobic bacteria and a reduction in lactobacillary flora (Simbar et al., 2008). The microorganisms involved in BV are very diverse and include *Gardnerella vaginalis, Mycoplasma hominis, Ureaplasma urealyticum, Mobiluncus* species, *Prevotella*

TABLE 19.2
Selected Essential Oils Derived from Medicinal, Food, and Spice Plants with Activity against *E. coli* Strains

Essential Oil	References
Anise (*Pimpinella anisum* L.)	Gülçin et al., 2003; Al-Bayati, 2008; Al-Daihan et al., 2013
Basil (*Ocimum basilicum* L.)	Hersch-Martínez et al., 2005; Wannissorn et al., 2005; Duarte et al., 2007; Hussain et al., 2008; Carović-Stanko et al., 2010; Runyoro et al., 2010
Celery (*Apium graveolens* L.)	Teixeira et al., 2013
Chamomile (*Matricaria recutita* L.)	Roby et al., 2013
Clove (*Syzygium aromaticum* [L.] Merrill & Perry)	Mahady et al., 2008; Lu et al., 2011
Coriander (*Coriandrum sativum* L.)	Delaquis et al., 2002; Oussalah et al., 2007
Eucalyptus (*Eucalyptus globulus* Labill)	Cimanga et al., 2002; Mulyaningsih et al., 2010; Elaissi et al., 2011; Bachir and Benali, 2012; Zonyane et al., 2013
Fennel (*Foeniculum vulgare* Mill.)	Diao et al., 2014; Rather et al., 2012
Frankincense (*Boswellia carterii* Birdwood.)	Van Vuuren et al., 2010
Juniper berry (*Juniperus communis* L.)	Hammer et al., 1999; Lesjak, 2011
Lemongrass (*Cymbopogon citratus* [DC.] Stapf.)	Onawunmia et al., 1984; Naik et al., 2010; Raut and Karuppayil, 2014
Palmarosa (*Cymbopogon martinii* [Roxb.] Wats.)	Oussalah et al., 2007
Rosemary (*Rosmarinus officinalis* L.)	Piccaglia et al., 1993; Božin et al., 2008; Zaouali et al., 2010; Jiang et al., 2011; Jordán et al., 2013; Ojeda-Sana et al., 2013; Teixeira et al., 2013; Barreto et al., 2014
Tea tree (*Melaleuca alternifolia* [Maiden & Betche] Cheel.)	Sailer et al., 1998; Warnke et al., 2013
Thyme (*Thymus vulgaris* L.)	Rota et al., 2008; El Bouzidi et al., 2013; Raut and Karuppayil, 2014

species, and other anaerobes, although no single bacterial agent consistently predominates (Weir, 2004). Therapeutic options for BV treatment are very scarce, and microorganism resistance is becoming an important constraint (Palmeira-de-Oliveira et al., 2013). Vulvovaginal candidosis (VVC), caused by *Candida* spp., is the second most frequent vaginal infection after BV (Palmeira-de-Oliveira et al., 2013). Considering that there is only a limited number of available antifungal drugs, resistance is increasing, indicating a great need for new therapeutic strategies.

Besides regular inhabitants of the vagina that can cause the infection, there are more than 20 pathogens that are transmissible through sexual intercourse. Trichomoniasis, caused by *Trichomonas vaginalis*, is the most common nonviral sexually transmitted disease in the world, with more than 173 million new cases every year (World Health Organization, 2001). The existing treatment for this infection (metronidazole therapy) has multiple side effects, including nausea, vomiting, metallic taste, and gastrointestinal upset, while resistance is increasing (Soper, 2004). *Chlamydia trachomatis*, an intracellular pathogen, is also one of the leading causes of sexually transmitted bacterial diseases in the world, with more than 92 million new cases every year (World Health Organization, 2001). Although *C. trachomatis* has been sensitive to several classes of antibiotics, such as tetracyclines, macrolides, and fluoroquinolones, recent reports have noted increasing resistance (Somani et al., 2000).

Viruses, herpes simplex virus type-2 (HSV-2 or genital herpes), and human papillomavirus (HPV), mostly spread through sexual contact, are common causes of vulvovaginitis. After primary infection, genital herpesvirus persists for life in a latent form in neurons of the host and periodically reactivates. Herpes simplex disease is predominantly treated with nucleosidic drugs (acyclovir and its derivatives), which are efficacious only when applied in the early stages of the disease. In addition, the resistance of virus strains to commonly used nucleosidic drugs is growing. Human papillomavirus (HPV) infection is a very common genital infection, as the majority of sexually active women are in contact and infected with this virus in their lifetime (Baseman and Koutsky, 2005). HPV is recognized as the main cause of cervical cancer in women (Arbyn et al., 2011). Systemic therapy for HPV infection is highly ineffective, with topical therapy being highly used. However, the frequently used topical therapy with cytotoxic agents has many adverse reactions, highlighting the need for new therapeutics with high activity but low toxicity (Stanley, 2012).

Essential oils (EOs) have been used traditionally as valuable therapies in the treatment of infectious diseases. Terpenes, especially monoterpene alcohols and phenols, are considered the most important antimicrobial compounds in essential oils (Knobloch et al., 1989). Numerous *in vitro* studies have proven the high potency of essential oils against genital pathogens. Specifically, it was shown that tea tree essential oil extracted from *Melaleuca* sp., dominantly containing terpinen-4-ol, 1,8-cineole, γ-terpinene, and α-terpinene, is highly active against *Candida* sp., *G. vaginalis*, and *T. vaginalis*, while probiotic bacteria are less sensitive to this oil, supporting its potential use in BV therapy. *Thymus* sp. and *Zataria multiflora* EOs, rich in thymol and carvacrol, are also very active against these pathogens (Palmeira-de-Oliveira et al., 2013; Sajed et al., 2013). Antiparasitic activity against *T. vaginalis* was also proven for *Lavandula* and *Ocimum basilicum* essential oil (Moon et al., 2006; Ezz Eldin and Badawy, 2015). Božin et al. (2008) found that essential oils of two varieties of *Achilea millefolium* (var. *colina* and var. *pannonica*) show a very high antimicrobial effect on several bacterial strains isolated from the genital tract of female patients (*Staphylococcus aureus*, *Streptococcus pneumonia*, *Streptococcus agalactiae*, *Streptococcus viridians*, *Streptococcus pyogenes*), even though they have completely different chemical compositions (β-pinene, chamazulene, and E-caryophyllene are dominant in *A. colina*, while 1,8-cineole and camphor are the most abundant in *A. pannonica*). Furthermore, *Origanum vulgare*, *Satureja montana*, and *Satureja hortensis* EOs, which are characterized by a high amount of carvacrol, are potent anticandidal agents (Tampieri et al., 2005; Sajed et al., 2013). Additionally, essential oils of *Mentha* × *piperita* (rich in menthol, menthone, and 1,8-cineole), *Cuminum cyminum* (cuminic alcohol, γ-terpinene, and cuminic aldehyde), and *Foeniculum vulgare* (fenchone and anethole) demonstrate distinct anticandidal activity (Tampieri et al., 2005; Gavanji et al., 2015).

High antimicrobial activity against *Candida* sp. and *G. vaginalis* was also found for *Cymbopogon citrates* essential oil, commonly known as lemongrass oil, which is rich in aldehydes—citral, neral, and geranial (Schwiertz et al., 2006). *Cinnamomum verum* and *Syzygium aromaticum* EOs express strong anti-*Candida* activity as well, due to the presence of eugenol, which is known for antifungal properties (Tampieri et al., 2005; Pinto et al., 2009). Sessa et al. (2015) have shown that *Mentha suaveolens* essential oil is effective against *C. trachomatis*, whereby it not only deactivates infectious elementary bodies, but also inhibits chlamydial replication. Their study also revealed that *M. suaveolens* EO substantially reduces efficient doses of erythromycin. The studies show that essential oils, besides their antibacterial, antifungal, and antiparasitic effects, also possess great antiviral potential. Essential oils of anise, hyssop, thyme, ginger, chamomile, and sandalwood express virucidal activity against HSV-2, probably by interacting with the viral envelope (Koch et al., 2008). Furthermore, *Santolina insularis* essential oil possesses very high antiviral activity, probably due to its direct virucidal effect and inhibition of cell-to-cell transmission, while virus adsorption is not inhibited (De Logu et al., 2000). It was shown that peppermint oil is capable of exerting a direct virucidal effect on HSV-2 (Schuhmacher et al., 2003). Considering the lipophilic nature of the oil, which enables it to penetrate the skin, peppermint oil might be suitable for topical therapeutic use as a virucidal agent in recurrent herpes infection.

There are many commercially available herbal formulations for treatment of vaginal infections. However, most of them are over-the-counter products, since the number of *in vivo* animal studies and clinical trials confirming their safety and effectiveness are very limited. Although much has been made of the potential for tea tree oil to be used in the treatment of vaginal candidiasis, no clinical data have been published. However, results from an animal (rat) model of vaginal candidiasis support the use of tea tree oil for the treatment of this infection (Mondello et al., 2003).

19.5 GASTROINTESTINAL INFECTION

Gastrointestinal infections are viral, bacterial, or parasitic infections that cause gastroenteritis, an inflammation of the gastrointestinal tract involving both the stomach and the small intestine.

Nowadays, the most frequent cause of gastrointestinal infections is the Gram-negative bacteria *Helicobacter pylori*, which colonize the epithel of the gastric mucosa of more than half the world's population (Marshall and Warren, 1984). The infection with *H. pylori* is asymptomatic; however, it is necessary to eradicate the bacteria from the stomach mucosa since it represents a major cause of peptic ulcer disease and is associated with various digestive diseases, such as gastric carcinoma and primary gastric lymphoma (Parsonnet et al., 1991; Wotherspoon et al., 1991). The most frequent therapy recommended for the eradication of *H. pylori* is a combination of two antibiotics—amoxicillin and clarithromycin, together with a proton pump inhibitor (PPI); nevertheless, it provides unacceptably low therapy success (Graham and Fischbach, 2010).

As previously mentioned, essential oils are a convenient replacement for antibiotic therapies. The Gram-negative bacteria, like *H. pylori*, are considered less susceptible to the effect of essential oils and antibacterials generally, because of the outer membrane around the cell wall. Nevertheless, there have been reports about the *in vitro* activity of various essential oils against *H. pylori*. More than 60 different essential oils were tested against *H. pylori* in several different research experiments. Unfortunately, comparing the results is problematic because of the different methods used to assess the anti-*Helicobacter* activity of the oils. The commonly used methods are agar dilution (the results expressed as minimal inhibitory concentration [MIC]) and disk/well diffusion assay (the inhibition zone), but the incubation time varies from 24 h to 3–5 days, making the results hard to compare. Furthermore, in the experiments conducted, different *H. pylori* strains have been used, like commercial strains (CCUG, ATCC 700392, and ATCC 43504), clinical isolates, and mouse-adapted strains (P49 and SS1). The highest potential in targeting *H. pylori* was exhibited by the essential oils listed in the Table 19.3 (Bergonzelli et al., 2003; Ohno et al., 2003; Basile et al., 2006; Deriu et al., 2007; Esmaeili et al., 2012; Ozen et al., 2014).

Antimicrobial activity of essential oils is often attributed to the complexity of their chemical composition and synergistic or additive effect between components (Burt, 2004). For this reason, Simin et al. (2014) adopted an innovative approach and increased the total number of components by mixing the essential oils with the highest anti–*H. pylori* activity. A three-oil mixture of *Satureja hortensis*, *Origanum vulgare* subsp. *vulgare*, and *Origanum vugare* subsp. *hirtum* (MIC ~ 1 µl/ml) stands out as the most potent, indicating a synergistic effect of active components in these oils.

The main constituent of the essential oils responsible for the anti–*H. pylori* activity is a phenolic monoterpene: carvacrol. Its antimicrobial properties, particularly against Gram-negative bacteria, have been reported on several occasions (Helander et al., 1998). However, the overall inhibitory activity of the oils, against *H. pylori*, cannot be attributed solely to this compound, indicating that minor compounds may interact with carvacrol and increase its activity (Bergonzelli et al., 2003).

The effect of *Cymbopagon citratus* (lemongrass) essential oil against *H. pylori* was evaluated *in vivo*. This bacteria was completely eradicated in one of 10 mice (10%) treated with this oil, whereas the number of colonies in the mouse stomach

TABLE 19.3
Essential Oils with the Highest Anti–*H. pylori* Activity

Essential Oil	Inhibition Zone (cm)	References
Cinnamomum zeylanicum (cinnamon bark)	4.5	Bergonzelli et al., 2003
Cymbopagon citratus (lemongrass)	3.2	
Lippia citriodora (vervein)	2.9	
Citrus paradisi (white grapefruit)	2.9	
Eugenia caryophyllus (clove leaf)	2.5	
Satureja montana (savory)	2.5	
	MIC (µg/ml)	
Myrtus communis (myrtle)	1–7.5	Deriu et al., 2007
Tymus vulgaris (thyme)	10.8	Esmaeili et al., 2012

was reduced in all cases (Ohno et al., 2003). The effect of essential oils against *H. pylori* colonizing the human stomach was reported by Donatini (2014). Over a 6-week period, 25 patients were treated with a combination of essential oils *Thymum vulgaris*, *Mentha piperata*, *Syzygium arometicum*, *Origanum vulgare*, and *Cinnamomum verum*, fixed on *Laetiporus sulfureus* (edible fungi). After the treatment, 33.3% of the patients showed a negative *H. pylori* test, indicating complete eradication.

Food-associated infections of the gastrointestinal tract occur after consumption of food contaminated with various bacterial pathogens, the most common being *Staphylococcus aureus*, *Campylobacter jejuni*, *Listeria monocytogenes*, *Salmonella enterica*, and *Escherichia coli* O157. Symptoms include diarrhea, vomiting, and abdominal pain, followed by dehydration. These infections are self-limited and resolve within a few days; however, they are potentially serious in infant and elderly populations. Therefore, a great number of investigations have been conducted to evaluate the potential of the essential oils in preventing food spoilage by these pathogens. The essential oils most commonly used in food preservation are isolated from *Mentha* spp., *Origanum* spp., and *Citrus* spp. These oils have been incorporated into human diets since ancient times, because of their flavor and food preservation properties (Rivera Calo et al., 2015). *Origanum vulgare* oil inhibits the growth of *E. coli* and the pathogens belonging to genera *Bacillus* and *Staphylococcus* (Sahin et al., 2004; Mimica-Dukić and Božin, 2007; de Barros et al., 2009). Additionally, it suppresses the synthesis of staphylococcal enterotoxins responsible for the majority of unpleasant food poisoning symptoms (de Souza et al., 2010). From the *Citrus* oils, bergamot oil (*Citrus bergamia*) exhibited the highest inhibitory activity against *L. monocytogenes*, *S. aureus*, *Bacillus cereus*, *E. coli* O157, and *C. jejuni* (Fisher and Phillips, 2006). Essential oils isolated from *Mentha* species (*M. aquatica*, *M. longifolia*, and *M. piperita*) exhibited strong inhibitory activity against *E. coli*. Apart from this, *M. piperita* essential oil was active against a multiresistant strain of *Shigella sonei*, the Gram-negative bacteria that cause shigellosis (Mimica-Dukić et al., 2003a). Interestingly, when examining 96 essential oils against the most common food pathogens, the results indicate a diverse mechanism of antimicrobial activity among essential oils and different bacterial susceptibility. For example, it was found that the growth of *L. monocytogenes*, *S. enterica*, and *E. coli* O157:H7 was inhibited by the same essential oils (thyme, oregano, bay leaf, clove bud, cinnamon, and allspice oils), while *C. jejuni* showed susceptibility to completely different oils (ginger root, jasmine, carrot seed, celery seed, and orange bitter oils) (Friedman et al., 2002).

So far, the aforementioned essential oils have been proposed only as food additives, to prevent contamination and prolong a product's shelf life, rather than as a substitute for antibiotic therapy for food pathogen infections (Rivera Calo et al., 2015).

19.6   SKIN INFECTIONS

19.6.1   BACTERIAL INFECTIONS

The most common bacterial skin infections include impetigo, cellulitis, and ecthyma (all caused by *Staphylococcus aureus* or *Streptococcus pyogenes*), erysipelas

(*S. pyogenes*), folliculitis (*S. aureus*, *Pseudomonas aeruginosa*, or some abiotic factors), and furunculosis or carbunculosis (*S. aureus*) (Hall and Hall, 2009).

Staphylococcus aureus is a Gram-positive bacterium that is a part of normal nasal microbiota in many humans, permanently inhabiting 20% of the population and intermittently another 60% (Kluytmans et al., 1997). However, it can spread to other parts of the body and, if skin or mucosal barriers have been breached (e.g., during surgery), cause various symptoms, from minor skin disturbances to life-threatening deep tissue and systemic diseases, including necrotizing fasciitis, pneumonia, meningitis, and sepsis. While initial treatments with penicillin in the 1940s were met with success, resistant strains soon emerged. Attempts to overcome this problem by the use of methicillin were only partially successful, due to the development of methicillin-resistant *Staphylococcus aureus* (MRSA) strains, nowadays widespread in the community, having been previously restricted to certain populations, such as hospital patients (Chambers, 2001; Hall and Hall, 2009). The use of more efficient, non-β-lactame antibiotics has issues that include toxicity, developing resistance, and the need for oral or intravenous administration. Thus, a new, safe, and efficient topical anti-*Staphylococcus* therapy is eagerly sought out.

The constantly decreasing efficacy of established antibiotics poses a serious threat to public health. Plant extracts and essential oils represent promising alternatives or adjuvants to conventional antibiotics in the treatment of skin infections, thanks to the antimicrobial properties of their constituents—terpenoids and phenolic compounds. In addition, many patients show a preference for natural drugs over synthetic antibiotics, and are well accustomed to essential oils as part of personal hygiene and skin care products (usually being used as fragrances or anti-inflammatory agents).

Numerous oils were tested against bacteria, including skin disease–causing species. Gram-negative bacteria generally showed higher susceptibility, but the growth of Gram-positive species, including antibiotic-resistant strains, was also inhibited by low concentrations of essential oils, with MICs typically in the sub-µl/ml range (D'Arrigo et al., 2010; Qiu et al., 2011; Solórzano-Santos and Miranda-Novales, 2012). For example, tea tree (*Melaleuca alternifolia*, Myrtaceae) oil, with terpinen-4-ol (40%), γ-terpinen (13%), and p-cymene (13%) as dominant components, was found to inhibit growth of *S. aureus* at the 5 µl/ml level (D'Arrigo et al., 2010). Some other oils were effective against this resistant bacterium at even lower concentrations: for wild ginger *Alpinia pahangensis*, Zingiberaceae (containing 12% γ-selinene and 11% β-pinene), the MIC was 80–310 µg/ml (Awang et al., 2011); for *Zataria multiflora*, Lamiaceae (39% thymol, 15% carvacrol), 0.25–1 µl/ml (Mahboubi and Bidgoli, 2010); for perilla, *Perilla frutescens*, Lamiaceae, 0.2–0.8 µl/L (Qiu et al., 2011); and for ambar, *Hofmeisteria schaffneri*, Asteraceae (~65% thymol esters), 48–192 µg/ml. No activity was observed toward Gram-negative species (Pérez-Vásquez et al., 2011). Other oils that inhibited *S. aureus* growth include *Lavandula angustifolia* (37% linalyl acetate, 29% linalool), *L. latifolia* (39% linalool, 28% 1,8-cineole, 15% camphor), and other lavender species (Roller et al., 2009); *Thymus vulgaris* (48% thymol, 16% p-cymene, 15% γ-terpinene) and *Eucalyptus globulus* (47% 1,8-cineole, 18% spathulenol) (Tohidpour et al., 2010); oregano, *Origanum vulgare*, Lamiaceae

(25% thymol, 14% carvacrol) (Nostro et al., 2007); *Juniperus macrocarpa*, Cupressaceae (49% α-pinene, 18% germacrene D) (Lesjak et al., 2014); *Achillea collina* (22% β-pinene, 15% β-caryophyllene, 11% 1,8-cineole) and *Achillea pannonica*, Apiaceae (40% 1,8-cineole, 11% camphor, 11% germacrene D) (Božin et al., 2008); and many others (Warnke et al., 2009). Essential oils of *Ocimum basilicum*, *Origanum vulgare*, *Thymus vulgaris*, *Melissa officinalis*, *Eucalyptus gunnii*, *Rosmarinus officinalis* and *Salvia officinalis* were found to be effective against several bacterial species, including *Pseudomonas aeruginosa*, *S. aureus*, and *Staphylococcus epidermidis*, some acting even on penicillin-resistant strains (Mimica-Dukić et al., 2004; Božin et al., 2006, 2007; Bugarin et al., 2014).

In essential oil combinations with conventional antibiotics, synergistic effects were sometimes observed, with a significant decrease of MIC against multidrug-resistant *S. aureus* strains. For example, *Zataria multiflora* oil showed synergism with vancomycin toward MRSA, with fractional inhibitory concentration (FIC) indices of 0.2 and 0.12 for oil and antibiotic, respectively (Mahboubi and Bidgoli, 2010). Some oils exhibited different adjuvant effects. For example, tea tree oil did not significantly decrease the MIC value of antibiotic tobramycin toward *S. aureus* (FIC = 0.62), but did exhibit significant postantibiotic sub-MIC effect, that is, prolonged the bacterial growth suppression period at an antibiotic concentration below MIC (D'Arrigo et al., 2010).

Essential oil components may also influence the production of toxins responsible for toxic shock syndrome and necrotic effects, even at sub-MIC concentrations. For example, oil of *Perilla frutescens*, Lamiaceae, was found to reduce secretion of hemolytic agents (hemolysins and α-toxin) and superantigens (SEA, SEB, and TSST-1) by *S. aureus*, as opposed to β-lactam antibiotics (Qiu et al., 2011).

While there is a growing body of evidence that essential oils and plant extracts exhibit significant antimicrobial effects *in vitro*, clinical studies are scarce and results are often inconclusive due to inadequate experimental design (Caelli et al., 2000; Martin and Ernst, 2003; Solórzano-Santos and Miranda-Novales, 2012). However, it seems that at least some oils show efficacy similar to that of commercial antibiotics. Tea tree oil, one of the most investigated, was comparable to triclosan-, mupirocin-, and chlorhexidine-based therapies when applied topically as an ointment or body wash (Caelli et al., 2000; Dryden et al., 2004).

In addition to direct antimicrobial activity, essential oils can be used to facilitate the action of other medicaments. Namely, antiseptic agents such as chlorhexidine exhibit restricted skin penetration, their action being limited to the upper layers of the skin. At the same time, microorganisms (such as *Candida* spp. and *Propionibacterium* spp.) in lower layers such as the sebaceous glands and hair follicles remain unaffected and can cause infection following skin damage, for example, surgery. Essential oils, with their ability to enhance penetration of both hydrophilic compounds (through reversible, nondamaging disruption of intercellular and membrane lipids) and lipophylic compounds (through diffusion coefficient increase), demonstrated promising potential as natural and safe transdermal drug delivery vehicles (Aqil et al., 2007; Karpanen et al., 2008, 2010). One of the most efficient compounds with regard to penetration enhancement is menthol, but the effect was also observed for 1,8-cineole (especially abundant in eucalyptus oil), terpineol, limonene, linalool, nerolidol, farnesol, and so forth, in concentrations as low as 1%–5% (Aqil et al., 2007; Karpanen et al., 2010).

19.6.2 Fungal and Yeast Infections

Fungal skin infections (dermatophytoses) are classified according to the infected area—tinea capitis (scalp), tinea corporis (trunk), tinea pedis (feet), and forth. They are caused by three fungal genera: *Microsporum*, *Trichophyton*, and less commonly, *Epidermophyton*, with regional and temporal variations in exact species causing a specific disease. In addition to these genera (commonly known as dermatophytes), some yeasts can also cause mycoses, including *Malassezia* spp. (seborrhoeic dermatitis, dandruff, and pityriasis versicolor) and *Candida* spp. (candidiasis). A number of antifungal agents are available, including ketoconazole, griseofulvin, and fluconazole. While skin infections are usually treated topically, chronic diseases may require oral administration of antifungals, with associated risks of hepatotoxicity and other side effects that, in addition to the emergence of resistant strains, pose difficulty in effective treatment of mycoses (Devkatte et al., 2005; Hall and Hall, 2009). Essential oils thus represent a viable alternative, since it is known that dermatophytes and other pathogenic fungi are susceptible to the action of both terpenoid- and phenylpropanoid-rich oils.

Numerous oils were tested *in vitro* for their antifungal activity (Raut and Karuppayil, 2014), mostly against *Candida* species. In one study (Devkatte et al., 2005), a total of 38 essential and fatty oils were assayed versus *Candida albicans* strains, with 25 showing appreciable fungicidal activity. Lemongrass, clove leaf, cinnamon, Japanese mint, geranium, motiarosha, and ginger grass oil were found to be the most effective, with concentrations of 0.01%–0.12% completely inhibiting the growth of fluconazole-susceptible and -resistant strains alike. In another study (Hammer et al., 1998), 24 essential oils were investigated against seven *Candida* species. Sandalwood oil (*Santalum album*, Santalales) was the most potent, with a MIC of 0.06%, but lemongrass (*Cymbopogon citratus*), spearmint (*Mentha spicata*), oregano (*Origanum vulgare*), bay (*Pimenta racemosa*), and clove (*Syzigium aromaticum*) oil showed similar activity (MIC = 0.12%). Other investigated oils include juniper berry oil, *Juniperus communis*, Cupressaceae, with MICs of 0.78%–2% against *Candida* spp. and 0.39%–2% against *Microsporum* and *Trichophyton* dermatophytes (Pepeljnjak et al., 2005); two species of eucalyptus, *E. robusta* and *E. saligna*, Myrtaceae (Sartorelli et al., 2007); and 30 species including eucalyptus (*Eucalyptus globulus*, Myrtaceae), peppermint (*Mentha piperita*, Lamiaceae), ginger grass (*Cymbopogon martinii*, Poaceae), and clove (*Syzigium aromaticum*, Myrtaceae) as the most active, with MICs in the range of 0.08%–0.35% (Agarwal et al., 2008). In addition, it was found that essential oils such as cardamom and boswella can exhibit synergistic effects in combination with conventional antifungal drugs such as fluconazole (Rabadia et al., 2011). Essential oil obtained from the seeds of *Foeniculum vulgarae* exhibited strong antifungal activity, especially against different *Aspergillus* sp., and is therefore suitable to be used in the food industry for preventing *Aspergillus* contamination and mycotoxin production, as well as fungal infections of the skin, hair, and nails caused by dermathophytes (Mimica-Dukić et al., 2003b). *Ocimum basilicum, Origanum vulgare, Thymus vulgaris, Melissa officinalis, Rosmarinus officinalis,* and *Salvia officinalis* essential oils were also effective against *Candida albicans, Epidermophyton floccosum, Microsporum canis, Trichophyton mentagrophytes* var. *mentagrophytes, Trichophyton rubrum,* and *Trichophyton tonsurans* (Mimica-Dukić et al., 2004; Božin et al., 2006, 2007).

Despite the evident activity, the use of essential oils in dermatophytoses and other mycoses treatment is still very limited, notable exceptions being tea tree oil (*Melaleuca alternifolia,* Myrtaceae) and rosemary oil (*Rosmarinus officinalis,* Lamiaceae) (Devkatte et al., 2005). The lack of widespread use in medical practice is a result of the scarcity of clinical trials. The majority of studies focused on tea tree oil use in treatment of tinea pedis (athlete's foot) and onychomycosis (Tong et al., 1992; Buck et al., 1994; Satchell et al., 2002). Tea tree oil demonstrated weaker effects toward tinea pedis than the synthetic antifungal agent tolnaftate, but significantly better than placebo. The effects toward onychomycosis were comparable to those of the synthetic drug clotrimazole. In all trials, several patients treated with essential oil reported side effects. A study on the application of bitter orange oil (*Citrus auranthium,* Rutaceae) in the treatment of tinea corporis, tinea cruris, and tinea pedis (Ramadan et al., 1996) was also conducted, showing promising results, but the quality of data is limited due to small sample size.

19.7 VIRAL INFECTIONS

Viruses are infectious agents that replicate only inside the living cells of other organisms (animals, plants, and microorganisms). Several hundred different viruses infect humans, and they often spread via respiratory and enteric excretions. Some viruses are transmitted sexually and through transfer of blood or through transplantation of tissue, and some are transmitted via different vectors (rodents, arthropods, and bats). For humans, the herpes simplex viruses (HSV-1 and -2) are pathogenic. Herpesvirus type-1 is an enveloped DNA virus in the Herpesviridae family that is widespread in the human population (Pilau et al., 2011). Among HSV-related diseases, genital herpes (commonly caused by HSV-2) is an important sexually transmitted disease. HSV infections can cause serious systemic illnesses in immunocompromised patients. Also, HSV is involved in some ocular diseases, which may lead to blindness (herpetic stromal keratitis) (Khan et al., 2005). The other members of herpesviruses causing different illnesses are HHV-3 (varicella zoster virus), HHV-4 (Epstein-Barr virus), HHV-5 (cytomegalovirus), HHV-6, HHV-7, and HHV-8 (Mukhtar et al., 2008). Other groups of viruses that are frequently transmitted through the fecal–oral route are noroviruses (NoVs), hepatitis A virus (HAV), and rotaviruses (RoVs). Viral hepatitis (inflammation of the liver) is caused by different viruses (named A, B, C, D, and E). Types B and C lead to chronic disease in hundreds of millions of people worldwide. It is estimated that 13 million people live with chronic hepatitis B, and 15 million people are infected with hepatitis C (Hope et al., 2014). The human rotavirus is one of the most common causes of gastroenteritis and severe diarrheas. It is a nonenveloped virus with a double-stranded RNA segmented genome.

Plants have been a valuable source of biologically active isolates for centuries. One of the first systematic attempts to spot plants with anti-influenza A activity (among

142 plant extracts screened) was published in the *Journal of General Microbiology* in 1952 (Chantrill et al., 1952; Mukhtar et al., 2008). Since then, numerous studies have confirmed the antiviral potential of medicinal plants, but much more scientific data refer to investigation of plant extracts than essential oils. Still, the antiviral effect of essential oils was tested on a wide range of viral pathogens, and they exhibited stronger antiviral activity on enveloped viruses, due to the lipophilic nature of essential oil constituents.

According to Astani et al. (2011), star anise essential oil as well as phenylpropanoids and sesquiterpenoids (especially β-caryophyllene) showed strong antiviral activity against herpes simplex virus type-1 *in vitro*. High antiviral activity was obtained when herpesvirus was incubated with EO (or isolated compounds) prior to host cell infection, interacting directly with free virus particles. Pretreatment of cells with drugs had no effect on viral infectivity during intracellular replication. Comparing inhibitory effects against herpes simplex virus (HSV-1) of several essential oils (from eucalyptus, tea tree, and thyme) with the antiviral potential of their major monoterpenic compounds, Astani et al. (2010) concluded that the complex mixtures of the essential oils seem to be superior and preferable to single compounds. Tea tree oil, which is able to penetrate the skin, can be a promising topical therapeutic agent, as it has already been successfully applied in labial herpes infections. According to Armaka et al. (1999), isoborneol was singled out as a very propitious compound for inhibiting the HSV-1 life cycle (completely inhibiting viral replication, without affecting viral adsorption). Based on experimental results that two viral glycoproteins (gB and gD) were not present on fully matured virus if it was replicated in the presence of isoborneol, it was concluded that isoborneol specifically inhibited glycosylation of polypeptides.

Based on the results of Cermelli et al. (2008), *Eucalyptus globulus* essential oil showed a mild antiviral activity against a strain of mumps virus (MV), but no activity against a strain of adenovirus. Both pathogens were isolated from patients with respiratory tract infections. As herpesviruses, MVs are also enveloped viruses, so it can be speculated that this antiviral activity is due to a direct action on virus particles during the extracellular phase of the virus cycle.

Duschatzky et al. (2005) used seven different essential oils isolated from aromatic plants collected in Argentina, to evaluate their antiviral activity against HSV-1 and two RNA-viruses lacking any effective chemotherapeutic agents: arenavirus Junin causing hemorrhagic fever and dengue virus (an arthropod-borne virus). Results showed an effective inhibition against JUNV, of all examined essential oils. By using a radiolabeled virion binding assay, the authors tried to gain more insight into the mechanism of antiviral action. Since JUNV virions inactivated by some essential oils did not change their binding ability to Vero cells, it was presumed that glycoproteins in the envelope were affected by the oil treatment.

An extent of antiviral activity on norovirus surrogate suspensions (murine norovirus [MNV-1] and feline calicivirus [FCV]) has been observed using EOs of clove (*Eugenia caryophyllus*), oregano (*Origanum compactum*), and zataria (*Zataria multiflora* Boiss) (Elizaquível et al., 2013). Obtained results highlighted their potential as biopreservatives to improve food safety.

Based on results of Garozzo et al. (2009), the essential oil of tea tree (*Melaleuca alternifolia*, Myrtaceae) and some of its components (terpinen-4-ol, terpinolene, and α-terpineol) exhibited an inhibitory effect on influenza virus A/PR8 replication, while some other components (α-terpinene, p-cymene, and γ-terpinene) were completely ineffective. Although antiviral activity of the tested compounds was evaluated against polio 1, ECHO 9, Coxsackie B1, adeno 2, HSV-1, and HSV-2 viruses, they proved to be ineffective.

Pilau et al. (2011) conducted a thorough antiviral investigation of Mexican oregano (*Lippia graveolens*) essential oil and its major compound, carvacrol, against different human and animal viruses, of which five are classified as DNA viruses (acyclovir-resistant herpes simplex virus type-1 [ACVR-HHV-1], acyclovir-sensitive HHV-1, and bovine herpesvirus type-1, type-2, and type-5 [BoHV-1, BoHV-2, and BoHV-5]) and three as RNA viruses (human respiratory syncytial virus [HRSV], human rotavirus [RV], and bovine viral diarrhea virus [BVDV]). Examined essential oil showed a broader spectrum of action than carvacrol, but carvacrol alone exhibited high antiviral activity against RV. There also were differences in the stage of virus infection when the drug was more active, meaning essential oil was able to inhibit viruses before, but also after virus inoculation, while carvacrol was effective only when added after virus inoculation.

The effect of carvacrol on enteric viruses (hepatitis A virus and two norovirus surrogates—murine norovirus and feline calicivirus) was evaluated by Sánchez et al. (2015). Obtained results suggest that carvacrol slightly affects HAV infectivity. For the two noroviruses, carvacrol had the strongest antiviral effect at 37°C and was still active at refrigerated temperatures—highlighting its potential as an inexpensive natural alternative to reduce viral contamination and therefore improve the safety of fresh-cut products.

19.8   SAFETY ISSUES

Essential oils are often considered to exhibit no skin toxicity at all (Okabe et al., 1990), and to the general public they can appear to be natural and thus safe. However, it should be noted that essential oils consist of numerous compounds affecting multiple targets in cells (Bakkali et al., 2008; Raut and Karuppayil, 2014), especially biological membranes (thus disrupting ion homeostasis and energy production). The cytotoxic effects are especially observed for alcohols, aldehydes, and phenols. While these effects are responsible for desired antimicrobial activity, they can also result in adverse reactions toward the host, ranging from short-term irritation to phototoxicity, organ toxicity (e.g., neuro-, hepato-, or nephrotoxicity), carcinogenicity, and teratogenicity. It should be noted that for skin infections, especially localized ones, topical application may be sufficient, thus usually avoiding the systemic effects associated with other application routes (oral, intravenous). However, the potential for toxic effect still exists; for example, depression, weakness, and muscle tremors were observed in cats and dogs treated with tea tree oil, one of the most common essential oils in skin infection therapy, the symptoms disappearing after stopping the application (Villar et al., 1994). Thus, the safety of each essential oil for human application needs to be evaluated. Numerous studies were conducted to assess the effects of essential oils and isolated components on mammals (Vigan, 2010; Raut and Karuppayil, 2014), documenting the carcinogenic effects of some phenols such as estragole and methyl iso-eugenol from tarragon, anise, basil, and fennel; hepatotoxic effects of pulegone and menthofuran from *Mentha pulegium*; phototoxicity and allergenic effects of many terpenoids and phenols; and dermatonecrotic effects of lemon myrtle (*Backhousia citriodora*) essential oil (Hayes and Marković, 2003).

REFERENCES

Agarwal, Vishnu, Priyanka Lal, and Vikas Pruthi. Prevention of *Candida albicans* biofilm by plant oils. *Mycopathologia* 165 (2008): 13–9.

Al-Bayati, Firas A. Synergistic antibacterial activity between *Thymus vulgaris* and *Pimpinella anisum* essential oils and methanol extracts. *Journal of Ethnopharmacology* 116 no. 3 (2008): 403–6.

Al-Daihan, Sooad, Manar Al-Faham, Nora Al-Shawi, Rawan Almayman, Amal Brnawi, Seema Zargar, and Ramesa Shafi Bhat. Antibacterial activity and phytochemical screening of some medicinal plants commonly used in Saudi Arabia against selected pathogenic microorganisms. *Science* (Journal of King Saud University) 25 no. 2 (2013): 115–20.

Aleksić, Verica, Neda Mimica-Dukić, Nataša Simin, Nataša Stanković-Nedljković, and Petar Knežević. Synergetic effect of *Myrtus communis* L., essential oils and conventional antibiotics against multi-resistant *Acinetobacter baumannii* wound isolates. *Phytomedicine* 21 no. 12 (2014): 1666–74.

Amalaradjou, Mary Anne Roshni, and Kumar Venkitanarayanan. Natural approaches for controlling urinary tract infections. In *Urinary Tract Infections*. In Tech, Rijeka, Croatica, 2011.

Aqil, Mohammed, Abdul Ahad, Yasmin Sultana, and Asgat Ali. Status of terpenes as skin penetration enhancers. *Drug Discovery Today* 12 no. 23–24 (2007): 1061–7.

Arbyn, Marc, Xavier Castellsagué, Silvia de Sanjosé et al. Worldwide burden of cervical cancer in 2008. *Annals of Oncology* 22 (2011): 2675–86.

Armaka, Maria, Eleni Papanikolaou, Afroditi Sivropoulou, and Minas Arsenakis. Antiviral properties of isoborneol, a potent inhibitor of herpes simplex virus type 1. *Antiviral Research* 43 (1999): 79–92.

Arroll, Bruce. Antibiotics for upper respiratory tract infections: An overview of Cochrane reviews. *Respiratory Medicine* 99 (2005): 255–61.

Astani, Akram, Jürgen Reichling, and Paul Schnitzler. Comparative study on the antiviral activity of selected monoterpenes derived from essential oils. *Phytotheraphy Research* 24 (2010): 673–9.

Astani, Akram, Jürgen Reichling, and Paul Schnitzler. Screening for antiviral activities of isolated compounds from essential oils. *Evidence-Based Complementary and Alternative Medicine* (2011), article ID 253643.

Awang, Khalijah, Halijah Ibrahim, Devi Rosmy Syamsir, Mastura Mohtar, Rasadah Mat Ali, and Nor Azah Mohamad Ali. Chemical constituents and antimicrobial activity of the leaf and rhizome oils of *Alpinia pahangensis* Ridl., an endemic wild ginger from peninsular Malaysia. *Chemistry and Biodiversity* 8 (2011): 668–73.

Bachir, Raho G., and Mechaal Benali. Antibacterial activity of the essential oils from the leaves of *Eucalyptus globulus* against *Escherichia coli* and *Staphylococcus aureus*. *Asian Pacific Journal of Tropical Biomedicine* 2 no. 9 (2012): 739–42.

Bakkali, Fadil, Simone Averbeck, Dietrich Averbeck, and Mouhamed Idaomar. Biological effects of essential oils: A review. *Food and Chemical Toxicology* 46 (2008): 446–75.

Barreto, Humberto M., Edson C. Silva Filho, Edeltrudes De O. Lima et al. Chemical composition and possible use as adjuvant of the antibiotic therapy of the essential oil of *Rosmarinus officinalis* L. *Industrial Crops and Products* 59 (2014): 290–4.

Baseman, Janet G., and Laura A. Koutsky. The epidemiology of human papillomavirus infections. *Journal of Clinical Virology* 32 Suppl (2005): S16–24.

Basile, Adriana, Felice Senatore, Rosalba Gargano et al. Antibacterial and antioxidant activities in *Sideritis italica* (Miller) Greuter et Burdet essential oils. *Journal of Ethnopharmacology* 107 (2006): 240–8.

Bergonzelli, Gabriela E., Dominique Donnicola, Nadine Porta, and Irène E. Corthesy-Theulaz. Essential oils as components of a diet-based approach to management of *Helicobacter* infection. *Antimicrobial Agents and Chemotherapy* 47 no. 10 (2003): 3240–6.

Blumenthal, Mark. *The Complete German Commission E Monographs*. Austin, TX: American Botanical Council, 1999.

Božin, Biljana, Neda Mimica-Dukić, Nataša Simin, and Goran Anačkov. Characterization of essential oils of some Lamiaceae species and the antimicrobial and antioxidant activities of entire oils. *Journal of Agricultural and Food Chemistry* 54 (2006): 1822–8.

Božin, Biljana, Neda Mimica-Dukić, Isidora Samojlik, Emilija Jovin. Antimicrobial and antioxidant properties of rosemary and sage (*Rosmarinus officinalis* L. and *Salvia officinalis* L.) essential oil. *Journal of Agricultural and Food Chemistry* 55 (2007): 7879–85.

Božin, Biljana, Neda Mimica-Dukić, Mirjana Bogavac et al. Chemical composition, antioxidant and antibacterial properties of *Achillea collina* Becker ex Heimerl s.l. and *A. pannonica* Scheele essential oils. *Molecules* 13 (2008): 2058–68.

Bruneton, Jean-Noel. *Pharmacognosy, Phytochemistry, Medicinal Plants*, 2nd ed. London: Intercept Ltd., 1999.

Buck, David S., David M. Nidorf, and John G. Addino. Comparison of two topical preparations for the treatment of onychomycosis: *Melaleuca alternifolia* (tea tree) oil and clotrimazole. *Journal of Family Practice* 38 no. 6 (1994): 601–5.

Bueno, Juan, Patricia Escobar, Jairo René Martínez, Sandra Milena Leal, and Elena Stashenko. Composition of three essential oils, and their mammalian cell toxicity and antimycobacterial activity against drug-resistant tuberculosis and nontuberculous mycobacteria strains. *Natural Product Communications* 6 (2011): 1743–8.

Bugarin, Dušan, Slavenko Grbović, Dejan Orčić, Dragana Mitić-Ćulafić, Jelena Knežević-Vukčević, and Neda Mimica-Dukić. Essential oil of *Eucalyptus gunnii* Hook. as a novel source of antioxidant, antimutagenic and antibacterial agents. *Molecules* 19 (2014): 19007–20.

Burt, Sara. Essential oils: Their antibacterial properties and potential applications in foods— A review. *International Journal of Food Microbiology* 94 (2004): 223– 53.

Caelli, M., Jenny E. Porteous, Christine F. Carson, Richard Heller, and Thomas V. Riley. Tea tree oil as an alternative topical decolonization agent for methicillin-resistant *Staphylococcus aureus*. *Journal of Hospital Infection* 46 (2000): 236–7.

Carović-Stanko, Klaudija, Sandi Orlić, Olivera Politeo et al. Composition and antibacterial activities of essential oils of seven *Ocimum* taxa. *Food Chemistry* 119 no. 1 (2010): 196 201.

Cermelli, Claudio, Anna Fabio, Giuliana Fabio, and Paola Quaglio. Effect of eucalyptus essential oil on respiratory bacteria and viruses. *Current Microbiology* 56 (2008): 89–92.

Chambers, Henry F. The changing epidemiology of *Staphylococcus aureus*? *Emerging Infectious Diseases* 7 no. 2 (2001): 178–82.

Chantrill, B.H., Charles Edward Coulthard, Dickinson, L., Inkley, G.W., Morris, W., and Pyle, A.H. The action of plant extracts on a bacteriophage of *Pseudomonas pyocyanea* and on influenza A virus. *Journal of General Microbiology* 6 (1952): 74–84.

Chen, Chi-Yu, Yen-Hsu Chen, Po-Liang Lu, Wei-Ru Lin, Tun-Chieh Chen, and Chun-Yu Lin. Proteus mirabilis urinary tract infection and bacteremia: Risk factors, clinical presentation, and outcomes. *Journal of Microbiology, Immunology and Infection* 45 no. 3 (2012): 228–36.

Cimanga, Kanyanga, Sandra Apers, Tess de Bruyne et al. Chemical composition and antifungal activity of essential oils of some aromatic medicinal plants growing in the Democratic Republic of Congo. *Journal of Essential Oil Research* 14 no. 5 (2002): 382–7.

Couladis, Maria, Olga Tzakou, Sebastijan Kujundžić, Marina Soković, Neda Mimica-Dukić. Chemical analysis and antifungal activity of *Thymus striatus*. *Phytotherapy Research* 18 (2004): 40–2.

D'Arrigo, Manuela, Giovanna Ginestra, Giuseppina Mandalari, P.M. Furneri, and G. Bisignano. Synergism and postantibiotic effect of tobramycin and *Melaleuca alternifolia* (tea tree) oil against *Staphylococcus aureus* and *Escherichia coli*. *Phytomedicine* 17 (2010): 317–22.

Dasaraju, Purushothama, and Chien Liu. Infections of the Respiratory System. *In Medical Microbiology*, ed. S. Baron. 4th ed. Galveston: University of Texas Medical Branch, 1996, chap. 93.

de Barros, Jefferson Carneiro, Maria Lúcia da Conceicao, Nelson Justino Gomes Neto et al. Interference of *Origanum vulgare* L. essential oil on the growth and some physiological characteristics of *Staphylococcus aureus* strains isolated from foods. *LWT—Food Science and Technology* 42 no. 6 (2009): 1139–43.

Delaquis, J. Pascal, Kareen Stanich, Benoit Girard, and G. Mazza. Antimicrobial activity of individual and mixed fraction of dill, celandra, coriander and eucalyptus essential oil. *International Journal of Food Microbiology* 74 (2002): 101–9.

De Logu, Alessandro, Giuseppe Loy, Maria L. Pellerano, Leonardo Bonsignore, and Maria L. Schivo. Inactivation of HSV-1 and HSV-2 and prevention of cell-to-cell virus spread by *Santolina insularis* essential oil. *Antiviral Research* 48 (2000): 177–85.

Deriu, Antonella, Giovanna Branca, Paola Molicotti et al. In vitro activity of essential oil of *Myrtus communis* L. against *Helicobacter pylori*. *International Journal of Antimicrobial Agents* 30 (2007): 562–5.

de Souza, Evandro Leite, Jefferson Carneiro de Barros, Carlos Eduardo Vasconcelos de Oliveira, and Maria Lucia da Conceicao. Influence of *Origanum vulgare* L. essential oil on enterotoxin production, membrane permeability and surface characteristics of *Staphylococcus aureus*. *International Journal of Food Microbiology* 137 no. 2–3 (2010): 308–11.

Devkatte, Anupama N., Gajanan B. Zore, and S. Mohan Karuppayil. Potential of plant oils as inhibitors of *Candida albicans* growth. *FEMS Yeast Research* 5 (2005): 867–73.

Diao, Wen-Rui, Qing-Ping Hu, Hong Zhang, and Jian-Guo Xu. Chemical composition, antibacterial activity and mechanism of action of essential oil from seeds of fennel (*Foeniculum vulgare* Mill.). *Food Control* 35 no. 1 (2014): 109–16.

Donatini, Bruno. Étude randomisée comparant l'efficacité d'Hericium erinaceusversus huiles essentielles sur *Helicobacter pylori* (HP) [Randomized study comparing the efficacy of Hericium versus essential oils against *Helicobacter pylori* (HP) infection]. *Phytothérapie* 12 (2014): 3–5.

Dryden, Matthew, Sue Dailly, and M. Crouch. A randomized, controlled trial of tea tree topical preparations versus a standard topical regimen for the clearance of MRSA colonization. *Journal of Hospital Infection* 56 (2004): 283–6.

Duarte, Marta Cristina Teixeira, Ewerton Eduardo Leme, Camila Delarmelina, Andressa Almeida Soares, Glyn Mara Figueira, and Adilson Sartoratto. Activity of essential oils from Brazilian medicinal plants on *Escherichia coli*. *Journal of Ethnopharmacology* 111 no. 2 (2007): 197–201.

Duschatzky, B. Claudia, Mirta L. Possetto, Laura B. Talarico et al. Evaluation of chemical and antiviral properties of essential oils from South American plants. *Antiviral Chemistry and Chemotherapy* 16 (2005): 247–51.

Elaissi, Ameur, Karima Hadj Salah, Samia Mabrouk, Khouja Mohamed Larbi, Rachid Chemli, and Fethia Harzallah-Skhiri. Antibacterial activity and chemical composition of 20 eucalyptus species' essential oils. *Food Chemistry* 129 no. 4 (2011): 1427–34.

El Bouzidi, Laila, Chaima Alaoui Jamali, Khalid Bekkouche et al. Chemical composition, antioxidant and antimicrobial activities of essential oils obtained from wild and cultivated Moroccan *Thymus* species. *Industrial Crops and Products* 43 no. 1 (2013): 450–6.

Elizaquível, Patricia, Maryam Azizkhani, Rosa Aznar, and Gloria Sánchez. The effect of essential oils on norovirus surrogates. *Food Control* 32 (2013): 275–8.

Esmaeili, Davood, Ashraf Mohabati-Mobarez, and Abolghasem Tohidpour. Anti-*Helicobacter pylori* activities of Shoya powder and essential oils of *Thymus vulgaris* and *Eucalyptus globulus*. *Open Microbiology Journal* 6 (2012): 65–9.

Ezz Eldin, Hayam M., and Abeer F. Badawy. In vitro anti-*Trichomonas vaginalis* activity of *Pistacia lentiscus* mastic and *Ocimum basilicum* essential oil. *Journal of Parasitic Diseases* (2015): in press. doi: 10.1007/s12639-013-0374-6.

Fisher, Katie, and Carol A. Phillips. The effect of lemon, orange and bergamot essential oils and their components on the survival of *Campylobacter jejuni*, *Escherichia coli* O157, *Listeria monocytogenes*, *Bacillus cereus* and *Staphylococcus aureus* in vitro and in food systems. *Journal of Applied Microbiology* 101 (2006): 1232–40.

Friedman, Mendel, Philip R. Heinka, and Robert E. Mendrell. Bactericidal activities of plant essential oils and some of their isolated constituents against *Campylobacter jejuni*, *Escherichia coli*, *Listeria monocytogenes*, and *Salmonella enterica*. *Journal of Food Protection* 65 no. 10 (2002): 1545–60.

Gales, Ana C., Ronald N. Jones, Kelley A. Gordon et al. Activity and spectrum of 22 antimicrobial agents tested against urinary tract infection pathogens in hospitalized patients in Latin America: Report from the second year of the SENTRY Antimicrobial Surveillance Program (1998). *Journal of Antimicrobial Chemotherapy* 45 no. 3 (2000): 295–303.

Garozzo, Adriana, Rossella Timpanaro, Benedetta Bisignano, Pio Maria Furneri, Giuseppe Bisignano, and Angelo Castro. In vitro antiviral activity of *Melaleuca alternifolia* essential oil. *Letters in Applied Microbiology* 49 (2009): 806–8.

Garozzo, Adriana, Rossella Timpanaro, Stivala Aldo, Giuseppe Bisignano, and Angelo Castro. Activity of *Melaleuca alternifolia* (tea tree) oil on influenza virus A/PR/8: Study on the mechanism of action. *Antiviral Research* 89 (2011): 83–8.

Gavanji, Shahin, Sayed R. Zaker, Zahra G. Nejad, Azizollah Bakhtari, Elham S. Bidabadi, and Behrouz Larki. Comparative efficacy of herbal essences with amphotricin B and ketoconazole on *Candida albicans* in the in vitro condition. *Integrative Medicine Research* 4 (2015): 112–8.

Graham, David Y., and Lori Fischbach. *Helicobacter pylori* treatment in the era of increasing antibiotic resistance. *Gut* 59 (2010): 1143–53.

Gülçin, Ilhami, Münir Oktay, Ekrem Kireçci, and Ö Irfan Küfrevioğlu. Screening of antioxidant and antimicrobial activities of anise (*Pimpinella anisum* L.) seed extracts. *Food Chemistry* 83 no. 3 (2003): 371–82.

Hall, John C., and Brian J. Hall. *Skin Infections: Diagnosis and Treatment*. Cambridge: Cambridge University Press, 2009.

Hammer, Katherine A., Christine F. Carson, and Thomas V. Riley. In-vitro activity of essential oils, in particular *Melaleuca alternifolia* (tea tree) oil and tea tree oil products, against *Candida* spp. *Journal of Antimicrobial Chemotherapy* 42 (1998): 591–5.

Hammer, Katherine A., Christine F. Carson, and Thomas V. Riley. Antimicrobial activity of essential oils and other plant extracts. *Journal of Applied Microbiology* 86 (1999): 985–90.

Harkenthal, Michael, Gerlinde Layh-Schmitt, and Jürgen Reichling. Effect of Australian tea tree oil on the viability of the wall-less bacterium *Mycoplasma pneumoniae*. *Pharmazie* 55 (2000): 380–4.

Hayes, Amanda, and Boban Marković. Toxicity of Australian essential oil *Backhousia citriodora* (lemon myrtle). Part 2. Absorption and histopathology following application to human skin. *Food and Chemical Toxicology* 41 no. 10 (2003): 1409–16.

Hedayat, Kamyar. Essential oil diffusion for the treatment of persistent oxygen dependence in a three-year-old child with restrictive lung disease with respiratory syncytial virus pneumonia. *Explore* 4 (2008): 264–6.

Heinrich, Michael, Joanne Barnes, Simon Gibbons, and Elizabeth M. Williamson. *Fundamentals of Pharmacognosy and phytotherapy.* Edinburgh: Elsevier, Churchill Livingstone, 2012.

Helander, Ilkka M., Hanna-Leena Alakomi, Kyosti Latva-Kala et al. Characterization of the action of selected essential oil components on Gram-negative bacteria. *Journal of Agricultural and Food Chemistry* 46 (1998): 3590–5.

Hersch-Martínez, Paul, Blanca E. Leaños-Miranda, and Fortino Solórzano-Santos. Antibacterial effects of commercial essential oils over locally prevalent pathogenic strains in Mexico. *Fitoterapia* 76 no. 5 (2005): 453–7.

Hope, Vivian D., Irina Eramova, Daniel Capurro, and Martin C. Donoghoe. Prevalence and estimation of hepatitis B and C infections in the WHO European region: A review of data focusing on the countries outside the European Union and the European Free Trade Association. *Epidemiology and Infection* 142 (2014): 270–86.

Howard, David H., Douglas R. Scott II, Randall Packard, and DeAnn Jones. The global impact of drug resistance. *Clinical Infectious Diseases* 36 no. 1 (2003): S4–10.

Hussain, Abdullah Ijaz, Farooq Anwar, Syed Tufail Hussain Sherazi, and Roman Przybylski. Chemical composition, antioxidant and antimicrobial activities of basil (*Ocimum basilicum*) essential oils depends on seasonal variations. *Food Chemistry* 108 no. 3 (2008): 986–95.

Inouyea, Shigeharu, Toshio Takizawb, and Hideyo Yamaguchia. Antibacterial activity of essential oils and their major constituents against respiratory tract pathogens by gaseous contact. *Journal of Antimicrobial Chemotherapy* 47 (2001): 565–73.

Jiang, Yang, Nan Wu, Yu-Jie Fu et al. Chemical composition and antimicrobial activity of the essential oil of rosemary. *Environmental Toxicology and Pharmacology* 32 no. 1 (2011): 63–8.

Johansen, Bjerklund Truls E., Rasmus Nilsson, Zafer Tandogdu, and Florian Wagenlehner. Clinical presentation, risk factors and use of antibiotics in urinary tract infections. *Surgery* (Oxford) 32 no. 6 (2014): 297–303.

Jordán, Maria J., Vanesa Lax, Maria C. Rota, Susana Lorán, and José A. Sotomayor. 2013. Effect of the phenological stage on the chemical composition, and antimicrobial and antioxidant properties of *Rosmarinus officinalis* L. essential oil and its polyphenolic extract. *Industrial Crops and Products* 48 (2013): 144–52.

Karpanen, Tarja J., Tony Worthington, E.R. Hendry, Barbara R. Conway, and Peter A. Lambert. Antimicrobial efficacy of chlorhexidine digluconate alone and in combination with eucalyptus oil, tea tree oil and thymol against planktonic and biofilm cultures of *Staphylococcus epidermidis*. *Journal of Antimicrobial Chemotherapy* 62 (2008): 1031–6.

Karpanen, Tarja J., Barbara R. Conway, Tony Worthington, Anthony C. Hilton, Tom S.J. Elliott, and Peter A. Lambert. Enhanced chlorhexidine skin penetration with eucalyptus oil. *BMC Infectious Diseases* 24 (2010): 278–83.

Khan, Mahmud Tareq Hassan, Arjumand Ather, Kenneth D. Thompson, and Roberto Gambari. Extracts and molecules from medicinal plants against herpes simplex viruses. *Antiviral Research* 67 (2005): 107–19.

Kluytmans, Jan, Alex Van Belkum, and Henry Verbrugh. Nasal carriage of *Staphylococcus aureus*: Epidemiology, underlying mechanisms, and associated risks. *Clinical Microbiology Reviews* 10 no. 3 (1997): 505–20.

Knobloch, Karl, Alexander Pauli, Bernard Iberl, Hildegunde Weigand, and Norbert Weis. Antibacterial and antifungal properties of essential oil components. *Journal of Essential Oil Research* 1 (1989): 119–28.

Koch, Christine, Jürgen Reichling, Jürgen Schneele, and Paul Schnitzler. Inhibitory effect of essential oils against herpes simplex virus type 2. *Phytomedicine* 15 (2008): 71–8.

Lesjak, Marija. Biopotential and chemical characterization of extracts and essential oils of *Juniperus* L. (Cupressaceae) species. PhD thesis, University of Novi Sad, Novi Sad, Serbia, 2011.

Lesjak, Marija M., Ivana N. Beara, Dejan Z. Orčić, Petar N. Knežević, Nataša Đ. Simin, Svirčev Đ. Emilija, and Neda M. Mimica-Dukić. Phytochemical composition and antioxidant, anti-inflammatory and antimicrobial activities of *Juniperus macrocarpa* Sibth. et Sm. *Journal of Functional Foods* 7 (2014): 257–68.

Liao, Qingjiao, Zhengxu Qian, Rui Liu, Liwei An, and Xulin Chen. Germacrone inhibits early stages of influenza virus infection. *Antiviral Research* 100 (2013): 578–88.

Lu, Fei, Yi Cheng Ding, Xing Qian Ye, and Yu Ting Ding. 2011. Antibacterial effect of cinnamon oil combined with thyme or clove oil. *Agricultural Sciences in China* 10 no. 9 (2011): 1482–7.

Mahady, Gail B., Yue Huang, Brian J. Doyle, and Tracie Locklear. Natural products as antibacterial agents. *Studies in Natural Products Chemistry* 35 no. C (2008): 423–44.

Mahboubi, M., and F. Ghazian Bidgoli. Antistaphylococcal activity of *Zataria multiflora* essential oil and its synergy with vancomycin. *Phytomedicine* 17 (2010): 548–50.

Marshall, Barry, and Robin J. Warren. Unidentified curved bacilli in the stomach of patients with gastritis and peptic ulceration. *Lancet* 232 (1984): 1311–5.

Martin, Karen W., and Edzard Ernst. Herbal medicines for treatment of bacterial infections: A review of controlled clinical trials. *Journal of Antimicrobial Chemotherapy* 51 (2003): 241–6.

Medina-Polo, Jose, Felix Guerrero-Ramos, Santiago Pérez-Cadavid et al. Community-associated urinary infections requiring hospitalization: Risk factors, microbiological characteristics and patterns of antibiotic resistance. *Actas Urológicas Españolas* (English edition) 39 no. 2 (2015): 104–11.

Mimica-Dukić, Neda, and Biljana Božin. Essential oil from Lamiaceae species as promising antioxidant and antimicrobial agents. *Natural Product Communication* 2 no. 4 (2007): 445–52.

Mimica-Dukić, Neda, and Biljana Božin. *Mentha* L. (Lamiaceae) as promising sources of bioactive secondary metabolites. *Current Pharmaceutical Design* 14 (2008): 141–50.

Mimica-Dukić, Neda, Biljana Božin, Marina Soković, Biserka Mihajlović, and Milan Matavulj. Antimicrobial and antioxidant activities of three *Mentha* L. species essential oils. *Planta Medica* 69 (2003a): 413–9.

Mimica-Dukić, Neda, Sebastijan Kujundžić, Marina Soković, and Maria Couladis. Essential oil composition and antifungal activity of *Foeniculum vulgare* Mill. obtained by different distillation conditions. *Phytotherapy Research* 17 (2003b): 368–71.

Mimica-Dukić, Neda, Biljana Božin, Marina Soković, and Nataša Simin. Antimicrobial and antioxidant activity of *Melissa officinalis* (Lamiaceae) essential oil. *Journal of Agricultural and Food Chemistry* 52 (2004): 2485–9.

Mimica-Dukić, Neda, Dušan Bugarin, Slavenko Grbović, Dragana Mitić-Ćulafić, Branka Vuković-Gačić, Dejan Orčić, Emilija Jovin, and Maria Couladis. Essential oil of *Myrtus communis* L. as a potential antioxidant and antimutagenic agents. *Molecules* 5 no. 4 (2010): 2759–70.

Mišan, Aleksandra, Neda Mimica-Dukić, Marijana Sakač et al. Antioxidant activity of medicinal plant extracts in cookies. *Journal of Food Science* 76 no. 9 (2011): 239–44.

Mondello, Francesca, Flavia De Bernardis, Antonietta Girolamo, Giuseppe Salvatore, and Antonio Cassone. In vitro and in vivo activity of tea tree oil against azole-susceptible and -resistant human pathogenic yeasts. *Journal of Antimicrobial Chemotherapy* 51 (2003): 1223–9.

Moon, Therese, Jenny M. Wilkinson, and Heather M. Cavanagh. Antiparasitic activity of two *Lavandula* essential oils against *Giardia duodenalis, Trichomonas vaginalis* and *Hexamita inflata. Parasitology Research* 99 (2006): 722–8.

Mukhtar, Muhammad, Mohammad Arshad, Mahmood Ahmad, Roger Pomerantz, Brian Wigdahl, and Zahida Parveen. Antiviral potentials of medicinal plants. *Virus Research* 131 (2008): 111–20.

Mulyaningsih, Sri, Frank Sporer, Stefan Zimmermann, Jürgen Reichling, and Michael Wink. Synergistic properties of the terpenoids aromadendrene and 1,8-cineole from the essential oil of *Eucalyptus globulus* against antibiotic-susceptible and antibiotic-resistant pathogens. *Phytomedicine* 17 no. 13 (2010): 1061–6.

Naik, Mohd Irfan, Bashir Ahmad Fomda, Ebenezar Jaykumar, and Javid Ahmad Bhat. Antibacterial activity of lemongrass (*Cymbopogon citratus*) oil against some selected pathogenic bacterias. *Asian Pacific Journal of Tropical Medicine* 3 no. 7 (2010): 535–8.

Newman, David J., Gordon M. Cragg, and Kenneth M. Snader. Natural products as sources of new drugs over the period 1981–2002. *Journal of Natural Product* 66 (2003): 1022–37.

NICE Clinical Guideline 69. Respiratory tract infections: Antibiotic prescribing. Prescribing of antibiotics for self-limiting respiratory tract infections in adults and children in primary care. London: National Institute for Health and Clinical Excellence, 2008.

Nostro, Antonia, Andrea Sudano Roccaro, Giuseppe Bisignano et al. Effects of oregano, carvacrol and thymol on *Staphylococcus aureus* and *Staphylococcus epidermidis* biofilms. *Journal of Medical Microbiology* 56 (2007): 519–23.

Ohno, Tomoyuki, Masakazu Kita, Yoshio Yamaoka et al. Antimicrobial activity of essential oils against *Helicobacter pylori. Helicobacter* 8 no. 3 (2003): 207–15.

Ojeda-Sana, Adriana M., Catalina M. van Baren, Miguel A. Elechosa, Miguel A. Juárez, and Silvia Moreno. New insights into antibacterial and antioxidant activities of rosemary essential oils and their main components. *Food Control* 31 no. 1 (2013): 189–95.

Okabe, Hideaki, Yasuko Obata, Kozo Takayama, and Tsuneji Nagai. Percutaneous absorption enhancing effect and skin irritation of monocyclic monoterpenes. *Drug Design and Delivery* 6 (1990): 229–38.

Onawunmia, Grace O., Wolde-Ab Yisak, and E.O. Ogunlana. Antibacterial constituents in the essential oil of *Cymbopugon citratus* (DC.) Stapf. *Journal of Ethnopharmacology* 12 (1984): 279–86.

Oussalah, Mounia, Stéphane Caillet, Linda Saucier, and Monique Lacroix. Inhibitory effects of selected plant essential oils on the growth of four pathogenic bacteria: *E. coli* O157:H7, *Salmonella typhimurium, Staphylococcus aureus* and *Listeria monocytogenes. Food Control* 18 no. 5 (2007): 414–20.

Ozen, Filiz, Fatma Y. Ekinci, and May Korachi. The inhibition of *Helicobacter pylori* infected cells by *Origanum minutiflorum. Industrial Crops and Products* 58 (2014): 329–34.

Palmeira-de-Oliveira, Ana, Branca M. Silva, Rita Palmeira-de-Oliveira, José Martinez-de-Oliveira, and Lígia R. Salgueiro. Are plant extracts a potential therapeutic approach for genital infections? *Current Medicinal Chemistry* 20 (2013): 2914–28.

Parsonnet, Julie, Gary D. Friedman, Daniel P. Vandersteen et al. *Helicobacter pylori* infection and the risk of gastric carcinoma. *New England Journal of Medicine* 325 (1991): 1127–31.

Pepeljnjak, Stjepan, Ivan Kosalec, Zdenka Kalođera, and Nikola Blažević. Antimicrobial activity of juniper berry essential oil (*Juniperus communis* L., Cupressaceae). *Acta Pharmaceutica* 55 (2005): 417–22.

Pérez-Vásquez, Araceli, Santiago Capella, Edelmira Linares, Robert Bye, Guadalupe Angeles-López, and Rachel Mata. Antimicrobial activity and chemical composition of the essential oil of *Hofmeisteria schaffneri*. *Journal of Pharmacy and Pharmacology* 63 (2011): 579–86.

Piccaglia, Roberta, Mauro Marotti, Enrico Giovanelli, Stanley G. Deans, and Elizabeth Eaglesham. Antibacterial and antioxidant properties of Mediterranean aromatic plants. *Industrial Crops and Products* 2 no. 1 (1993): 47–50.

Pilau, Marciele Ribas, Sydney Hartz Alves, Rudi Weiblen, Sandra Arenhart, Ana Paula Cueto, and Luciane Teresinha Lovato. Antiviral activity of the *Lippia graveolens* (Mexican oregano) essential oil and its main compound carvacrol against human and animal viruses. *Brazilian Journal of Microbiology* 42 (2011): 1616–24.

Pinto, Eugenia, Luís A. Vale-Silva, Carlos Cavaleiro, and Ligia R. Salgueiro. Antifungal activity of the clove essential oil from *Syzygium aromaticum* on *Candida*, *Aspergillus* and dermatophyte species. *Journal of Medical Microbiology* 58 (2009): 1454–62.

Qiu, Jiazhang, Xiaoran Zhang, Mingjing Luo et al. Subinhibitory concentrations of perilla oil affect the expression of secreted virulence factor genes in *Staphylococcus aureus*. *PLoS One* 6 no. 1 (2011): 1–8.

Rabadia, Alpa Gopal, Sheela D. Kamat, and Dilip V. Kamat. Antifungal activity of essential oils against fluconazole resistant fungi. *International Journal of Phytomedicine* 3 (2011): 506–10.

Ramadan, Wafaà, Basma Mourad, Suzan Ibrahim, and Fatma Sonbol. Oil of bitter orange: New topical antifungal agent. *International Journal of Dermatology* 35 no. 6 (1996): 448–9.

Rather, Manzoor, Bilal A. Dar, Shahnawaz N. Sofi, Bilal A. Bhat, and Mushtaq A. Qurishi. *Foeniculum vulgare*: A comprehensive review of its traditional use, phytochemistry, pharmacology, and safety. *Arabian Journal of Chemistry* (King Saud University) (2012): in press doi:10.1016/j.arabjc.2012.04.011.

Raut, Jayant Shankar, and Sankunny Mohan Karuppayil. A status review on the medicinal properties of essential oils. *Industrial Crops and Products* 62 (2014): 250–64.

Rivera Calo, Juliany, Philip G. Crandall, Corliss A. O'Bryan, and Steven C. Ricke. Essential oils as antimicrobials in food systems: A review. *Food Control* 54 (2015): 111–9.

Roby, Mohamed Hussein Hamdy, Mohamed Atef Sarhan, Khaled Abdel Hamed Selim, and Khalel Ibrahim Khalel. Antioxidant and antimicrobial activities of essential oil and extracts of fennel (*Foeniculum vulgare* L.) and chamomile (*Matricaria chamomilla* L.). *Industrial Crops and Products* 44 (2013): 437–45.

Roller, Sibel, Nina Ernest, and Jane Buckle. The antimicrobial activity of high-necrodane and other lavender oils on methicillin-sensitive and -resistant *Staphylococcus aureus* (MSSA and MRSA). *Journal of Alternative and Complementary Medicine* 15 no. 3 (2009): 275–9.

Rota, María C., Antonio Herrera, Rosa M. Martínez, Jose A. Sotomayor, and María J. Jordán. Antimicrobial activity and chemical composition of *Thymus vulgaris*, *Thymus zygis* and *Thymus hyemalis* essential oils. *Food Control* 19 no. 7 (2008): 681–7.

Runyoro, D., O. Ngassapa, K. Vagionas, N. Aligiannis, K. Graikou, and I. Chinou. 2010. Chemical composition and antimicrobial activity of the essential oils of four *Ocimum* species growing in Tanzania. *Food Chemistry* 119 no. 1 (2010): 311–6.

Saad, Nizar, Christian Muller, and Annelise Lobstein. Major bioactivities and mechanism of action of essential oils and their components. *Flavour and Fragrance Journal* 28 (2013): 269–79.

Sahin, Fikrettin, Medine Güllüce, Dimitra Daferera et al. Biological activities of the essential oils and methanol extract of *Origanum vulgare* ssp. *vulgare* in the eastern Anatolia region of Turkey. *Food Control* 15 no. 7 (2004): 549–57.

Sailer, Reinhard, Tobias Berger, Jurgen Reichling, and Michael Harkenthal. Pharmaceutical and medicinal aspects of Australian tea tree oil. *Phytomedicine* 5 no. 6 (1998): 489–95.

Sajed, Hassan, Amirhossein Sahebkar, and Mehrdad Iranshahi. *Zataria multiflora* Boiss. (Shirazi thyme): An ancient condiment with modern pharmaceutical uses. *Journal of Ethnopharmacology* 145 (2013): 686–98.

Samojlik, Isidora, Slobodan Petkovic, Neda Mimica-Dukić, and Biljana Božin. Acute and chronic pretreatment with essential oil of peppermint (*Mentha × piperita* L., Lamiaceae) influences drug effects. *Phytotherapy Research* 26 no. 6 (2012): 820–5.

Sánchez, César, Rosa Aznar, and Gloria Sánchez. The effect of carvacrol on enteric viruses. *International Journal of Food Microbiology* 192 (2015): 72–6.

Sartorelli, Patrícia, Alexandre Donizete Marquioreto, Adriana Amaral-Baroli, Marcos Enoque L. Lima, and Paulo Roberto H. Moreno. Chemical composition and antimicrobial activity of the essential oils from two species of *Eucalyptus*. *Phytotherapy Research* 21 (2007): 231–3.

Satchell, Andrew C., Anne Saurajen, Craig Bell, and Ross St. C. Barnetson. Treatment of interdigital tinea pedis with 25% and 50% tea tree oil solution: A randomized, placebo-controlled, blinded study. *Australasian Journal of Dermatology* 43 no. 3 (2002): 175–8.

Schuhmacher, A., Jürgen Reichling, and Paul Schnitzler. Virucidal effect of peppermint oil on the enveloped viruses herpes simplex virus type 1 and type 2 in vitro. *Phytomedicine* 10 (2003): 504–10.

Schwiertz, Andreas, C. Duttke, J. Hild, and Hanne J. Muller. In vitro activity of essential oils on microorganisms isolated from vaginal infections. *International Journal of Aromatherapy* 16 (2006): 169–74.

Sessa, Rosa, Marisa Di Pietro, Fiorenzo De Santis, Simone Filardo, Rino Ragno, and Letizia Angiolella. Effects of *Mentha suaveolens* essential oil on *Chlamydia trachomatis*. *Biomed Research International* (2015): Article ID 508071. doi: dx.doi.org /10.1155/2015/508071.

Sherry, Eugene, and Patrick Warnke. Successful use of an inhalational phytochemical to treat pulmonary tuberculosis: A case report. *Phytomedicine* 11 (2004): 95–7.

Simbar, Masoumeh, Zohreh Azarbad, Faraz Mojab and Hamid Alavi Majd. A comparative study of the therapeutic effects of the *Zataria multiflora* vaginal cream and metronidazole vaginal gel on bacterial vaginosis. *Phytomedicine* 15 (2008): 1025–31.

Simin, Nataša, Marija Lesjak, Petar Knezević et al. Synergistic effect of selected essential oils against *Helicobacter pylori*. In *International Symposium: Natural Products and Drug Discovery—Future Perspectives*, Vienna, Austria, November 13–14, 2014, p. 57.

Solórzano-Santos, Fortino, and Maria Guadalupe Miranda-Novales. Essential oils from aromatic herbs as antimicrobial agents. *Current Opinion in Biotechnology* 23 no. 2 (2012): 136–41.

Somani, Jyoti, Vinod B. Bhullar, Kimberly A. Workowski, Carol E. Farshy, and Carolyn M. Black. Multiple drug-resistant *Chlamydia trachomatis* associated with clinical treatment failure. *Journal of Infectious Diseases* 181 (2000): 1421–7.

Soper, David. Trichomoniasis: Under control or undercontrolled? *American Journal of Obstetrics and Gynecology* 190 (2004): 281–90.

Stanley, Margaret A. Genital human papillomavirus infections: Current and prospective therapies. *Journal of General Virology* 93 (2012): 681–91.

Stein, Raimund, Hasan S. Dogan, Piet Hoebeke et al. 2015. Urinary tract infections in children: EAU/ESPU guidelines. *European Urology* 67 no. 3 (2015): 546–58.

Stothers, Lynn. Cranberry and other dietary supplements for the treatment of urinary tract infections in aging women. In *Complementary and Alternative Therapies and the Aging Population*, 179–91. Oxford: Academic Press, 2009.

Tampieri, Maria P.A., Roberta Galuppi, Fabio Macchioni et al. The inhibition of *Candida albicans* by selected essential oils and their major components. *Mycopathologia* 159 (2005): 339–45.

Teixeira, Bárbara, António Marques, Cristina Ramos et al. 2013. Chemical composition and antibacterial and antioxidant properties of commercial essential oils. *Industrial Crops and Products* 43 no. 1 (2013): 587–95.

Tohidpour, Abolghasem, Morteza Sattari, Reza Omidbaigi, Abbas Yadegar, and Javad Nazemi. Antibacterial effect of essential oils from two medicinal plants against methicillin-resistant *Staphylococcus aureus* (MRSA). *Phytomedicine* 17 (2010): 142–5.

Tong, Melinda M., Phillip M. Altman, and Ross St. C. Barnetson. Tea tree oil in the treatment of tinea pedis. *Australasian Journal of Dermatology* 33 no. 3 (1992): 145–9.

Van Vuuren, Sandy F., Guy P.P. Kamatou, and Alvaro M. Viljoen. Volatile composition and antimicrobial activity of twenty commercial frankincense essential oil samples. *South African Journal of Botany* 76 no. 4 (2010): 686–91.

Vigan, Martine. Essential oils: Renewal of interest and toxicity. *European Journal of Dermatology* 20 no. 6 (2010): 685–92.

Villar, David, M.J. Knight, Steven Hansen, and William Buck. Toxicity of *Melaleuca* oil and related essential oils applied topically on dogs and cats. *Veterinary and Human Toxicology* 36 (1994): 139–42.

Wang, Guangyi, Weiping Tang, and Robert R. Bidigare. Terpenoids as therapeutic drugs and pharmaceutical agents. In *Natural Products: Drug Discovery and Therapeutic Medicine*, ed. L. Zhang and Demain, 197–227. Totowa, NJ: Humana Press, 2005.

Wannissorn, Bhusita, Siripen Jarikasem, Thammathad Siriwangchai, and Sirinun Thubthimthed. Antibacterial properties of essential oils from Thai medicinal plants. *Fitoterapia* 76 no. 2 (2005): 233–6.

Warnke, Patrick H., Stephan T. Becker, Rainer Podschun et al. The battle against multi-resistant strains: Renaissance of antimicrobial essential oils as a promising force to fight hospital-acquired infections. *Journal of Cranio-Maxillofacial Surgery* 37 (2009): 392–7.

Warnke, Patrick H., Alexander J.S. Lott, Eugene Sherry, Joerg Wiltfang, and Rainer Podschun. The ongoing battle against multi-resistant strains: In-vitro inhibition of hospital-acquired MRSA, VRE, pseudomonas, ESBL *E. coli* and *Klebsiella* species in the presence of plant-derived antiseptic oils. *Journal of Cranio-Maxillofacial Surgery* 41 no. 4 (2013): 321–6.

Weir, Erica. Bacterial vaginosis: More questions than answers. *Canadian Medical Association Journal* 171 (2004): 448.

World Health Organization. Global incidence and prevalence of selected curable sexually transmitted infections: Overview and estimates. Geneva, Switzerland: WHO, 2001.

Wotherspoon, Andrew C., Carlos Ortiz-Hidalgo, Mary R. Falzon, and Peter G. Isaacson. *Helicobacter pylori*-associated gastritis and primary B-cell gastric lymphoma. *Lancet* 338 (1991): 1175–6.

Wu, Qiao-Feng, Wei Wang, Xiao-Yan Dai et al. Chemical compositions and anti-influenza activities of essential oils from *Mosla dianthera*. *Journal of Ethnopharmacology* 139 (2012): 668–71.

Zai-Chang, Yang, Wang Bo-Chu, Yang Xiao-Sheng, and Wang Qiang. Chemical composition of the volatile oil from *Cynanchum stauntonii* and its activities of anti-influenza virus. *Colloids and Surfaces B: Biointerfaces* 43 (2005): 198–202.

Zanetti, Stefania, Sara Cannas, Paola Molicotti et al. Evaluation of the antimicrobial properties of the essential oil of *Myrtus communis* L. against clinical strains of *Mycobacterium* spp. *Interdisciplinary Perspectives on Infectious Diseases* 2010 (2010): 1–3.

Zaouali, Yosr, Taroub Bouzaine, and Mohamed Boussaid. Essential oils composition in two *Rosmarinus officinalis* L. varieties and incidence for antimicrobial and antioxidant activities. *Food and Chemical Toxicology* 48 no. 11 (2010): 3144–52.

Zenati, Fatima, Fethi Benbelaid, Abdelmounaim Khadir, Chafika Bellahsene, and Mourad Bendahou. Antimicrobial effects of three essential oils on multidrug resistant bacteria responsible for urinary infections. *Journal of Applied Pharmaceutical Science* 4 no. 11 (2014): 15–8.

Zhao, Chunzhen, Jianbo Sun, Chunyan Fang, and Fadi Tang. 1,8-Cineol attenuates LPS-induced acute pulmonary inflammation in mice. *Inflammation* 37 (2014): 566–72.

Zonyane, S., Sandy Freda Reda Van Vuuren, and Nokwanda P. Makunga. Antimicrobial interactions of Khoi-San poly-herbal remedies with emphasis on the combination: *Agathosma crenulata*, *Dodonaea viscosa* and *Eucalyptus globulus*. *Journal of Ethnopharmacology* 148 no. 1 (2013): 144–51.

Section V

Regulatory Issues

20 Regulatory Issues in Aromatherapy

Gioacchino Calapai

CONTENTS

20.1 INTRODUCTION

Essential oils have been described as "the volatile, organic constituents of fragrant plant matter and contribute to both flavor and fragrance and are extracted either by distillation or by cold pressing (expression)" (Tisserand and Balacs, 1995). Physician Avicenna (Abu Ali al-Hussein Ibn Abdallah Ibn Sina, 980–1037) from Persia invented the process of distillation, starting the history of the distillation of essential oils (Tisserand, 1988). Frenchman René Maurice Gattefossé, in the 1920s, coined the term *aromatherapy*; aromatherapy is today considered a subcategory of herbal medicine (or phytotherapy). Since the 1980s, the popularity of aromatherapy has widely increased in the Western world. Aromatherapy encompasses the use of essential oils derived from different types of plant sources for a variety of applications. Generally, the whole fresh plant (not crushed or powdered) is used for the essential oil distillation process.

Most commonly, essential oils are applied topically in diluted forms; other times they are applied with a carrier oil as part of massage therapy to manipulate the soft tissue of the body, or by using an incense burner for inhalation of the aroma. Oils may be inhaled by adding a few drops to steaming water; thereafter, an atomizer or humidifier spreads the aroma throughout the room. Certain essential oils are also ingested through teas, whereas others can be added to bathwater or pillows, or used to make ointments, creams, and compresses. Some aromatherapists argue that the use of certain herbs in food can also be considered part of aromatherapy (Boehm et al., 2012).

A specific policy for aromatherapy does not exist in the European Union or United States. For this reason, from the regulatory point of view, health professionals working in the field of aromatherapy should refer to the regulatory framework for herbal medicine.

20.2 REGULATORY ISSUES

The practice of aromatherapy is currently an unregulated and unlicensed field. This situation reflects the practice of aromatherapy as well as the manufacture of aromatherapy products. As a whole, the industry seeks to comply with current safety and standards of practice and to stay informed about potential impending regulations with regards to manufacturing aromatherapy-based products.

Aromatherapy is generally an unlicensed profession in most parts of the world. For this reason, many practitioners obtain a license in other fields presenting an affinity with aromatherapy, for example, esthetics, naturopathy, and acupuncture. As regards the products, since in each country there is no legislation for products used in aromatherapy, they must be classified according to the most appropriate regulatory framework. It is the responsibility of companies that place any products on the market to correctly identify for themselves which laws apply to their products. It is noteworthy that generally, in the legislation of various countries, whether a product is a cosmetic or a drug under the law is determined by its intended use. Worldwide, different laws and regulations apply to each type of product (Miroddi et al., 2013).

20.2.1 HERBAL MEDICINAL PRODUCTS

In the United States, herbal medicinal products can be prescription drugs or over-the-counter drugs. Categorization of herbal medicinal products is based on intended use, safety, regulatory status, and degree of characterization (Schmidt et al., 2008). Obtaining a license for the market requires rigorous testing, including three distinct phases of clinical testing to ensure safety and efficacy, and close scrutiny by the Food and Drug Administration (FDA). About 25% of the licensed drugs in the United States are based on plant-derived products (Regulation EC No. 1924/2006). Pure compounds isolated from plants and subjected to the same testing as synthetic pharmaceuticals can be licensed as conventional drugs (Butler, 2004).

Guidelines for registration of botanical drugs in the United States were released in 2004. Herbal medicinal products are evaluated for safety and clinical efficacy, just as conventional drugs are; however, the process for authorization of market introduction of herbal medicinal products can be accelerated on the basis of the empiric knowledge of safety derived from data coming from observation in human use. To summarize, when licensed as drugs, herbal medicinal products are produced under the same strictly regulated conditions as conventional pharmaceuticals (Hasler, 2008; Schmidt et al., 2008). Many essential oils are considered by the FDA to be not only therapeutic but also safe and certified as generally recognized as safe (GRAS) or a food additive. *GRAS* is the term used by the FDA to define a chemical or substance added to food that has been evaluated by experts. GRAS substances are exempt from the usual food additive tolerance requirements. Essential oils, oleoresins (solvent-free), and natural extractives (including distillates) that are generally recognized as safe for their intended use by the FDA are listed on the FDA's website. In the European Union (EU), after years of commercialization of plants with medicinal properties through the food supplement market, the Directive 24/EC/2004 was delivered (came into force in April 2011). This legislation aimed to protect public health and secure the free movement of herbal products within the EU. It is the current policy regulating the use of herbal medicines in phytotherapy in European countries (Directive 2004/24/EEC). Directive 2004/24/EC establishes that "herbal medicines are any medicinal product exclusively containing, as active ingredients, one or more herbal substance, one or more herbal preparation or more such herbal substances in combination with one or more such herbal preparations." Directive 2004/24/EC defines what are herbal preparations, including essential oils, as follows: "Herbal preparations: preparations obtained by subjecting herbal substances to treatments such as extraction, distillation, expression, fractionation, purification, concentration or fermentation. These include comminuted or powdered herbal substances, tinctures, extracts, essential oils, expressed juices and processed exudates." Thus, according to this European directive, essential oils are fully considered herbal preparations. Consequently, essential oils showing medicinal properties and marketed as herbal medicinal products are subjected to the 24/EC/2004. This legislation amended the previous 2001/83/EC (Directive 2001/83/EC) by establishing that herbal medicinal products released in the market need authorization as well as drugs. However, authorization implies a simplified registration, delivered after undergoing an evaluation procedure with minor cost compared to that for synthetic drugs (Directive 2004/24/EEC). The 2004/24/EC establishes that in European countries, for the registration of herbal medicinal products, companies refer to one unique set of information on an herbal substance or herbal preparation purchased through the community monograph drawn by the ad hoc committee Herbal Medicinal Products Committee (HMPC) of the European Medicines Agency (EMA) (London). Community herbal monographs comprise the scientific opinion of the HMPC on safety and efficacy data concerning an herbal substance. For any single plant and each herbal preparation (including essential oils), the set of information contained in the monograph comprises clinical and safety aspects (Calapai and Caputi, 2007). The EMA delivered a reflection paper highlighting the aspects related to the nature and specific production processes of essential oils. In the reflection paper it declared that essential oils are considered active substances in herbal medicinal products (HMPs) for both human and veterinary use and in traditional herbal medicinal products (THMPs) for human use. According to the 2004/24/EC, essential oils are herbal preparations (EMA, 2014). In the United States, medicinal plants are categorized according to their intended use, safety, regulatory status, and degree of characterization. The FDA considers essential oils as either cosmetics or drugs, depending on their intended use. FDA decisions concerning the regulation of essential oils are made on a case-by-case basis according to the request of the applicant (Schmidt et al., 2008). Fragrance products based on essential oils are sometimes marketed with claims or implications that their use will improve personal well-being in a variety of ways, such as "strengthening the body's self-defense mechanisms." These are also known as behavioral fragrance or aromatherapy products. Traditionally, the FDA considered perfumes as cosmetics; the Federal Food, Drug, and Cosmetic Act (FD&C Act) defines cosmetics in part as articles intended to be applied to or introduced into the human body "for cleansing, beautifying, promoting attractiveness, or altering the appearance." Since products intended for use in the diagnosis, mitigation, treatment, or prevention of disease, and intended to affect the structure or any function of the body, are considered to be drugs by the FDA, this authority considers them new drugs requiring the FDA's premarket approval (FDA, 2014).

Drugs and cosmetics are both under the FDA's jurisdiction, but the legal requirements that apply to them differ. The claim that a perfume's aroma makes a person feel more attractive, in general, is considered a cosmetic claim and does not require FDA approval before the product is sold. But if a company advances an application requiring authorization for release in the market of a scent suggesting effectiveness as an aid to treat or prevent any condition or disease, or to affect the body's structure or function, such a claim may cause the product to be regulated as a drug, requiring premarket approval. The FDA makes decisions on a case-by-case basis. Advertising claims can be used to establish a product's intended use, and they are regulated by the Federal Trade Commission. Decisions on room fragrance systems (deodorizers and odor control) are the responsibility of the Consumer Products Safety Commission (FD&C Act, 2006). Products containing medicinal plants and licensed as drugs are prescription drugs or over-the-counter drugs. A license for these products requires rigorous evaluation, including the three distinct phases of clinical testing, to ensure safety and efficacy and close scrutiny by the FDA. In the United States, about 25% of the drugs used are based on plant-derived products; however, only pure compounds isolated from plants and subjected to the same rigorous evaluation as synthetic pharmaceuticals can be conventional drugs (Butler, 2004). The guidelines for registration of plant-derived drugs were released in 2004. Herbal medicinal product drugs are evaluated for safety and clinical efficacy under the same strictly regulated quality conditions as conventional drugs, but the process for them can be accelerated on the basis of the empiric knowledge of safety derived from observation in human use (Chinou et al., 2014).

20.2.2 Food Supplements

The use of medicinal plant products as food (or dietary) supplements comes from a long tradition where the consumption of herbal infusions, juices, elixirs, extracts, and essential oils had the objective to keep and promote health (Franz et al., 2011). In European legislation, the definition of *food* is contained in Regulation (EC) No. 178/2002. This law defines *food* (or *foodstuff*) as "any substance or product, whether processed, partially processed or unprocessed, intended to be, or reasonably expected to be ingested by humans." The definition of *food* includes drink (water included), chewing gum, and any other substance intentionally incorporated into the food during its manufacture, preparation or treatment (Regulation EC No. 178/2002).

Plant-derived products represent a principal ingredient, alone or in association with other substances, of dietary supplements. The food uses as supplements has been regulated by the Food Supplements Directive (FSD) 2002/46/EC, establishing the definition of *food supplements* as follows: "foodstuffs the purpose of which is to supplement the normal diet and which are concentrated sources of nutrients or other substances with a nutritional or physiological effect" (Directive 2002/46/EC). This definition expresses the concept that dietary supplements have no therapeutic function, whereas health-keeping functions are emphasized.

The food supplement context was further regulated through the delivery of "Regulation No. 1924/2006 of the European Parliament and of the Council of 20 December 2006 on Nutrition and Health Claims Made on Foods." It introduced the concept of *claim*, intended as "any message or representation which states, suggests or implies that a food has particular health characteristics." In this regulation, *health claim* has been defined as "any claim that states, suggests, or implies that a relationship exists between a food category, a food or one of its constituents and health." The aim of the regulation was to control the issue of intended health indications for food use through health claims. *Nutrition claims* (for products having nutritional properties) and *health claims* may be used in the labeling, presentation, and advertising of foods placed on the market in the EU only if they comply with the defined provisions. Use of a health claim needs to be authorized by the European Commission through the Standing Committee for Food Safety and Animal Health and a scientific assessment by the European Food Safety Authority (EFSA) to ensure that it is based on "generally-accepted scientific evidence, taking into account the totality of the available scientific data, and by weighing the evidence" (Regulation EC No. 1924/2006).

On the basis of exclusive support for physiological functions of food, this policy points out that claims have to recall the health-keeping and nontherapeutic role of food supplements. Regulation establishes that claims are also accepted in the case of "reduction of disease risk claims" intended as "any health claim that states, suggests or implies that the consumption of a food category, a food or one of its constituents significantly reduces a risk factor in the development of a human disease." To obtain authorization for a claim, companies have to produce an application to the member states, to accept or not according to the EFSA decisions. Whether available data for each claim are sufficient to substantiate the claim (on the basis of accepted scientific evidence) is a decision based on the scientific judgment of the EFSA. The EFSA makes a decision about the use of a claim after an accurate examination of the relevant scientific literature corroborating the requested claim (Silano et al., 2011).

In recent years, health claims for botanical products have become a crucial issue, since authorization of the great part of claims proposed for food supplements has been refused by the EFSA. Following this decision, strong criticism has been raised by companies, asking and suggesting for a softer regulatory approach. In particular, the objection is that it may be more difficult for consumers to fully understand, in the absence of health claims, the benefits, if any, associated with the consumption of a product (Silano et al., 2011).

Different rules in plant-derived products between Europe and the United States exist. Food supplements were previously defined in the United States by the Dietary Supplement Health and Education Act (DSHEA), released in 1994, as products taken by mouth that contain a dietary ingredient intended to supplement the diet. The DSHEA changed the marketing and legal climate for dietary supplements and herbs and enabled the exponential growth of product sales since that time. As defined by the DSHEA, a dietary supplement is a product other than tobacco that is intended to supplement the diet and contains one of the following dietary ingredients: a vitamin, a mineral, an herb or other botanical, an amino acid, a dietary substance to supplement the diet by increasing the total daily intake, or a concentrate, metabolite, constituent, extract, or combination of these ingredients (Cassileth et al., 2009).

The Nutrition Labeling and Education Act of 1990 gives the U.S. FDA the authority to regulate health claims on food labels (Nutrition Labeling and Education Act, 1990). The Nutrition Labeling and Education Act permits the use of health claims if there is evidence to support the claim and significant scientific agreement among qualified experts about the claim, and if the claim is not misleading. The FDA Modernization Act of 1997 permits manufacturers to use health claims based on authoritative statements by a scientific body of the U.S. government, such as the National Institutes of Health (FDA Modernization Act of 1997).

Three categories of claims can currently be used on food and dietary supplement labels in the United States: (1) health claims, (2) nutritional content claims, and (3) structure–function claims. Structure–function claims were authorized under the Dietary Supplement Health and Education Act of 1994 and describe the effect of a dietary supplement on the structure or function of the body. Health claims are authorized by the FDA only after a systematic review of scientific evidence (Hasler, 2008). Only studies conducted in healthy populations are considered, because health claims are directed to the general population or designated subgroups (e.g., elderly persons) and are intended to assist the consumer in maintaining healthful dietary practices. Health claims are limited to claims about risk reduction and cannot be about the diagnosis, cure, mitigation, or treatment of disease. The FDA exerts its oversight in determining, by means of the following acts, which nutritional content claims may be used on a label or in labeling: (1) the Nutrition Labeling and Education Act (NLEA) of 1990, by issuing a regulation authorizing a nutritional content claim, and (2) the FDA Modernization Act of 1997, by prohibiting or modifying by regulation a nutritional content claim. The NLEA required that the FDA issue regulations for authorizing the use of a health claim about a substance–disease relationship only when the significant scientific agreement standard was met (Ellwood et al., 2010).

In the United States, companies are responsible for the safety of their products and food supplements, including those containing botanicals, which do not need approval from the FDA before commercialization. Only in the case of the market introduction of new ingredients does legislation require a report including safety but not efficacy data. In conclusion, botanical products are generally sold in the United States as food supplements, with no particular authorization needed for their release in the market, but companies have to show the truthfulness of their claims (FDA, Qualified Health Claims, 2013).

20.3   CONCLUSIONS

Even though aromatherapy is not officially recognized as a single medical discipline, as it is for most clinical practices of herbal medicine (or phytotherapy), products containing essential oils are regulated by policy on plant-derived product introduction in the market. Essential oils are widely used as fragrances and flavorings in the cosmetic and food sectors. Usage within the pharmaceutical sector represents, in many cases, only a limited proportion of the commercial market. For these reasons, as above described, from a regulatory standpoint, essential oils present a number of particular issues similar to those of atypical substances when they are used as active pharmaceutical ingredients.

DISCLAIMER

Since 2008, G. Calapai has been one of the co-opted members of the Herbal Medicinal Products Committee of the European Medicines Agency (EMA) (London). For this reason, since this chapter is related to his work in EMA, according to the EMA policy on scientific publications, the following disclaimer is added: "The views expressed in this chapter are the personal views of the author and may not be understood or quoted as being made on behalf of or reflecting the position of the European Medicines Agency or one of its committees or working parties."

REFERENCES

Boehm, K., Bussing, A., and Ostermann, T. Aromatherapy as an Adjuvant Treatment in Cancer Care: A Descriptive Systematic Review. *Afr J Tradit Complement Altern Med* 9, 4 (2012): 503–18.

Butler, M.S. The role of natural product chemistry in drug discovery. *J Nat Prod* 67, 12 (2004): 2141–53.

Calapai, G., and Caputi, A.P. Herbal Medicines: Can We Do without Pharmacologist? *Evid Based Complement Alternat Med* 4, Suppl 1 (2007): 41–3.

Cassileth, B.R., Heitzer, M., and Wesa, K. The Public Health Impact of Herbs and Nutritional Supplements. *Pharm Biol* 47, 8 (2009): 761–7.

Chinou, I., Knoess, W., and Calapai, G. Regulation of Herbal Medicinal Products in the EU: An Up-to-date scientific review. *Phytochem Rev* 13 (2014): 539–45.

Ellwood, K.C., Trumbo, P.R., and Kavanaugh, C.J. How the US Food and Drug Administration Evaluates the Scientific Evidence for Health Claims. *Nutr Rev* 68, 2 (2010): 114–21.

FDA. 2014. http://www.fda.gov/Cosmetics/GuidanceRegulation/LawsRegulations/ucm074201 .htm (accessed July 30, 2015).

Franz, C., Chizzola, R., Novak, J., and Sponza, S. Botanical Species Being Used for Manufacturing Plant Food Supplements (PFS) and Related Products in the EU Member States and Selected Third Countries. *Food Funct* 2, 12 (2011): 720–30.

Hasler, C.M. Health Claims in the United States: An Aid to the Public or a Source of Confusion? *J Nutr* 138, 6 (2008): 1216S–20S.

Miroddi, M., Mannucci, C., Mancari, F., Navarra M., and Calapai, G. Research and Development for Botanical Products in Medicinals and Food Supplements Market. *Evid Based Complement Alternat Med* 2013 (2013): 649720.

Nutrition Labeling and Education Act. Public Law 101-535, U.S. Code Title 104, Section 2353, 1990.

Reflection Paper on Quality of Essential Oils as Active Substances in Herbal Medicinal Products/Traditional Herbal Medicinal Products. European Medicines Agency (EMA). http://www.ema.europa.eu/docs/en_GB/document_library/Scientific_guideline /2014/05/WC500166019.pdf (accessed July 7, 2014).

Regulation. Directive 2001/83/EC of the European Parliament and of the Council of November 6, 2001 on the Community Code Relating to Medicinal Products for Human Use. http://ec.europa.eu/health/files/eudralex/vol-1/dir_2001_83_consol_2012/dir_2001 _83_cons_2012_en.pdf (accessed July 7, 2014).

Regulation. Directive 2002/46/EC of 10 June 2002 on the Approximation of the Laws of the Member States Relating to Food Supplements. *Off J Eur Commun* L183 (2002): 51–57.

Regulation. Directive 2004/24/EEC of the European Parliament and of the Council of March 31, 2004 Amending, as Regards Traditional Herbal Medicinal Products, Directive 2001/83/EC on Community Code Relating to Medicinal Products for Human Use. *Off J Eur Commun* L136 (2004): 85–90.

Regulation. EC No. 178/2002 of the European Parliament and of the Council of January 28, 2002 Laying Down the General Principles and Requirements of Food Law, Establishing the European Food Safety Authority and Laying Down Procedures in Matters of Food Safety. *Off J Eur Commun* L31 (2002): 1–24.

Regulation. EC No. 1924/2006 of the European Parliament and of the Council of December 20, 2006 on Nutrition and Health Claims Made on Foods. *Off J Eur Union* (2007): 3–18.

Schmidt, B., Ribnicky D.M., Poulev A., Logendra S., Cefalu, W.T., and Raskin, I. A Natural History of Botanical Therapeutics. *Metabolism* 57 (2008): S3–9.

Silano, V., Coppens, P., Larranaga-Guetaria, A., Minghetti, P., and Roth-Ehrang, R. Regulations Applicable to Plant Food Supplements and Related Products in the European Union. *Food Funct* 2, 12 (2011): 710–9.

Tisserand, R. Essential Oils as Psychotherapeutic Agents. In S. Van Toller and G.H. Dodd (eds.), *Perfumery: The Psychology and Biology of Fragrance*. New York: Chapman & Hall 1988, pp. 167–80.

Tisserand, R., and Balacs, T. *Essential Oil Safety*. London: Churchill Livingstone, 1995.

U.S. Federal Food, Drug, and Cosmetic Act (FD&C Act). 2006. http://www.fda.gov/Regulatory Information/Legislation/FederalFoodDrugandCosmeticActFDCAct/default.htm (accessed July 7, 2014).

U.S. Food and Drug Administration (FDA). FDA Modernization Act of 1997 (FDAMA) Claims. http://www.fda.gov/RegulatoryInformation/Legislation/FederalFoodDrug andCosmeticActFDCAct/SignificantAmendmentstotheFDCAct/FDAMA/FullTextof FDAMAlaw/default.htm (accessed July 7, 2014).

U.S. Food and Drug Administration (FDA). Essential Oils, Oleoresins (Solvent-Free), and Natural Extractives (including Distillates). Code of Federal Regulations (CFR) Title 21, Section 182.20. Revised April 1, 2013. http://www.accessdata.fda.gov/scripts/cdrh /cfdocs/cfcfr/CFRSearch.cfm?fr=182.20 (accessed July 7, 2014).

U.S. Food and Drug Administration (FDA). Qualified Health Claims. 2013. http://www.fda .gov/food/ingredientspackaginglabeling/labelingnutrition/ucm2006877.htm (accessed July 7, 2014).

21 Pharmacovigilance and Phytovigilance for a Safe Use of Essential Oils

Alfredo Vannacci, Alessandra Pugi, Eugenia Gallo, Fabio Firenzuoli, and Alessandro Mugelli

CONTENTS

21.1 SURVEILLANCE SYSTEM OF DRUGS AND HERBAL MEDICINES

Preclinical and clinical studies have some limitations in the definition of the safety profile of a new drug. Information collected during these studies is incomplete for a variety of reasons. It is well known that animal tests are insufficiently predictive of human safety, and that clinical trials are affected by qualitative and quantitative limitations regarding the identification of possible adverse drug reactions (ADRs). From a quantitative perspective, clinical trials enroll a limited number of patients for a limited observational period, not sufficient to identify rare events. Study samples may also differ from population patients who are prescribed the drug in clinical practice. In clinical trials, patients are selected according to narrow inclusion and exclusion criteria, and since special groups are not often represented, insufficient information on them is provided. Finally, several conditions of use of the study drug may differ from clinical practice, among them the physiological status of the patients, presence of comorbidity, and polytherapy. Hence, the full safety profile of medicinal products can be fully appreciated only after the drugs have been placed on the market. It is therefore necessary, from a public health perspective, to complement the data available at the time of authorization with additional safety data that will only be available during the postmarketing phase.

In this frame, pharmacovigilance is defined as the science and activities relating to the detection, assessment, and prevention of adverse reactions to drugs currently available on the market. The major aims of a pharmacovigilance system are the early detection of unknown ADRs, the detection of an increased frequency of ADRs, the identification of risk factors for ADRs, and the dissemination of information on drugs' benefit–risks profiles to healthcare professionals and patients. The mainstay of a pharmacovigilance system is spontaneous reporting, which is the most cost-effective tool for drug safety evaluation in the postmarketing period. The suspicion of an ADR, meaning that there is at least a reasonable possibility of a causal relationship between a drug and an adverse event, should be a sufficient reason for reporting.

According to the new European legislation of pharmacovigilance (Directive 2010/84/EU), adopted in December 2010, the long-standing definition of *adverse reaction* was amended to also cover noxious and unintended effects. Presently, the term *adverse reaction* includes not only the effects derived from the authorized use of a medicinal product at normal doses, but also those from medication errors and uses outside the terms of the marketing authorization (off-label use), including misuse and abuse of the medicinal product.

The ultimate goal of pharmacovigilance is the identification of new risks or risks that have changed, with the aim of a better definition of the risk–benefit balance. The continuous monitoring of drug safety ensures that the benefit–risk ratio is always favorable for patient populations. Data derived from surveillance activities may impact regulatory decision making. In particular, the retrieved safety information may lead to labeling changes (e.g., warnings, precautions, and updated adverse reaction lists), enhanced pharmacovigilance activities (e.g., additional surveillance, registries, and observational studies), safety communications, prescribing actions (e.g., restricted use), or drug withdrawal from the market.

The use of herbal medicines (HMs) has grown enormously in Western countries in the past few decades and continues to expand rapidly across the world. According to the World Health Organization (WHO) definition, HMs include herbs, herbal materials, herbal preparations, and finished herbal products that contain as active ingredients parts of plants, other plant materials, or combinations; surveillance activity typical of pharmacovigilance is therefore extended to all those products (http://www.who.int/medicines/areas/traditional/definitions/en/).

Safety and efficacy, as well as quality control, of HMs have become important concerns for both health authorities and the public. Although HMs are often promoted as being safer than conventional drugs because they are deemed natural, they are not devoid of adverse reactions (ARs).

The need to monitor the possible ARs to HMs, in order to better understand their possible harms, led to the birth of a surveillance system of HMs. At the beginning of the twenty-first century, WHO published guidelines for pharmacovigilance of HMs to support the member states in strengthening or developing national monitoring programs of HMs. In this way, pharmacovigilance practices and tools previously developed for pharmaceutical medicines were extended to the HMs. As with conventional drugs, spontaneous reporting is essential for the notification of ARs by all healthcare professionals and, in some countries, consumers. A case report form should contain all information needed for the assessment of the case. In particular, the report should include elements related to the patient (age, sex, ethnic group, and medical history, if relevant), the adverse reaction (description, clinical investigation, start date, and outcome), and suspected products (name, active substance, manufacturer, dose, route of administration, period of assumption, and indication for use), for concomitant drugs, as well as other products or conditions. Health authorities should provide the report and make it easily available. Once filled out, healthcare professionals or consumers should submit the report to the national authorities, which finally forward it to the WHO Collaborating Center for International Drug Monitoring in Uppsala. The reporting of a suspected AR means that the reporter does not have the certainty of an association between the HM and the observed event, but only a suspicion. The causality is assessed on a case-by-case manner by the reporting centers.

Spontaneous reporting systems have some limitations that make it difficult to establish causality assessment and, more importantly, may cause an underestimation of the size of the problem, thus determining a lack of knowledge of a HM's safety profile. The most relevant limitations are the poor quality of some reports due to the lack of information and the widespread underreporting rate, which is likely to be greater for HMs than for conventional drugs. Because HMs are generally considered safe, consumers may not associate their use with the occurrence of ARs; they commonly fail to mention the use of such products to their physician or the use of other drugs to the providers of HMs. Many other reasons, such as fear of litigation, unawareness of the surveillance system, indifference, and lack of time, make healthcare professionals reluctant to report ARs for both drugs and HMs.

In the field of HMs, important issues regard the inadequate regulatory measures. Different from conventional drugs, many HMs are not licensed as prescription medicines, being instead merchandised as over-the-counter medications or dietary supplements. Hence, their quality, efficacy, and safety may not be properly assessed and evaluated by health authorities, and unfortunately, many products containing herbs do not require any medical prescription or supervision. Furthermore, in most European countries, the procedure for marketing authorization of dietary supplements is based on a simple notification system, with the lack of an exhaustive control on these kinds of products. Moreover, dietary supplement producers may autonomously decide what information (i.e., safety information and contraindications) should be present on the label and what should be omitted. As a consequence, some labels may be unclear, incomplete, or even omit plants or other xenobiotics actually present in the product. Similarly, some aromatherapy products are not subject to licensing regulation unless they are marketed as medicinal products. Finally, HMs are largely available to the public through uncontrolled distribution channels, such as websites, supermarkets, and vitamin stores, significantly contributing to their uncontrolled use. All these issues may pose a risk of ARs or interactions to consumers and must be taken into account in a surveillance system.

21.1.1   CLASSIFICATION OF ADVERSE REACTIONS TO DRUGS AND HERBAL MEDICINES

All medicinal products comprising HMs may potentially cause unexpected ARs. The ARs related to the use of HMs arise from the intrinsic toxicity of the plant, herb–drug or herb–herb interactions, or may be attributable to either poor product quality (presence of contaminants and adulterants) or improper use or prescription. Finally, the occurrence of ARs can be influenced by the consumer's status, such as age, gender, genetic predisposition, current disease, and treatment.

The classification of ARs proposed by Edwards and Aronson (2000) for conventional medicines can be equally applied to the HMs. According to them, ARs are classified as follows:

- Type A (augmented): Dose-related, predictable, and high-frequency reactions. Type A events are common because they are related to the principal or secondary pharmacological actions of the active compounds; the majority of cases are not serious and can be solved by reducing the dose or withdrawing the product.
- Type B (bizarre): Usually immunological and idiosyncratic-like reactions with a high risk of lethality. The unexpected effects are related to the pharmacological actions of the active compounds and are not dose dependent; therefore, they are difficult to predict. The causal relationship between the HMs and the ARs mainly depends on the time of onset. A future exposure to the drug should be avoided.
- Type C (chronic): Dose- and time-related events. The chronic use of some products may induce or contribute to the onset of new illness. The late onset of the reaction often makes the evaluation and identification of this kind of drug- or HM-related event difficult.
- Type D (delayed): Delayed events are usually dose related. They occur or become apparent some time after the use of the drug (i.e., teratogenesis or carcinogenesis). This kind of AR is not usually identified during clinical trials because it requires a long time to appear; for the same reason, it is often difficult to assess the causality role of the drug or HM.
- Type E (end): Uncommon reactions occurring after withdrawal of the drug. Some conditions, such as the sudden stop of drug administration, longtime therapy, and a short half-life of the drug, are required.
- Type F (failure): The unexpected failure of therapy is relatively common and often dose related. A common cause of type F reactions is drug interactions; therefore, it is necessary to consider a dose adjustment of the drug and the concomitant therapy.

With regard to HMs, ARs can also be classified as intrinsic or extrinsic effects. Intrinsic effects can be due to the composition of HMs and therefore to their pharmacological and toxicological properties. Generally, herbs can induce type A and B (predictable and unpredictable) reactions. Plants contain numerous chemical compounds, which may differ in the considered parts of the plant and may also vary in content and concentration, depending on several factors (climate, growing and storage conditions, time of harvest, and processing). For these reasons, it is difficult to ascribe events determined by complex HMs to a specific component of the products.

Finally, extrinsic effects are not related to the HMs themselves, but rather to issues in the manufacturing processes. For this reason, the lack of a proper regulation ensuring adherence to good manufacturing practices may result in poor quality products. The consequences may be different and range from a lack of standardization, contamination, substitution, and adulteration to incorrect or inappropriate preparation or labeling.

21.2 SPECIFIC PHARMACOVIGILANCE ISSUES OF HERBAL MEDICINES AND ESSENTIAL OILS

21.2.1 SAFETY ISSUES OF HERBAL MEDICINES

Although the efficacy of several medicinal herb products has been proved in different conditions, in some cases their safety profile is still questionable. Plants should be considered containers of many chemical entities with potential pharmacological activities, but not devoid of toxicological ones. Therefore, the use and management of such therapeutic tools should not be entrusted only to patient self-care. As with any other kind of therapy, we should always keep in mind the possibility of side effects, contraindications, drug interactions, and so forth. Even if some people still believe that products based on medicinal herbs are safe because they are natural, the use of many plants or plant extracts can induce adverse reactions caused by their very active principles. In addition, herbal products may interact with conventional therapies, resulting in serious adverse reactions.

The popularity of herbal medicines, deriving from the general opinion that they are safe and harmless, and therefore preferable to conventional drugs (Everett et al., 2005), may lead to different consequences: the rate of disclosure of herb use to clinicians is often poor, and herbal products are self-administered and often concurrent with prescribed medications, which may pose a risk of clinically relevant interactions to patients (Loman, 2003; McCan, 2006; Beshop, 2010). That is the reason why clinicians should investigate the use of herbal products during their routine clinical assessment, contextually informing their patients about possible risks and benefits. On the contrary, probably due to a lack of specific training, many doctors underestimate the use of herbal medicines and are not able to detect side effects associated with their use.

21.2.2 PHYTOVIGILANCE

Phytovigilance is the discipline that assesses the risk associated with the use of herbal products through the monitoring of adverse reactions. As with pharmacovigilance, its main instrument is spontaneous reporting, namely, the report by a healthcare professional or a citizen of the occurrence of an adverse reaction to herbal remedies. Since serious adverse reactions are often related to improper use of herbal remedies, lack of medical surveillance, or use in high-risk situations (children, elderly, and pregnancy), the proper use of herbal remedies should always be monitored by a doctor or an expert pharmacist.

Several factors may influence the risk of experiencing adverse events determined by herbal products. They are discussed in the following sections.

21.2.2.1 Type of Preparation

Herbal remedies can be prepared using the drug as it is, crushed and reduced to powder, or in the form of a crude extract, that is, an extract not undergoing additional processes (purification or concentration) after extraction. These products are unlikely to cause severe adverse reactions, if properly used.

Instead, when herbal remedies are prepared from concentrated extracts, purified, or enriched in active ingredients, the risk of adverse reaction increases. This is particularly true for essential oils, which in many cases are the richest possible form of plant extract, in terms of active principles.

As a general rule, concentrated and purified extracts are more toxic than raw ones. Of course, a treatment's safety also depends on the dose and frequency of dosing: higher doses and longer treatment courses increase the frequency and seriousness of side effects.

21.2.2.2 Contamination and Adulteration

In some cases, even when herbal products are used in the most appropriate mode, adverse reactions can still occur due to the presence in the final product of botanical, chemical, or microbiological contaminants. Such contamination may arise from accidental causes, such as the collection of the wrong plants with respect to those required, for a preparation error, or from deliberate adulteration. Several studies have, for example, shown that herbal products can contain conventional medications and hormonal substances (Vannacci et al., 2009; Gallo et al., 2012).

21.2.2.3 Patient Issues

The possibility for an herbal product to cause adverse reactions depends not only on the product itself, but also on the patient status. In some cases, patients may be at risk of developing adverse effects for reasons of age, sex, weight, neuroendocrine state, or particular physiological conditions (pregnancy, breastfeeding, etc.). For example, some essential oils with expectorant and antiseptic features may be irritating to the digestive tract (elderly and children) or even induce seizures (children). Children in particular may be highly sensitive to the effects of even low doses of concentrated plant extracts and may also be deficient in the ability to metabolize chemicals. Elderly people also show a higher risk of developing adverse reactions, mainly the risk of interactions with concurrent drug treatment and reduced detoxifying functions of the liver and kidney. Furthermore, herbal remedies are often used during pregnancy and lactation, even if no adequate study on the use of these products in those circumstances is available (Lapi et al., 2010), as well as in high-risk conditions such as in the perioperatory period (Lucenteforte et al., 2012).

21.2.2.4 Indirect Risks

Finally, herbal treatments practiced by a patient suffering from a serious disease, without professional counseling, may lead to the risk that an effective therapeutic approach is reduced, delayed, or replaced by a therapy whose efficacy is not known. This risk was recently increased by the abundance of misleading medical information on the web, with the possibility of buying herbal products over the Internet that may vary from harmless plants to dangerous ones (Maggini et al., 2013b).

21.2.3 SAFE USE OF ESSENTIAL OILS

Since medieval times, essential oils have been widely used and are known for their potential therapeutic activities; in particular, they are known to exert antibacterial, antiviral, fungicide, pesticide, and insecticide actions. By means of their medicinal properties and fragrance, essential oils are used in the fields of both cosmetics and healthcare, as well as in food industries for food conservation.

21.2.4 REGULATORY ISSUES

Essential oils are not marketed as drugs; they generally lack indications, safety data, and instructions for correct use; and they are therefore sometimes wrongly assumed by patients with the purpose of self-medication. Active ingredients are often highly concentrated, and this also explains their high toxicological potential. They can cause serious food poisonings even in small doses (5–10 ml) by acting on the gastrointestinal apparatus, cardiovascular system, kidneys, liver, and central nervous system.

From a regulatory point of view, it must be noted that essential oils are difficult to classify; for this reason, commercially available preparations usually belong to very different categories: foods, food supplements, air fresheners, perfumes, cosmetics, insect repellents, and others. For the same reason, many products are also inadequately labeled, presenting usually just a simple descriptive phrase, including the term *essential oil* or a fantasy name (such as "Essence of the Gnomes").

Lack of regulations for product marketing, lack of consumer information, and lack of in-depth studies on the safe use of essential oils, together with the heterogeneity of preparations available on the market, can be a cause of confusion and incorrect use of these products.

Although regulation is slightly different in different countries, a common ground should be defined: the label of an essential oil should clearly report the intended use (aroma, dietary supplement, cosmetic, fragrance, etc.), together with a clear indication of its functions and manner of use.

The poor regulation and the scarce controls of the natural products market is unfortunately one of the main causes leading consumers toward wrong use of essential oils, exposing them to a significant risk of poisoning. Some labels do not even clearly state if the product should be used externally or taken internally, leading to possible intoxications, with some essential oils with high concentrations of active ingredients that can be toxic even if ingested in small amounts. An overdose of these oils, whose therapeutic index is very low, can produce severe toxic consequences, especially on the gastrointestinal, genitourinary, cardiovascular, and central nervous systems. As a general rule, oral administration is highly discouraged in early childhood, pregnancy, lactation, and patients with liver or kidney failure.

Very relevant is the lack of clear legislation for the definition, use, production, marketing, and safety of essential oils; currently, information provided to buyers is scarce and uncertain, with consumers often fully relying on the false myth of the natural product that does not cause any kind of damage.

The European Medicines Agency (EMA) included some essential oils among the monographs of species that can be used in humans, indicating the recommended route of administration and dosage, but without specifying the need to dilute a product before taking it orally. To date, complete monographs are have been completed on anise oil, *Citrus bergamia* oil, *Cinnamomum* oil, clove oil, evening primrose oil, juniper oil, lavender oil, rosemary oil, and thyme oil. For all these products, the oral route is recommended, with a dosage of three to five drops, not exceeding two or three times per day for a maximum of 2 weeks (European Medicinal Agency, http://www.ema.europa.eu/ema/index.jsp?curl=pages/regulation/document_listing /document_listing_000212.jsp).

This category of natural products was implicated in many cases of acute poisoning, involving mostly children, some of whom presented severe clinical manifestations. In fact, compared to other preparations of plant-based products, active ingredients are highly concentrated in essential oils and can cause toxicity issues even in small doses. Considering the enormous confusion occurring among consumers, prescribers, and dispensers with regard to the proper use of plant-derived products, it becomes fundamental that essential oil marketing is more strictly controlled in terms of legislation, and that health authorities pay more attention to the information disseminated by manufacturing companies through media and advertising.

Currently, in many countries, including, for example, Italy, where this issue was investigated by our group (Maggini et al., 2013a), the marketing and labeling standards of essential oils are not adequate with regard to what is stated in the European directive. Frequently, some relevant information is missing, such as the part of the plant used (leaves, bark, or other), geographical origin, or botanical group. An element of ambiguity is also the fact that some different species or varieties are often indicated with the same traditional name; for example, the name *oregano* or *oregano oil* can indicate Greek oregano (*Origanum vulgare*), Spanish oregano (*Corydothymus capitatus*), Mexican oregano (*Lippia gaveolens*), or Turkish oregano (*Origanum onites*). The same problem can occur with many other plants, such as thymus, cedrus, or lemongrass. For this reason, the species used should be specified with the binomial Latin name, the only one that does not create ambiguity.

21.2.5 BIOLOGICAL VARIABILITY

Chemotypes are also very common among plants that contain essential oils. One of the best examples is thymus (*Timus vulgaris*) from the western Mediterranean. The species, morphologically homogeneous and with a stable karyotype, has seven different chemotypes: six in the dry valleys of the south of France (containing thymol, carvacrol, geraniol, linalool, and alfa terpineol) and Spain (containing cineol). The same phenomenon is observed for other species of thyme, but also for other Lamiaceae: the chemotypes of thymol and carvacrol have been found in some species of *Thymbra*, *Satureja*, *Majorana*, *Origanum*, and *Corydothymus*.

Oil composition also varies depending on many factors, including soil and environment, and can be precisely determined only by means of gas chromatography; for example, the essential oil of *Salvia officinalis* L. is particularly rich in the toxic compound thujone when prepared from plants growing in Estonia compared to plants coming from other parts of Europe (Vigane, 2012). The presence and concentration of toxic substances can also vary, depending on the time of collection, route of administration (oral, dermal, etc.), general health of the subject exposed (absorption and toxicity are maximum when skin is damaged), and additives used together with the oil.

From a pharmacological point of view, essential oils possess

- Common properties, related to their high concentration of principles and lipid solubility
- Specific actions, which depend on the composition of the species from which they derive and the extraction mode

21.2.6 TOXICOLOGICAL ISSUES OF ESSENTIAL OILS

Many reports of individual clinical cases related to adverse events or acute poisoning from essential oils are available in the medical literature, but strong structured epidemiological studies to highlight misuse of these products in the general population have not yet been published. In most cases of toxicity, consumers made an inappropriate use of essential oils, eventually determining unintentional poisonings.

Given that essential oils are widely used in the perfumery and cosmetic industry, many studies have been conducted on their potential toxicity (acutely and chronically) by topical application, with regard to risks of skin inflammation (mustard, thyme), sensitization (cinnamaldeide, saussurea), or phototoxicity (angelica, bergamot). The latter, in particular, is a relevant but underestimated issue with many essential oils, which may contain photoactive molecules such as furanocoumarins. For example, the essential oil of many plants from the genus *Citrus* contains psoralen, which binds to DNA when exposed to ultraviolet light, producing cytotoxic and highly mutagenic adducts (Hankinson et al., 2014). However, in the dark, the oil is not cytotoxic or mutagenic. Of course, cytotoxicity and phototoxicity depend on the type of molecules present in the oil and their compartmentalization in cells, producing different types of radicals according to light exposure. This is why occupational exposure is definitely one of the main causes of skin toxicity of essential oils, and one of the most frequent manifestations is allergic contact dermatitis, due to the fact that many of the components of the oils are potential allergens (Bleasel et al., 2002).

Unfortunately, establishing the exact pharmacological mechanism and determining the toxic dose of essential oils is extremely difficult, the main reason being the lack of information on active ingredients' content (titration, bioavailability, and pharmacodynamics). This makes it in some cases necessary to overestimate the possible risk, in order to ensure monitoring and an appropriate treatment in the event of clinical intoxication.

In this frame, several international study groups are trying to assess the toxicity of some components of the essential oils to determine their no adverse effect level (NOAEL), with the purpose of establishing standards to ensure safe use of these products (Vigane, 2012). Since essential oils are rich in highly fat-soluble molecules, they are able to easily and quickly penetrate biological membranes, possibly affecting the central nervous system (with mixed effects of depression and agitation), heart (with different effects depending on active substances), and liver and kidney (with possible parenchymal damage). Lipophilic substances are particularly irritants for skin and mucous tissues, especially of the digestive system, while highly volatile liquids are frequently the cause of intoxication by inhalation, causing irritation, dyspnea, and eventually chemical pneumonia. The toxic dose of essential oils, commonly expressed as LD_{50} in animals, is extremely variable; it is strictly dependent on exposure route and often not congruent with clinical features actually observed in humans. For example, in the case of camphor (*Cinnamonum camphora*) the LD_{50} values present in literature are very different in mouse and in rat and significantly higher than those observed in clinical cases of human acute intoxication: the very small amount of 30 mg/kg was in fact found to be fatal in a child, while adult fatal cases are reported for the amount of 50 mg/kg. A literature review showed that the worst cases of poisoning (most of which involved children) are due to a small number of essential oils: *Eugenia caryophyllus* C. (eugenol), *Eucalyptus globulus*, pennyroyal (pulegone), wintergreen (methyl salicylate), and *Crispum hortense* (apiolo). The neurotoxicity of oils containing tujone (*Tuhjia occidentalis*, *Salvia officinalis*, *Tanacetum vulgare*, and *Artemisia absintium*) or pinocamphone (*Hyssopus officinalis*) is well known: they can induce convulsions and sensorial and motorial alterations.

In 1994, American poison centers recorded 3185 calls regarding essential oils; among them, 1086 and 72 were related to mild and moderate cases, respectively. They were documented only in the four clinical cases of severe intoxication and one death for taking wintergreen oil (60 ml) that year (Bruneton, 2003).

In general, little clear information and reliable research is available in the field of essential oil safety, in particular regarding therapeutic dose and lethality of the essential oils.

Here we report a list of plants containing oils or combinations of volatile oils that have been linked in medical literature to toxic issues in humans.

21.2.6.1 Eucalyptus

Eucalyptus globulus oil is a traditional remedy for the relief of inflammatory conditions that affect the respiratory tract; it is quite inexpensive and can be easily found in many homes. Despite its high toxicity, cases of poisoning following ingestion are

rare. The almost fatal case of a 3-year-old child was reported; 30 minutes after ingestion of 10 ml of *Eucalyptus globulus* oil, the child showed hypotension and deep central nervous system (CNS) depression, progressing to coma. *Eucalyptus globulus* has
been linked to several cases of severe metabolic acidosis, hyporeflexya, depression
of the life signs, coma, cardiovascular failure, respiratory failure, and renal failure.
One case occurred after excessive ingestion of approximately 3 L of a mouthwash
containing volatile essential oils, including eucalyptol, menthol, and thymol (total
amount of essential oils ingested: 5.94 g). The safety threshold of *Eucalyptus globulus* oil for internal use in adults is estimated to be around 0.06–0.2 ml; amounts of
4–5 ml up to 30 ml can be fatal (Soo Hoo et al., 2003).

21.2.6.2   Geranium

A case of allergic contact cheilitis was described after exposure to *Pelargonium
capitatum* in an adult woman who applied on her lips a balsamic vinegar containing
geranium oil (Chang and Maibach, 1997).

21.2.6.3   Lavender

Lavandula officinalis oil is provided with a spasmolytic activity primarily due to its
largest constituent: linalool. *In vitro* studies have shown that its action is mediated by
an increase in intracellular cAMP and that the inhibition of the contraction is postsynaptic (Lis-Balchin and Hart, 1999). Consistently, exposure to or overdose of lavender
oil can cause CNS depression and ataxia, as well as hyperpigmentation and photosensitivity (Fetrow and Avila, 1999); the case of a 1-year-old child who developed ataxia
after ingestion of an unknown dose of *Lavandula officinalis* oil was also described
(Wilkinson, 1991). A long Japanese study (19 years) showed that 19.3% of exposures
to lavender oil result in contact dermatitis (Cavanagh and Wilkinson, 2002).

21.2.6.4   Thuja

Several cases of seizures following ingestion of *Thuja occidentalis* oil were reported;
in particular, a 7-month-old child developed seizures for 3 weeks after administration of the oil as a calming agent (Stafstrom, 2007)

21.2.6.5   Wormwood

Cases of acidosis, acute renal failure, rhabdomyolysis, visual changes, confusion,
and disorientation were reported after oral exposure or overdose of *Artemisia absintium* oil (Woolf, 1999).

21.2.6.6   Tea Tree Oil

Tea tree oil (TTO) is an extract of Australian *Melaleuca alternifolia* leaves, a popular ingredient of many over-the-counter healthcare products. It contains terpenes,
sesquiterpenes, hydrocarbons, and related oils with a minimum content of 30% ter-
pinen-4-ol and a maximum content of 15% 1,8-cineole. Adverse reactions to TTO
decrease with the minimization of 1,8-cineole content, which usually inverts the
proportion of terpinen-4-ol (Carson et al., 2006). This last component exerts antioxidant activity and has a broad spectrum of antimicrobial activity against bacterial,

viral, fungal, and protozoan infections, and it has the same activity as conventional treatment for cutaneous methicillin-resistant *Staphylococcus aureus* infections (Thompson et al., 2008). TTO is undoubtedly one of the oils responsible for the higher number of intoxication cases in medical literature; in particular, heartburn or stomachache, vomiting, neurological disorders, diarrhea, nausea, and contact dermatitis have been frequently reported.

As with most essential oils, a lethal dose for humans has not yet been established, while several studies have identified 1.9–2.6 ml/kg as the oral LD_{50} in rats (Southwell et al., 2006); rats treated with doses lower than 61.5 g/kg showed a decreased level of activity 72 hours after treatment, appearing ataxic and lethargic (Southwell et al., 2006). Although values determined in animal models do not necessarily correspond to human toxic levels, experimental data indicate a high oral toxicity of *Melaleuca alternifolia* oil.

It has been estimated that the concentrations of tea tree essential oil in commercial products can vary from 1% to 20%, so that doses of 5 and 15 ml, respectively, can be considered potentially toxic. Poisoning cases undoubtedly tend to be more dramatic in children than in adults because of their lower body weight; for example, a case of neurological disorder was described in a 2-year-old child who had drunk less than 10 ml of 100% pure essential oil of *Melaleuca alternifolia* (Jacobs and Hornfeldt, 1994). In adults, a case of a 12-hour coma, followed by 36 hours of hallucinations, was described after the assumption of about a half cup of tea with TTO, corresponding to a dose of about 0.5-1.0 ml/kg body weight. The patient reported abdominal pain and diarrhea for about 6 weeks after the event (Seawright, 1993).

A study conducted by the University of Denver (Colorado) and published in the *New England Journal of Medicine* (Henley et al., 2007) showed, based on laboratory evidence, that repeated topical applications of products containing essential oils of lavender and tea tree may have contributed to the development of gynecomastia in three male children. In fact, data obtained on human cell lines showed that both oils possess estrogenic and antiandrogenic activity (Henley et al., 2007).

Our group recently described the case of a 33-year-old woman who presented ataxia, nystagmus, tremors, concentration deficit, and diarrhea and a weight loss of 12 kg in 6 months. During the previous year, she had been using 100% tea tree oil daily (mistaken for a diluted solution), directly on the oral mucosa, to treat chronic gingivitis. She also presented allergic reactions with hives and bronchospasm (Lanzi et al., 2015).

No other data on the systemic toxicity of *Melaleuca alternifolia* essential oil in humans is available; however, available knowledge clearly demonstrates its toxicity after oral exposure. For this reason, tea tree oil ingestion should not be recommended. To avoid severe cases of intoxication, it would also be very useful to label all *M. alternifolia* products with a note reporting the obligations of keeping the product out of the reach of children and stating that it should not be taken for internal use.

REFERENCES

Bishop FL, Prescott P, Chan YK, Saville J, von Elm E, Lewith GT. Prevalence of complementary medicine use in pediatric cancer: A systematic review. *Pediatrics* 2010;125(4): 768–76. doi:10.1542/peds.2009-1775.

Bleasel N, Tate B, Rademaker M. Allergic contact dermatitis following exposure to essential oils. *Australas J Dermatol* 2002;43(3):211–3.

Bruneton J. *Pharmacognosie phytochimie plantes medicinales*. Lavoisier, Paris, 2003.

Carson CF, Hammer KA, Riley TV. *Melaleuca alternifolia* (tea tree) oil: A review of antimicrobial and other medicinal properties. *Clin Microbiol Rev* 2006;19:50–62.

Cavanagh HM, Wilkinson JM. Biological activities of lavender essential oil. *Phytother Res* 2002;16(4):301–8.

Chang YC, Maibach HI. Pseudo flautist's lip: Allergic contact cheilitis from geraniol. *Contact Dermatitis* 1997;37(1):39.

Edwards IR, Aronson, JK. Adverse drug reactions: Definitions, diagnosis, and management. *Lancet* 2000;356(9237):1255–9.

Everett LL, Birmingham PK, Williams GD, Brenn BR, Shapiro JH. Herbal and homeopathic medication use in pediatric surgical patients. *Paediatr Anaesth* 2005;15(6):455–60.

Fetrow CW, Avila JR. Professional's Handbook of Complementary and Alternative Medicines. Springhouse Corp, Springhouse PA, 1999.

Gallo E, Giocaliere E, Benemei S, Bilia AR, Karioti A, Pugi A, di Pirro M, Menniti-Ippolito F, Pieraccini G, Gori L, Mugelli A, Firenzuoli F, Vannacci A. Anything to declare? Possible risks for patients' health resulting from undeclared plants in herbal supplements. *Br J Clin Pharmacol* 2012;73(3):482–3.

Hankinson A, Lloyd B, Alweis R. Lime-induced phytophotodermatitis. *J Commun Hosp Intern Med Perspect* 2014;4(4).

Henley DV, Lipson N, Korach KS, Bloch CA. Prepubertal gynecomastia linked to lavender and tea tree oils. *N Engl J Med* 2007;356(5):479–85.

Jacobs MR, Hornfeldt CS. Melaleuca oil poisoning. *J Toxicol Clin Toxicol* 1994;32(4):461–64.

Lanzi C, Occupati B, Pracucci C, Gallo E, Vannacci A, Mannaioni G. Tea tree oil (*Melaleuca alternifolia*): Chronic misuse and neurological toxicity in a 33-year-old woman. *J Pharmacol Clin Toxicol* 2015;3(1):1038.

Lapi F, Vannacci A, Moschini M, Cipollini F, Morsuillo M, Gallo E, Banchelli G, Cecchi E, Di Pirro M, Giovannini MG, Cariglia MT, Gori L, Firenzuoli F, Mugelli A. Use, attitudes and knowledge of complementary and alternative drugs (CADs) among pregnant women: A preliminary survey in Tuscany. *Evid Based Complement Alternat Med* 2010;7(4):477–86.

Lis-Balchin M, Hart S. Studies on the mode of action of the essential oil of lavender (*Lavandula angustifolia* P. Miller). *Phytother Res* 1999;13(6):540–2.

Loman DG. The use of complementary and alternative health care practices among children. *J Pediatr Health Care* 2003;17(2):58–63.

Lucenteforte E, Gallo E, Pugi A, Giommoni F, Paoletti A, Vietri M, Lupi P, La Torre M, Diddi G, Firenzuoli F, Mugelli A, Vannacci A, Lapi F. Complementary and alternative drugs use among preoperative patients: A cross-sectional study in Italy. *Evid Based Complement Alternat Med* 2012;527238.

Maggini V, Gallo E, Pugi A, Benemei S, Mascherini V, Gori L, Mugelli A, Firenzuoli F, Vannacci A. Natural products labels and patient safety: A qualitative study to evaluate clinically relevant safety issues in pharmacy. *Res Complement Med* (Karger) 2013a;622(20, S1):32 (ICCMR 2013 abstract).

Maggini V, Gallo E, Vannacci A, Gori L, Mugelli A, Firenzuoli F. e-Phytovigilance for misleading herbal information. *Trends Pharmacol Sci* 2013b;34(11):594–5.

McCann LJ, Newell SJ. Survey of paediatric complementary and alternative medicine use in health and chronic illness. *Arch Dis Child* 2006;91:173–4. doi: 10.1136/adc.2004.052514.

Seawright A. Tea Tree Oil Poisoning—Comment. *Med J Australia* 1993;159(11–12):831.

Soo Hoo GW, Hinds RL, Dinovo, Renner SWJ. Fatal large-volume mouthwash ingestion in an adult: A review and the possible role of phenolic compound toxicity. *Intensive Care Med* 2003;18(3):150–5.

Southwell I, Leach DN, Lowe R, Pollack A. 2006. Quality assurance for tea tree oil safety investigative samples. Report to Rural Industries Research and Development Corporation, RIRDC, Kingston, ACT, publication no. 06/026, project no. Dan 241A.

Stafstrom CE. Seizures in 7-month-old child after exposure to the essential plant oil thuja. *Pediatr Neurol* 2007;37:446–8.

Thompson G, Blackwood B, McMullan R, Alderdice FA, Trinder TJ, Lavery GG, McAuley DF. A randomized controlled trial of tea tree oil (5%) body wash versus standard body wash to prevent colonization with methicillin-resistant *Staphylococcus aureus* (MRSA) in critically ill adults: Research protocol. *BMC Infect Dis* 2008;8:161.

Vannacci A, Lapi F, Baronti R, Gallo E, Gori L, Mugelli A, Firenzuoli F. Too much effectiveness from a herbal drug. *Br J Clin Pharmacol* 2009;67(4):473–4.

Vigane M. Essential oils: Renewal of interest and toxicity. *Eur J Dermatol* 2012;20(6):685–92.

Wilkinson HF. Childhood ingestion of volatile oils. *Med J Aust* 1991;154(6):430–1.

Woolf A. Essential oil poisoning. *J Toxicol Clin Toxicol* 1999;37(6):721–17.

Anna Loraschi and Marco Cosentino

CONTENTS

22.1 INTRODUCTION

Aromatherapy can be defined as treatment using odors, the inhalation of which can have beneficial effects on the users through their action on the limbic system in the brain and the usual hormonal pathways to their target sites (Lis-Balchin, 1999). The term *essential oil* was used for the first time in the sixteenth century by Paracelsus von Hohenheim, who referred to the effective component of a drug as "quinta essential" (Edris, 2007). The role of essential oils had been reduced, by the middle of the twentieth century, almost entirely to use in fragrances, cosmetics, and food flavourings, while their use in pharmaceutical preparations had declined (Edris, 2007).

Aromatherapy is a branch of complementary and alternative medicine (CAM), and large-scale surveys suggest that CAM has been increasing in popularity in Europe, North America, and Australia in recent years (Adams et al., 2011; Cooke and Ernst, 2000; Lis-Balchin, 1999), with a lifetime prevalence up to 85% and a current use prevalence up to 52% of the general population (Hunt et al., 2010; Robinson et al., 2007). However, studies specifically focused on aromatherapy use are scant (Mousley, 2005; Sibbritt et al., 2014) since the majority of the surveys have evaluated more broadly different CAM uses in a selected population.

22.2 PREVALENCE

22.2.1 GENERAL POPULATION

Aromatherapy appears to be becoming increasingly popular (Ernst and White, 2000; Robinson et al., 2007). Indeed, in a UK survey among almost 2700 adults, a rise in practitioner-provided aromatherapy has been estimated, from 0.1% in 1993 to 3.5% 5 years later (Thomas et al., 2001). In another UK survey, Ernst and White (2000) found a similar 12-month prevalence (3.5%). More recent data evaluating the overall use (self-prescription and practitioner provided; more than 7600 subjects surveyed in the UK) have shown higher values, since the lifetime prevalence seems to be up to 11%, while the 12-month prevalence interests are around 6% of the general population (Hunt et al., 2010).

Australian lifetime prevalence appears to be higher, at one-quarter of the general population in a survey among almost 500 subjects (Robinson et al., 2007).

According to a recent review of the literature evaluating 89 articles about CAM use, aromatherapy was the third most common choice among CAM users, soon after herbal medicine and homeopathy, and the average percentage value was one-quarter of all CAM in industrialized countries (Posadzki et al., 2013a).

In Table 22.1 the selected surveys that have evaluated the prevalence of aromatherapy are presented.

Hereafter we describe the use of aromatherapy in specific subgroups, the possibility of a hospital supply, the attitudes related to the user (the purpose of use, the factor associated, the source of information, and the disclosure to the health care provider) and the health care provider, and finally, the risks related to the use and limitation of the available data.

TABLE 22.1

Prevalence of Aromatherapy

Author	Year	Country	Sample	Method	Number of Respondents	Response Rate	% CAM	% Aromatherapy	Notes
General Population									
Hunt et al., 2010	2005	UK	General population	Household survey	7630	71%	Lifetime use: 44% 12-month use: 26.3%	Lifetime use: 11.2% 12-month use: 6% (500/7630)[a]	Aromatherapy was the second most frequent CAM
Thomas et al., 2001	1998	UK	General population	Postal self-completion questionnaires	2669	60%	12-month use: 10.6%	Lifetime use: 8.2% 12-month use: 3.5%	Data related to practitioner-provided treatment and excluded self-medication
Ernst et al., 2000	1999	UK	General adult population	Structured telephone interview	1204	–	12-month use: 20%	12-month use: 4.2% (51/1204)[a]	
Robinson et al., 2007	2005	Australia	General population	Postal self-completion questionnaires	459	40%	Lifetime use: 85%	Robinson et al., 2007	2005
Children									
Galicia-Connolly et al., 2014	2012	Canada	Neurologic pediatric patients attending two hospitals: Edmonton and Ottawa	Self-reported questionnaire	206	–	CAM overall use Edmonton: 78% Ottawa: 48%	Lifetime use: 6.8% (14/206)[a] Current use: 1.9% (4/206)[a]	Aromatherapy was the fourth most common CAM practice (16% of CAM) 53.8% of the users perceived helpfulness from aromatherapy treatment

(Continued)

TABLE 22.1 (CONTINUED)
Prevalence of Aromatherapy

Author	Year	Country	Sample	Method	Number of Respondents	Response Rate	% CAM	% Aromatherapy	Notes
					Children				
Adams et al., 2013	2012	Canada	Pediatric patients attending two hospitals: Edmonton and Ottawa	Self-reported questionnaire	926	95.9%	CAM overall use Edmonton: 71% Ottawa: 42%	Lifetime use: 6.6% (61/926)[a] Current use: 3.3% (31/926)[a]	Aromatherapy was the fourth most common CAM practice (16% of CAM)
Crawford et al., 2006	2004	UK	Pediatric inpatients and outpatients	Structured personal interviews	500	86.2%	12-month use: 41% Last-month use: 26%	12-month use: 2%[a]	Aromatherapy represented the third most common medicinal types of CAM (5%)
Simpson et al., 2001	1998	UK	Pediatric (<16 years) population	Self-reported questionnaire	904	79.7%	CAM overall use: 17.9%	Overall use: 6.2% (56/904)[a]	Aromatherapy was the second most common CAM (36.4%)
Lim et al., 2005	2004	Australia	Pediatric patients	Face-to-face interview	509	–	12-month use: 51% Last month use: 30%	12-month use: 3.6%[a]	Aromatherapy was the most common nonmedicinal CAM used (7%)

(Continued)

TABLE 22.1 (CONTINUED)
Prevalence of Aromatherapy

Author	Year	Country	Sample	Method	Number of Respondents	Response Rate	% CAM	% Aromatherapy	Notes
					Elderly				
Cherniack et al., 2008	2003–2005	United States	Ambulatory geriatric patients	Questionnaire completed before the visit	338	–	Current use: 42.6%	Current use: 2.1%	
Andrews, 2002	2000–2001	UK	GPs' ambulatory patients aged 60 or more	Questionnaire completed before the visit	144	64.5%	–	12-month use: 8.0%	Aromatherapy was the fifth most common CAM (30%)
					Women				
Sibbrit et al., 2014	2009	Australia	Sample of women aged 31–36	Self-reported questionnaire; part of the Australian Longitudinal Study on Women's Health	8200 (804 pregnant)	41%	–	Current use: 17.9% in pregnant 21.3% in nonpregnant	Self-prescribed aromatherapy was used by 15.2% of pregnant women and 17.5% of nonpregnant
Adams et al., 2001	2009	Australia	Women	Self-reported questionnaire, substudy of the Australian Longitudinal Study on Women's Health	1800	85%	12-month use: 90.%	12-month use: 23.9%	Aromatherapy was the fourth most common CAM used

(Continued)

TABLE 22.1 (CONTINUED)
Prevalence of Aromatherapy

Author	Year	Country	Sample	Method	Number of Respondents	Response Rate	% CAM	% Aromatherapy	Notes
					Women				
Skouteris et al., 2008	2005	Australia	CAM use in previous 8 weeks of pregnancy	Postal self-completion questionnaires	321	–	73%	18%	
Bishop et al., 2011	1991–1992	UK	Pregnant women	Postal self-completion questionnaires	14,115	97%	Any use during pregnancy: 26.7%	Any use during pregnancy: 0.51	The use of CAM increased from 6% in the first trimester to 12.4% in the second and 26.3% in the third Aromatherapy use was 0.09 in the first trimester, 0.30 in the second, and 0.27 in the third
					Other Subgroups				
Kalaaji et al., 2012	2010	United States	Dermatologic patients	Questionnaire completed before the visit	300	–	12-month use: 82%	12-month use: 10%	

(Continued)

TABLE 22.1 (CONTINUED)
Prevalence of Aromatherapy

Author	Year	Country	Sample	Method	Number of Respondents	Response Rate	% CAM	% Aromatherapy	Notes
					Other Subgroups				
Van Tilburg et al., 2008	2001–2002	United States	Patients with functional bowel disorders	Email questionnaire	1770	59%	Overall last 3 months of use: 35.0%	Last 3 months of use in Irritable bowel syndrome: 7.2% Functional constipation: 5.7% Functional abdominal pain: 5.6% Functional diarrhea: 3.3%	
Blanc et al., 2001	1999	United States	Asthma or rhinosinusitis with concomitant asthma patients	Structured telephone interview	300	77.7%	12-month use: 42%	12-month use: 14.7%	

(Continued)

TABLE 22.1 (CONTINUED)
Prevalence of Aromatherapy

Author	Year	Country	Sample	Method	Number of Respondents Other Subgroups	Response Rate	% CAM	% Aromatherapy	Notes
Shakeel et al., 2010	2005–2006	UK	Othorhinolaryng-ology patients	Questionnaire completed before the visit	1789	73%	12-month use: 60%	12-month use: 9.5% (170/1,789)[a]	Aromatherapy was used for relaxation (33), stress/anxiety (25), general health (21), musculoskeletal (18), rhinosinusitis (18), depression (4), insomnia (2), Meniere's disease (1), earache (1), childbirth (1), and missing (57)
Nicolaou and Johnston, 2004	2002	UK	Patients of contact dermatitis clinic	Face-to-face interview	109	100%	Current use: 10% Overall use: 30%	Current use: 5.5% (6/109)[a]	Aromatherapy represented the second most common CAM used (18%)
Ferry et al., 2002	2001	UK	Parkinsonian patients	Face-to-face interview	80	90%	Current use: 54%	Current use: 10% (8/80)[a]	Aromatherapy represented the second most frequent CAM used (14%) (Continued)

TABLE 22.1 (CONTINUED)
Prevalence of Aromatherapy

Author	Year	Country	Sample	Method	Number of Respondents	Response Rate	% CAM	% Aromatherapy	Notes
					Other Subgroups				
Lewith et al., 2002	2001	UK	Adult cancer patients	Questionnaire completed before the visit	162	60%	Current use: 32%	Current use: 19.1%	More hospice patients, 70% (19/27), were receiving aromatherapy than the out patients (5%, 4/79) or inpatients (14%, 8/56)
Sinha and Efron, 2005	2003	Australia	ADHD patients 5–17 years	Postal self-completion questionnaires	75	71.4%	Lifetime use: 67.6%	Lifetime use: 17.3% (13/75)[a]	Aromatherapy represented the third most common CAM used (26% of CAM users) 38.5% found aromatherapy helpful

[a] Based on data presented in the study.

22.2.2 Subgroups

22.2.2.1 Children

The use of CAM in general is quite frequent among pediatric patients, especially in children with chronic diseases such as cystic fibrosis, cancer, and asthma, with a CAM use ranging from 11% to 80% (Neuhouser et al., 2001; Sawni and Thomas, 2007; Sawyer et al., 1994) and a prevalence in primary care pediatrics of 5%–21% (Crawford et al., 2006; Galicia-Connolly et al., 2014; Lim et al., 2005; Sawni and Thomas, 2007; Simpson and Roman, 2001).

A recent survey on CAM use in almost 1000 pediatric Canadian patients showed that aromatherapy was the fourth most common CAM practice (16% of all CAM), with a lifetime use prevalence of 6.6% (Adams et al., 2013). When restricted to the neurological subgroup of the same patients, the prevalence values remained similar and more details were offered about the singular CAM (Galicia-Connolly et al., 2014). For instance, 53.8% of the users perceived helpfulness from aromatherapy treatment.

These features are in accordance with a systematic review of the literature about CAM use in the pediatric population in the UK, according to which aromatherapy was the third most common CAM, representing an average of 19% of all CAM used (Posadzki et al., 2013b).

22.2.2.2 Elderly

The rapid growth of CAM use in the last decades also affected elderly subjects, with rates of use up to 90% in the United States, and should be related to the higher risks of comorbidities and chronic diseases (Cherniack et al., 2008; Ness et al., 2005; Wilson and Andrews, 2004).

According to a U.S. survery among 338 ambulatory patients, the use of aromatherapy was 2.1% (Cherniack et al., 2008). In another survey performed among 144 UK patients, the prevalence of use within the previous year raised to 8%, and aromatherapy was preferred by one-third of CAM users (Andrews, 2002).

22.2.2.3 Women

In a large cohort of 8200 women aged 31–36 years, part of the Australian Longitudinal Study on Women's Health (ALSWH), the prevalence of aromatherapy use was similar between pregnant and nonpregnant women (18% vs. 21%), suggesting that during pregnancy women are not reducing or forgoing aromatherapy use (Sibbritt et al., 2014). Due to the fact that aromatherapy oil use was self-prescribed in 15% of pregnant women, these women may be unaware of the potential risks.

These prevalence data are in accordance with a cross-sectional subgroup of the ALSWH among 1800 Australian women, among which the 12-month use of aromatherapy oils was almost 24% (Adams et al., 2011).

In another survey involving more than 14,000 UK women, a very low prevalence in pregnancy was observed since the use of aromatherapy occurred in less than 1% of the respondents (Bishop et al., 2011). Aromatherapy use showed a slight increase during the trimesters and lavender oil was the most common essential oil used (20 out of 72 users), followed by eucalyptus (15 cases), peppermint or spearmint (10), neroli (5), and chamomile (4) (Bishop et al., 2011).

22.2.2.4 Other Subgroups

Other surveys on CAM use also evaluated aromatherapy in subgroups represented by patients suffering from chronic diseases, surgery patients, and so forth (Table 22.1).

22.3 HOSPITAL SUPPLY

The availability of CAM in the national health system and the potential reimbursement should influence use in that country (Posadzki et al., 2013a).

Consumer demand has led to considerable support for CAM to be provided by national health care systems, and as a consequence, the number of hospitals offering CAM appears to have risen (Carruzzo et al., 2013).

In an annual survey of hospitals, the American Hospital Association reported the proportion of hospitals using CAM has increased from 7.7% in 1999 to 37.7% in 2008 (Salomonsen et al., 2011).

Northern Europe has been reported to have the highest rate of CAM offered: about 50% of Norwegian and one-third of Danish hospitals offer CAM to their patients (Salomonsen et al., 2011).

According to a recent Swiss study, 19 of out 37 surveyed hospitals used CAM, and in particular, aromatherapy was used in 11% (4/37) of palliative care units, 11% (4/37) of gynecology–obstetrics, and 5% (2/37) of the orthopedic departments (Carruzzo et al., 2013).

This rate is similar to that found by another hospital survey (Lewith et al., 2001) among almost 2800 UK physicians, according to which aromatherapy was used by the clinical team in 14.3% of cases.

Aromatherapy has been reportedly available within 50% of obstetric departments in Germany (70/138) (Münstedt et al., 2009), in which it was largely delivered by midwives alone (>90%).

In addition, a CAM service expressly devoted to aromatherapy was introduced in a maternity unit in the UK (Mousley, 2005) in 2000, offering antenatal and postnatal usage and aroma massage classes. The service was supervised by aromatherapist midwives, and the essential oils most used were lavender and frankincense.

22.4 PURPOSE OF USE

Similar to other CAM, aromatherapy is used to improve the quality of life (wellness and well-being issues) and prevent illness.

In a survey among 66 CAM health care providers, the top five most common indications for aromatherapy were represented by anxiety and stress, muscular-skeletal problems, insomnia, headaches and migraines, and hormonal problems. Other common conditions included respiratory problems (including asthma), arthritis and rheumatism, depression, skin problems (including eczema), chronic fatigue, rhinosinusitis, constipation, multiple sclerosis, cancer, and HIV (Long et al., 2001).

When aromatherapy is supplied by the health care system, it is also used in palliative care units for cancer patients (Lewith et al., 2001).

In midwifery practice, it may be used for nausea, vomiting, relaxation, back pain, perineal discomfort, and postnatal depression (Allaire et al., 2000; Hall et al., 2012). Pregnant women may seek CAM, including aromatherapy, to reduce any potential effects on fetal development as an alternative to conventional treatments, especially in the case of hay fever, allergy, and urinary tract infections (Furlow et al., 2008; Hall et al., 2011; Sibbrit et al., 2014).

When supplied in obstetric departments, aromatherapy may be offered mainly for prophylaxis (58.5%), but in 40% of departments it is available for both prophylaxis and to treat clinical problems (Münstedt et al., 2009).

The use of essential oils, as other CAM, should be a consequence of self-medication because it allows people to gain a sense of control over their health problems, especially chronic diseases, and have an active role in the treatment choice (Robinson et al., 2007; Wilson and Andrews, 2004).

In addition, a substantial proportion of aromatherapy use may be reported to be for reasons not directly associated with health care or health behavior, such as prizes, gifts, beauty salon treatments, to feel good, and so forth (Thomas et al., 2001).

22.5   FACTORS ASSOCIATED

The use of CAM appears to be higher among adults and children with chronic medical problems, indicating that conventional medical therapies alone are often not enough when dealing with chronic medical problems, and that use of CAM adjunctively might be an option (Sawni and Thomas, 2007).

CAM appears to be influenced by some sociodemographic characteristics and seems to be used more by women, by the below-60 age groups, and by users with tertiary-level education (Robinson et al., 2007). Women, in particular, are more proactive in their health care behaviors and are often the main caregiver within the family when health care issues arise (Bell, 2005; Lee, 1998; McMurray, 2003; Robinson et al., 2007).

Accordingly, in an Australian survey among almost 500 subjects (general population), when specifically analyzed, young age (odds ratio [OR] = 12.25 among 18–40 vs. >60 years, 95% confidence interval [CI] = 5.77–25.99; $p < .001$) appears to be associated with a higher frequency of aromatherapy use, and male subjects appear to be less prone to aromatherapy use (OR = 0.22, 95% CI = 0.12–0.40; $p < .001$) (Robinson et al., 2007).

22.6   SOURCE OF INFORMATION

Though, unfortunately, no specific data are available for aromatherapy, the most common sources of information for CAM are represented by families (more than 63.7%), pharmacists (44.4%), books (38.7%), and the Internet (37.1%) (Galicia-Connolly et al., 2014). In addition, the most trusted sources are physicians, followed by pharmacists and CAM providers (Adams et al., 2013; Galicia-Connolly et al., 2014).

These features support a high proportion of self-prescribing, rather than seeking professional guidance for CAM use.

22.7 HEALTH CARE DISCLOSURE ABOUT CAM USE

Although health care providers appear to be considered the most trusted sources for CAM information, the rate of disclosure is often poor and may be as low as 20% due to concerns about a potential negative response by the physician or the belief that he or she did not need to know about it (Adams et al., 2013; Galicia-Connolly et al., 2014; Lim et al., 2005; Perry and Dowrick 2000; Wilson and Andrews, 2004).

This lack of disclosure may potentially put a patient's health at risk, exposing him or her to unwanted adverse reactions (see Section 22.10).

Moreover, doctors and other caregivers, such as nurses, do not routinely ask about CAM; indeed, if many patients fail to discuss using CAM with their health care professionals, it is often because the health care professionals do not ask the patients appropriate questions while obtaining medical histories (Cherniack et al., 2008). In addition, the health care professionals may record this information in patients' charts in a few cases (35%) (Wilson and Andrews, 2004).

22.8 HEALTH CARE PROFESSIONALS' ATTITUDES AND KNOWLEDGE

22.8.1 Physicians

There is a rising interest, awareness, and communication about CAM among physicians, and this may be reflective of the growing trend in use by the general population (Sawni and Thomas, 2007; Wong and Neill, 2001). Physicians appear to not see CAM as preventative or simply as a fashionable trend or as a treatment of last resort and believe that CAM should be subject to more accurate scientific testing (Lewith et al., 2001). Younger physicians, specially if female (up to six times), seem to have a more positive approach to CAM in terms of use and belief of effectiveness (Furlow, 2008; Wahner-Roedler et al., 2014).

Several studies assessing attitudes, beliefs, and use of CAM by primary care physicians in Europe and North America report that 10%–80% of physicians expressed an interest in CAM, want more education on CAM, have a positive attitude toward CAM, and consider referring patients for CAM (Sawni and Thomas, 2007).

As a consequence, there is an increasing need for knowledge and training in CAM and the need for more education on it (Sawni and Thomas, 2007).

Attitudes and knowledge appear to be improved by educational interventions, and a recent survey involving almost 200 U.S. physicians has shown a more positive attitude toward CAM and increased willingness to use CAM to address patient care needs after attending educational events (Wahner-Roedler et al., 2014).

In particular, pediatrician attitudes are usually positive toward CAM (Sawni and Thomas, 2007). According to a UK survey among general pediatric doctors (49 respondents), the use of CAM is relatively common in pediatric doctors and their families, and around one-third of them have received a little formal CAM education (Fountain-Polley et al., 2007). Indeed, in a survey among almost 700 pediatricians, only 2.3% were not able to name any kind of CAM, and aromatherapy—the fourth most popular CAM—was named in more than one-third of the cases. These findings are in accordance with a U.S. survey of almost 700 pediatricians (Sawni and Thomas, 2007): 2.5% of the surveyed subjects practiced aromatherapy, 20% used it for self or family, and 5% referred it (Sawni and Thomas, 2007). Aromatherapy was generally perceived as effective (26%) and safe (49%), and only 4% of the surveyed pediatricians considered it potentially harmful (Sawni and Thomas, 2007).

Another specialization with a general positive attitude toward CAM is represented by obstetrician–gynecology physicians. According to a U.S. survey among 400 obstetrician–gynecology physicians, 32.3% of them endorsed, provided, or referred aromatherapy and 13.6% perceived aromatherapy as highly or moderately effective (Furlow et al., 2008).

22.8.2 MIDWIFE KNOWLEDGE

CAM in general and aromatherapy use are widespread in midwifery practice, and may represent up one-third of CAM used in women (Allaire et al., 2000). Rather than rejecting conventional medicine, midwives appear to be integrating CAM with conventional therapy in order to reduce the need for medical intervention (Hall et al., 2012).

In fact, midwives represent the prime movers in CAM provision and usually deliver the therapy (Münstedt et al., 2009) and represent an important source of aromatherapy advice (especially for pain relief during birth) in maternity departments. Therefore, it is important to warrant a good level of CAM training among midwives in order to promote the effective and safe use of aromatherapy and other CAM in vulnerable categories such as pregnant women (Muñoz-Sellés et al., 2013).

22.8.3 CAM PRACTITIONERS

In a UK survey, the majority of the 200 CAM practitioners interviewed stated that they had not had adequate training in evidence-based medicine (EBM) (Hadley et al., 2008).

Indeed, a report from the UK House of Lords has recommended that every therapist working in CAM should have a clear understanding of the principles of EBM in order to base their decisions about health care on the best available, current, valid, and relevant evidence (Hadley et al., 2008).

22.9 ASSOCIATION FOR AROMATHERAPHY

Several associations for aromatherapy have been created at both the national and international levels with the aim to develop and maintain education standards for the aromatherapy profession.

22.9.1 INTERNATIONAL ASSOCIATION

The International Federation of Aromatherapists (IFA) is the first and largest governing body for professional aromatherapy and aromatherapists worldwide (http://www.ifaroma.org/it/home/).

22.9.2 European Association

The Aromatherapy Trade Council is the trade association for the specialist aromatherapy essential oil trade, and represents manufacturers and suppliers of aromatherapy products as well as the interest of consumers in the United Kingdom (http://www.a-t-c.org.uk/).

The Italian Society for the Research on Essential Oils (Società Italiana per la Ricerca sugli Oli Essenziali [SIROE]) aims to promote research and information events about essential oil use (http://www.siroe.it/).

22.9.3 North American Association

The National Association for Holistic Aromatherapy (NAHA) is a leading aromatherapy organization in the United States and internationally (https://www.naha.org/about/mission/).

The Canadian Federation of Aromatherapists was established to foster continuing growth, quality, and high standards of education and practice within the aromatherapy profession and provide ongoing information about the quality of aromatherapy products and services to the public (http://cfacanada.com/about/).

22.9.4 Australian Association

The International Aromatherapy and Aromatic Medicine Association, formerly the IFA Australia branch, is the leading independent non-profit professional association dedicated to support aromatherapy practitioners in Australia and overseas (http://www.iaama.org.au/).

22.10 RISKS

Despite many assertions to the contrary, aromatherapy is not free from the potential to cause harm (Posadzki et al., 2013a), especially in vulnerable groups such as children, elderly patients, and pregnant women. For instance, jasmine, juniper, peppermint, clove, cedarwood, sage, and rosemary essential oils should be avoided during pregnancy, with some of them possessing abortifacent properties (Sibbrit et al., 2014).

Essential oils usually should not be taken internally, as many of them are poisonous. Though acute, subacute, and chronic toxicities following essential oil administration have been reported (Pisseri et al., 2008), use of the most common essential oils in massage is seldom dangerous, as they have low systemic toxicity, especially when used at a maximum concentration of 3%–4% in a carrier oil dilution (provided they are not adulterated). However, their safety during pregnancy, childbirth, and for babies has not been clearly demonstrated.

In dermatological prescriptions, local reactions such as sensitization leading to contact dermatitis are frequently observed. The reaction is developed early, and its severity depends on the amount of the irritant substance. Essential oils containing a high ratio of phenols, such as *Citrus lemon*, *Origanum vulgaris*, and *Thymus vulgaris*, can yield a skin irritation (Pisseri et al., 2008).

The danger is that most novel and unusual essential oils, plant extracts, and phytols, including chemotypes, have not been tested for toxicity, especially on the skin (Lis-Balchin, 1999; Münstedt et al., 2009).

For instance, adverse reactions attributed to the *Croton* species include inflammation of the skin, reddening, edema, swelling, and vesicles. If splashed into the eye or the eye is rubbed with a contaminated hand, inflammation of the cornea and conjunctiva occurs, leading to possible blindness. Oral intake causes gastroenteritis, vomiting, and diarrhea (Lis-Balchin, 1999).

The additional risk is due to the fact that many of these new products are introduced by people with no scientific knowledge or pharmacognostic, pharmacological, or medical training (Lis-Balchin, 1999).

Several components of the essential oils present a dose-dependent systemic toxicity. The phenolic terpenes can be caustic, leading to irritation and lesions to the intestinal mucous membrane. Some ketones have a strong neurotoxicity and may be accumulated in the organism. The nonoxigenated terpenes cause blistering of the skin and mucous membranes. Moreover, in the case of inappropriate cutaneous applications at very high dosages, symptoms such as depression, incoordination, and muscular tremors are found for essential oils such as pure tea tree oil (Pisseri et al., 2008).

In addition, safety guidelines have been provided by NAHA that include avoiding the use of photosensitizing essential oils prior to going into a sun tanning booth or the sun and keeping essential oils away from direct contact with flames, since they are highly flammable substances (https://www.naha.org/explore-aromatherapy/safety/general-safety-guidelines/).

Though the actual frequency remains unknown, a systematic review of the adverse effects associated with aromatherapy collected a total of 71 cases of adverse events associated with aromatherapy, ranging from mild to severe (one fatality included). The most common adverse effect was dermatitis. Lavender, peppermint, tea tree oil, and ylang-ylang were the most common essential oils responsible for adverse effects (Posadzki et al., 2012).

Novel essential oils or herb oils should not be used or used carefully, as these have not been tested and may be potentially dangerous, especially to babies, young children, expectant and nursing mothers, and elderly subjects (Lis-Balchin, 1999).

22.11   LIMITS AND PERSPECTIVES

Prevalence data appear to be widely variable due to the fact that they are clearly affected by the methodological quality (which is often very limited), sample size, response rate, survey design, and apparent differences between countries (Hunt et al., 2010; Posadzki et al., 2013a).

A low response rate, for instance, may determine falsely high prevalence rates due to the fact that who failed to respond may have less interest in CAM (Posadzki et al., 2013a). Data based on self-reports are subject to recall bias, while the risk is lower through face-to-face interview (Hunt et al., 2010). There is no universally accepted definition of CAM; therefore, different surveys may evaluate the use of different CAM options. In addition, most of the surveys have used different frame times (i.e., current, past 12 months, or lifetime use). Moreover, the majority of the surveys have not been formally validated, and therefore they did not necessarily evaluate what they aimed to measure (Posadzki et al., 2013a).

Therefore, surveys specifically devoted to aromatherapy use in a representative sample should overcome this gap and will allow a better evaluation of the actual incidence of the use of essential oils and the related details (knowledge, attitudes, related factors, etc.).

22.12 CONCLUSIONS

Aromatherapy is a popular CAM, and its use is becoming more common within the health services. In general, it appears that aromatherapy is used to promote wellness and well-being. Other purposes of aromatherapy use are as complementary treatment for chronic conditions where unmet needs are still present and in the vulnerable category as an alternative to conventional treatment considered too toxic, and as a way to take an active part in the therapeutic path.

CAM also appears to be gaining acceptance among conventionally trained physicians. Health professionals should be aware that CAM use is widespread and ask their patients about its use and be alert for possible side effects. Although health care providers are often considered the most trusted sources for CAM information, its use is often undisclosed.

Therefore, physicians should routinely inquire about CAM use since concurrent treatments need to be assessed, especially in vulnerable subjects such as children, the elderly, and pregnant women. Moreover, after improving their knowledge about CAM, their patients may feel more comfortable in disclosing CAM use and may receive more information about CAM from a trustworthy source.

With the increasing demand and use of CAM by the general population, it is fundamental that health care professionals can make informed decisions when advising or referring their patients who wish to use CAM.

REFERENCES

Adams, J., Sibbritt, D., Broom A.A. et al. A comparison of complementary and alternative medicine users and use across geographical areas: A national survey of 1,427 women. *BMC Complement Altern Med* 11 (2011): 85.

Adams, D., Dagenais, S., Clifford T. et al. Complementary and alternative medicine use by pediatric specialty outpatients. *Pediatrics* 131 (2013): 225–32.

Allaire, A.D., Moos, M.-K., and Wells, S.R. Complementary and alternative medicine in pregnancy: A survey of North Carolina certified nurse-midwives. *Obstet Gynecol* 95 (2000): 19–23.

Andrews, G.J. Private complementary medicine and older people: Service use and user empowerment. *Ageing Soc* 22 (2002): 343–68.

Bishop, J.L., Northstone, K., Green, J.R., and Thompson, E.A. The use of complementary and alternative medicine in pregnancy: Data from the Avon Longitudinal Study of Parents and Children (ALSPAC). *Complement Ther Med* 19 (2011): 303–10.

Blanc, P.D., Trupin, L., Earnest, G., Katz, P.P., Yelin, E.H., and Eisner, M.D. Alternative therapies among adults with a reported diagnosis of asthma or rhinosinusitis. *Chest* 120 (2001): 1461–67.

Carruzzo, P., Graz, B., Rodondi, P.-Y., and Michaud, P.-A. Offer and use of complementary and alternative medicine in hospitals of the French-speaking part of Switzerland. *Swiss Med Wkly* 143 (2013): w13756.

Cherniack, E.P., Ceron-Fuentes, J., Florez, H., Sandals, L., Rodriguez, O., and Palacios, J.C. Influence of race and ethnicity on alternative medicine as a self-treatment preference for common medical conditions in a population of multi-ethnic urban elderly. *Complement Ther Clin Pract* 14 (2008): 116–23.

Cooke, B., and Ernst, E. Aromatherapy: A systematic review. *Br J Gen Pract* 50 (2000): 493–96.

Crawford, N.W., Cincotta, D.R., Lim, A., and Powell, C.V.E. A cross-sectional survey of complementary and alternative medicine use by children and adolescents attending the University Hospital of Wales. *BMC Complement Altern Med* 2 (2006): 16.

Edris, A.E. Pharmaceutical and therapeutic potentials of essential oils and their individual volatile constituents: A review. *Phytother Res* 21 (2007): 308–23.

Ernst, E., and White, A. The BBC survey of complementary medicine use in the UK. *Complement Ther Med* 8 (2000): 32–36.

Ferry, P., Johnson, M., and Wallis, P. Use of complementary therapies and non-prescribed medication in patients with Parkinson's disease. *Postgrad Med J* 78 (2002): 612–14.

Fountain-Polley, S., Kawai, G., Goldstein, A., and Ninan, T. Knowledge and exposure to complementary and alternative medicine in paediatric doctors: A questionnaire survey. *BMC Complement Altern Med* 7 (2007): 38.

Furlow, M.L., Patel, D.A., Sen, A., and Liu, J.R. Physician and patient attitudes towards complementary and alternative medicine in obstetrics and gynecology. *BMC Complement Altern Med* 8 (2008): 35.

Galicia-Connolly, E., Adams, D., Bateman, J. et al. CAM use in pediatric neurology: An exploration of concurrent use with conventional medicine. *PLoS One* 9 (2014): e94078.

Hadley, J., Hassan, I., and Khan, K.S. Knowledge and beliefs concerning evidence-based practice amongst complementary and alternative medicine health care practitioners and allied health care professionals: A questionnaire survey. *BMC Complement Altern Med* 8 (2008): 45.

Hall, H.G., Griffiths, D.L., and McKenna, L.G. The use of complementary and alternative medicine by pregnant women: A literature review. *Midwifery* 27 (2011): 817–24.

Hall, H.G., Griffiths, D.L., and McKenna, L.G. Midwives' support for Complementary and Alternative Medicine: A literature review. *Women Birth* 25 (2012): 4–12.

Hunt, K.J., Coelho, H.F., Wider, B. et al. Complementary and alternative medicine use in England: Results from a national survey. *Int J Clin Pract* 64 (2010): 1496–502.

Lewith, G.T., Hyland, M., and Gray, S.F. Attitudes to and use of complementary medicine among physicians in the United Kingdom. *Complement Ther Med* 9 (2001): 167–72.

Lewith, G.T., Broomfield, J., and Prescott, P. Complementary cancer care in Southampton: A survey of staff and patients. *Complement Ther Med* 10 (2002): 100–6.

Lim, A., Cranswick, N., Skull, S., and South, M. Survey of complementary and alternative medicine use at a tertiary children's hospital. *J Paediatr Child Health* 41 (2005): 424–27.

Lis-Balchin, M. Possible health and safety problems in the use of novel plant essential oils and extracts in aromatherapy. *J R Soc Promot Health* 119 (1999): 240–43.

Long, L., Huntley, A., and Ernst, E. Which complementary and alternative therapies benefit which conditions? A survey of the opinions of 223 professional organizations. *Complement Ther Med* 9 (2001): 178–85.

Mousley, S. Audit of an aromatherapy service in a maternity unit. *Complement Ther Clin Pract* 11 (2005): 205–10.

Muñoz-Sellés, E., Vallès-Segalés, A., and Goberna-Tricas, J. Use of alternative and complementary therapies in labor and delivery care: A cross-sectional study of midwives' training in Catalan hospitals accredited as centers for normal birth. *BMC Complement Altern Med* 13 (2013): 318.

Münstedt, K., Brenken, A., and Kalder, M. Clinical indications and perceived effectiveness of complementary and alternative medicine in departments of obstetrics in Germany: A questionnaire study. *Eur J Obstet Gynecol Reprod Biol* 146 (2009): 50–54.

Ness, J., Cirillo, D.J., Weir, D.R., Nisly, N.L., and Wallace, R.B. Use of complementary medicine in older Americans: Results from the health and retirement study. *Gerontologist* 45 (2005): 516–24.

Neuhouser, M.L., Patterson, R.E., Schwartz, S.M., Hedderson, M.M., Bowen, D.J., and Standish, L.J. Use of alternative medicine by children with cancer in Washington state. *Prev Med* 33 (2001): 347–54.

Nicolaou, N., and Johnston, G.A. The use of complementary medicine by patients referred to a contact dermatitis clinic. *Contact Dermatitis* 51 (2004): 30–33.

Perry, R., and Dowrick, C.F. Complementary medicine and general practice: An urban perspective. *Complement Ther Med* 8 (2000): 71–75.

Pisseri, F., Bertoli, A., and Pistelli, L. Essential oils in medicine: Principles of therapy. *Parassitologia* 50 (2008): 89–91.

Posadzki, P., Alotaibi, A., and Ernst, E. Adverse effects of aromatherapy: A systematic review of case reports and case series. *Int J Risk Saf Med* 24 (2012): 147–61.

Posadzki, P., Watson, L.K., Alotaibi, A., and Ernst, E. Prevalence of use of complementary and alternative medicine (CAM) by patients/consumers in the UK: Systematic review of surveys. *Clin Med* 13 (2013a): 126–31.

Posadzki, P., Watson, L., Alotaibi, A., and Ernst, E. Prevalence of complementary and alternative medicine (CAM) use in UK paediatric patients: A systematic review of surveys. *Complement Ther Med* 21 (2013b): 224–31.

Robinson, A., Chesters, J., and Cooper, S. People's choice: Complementary and alternative medicine modalities. *Complement Health Pract Rev* 12 (2007): 99–118.

Salomonsen, L.J., Skovgaard, L., la Cour, S., Nyborg, L., Launsø, L., and Fønnebø, V. Use of complementary and alternative medicine at Norwegian and Danish hospitals. *BMC Complement Altern Med* 11 (2011): 4.

Sawni, A., and Thomas, R. Pediatricians' attitudes, experience and referral patterns regarding complementary/alternative medicine: A national survey. *BMC Complement Altern Med* 7 (2007): 18.

Sawyer, M.G., Gannoni, A.F., Toogood, I.R., Antoniou, G., and Rice, M. The use of alternative therapies by children with cancer. *Med J Aust* 160 (1994): 320–22.

Shakeel, M., Trinidade, A., and Ah-See, K.W. Complementary and alternative medicine use by otolaryngology patients: A paradigm for practitioners in all surgical specialties. *Eur Arch Otorhinolaryngol* 267 (2010): 961–71.

Sibbritt, D.W., Catling, C.J., Adams, J., Shaw, A.J., and Homer, C.S.E. The self-prescribed use of aromatherapy oils by pregnant women. *Women Birth* 27 (2014): 41–45.

Simpson, N., and Roman, K. Complementary medicine use in children: Extent and reasons. A population-based study. *Br J Gen Pract* 51 (2001): 914–16.

Sinha, D., and Efron, D. Complementary and alternative medicine use in children with attention deficit hyperactivity disorder. *J Paediatr Child Health* 41 (2005): 23–26.

Skouteris, H., Wertheim, E.H., Rallis, S., Paxton, S.J., Kelly, L., and Milgrom, J. Use of complementary and alternative medicines by a sample of Australian women during pregnancy. *Aust NZ J Obstet Gynaecol* 48 (2008): 384–90.

Thomas, K.J., Nicholl, J.P., and Coleman, P. Use and expenditure on complementary medicine in England: A population based survey. *Complement Ther Med* 9 (2001): 2–11.

Wahner-Roedler, D.L., Lee, M.C., Chon, T.Y., Cha, S.S., Loehrer, L.L., and Bauer, B.A. Physicians' attitudes toward complementary and alternative medicine and their knowledge of specific therapies: 8-year follow-up at an academic medical center. *Complement Ther Clin Pract* 20 (2014): 54–60.

Wilson, K.D., and Andrews, G.J. Complementary medicine and older people: Past research
    and future directions. *Complement Ther Nurs Midwifery* 10 (2004): 80–91.
Wong, H.C.G., and Neill, J.C. Physician use of complementary and alternative medicine
    (CAM) literature. *Complement Ther Med* 9 (2001): 173–77.

WEB REFERENCES

Aromatherapy Council: http://www.a-t-c.org.uk/.
Canadian Federation of Aromatherapists: http://cfacanada.com/about/.
International Aromatherapy and Aromatic Medicine Association: http://www.iaama.org.au/.
International Federation of Aromatherapists: http://www.ifaroma.org/it/home/.
Italian Society for the Research on Essential Oils: http://www.siroe.it/.
National Association for Holistic Aromatherapy: https://www.naha.org/about/mission/.

Index

Page numbers followed by f and t indicate figures and tables, respectively.

Printed and bound by CPI Group (UK) Ltd, Croydon, CR0 4YY

24/10/2024

01779068-0001